DERMATOLOGY
Just the Facts

Francisco A. Kerdel, BSc, MBBS

Professor of Clinical Dermatology
Department of Dermatology and Cutaneous Surgery
University of Miami School of Medicine
Chief of Dermatology
Cedars Medical Center
Miami, Florida

Francisco Jimenez-Acosta, MD

Chief of Dermatology Services
Clinica San Roque
Las Palmas Gran Canaria
Canary Islands, Spain

McGraw-Hill

Medical Publishing Division

New York   Chicago   San Francisco   Lisbon   London   Madrid   Mexico City
Milan   New Delhi   San Juan   Seoul   Singapore   Sydney   Toronto

Dermatology
Just the Facts

1 2 3 4 5 6 7 8 9 0   CUS/CUS   0 9 8 7 6 5 4 3

ISBN 0-07-139143-6

Notice

Medicine is an ever-changing science. As new research and clinical experience broaden our knowledge, changes in treatment and drug therapy are required. The authors and the publisher of this work have checked with sources believed to be reliable in their efforts to provide information that is complete and generally in accord with the standards accepted at the time of publication. However, in view of the possibility of human error or changes in medical sciences, neither the authors nor the publisher nor any other party who has been involved in the preparation or publication of this work warrants that the information contained herein is in every respect accurate or complete, and they disclaim all responsibility for any errors or omissions or for the results obtained from use of the information contained in this work. Readers are encouraged to confirm the information contained herein with other sources. For example and in particular, readers are advised to check the product information sheet included in the package of each drug they plan to administer to be certain that the information contained in this work is accurate and that changes have not been made in the recommended dose or in the contraindications for administration. This recommendation is of particular importance in connection with new or infrequently used drugs.

This book was set in Times New Roman by Macmillan India. The editors were Darlene Cooke, Michelle Watt, and Mary Bele. The production supervisor was Lisa Mendez. The cover designer was Aimee Nordin. The index was prepared by Ben Tedoff. Von Hoffmann Graphics was printer and binder.

This book is printed on acid-free paper.

Library of Congress Cataloging-in-Publication Data

Kerdel, Francisco A.
    Dermatology : just the facts / Francisco A. Kerdel, Francisco Jimenez-Acosta.
        p. cm.
    Includes bibliographical references and index.
    ISBN 0-07-139143-6 (softcover)
        1. Dermatology—Outlines, syllabi, etc. 2. Skin—Diseases—Outlines, syllabi, etc. I. Jimenez-Acosta, Francisco. II. Title.
RL74.3.K475 2003
616.5′0076—dc21
                                       2002044455

To Isabella, Christina, and Franz
(FAK)

To Inma, Carla, and Francisco
(FJA)

CONTENTS

CONTRIBUTORS

Javier Alonso-Llamazares, MD, Attending Physician, Department of Dermatology, Hospital Severo Ochoa, Madrid, Spain

Ysabel M. Bello, MD, Dermatology Resident, Department of Dermatology and Cutaneous Surgery, University of Miami School of Medicine, Cedars Medical Center, Miami, Florida

Rafael Botella-Estrada, MD, Dermatology Consultant, Department of Dermatology, Instituto Valenciano de Oncologia, Valencia, Spain

Jeffrey Callen, MD, Professor of Medicine (Dermatology), Chief, Division of Dermatology, University of Louisville, Louisville, Kentucky

Manuel Cruces, MD, Chief of Dermatology Service, Centro Dermatologico, Placeres (Pontevedra), Spain

Deborah Cummins, BS, Medical Student, Division of Dermatoimmunology, Department of Dermatology, Johns Hopkins Medical Institutions, Baltimore, Maryland

Anna Drosou, MD, Dermatology Resident, Department of Dermatology and Cutaneous Surgery, University of Miami School of Medicine, Miami, Florida

Karynne O. Duncan, MD, Assistant Professor of Dermatology and Internal Medicine, Department of Dermatology, University of Colorado Health Sciences Center, Denver, Colorado

Boni E. Elewski, MD, Professor of Dermatology, University of Alabama at Birmingham, The Eye Foundation Professional Building, Birmingham, Alabama

Joseph C. English III, MD, Assistant Professor of Dermatology, Department of Dermatology, University of Virginia Health System, Charlottesville, Virginia

Anna F. Falabella, MD, Assistant Professor of Dermatology, University of Miami School of Medicine, Miami, Florida

Jo-David Fine, MD, MPH, Dermatology Associates of Kentucky, Professor of Medicine (Dermatology), University of Kentucky College of Medicine, Head, National Epidermolysis Bullosa Registry, Lexington, Kentucky

Angeles Flórez, MD, Attending Dermatologist, Hospital Provincial, CHOP, Pontevedra, Spain

Gloria P. Jiménez, MD, Clinical Research Fellow, Department of Dermatology and Cutaneous Surgery, University of Miami School of Medicine, Cedars Medical Center, Miami, Florida

Francisco Jimenez-Acosta, MD, Chief of Dermatology Services, Clinica San Roque, Las Palmas Gran Canaria, Canary Islands, Spain

Francisco A. Kerdel, BSc, MBBS, Professor of Clinical Dermatology, Department of Dermatology and Cutaneous Surgery, University of Miami School of Medicine, Chief of Dermatology, Cedars Medical Center, Miami, Florida

Robert S. Kirsner, MD, Associate Professor, Department of Dermatology and Cutaneous Surgery, Epidemiology and Public Health, University of Miami School of Medicine, Chief of Dermatology, Veterans Administration Medical Center, Miami, Florida

Melissa C. Lazarus, MD, Resident, Department of Dermatology and Cutaneous Surgery, University of Miami School of Medicine, Cedars Medical Center, Miami, Florida

Lela A. Lee, MD, Professor of Dermatology and Medicine, University of Colorado School of Medicine, Chief of Dermatology, Denver Health Medical Center, Denver, Colorado

Cheryl L. Lonergan, BA, BSN, Medical Student, Department of Dermatology, University of Virginia Health System, Charlottesville, Virginia

Chetan Maingi, MD, CPT USA MC, Dermatology Resident, Brooke Army Medical Center, San Antonio Uniformed Services Health Education Consortium, Fort Sam Houston, Texas

Jeffrey J. Meffert, MD, Col USAF MC, Program Director, Dermatology, San Antonio Uniformed Services Health Education Consortium, Dermatology MCHE-DD, Fort Sam Houston, Texas

H. Carlos Nousari, MD, Chairman, Department of Dermatology, Director, Division of Dermatopathology and Immunodermatology, Cleveland Clinic Florida, Weston, Florida

Marianne O'Donoghue, MD, Associate Professor, Rush Presbyterian-St. Luke Medical Center, Oak Brook, Illinois

Sandra P. Osswald, MD, LtCol USAF MC, Staff Dermatologist, Brooke Army Medical Center, San Antonio Uniformed Services Health Education Consortium, Fort Sam Houston, Texas

Theresa R. Pacheco, MD, Assistant Professor of Dermatology, University of Colorado School of Medicine, Denver, Colorado

Enrique Poblet, MD, Staff Pathologist, Hospital General Universitario de Albacete, Associate Professor of Pathology, Universidad de Castilla-La Mancha, Spain

Ramón M. Pujol, MD, Head of Section, Department of Dermatology, Hospital del Mar, Barcelona, Spain

Adrienne Rencic, MD, PhD, Attending Dermatologist, Mercy Medical Center, Clinical Instructor, University of Maryland Medical Center, Baltimore, Maryland

Luis Requena, MD, Associate Chief of Dermatology, Fundación Jiménez Díaz, Associate Professor of Dermatology, Universidad Autónoma de Madrid, Madrid, Spain

Alfredo C. Rivadeneira, MD, Assistant Professor of Rheumatology, University of North Carolina, Chapel Hill, North Carolina

Georgette Rodriguez, MD, Dermatology Resident, Department of Dermatology and Cutaneous Surgery, University of Miami School of Medicine, Miami, Florida

Paolo Romanelli, MD, Assistant Professor, Department of Dermatology and Cutaneous Surgery, University of Miami School of Medicine, Miami, Florida

Franco Rongioletti, MD, Associate Professor of Dermatology, Department of Dermatology, University of Genova, Genova, Italy

Evaristo Sánchez-Yus, MD, Professor of Dermatology, Department of Dermatology, Hospital Clínico San Carlos, Universidad Complutense de Madrid, Madrid, Spain

Onofre Sanmartín, MD, Dermatology Consultant, Department of Dermatology, Instituto Valenciano de Oncologia, Valencia, Spain

Jay L. Viernes, MD, LtCol USAF MC, Staff Dermatologist, Wilford Hall Medical Center, San Antonio Uniformed Services Health Education Consortium, Fort Sam Houston, Texas

Justin J. Vujevich, MD, Cosmetic Dermatology Research Fellow, Department of Dermatology and Cutaneous Surgery, University of Miami School of Medicine, Cedars Medical Center, Miami, Florida

Esperanza C. Welsh, MD, Dermatology Resident, Department of Dermatology and Cutaneous Surgery, University of Miami School of Medicine, Cedars Medical Center, Miami, Florida

Martin N. Zaiac, MD, Director of Dermatology, Mount Sinai Hospital, Miami Beach, Florida, Associate Clinical Faculty, Department of Dermatology and Cutaneous Surgery, University of Miami, Miami, Florida

PREFACE

The impetus for writing this book originated when one of the editors (FAK) held the position of President of the Medical Dermatology Society (US). At the time, it was felt that a publication originating from the Society would enhance visibility and benefit the group. The concept was approved by most of the members and indeed many of the authors are current members of the Medical Dermatology Society. This book is to some degree the product of the Medical Dermatology Society and if the book is successful in promoting the Society, then we will feel that we have accomplished what we set out to do.

We had planned to publish a simple dermatology book which could be translated to many languages over a decade ago. Even though substantial effort was dedicated to the project, the publishing of a book never came to fruition. Through this book, we have been able to finish this project that had the longest gestation period on record.

We wish to acknowledge the Medical Dermatology Society for their support and to the individual authors who participated in the writing of this book. We would also like to thank Veronica A. Montoto for her efforts in reformatting and correcting the individual manuscripts. In addition, we would like to thank Leslie Baumann, MD, who was our initial contact with McGraw-Hill, and Darlene Cooke for believing that the work could be accomplished. Our gratitude is also extended to Professor Renzo Romanelli for helping review the manuscript.

Francisco A. Kerdel, BSc, MBBS
Francisco Jimenez-Acosta, MD

1 PAPULOSQUAMOUS DISORDERS

Lela A. Lee
Theresa R. Pacheco

PSORIASIS

EPIDEMIOLOGY

- Psoriasis occurs in about 2% of the U.S. population.
- There are two peaks of onset, one in the third decade and one in the sixth decade. However, psoriasis may begin at any age.
- Onset in childhood portends more severe disease.
- Psoriatic arthritis occurs in 5% or more of patients with psoriasis.

PATHOPHYSIOLOGY

- Psoriasis is a multigenetic disease with environmental triggers. If one parent is affected, about 8% of offspring will develop psoriasis. If two parents are affected, about 40% will be affected.
- Triggers include trauma to the skin, such as a surgical incision, and infection, notably streptococcal infection.
- Considerable evidence implicates T lymphocytes as crucial to the initiation of a psoriatic lesion.
- Psoriasis has a T_H1 phenotype, with potential contributions from the T_H1-type cytokines TNF-α, IL-2, IFN-γ, IL-12, and IL-18. In addition, IL-8 may promote keratinocyte proliferation, recruit inflammatory cells to the skin, and stimulate angiogenesis.
- The importance of T cells in the pathophysiology of psoriasis is highlighted by the effectiveness of therapeutic interventions that target T-cell activation, T-cell proliferation, or migration of T cells into the skin, or that target T_H1-type cytokines.

CLINICAL FEATURES

- Untreated psoriatic lesions are typically sharply demarcated plaques with silvery scale on an erythematous base. When the scale is removed by scraping, small drops of blood appear on the erythematous base, a finding called the Auspitz sign. In some cases, lesions may follow trauma to the skin, such as a scratch or surgical incision. The occurrence of psoriasis along an area of injury to the skin is called the Koebner phenomenon.
- The lesions are not usually pruritic, but may be.
- Exacerbating factors include HIV, heavy alcohol use, use of certain medications such as lithium and beta blockers, and stress. Psoriasis is apt to be worse in climates with relatively little sunshine.
- A severe exacerbation of psoriasis may occur upon withdrawal of systemic steroids, particularly if the systemic steroids have been administered over a long period.
- Psoriasis has many phenotypes, the most common of which is chronic plaque psoriasis. Other phenotypes include guttate, erythrodermic, generalized pustular, and localized pustular psoriasis.
- In chronic plaque psoriasis, large plaques occur predominantly on the elbows, knees, scalp, retroauricular skin, umbilicus, and gluteal cleft. Lesions may occur much more widely over virtually all the skin surface, although the most sun-exposed areas are generally the least likely to be affected. Occasionally, there is a predominance of lesions in intertriginous areas, and in those areas scaling may be inapparent.
- Guttate psoriasis is often associated with a preceding streptococcal infection. Lesions are small, numerous, and widespread, particularly over the trunk and proximal extremities.
- Erythrodermic and generalized pustular psoriasis are dramatic forms of psoriasis. Erythrodermic psoriasis consists of widespread erythema and scale, with erythema over most of the body surface being the predominant finding. High-output cardiac failure may occur in susceptible individuals. In generalized pustular psoriasis, the lesions may appear acutely and be associated with fever, leukocytosis, and debility.
- Localized pustular psoriasis often occurs on hands and feet, and may produce significant functional impairment.
- Nail involvement is common. Pitting of the nails, yellowish discolorations called oil spots, diffuse onychodystrophy, or even loss of the nail may occur.
- Psoriatic arthritis may occur as asymmetric peripheral joint disease, symmetric peripheral joint disease, axial disease, tenosynovitis, and enthesopathy. The most

common type of arthritis is peripheral asymmetric oligoarthritis involving small joints of the hands and feet, large joints of the legs, or both. Although there is some correlation between severity of psoriatic skin lesions and arthritis, arthritis may occur in patients who have minimal skin findings, and the courses of the arthritis and the skin disease are not parallel.

HISTOPATHOLOGY

• The histologic findings vary depending on the stage and phenotype of the lesion. In typical plaque psoriasis, the early findings consist of dilated capillaries and perivascular mononuclear cells. As the lesion matures, there is dramatic epidermal hyperplasia, which is associated with elongation of the rete ridges and thinning of the suprapapillary plates. This brings the congested blood vessels close to the surface and accounts for the Auspitz sign when the scale is removed. Because of the rapid turnover of cells, there is no stratum granulosum, but nuclei may be observed in the stratum corneum (parakeratosis). Characteristically, there are neutrophils in the superficial epidermis.

DIAGNOSIS AND DIFFERENTIAL

• The diagnosis of chronic plaque psoriasis is usually not difficult and is typically made on clinical grounds alone. In difficult cases, and in particular in patients with the erythrodermic form, skin biopsy may be helpful in narrowing the diagnostic possibilities.
• Lesions of nummular eczema may be difficult to distinguish from those of chronic plaque psoriasis. In some instances, the differential diagnosis of chronic plaque psoriasis includes seborrheic dermatitis, cutaneous lupus, pityriasis rubra pilaris, dermatophytosis, or cutaneous T-cell lymphoma.
• The differential diagnosis of guttate psoriasis may include pityriasis rosea, secondary syphilis, and parapsoriasis.
• Erythrodermic psoriasis may be difficult to distinguish clinically from drug eruption, pityriasis rubra pilaris, cutaneous T-cell lymphoma, and severe atopic dermatitis.
• Psoriatic lesions of the nail may be mistaken for fungal infection. Close attention to the nail morphology, and in some cases sampling of the nail for microscopic examination and culture, can help differentiate.
• If the patient has a single psoriasis-like lesion, particularly if it is in an atypical location, the diagnosis

of squamous cell carcinoma-in-situ should be considered.

TREATMENT

• Psoriasis is a condition with many, quite distinct treatment options available. Patients who have persistent, disabling, and/or extensive disease are best managed by a physician familiar with the full range of treatment options, including their benefits and side effects.
• Topical therapy or phototherapy is preferred for most patients, as side effects are minimized. Both topical and phototherapy may be quite helpful, even for patients with extensive skin involvement.
• Combination therapies are frequently used.
• Topical medications in frequent use are corticosteroids, tar, anthralin, calcipotriene, and tazarotene. Salicylic acid is sometimes employed to decrease scaling.
• Topical medications differ in ease of use, expense, and duration of remission. Periods of remission may refer either to periods during which there are no psoriatic lesions visible or periods where the psoriasis is still present but of minor severity by comparison to the pre-treatment severity.
• Among topical therapies administered as monotherapy, the duration of remission appears to be better for anthralin and tazarotene than steroids and calcipotriene.
• Topical steroids are easy to use, but cutaneous side effects may be limiting in some patients.
• Tar is often effective but may stain clothing and have an unpleasant odor.
• Anthralin is convenient to use for patients who follow directions closely. Short-contact (from a few minutes up to an hour) anthralin is preferred, as the short contact regimen decreases the likelihood of irritation.
• Calcipotriene is convenient to use and has efficacy comparable to a high-potency topical steroid.
• Tazarotene is convenient to use. It may be irritating to the skin, but the cream preparations are better tolerated than the gels.
• Phototherapy may be administered using natural sunlight, UVB, narrowband UVB, or PUVA (psoralen plus UVA). Many factors are considered when determining which type of phototherapy to use. Natural sunlight is obviously the least expensive.
• Systemic therapy is reserved for patients with extensive or disabling disease. The most commonly used systemic therapies are methotrexate, retinoids (particularly acitretin), and cyclosporine. A limitation of methotrexate and retinoids is their potential for hepatotoxicity. In addition, retinoids are teratogenic, and

are generally not used to treat psoriasis in women of childbearing potential. Cyclosporine has a potential for nephrotoxicity.

- There are a host of other therapies that have been used successfully for psoriasis, including 6-thioguanine, hydroxyurea, tacrolimus, mycophenolate mofetil, and topical 5-fluorouracil.
- Newer or experimental therapies for psoriasis include immune-modulating agents such as etanercept (which binds the TNF-α receptor), infliximab (which binds TNF-α), IL-10 (which inhibits T_H1-type cytokine production), and molecules that block the interactions of B7 and CD28, LFA1 and ICAM-1, or CD2 and LFA3.
- The National Psoriasis Foundation is an excellent resource for patient education.

REFERENCES

Gottlieb AB. Psoriasis: Immunopathology and immunomodulation. *Dermatol Clin.* 2001;19:649.

Koo J, Lebwohl M. Duration of remission of psoriasis therapies. *J Am Acad Dermatol.* 1999;41:51.

Lebwohl M, Ali S. Treatment of psoriasis. Part 1. Topical therapy and phototherapy. *J Am Acad Dermatol.* 2001;45:487.

SEBORRHEIC DERMATITIS

EPIDEMIOLOGY

- Seborrheic dermatitis is an exceedingly common condition and is usually not an indicator of underlying internal disease.
- Patients with HIV or with neurologic disease such as Parkinson's disease have an increased prevalence and severity.

PATHOPHYSIOLOGY

- The cause is unknown.
- Some evidence implicates *Malassezia furfur*, but there is not a definitive link.

CLINICAL FEATURES

- There is scaling, which is often greasy in appearance, and erythema, which ranges widely in severity from imperceptible to severe.
- Lesions have a symmetric distribution and a predilection for scalp, retroauricular skin, nasolabial area, eyebrows, eyelids, beard area, midchest, and intertriginous skin.
- Tinea amiantacea is a name given to describe thick scaling adhering to the proximal portions of hairs and often binding them together; tinea amiantacea is not a dermatophyte infection.

HISTOPATHOLOGY

- Findings include moderate acanthosis, a mild perivascular mononuclear cell infiltrate, mild spongiosis, parakeratosis, and often some neutrophils at the follicular ostia.

DIAGNOSIS AND DIFFERENTIAL

- Diagnosis is made by clinical examination; skin biopsy is usually unnecessary and nondiagnostic.
- Consider checking HIV in a patient with otherwise unexplained, severe seborrheic dermatitis.
- Differential diagnosis may include psoriasis, atopic dermatitis, rosacea, and perioral dermatitis.
- Scalp psoriasis and seborrheic dermatitis may be indistinguishable. Features more suggestive of psoriasis are discrete, sharply marginated, erythematous, scaly plaques with intervening areas of normal-appearing scalp.
- Although dermatophyte infection of the scalp is common in children, tinea capitis is uncommon in immunocompetent adults and is usually not a likely diagnostic consideration.

TREATMENT

- Medicated shampoo is sufficient for most individuals with the condition limited to the scalp. Shampoo may also be used for scaling in eyebrows and other hairy sites such as the moustache and midchest.
- Seborrhea shampoos may contain ketoconazole, tar, sulfur, selenium sulfide, or zinc pyrithione. Currently, these shampoos are available in the United States without a prescription.
- Shampoos or solutions containing a keratolytic agent such as salicylic acid may be helpful to decrease thick scale in the scalp.
- Shampooing daily to every other day is beneficial, as infrequent shampooing may contribute to seborrhea.

- Because medicated shampoos tend to be more expensive than nonmedicated shampoos, and some medicated shampoos may have a somewhat unpleasant odor, it is often acceptable to alternate the use of nonmedicated shampoos with medicated shampoos. The frequency of use of medicated shampoo necessary to keep the condition under control may be determined empirically.
- For inflamed skin, topical steroids are often used. In the scalp, steroid solutions such as fluocinolone or fluocinonide topical solution used once daily after shampooing may be helpful. On the facial skin or intertriginous areas, twice to thrice daily non-prescription-strength hydrocortisone cream may suffice. If prescription strength steroid is needed, a steroid should be chosen from the low-potency category in order to minimize the likelihood of adverse cutaneous reactions on the face or intertriginous skin.
- Other topical treatments that have been used include imidazole creams, metronidazole, and ciclopirox.

REFERENCES

Myskowski PL, Ahkami R. Dermatologic complications of HIV infection. *Med Clin North Am.* 1996;80:1415.

Pierard-Franchimont C, Pierard GE, Arrese JE, De Doncker P. Effect of ketoconazole 1% and 2% shampoos on severe dandruff and seborrhoeic dermatitis: Clinical, squamometric and mycological assessments. *Dermatology.* 2001;202:171.

LICHEN PLANUS AND LICHEN NITIDUS

EPIDEMIOLOGY

- The incidence of lichen planus is not known precisely, but may be about 0.5%.
- Most cases occur in the fourth to sixth decades, but all ages may be affected.

PATHOPHYSIOLOGY

- The histologic findings of a lymphocytic infiltrate with damage to basal cells of the epidermis suggest the possibility of cytotoxicity of basal cells mediated by lymphocytes. There is no evidence that lichen planus is mediated by autoantibodies.
- An association with hepatitis C has been reported in many studies, most commonly in patients with erosive mucosal lesions.

CLINICAL FEATURES

- The characteristic skin lesions are flat-topped, violaceous, polygonal papules, typically rather small in diameter and with a thin, transparent scale.
- Pruritus is extremely common and often intense.
- The above characteristics may be remembered as *p*lanar (flat-topped), *p*urple, *p*olygonal, *p*ruritic *p*apules.
- Lesions are symmetric and occur predominantly on the extremities, with the wrists and flexural areas of arms and legs most likely to be affected, and the trunk and neck occasionally affected. The shaft of the penis is commonly involved.
- The Koebner phenomenon may be observed (see the section on psoriasis earlier in this chapter).
- Oral lesions may occur either coincident with skin lesions or as an isolated finding. Oral lesions often consist of lacy white papules or erosions, although other phenotypes may be observed. The buccal and gingival mucosa and the tongue are often involved. Other mucosal surfaces, particularly genital mucosa, may be affected.
- A small but increased risk for oral squamous cell carcinoma has been reported in patients who have oral lichen planus.
- Nails are affected in a minority of patients. Typical findings are ridging, thinning, distal splitting, and dorsal pterygium. Permanent loss of the nails may occur.
- There are several clinical variants of lichen planus. These include actinic, follicular, erosive, ulcerative, bullous, atrophic, hypertrophic, palmoplantar, annular, and linear lichen planus, and lichen planus-lupus overlap syndrome.
- Lichen planus usually resolves in 1 or 2 years, but relapses may occur. Oral lesions appear to have a longer duration.
- Lichen-planus-like, or lichenoid, eruptions may result from exposure to certain medications or metals. The lesions tend to be somewhat larger in diameter than those of classic lichen planus and the distribution is more often on sun-exposed skin, but it may not be possible to distinguish a lichenoid drug eruption from lichen planus in every case. Some of the drugs that have been reported to induce a lichenoid eruption are gold, beta blockers, captopril, penicillamine, antimalarials, thiazide diuretics, furosemide, and spironolactone. Certain dental materials have been noted to induce oral lichenoid eruptions.
- Lichen nitidus is a condition consisting of numerous pinpoint, flesh-colored or pink, round papules with minimal scale. Most common sites of involvement are the flexural surfaces of the arms and wrists, abdomen, breasts, and genital area. Lesions are usually

asymptomatic. Histology is distinctive. A relationship between lichen nitidus and lichen planus has been proposed, as some patients with lichen planus also have lesions of lichen nitidus, but the relationship of these two conditions has not been definitively established.

HISTOPATHOLOGY

- Lichen planus is characterized by apoptotic damage of basal keratinocytes, a dense band-like infiltrate of mononuclear cells at the dermal–epidermal interface, wedge-shaped hypergranulosis, orthokeratosis, and elongation of rete ridges in a saw-toothed pattern.
- Immunofluorescent examination of lichen planus lesions shows the apoptotic keratinocytes staining heavily with IgM and often IgG, IgA, C3, and fibrin. Fibrinogen deposits in a shaggy pattern at the dermal-epidermal junction are characteristic.
- Lichen nitidus has a well-circumscribed, dense infiltrate of mononuclear cells in a widened dermal papilla. Above the infiltrate there is epidermal thinning, basal cell damage, loss of the granular layer, and parakeratosis. At the lateral aspects of the infiltrate, the rete ridges point toward the infiltrate, giving the appearance of arms enveloping the infiltrate.

DIAGNOSIS AND DIFFERENTIAL

- The differential may include other papulosquamous diseases such as dermatitis, lichen simplex, and psoriasis, but these are usually distinguishable by clinical examination.
- Skin biopsy may be quite helpful in establishing a definitive diagnosis, as the histologic findings are distinctive. In cases of typical cutaneous lichen planus, a biopsy may not be necessary.
- Findings on immunofluorescent examination of tissue are non-diagnostic, but may nevertheless provide supportive information and may help distinguish lichen planus from autoantibody-associated diseases. This is particularly the case in oral lichen planus, where the differential diagnosis may include pemphigus or pemphigoid syndromes.
- The histologic findings of lichenoid graft-versus-host disease, lichenoid keratosis, and lichenoid drug eruption may resemble those of lichen planus.
- Lichen planus lesions of the nail may be mistaken for fungal infection. Close attention to the nail morphology, and in some cases sampling of the nail for microscopic examination and culture, can help distinguish.
- Lesions of lichen nitidus may resemble flat warts, follicular eczema, or keratosis pilaris.

TREATMENT

- Lichen planus is often poorly responsive to therapy. Anecdotal reports of responses to specific therapies are difficult to evaluate, given that the disease spontaneously remits.
- In selecting therapy, potential side effects must be weighed against potential benefits. Topical corticosteroids are often the first agent to be used for cutaneous lichen planus and are usually well tolerated. The potential side effects of systemic steroids usually outweigh potential benefits. Presently, topical tacrolimus has proven useful in oral lichen planus.
- Phototherapy with UVB or PUVA has been used for cutaneous lesions.
- Oral antihistamines may be helpful for decreasing pruritus.
- For disabling oral lesions, systemic retinoids have been used, as has cyclosporine.
- If lichenoid drug eruption is in the differential, consider discontinuing the possible inciting agent.
- Lichen nitidus usually does not require therapy.

REFERENCES

Chan ES, Thornhill M, Zakrzewska J. Interventions for treating oral lichen planus. *Cochrane Database Syst Rev.* 2000; CD001168.
Eisen D. The clinical features, malignant potential, and systemic associations of oral lichen planus: A study of 723 patients. *J Am Acad Dermatol.* 2002;46:207.

PITYRIASIS ROSEA

EPIDEMIOLOGY

- The incidence of pityriasis rosea (PR) has been reported to be 0.75 per 100 dermatologic patients.
- The peak incidence is in the 20- to 24-year-old age group, with a majority of cases occurring between the ages of 10 and 35.
- The disease is more common in the spring and fall.

PATHOPHYSIOLOGY

- PR is a common, acute, self-limited papulosquamous eruption of unknown cause.
- An infectious, possibly viral, etiology has been proposed and extensively investigated. To date, no specific virus has been conclusively associated with PR.

CLINICAL FEATURES

- The eruption has a characteristic pattern. A single, sharply-defined thin oval plaque (herald patch) first appears, followed by numerous similar-appearing, smaller lesions.
- Most cases have a truncal distribution with sparing of the face, palms, and soles. In approximately 10% of cases, an inverse distribution involving mainly the extremities is seen.
- The rash lasts from 1 to 8 weeks in 80% of the patients with most patients having the rash for about 5 weeks.
- The eruption is usually asymptomatic, but pruritus can occur.

HISTOPATHOLOGY

- There is focal spongiosis with mounds of parakeratosis and a superficial perivascular lymphocytic infiltrate.

DIAGNOSIS AND DIFFERENTIAL

- Differential diagnoses to consider include tinea and secondary syphilis. In selected cases, other papulosquamous disorders may be in the differential diagnosis. Tinea is more likely to be considered when PR is in the isolated, herald patch stage. A scraping of scale to examine for fungus can be helpful.
- Secondary syphilis is more likely to be considered when the eruption is extensive. Secondary syphilis is characterized by discrete pink macules or pink papules with a fine scale distributed over the trunk, and is associated with lymphadenopathy, low-grade fever, malaise, and arthralgias. Skin lesions erupt 3- to 6 weeks after the appearance of the primary chancre. Clinically, secondary syphilis can be differentiated from PR by documenting involvement of the palms and soles, lymphadenopathy, systemic symptoms, and a positive serologic test for syphilis (RPR or VDRL).
- A biopsy specimen is helpful to confirm the diagnosis of PR in atypical cases.

TREATMENT

- Treatment of PR is only required if the lesions are symptomatic. Topical steroids and antihistamines may help relieve pruritus.
- Ultraviolet radiation treatment (UVB or sun exposure) may be helpful in some patients.

REFERENCES

Hartley AH. Pityriasis rosea. *Pediatr Rev.* 1999;20:266.
Nelson JS, Stone MS. Update on selected viral exanthems. *Acta Derm Venereol.* 1999;79:405.

PITYRIASIS RUBRA PILARIS

EPIDEMIOLOGY

- The incidence of pityriasis rubra pilaris (PRP) is not known precisely, but it is quite uncommon.
- PRP occurs equally among male and female patients.
- There are two peaks of onset of the acquired form of PRP, one in the first decade and one in the fifth decade. However, PRP may begin at any age.
- Additionally, there is a familial autosomal dominant form of PRP, which begins in early childhood.

PATHOPHYSIOLOGY

- PRP is a rare disease in which the primary abnormality may be hyperproliferation of the epidermis.
- Vitamin A deficiency or abnormal vitamin A metabolism has been postulated to contribute to the disease, but evidence to support this hypothesis is lacking.

CLINICAL FEATURES

- Five variants have been described. The five categories are the classical adult type, atypical adult type, classical juvenile type, circumscribed juvenile type, and atypical juvenile type. The classical adult type is the most common.
- Orange-red or salmon-colored scaling plaques with sharp borders characterize PRP. There are often areas of uninvolved skin referred to as "islands of sparing."
- The eruption begins on the head and neck and may expand to involve virtually the entire body, resulting in erythroderma.
- The palms and soles become thickened and yellow, resulting in a well-demarcated palmoplantar keratoderma called the "PRP sandal."
- Follicular hyperkeratosis is commonly seen on the dorsal aspects of the proximal phalanges, elbows, and wrists.
- Nail changes include distal yellow-brown discoloration with subungual hyperkeratosis. Complete loss of the nail can occur in severe cases.

- The eruption is usually asymptomatic, but pruritus can occur.
- Prognosis is variable, but about 80% of patients clear spontaneously in several years.

HISTOPATHOLOGY

- There is mild acanthosis without thinning of the suprapapillary plates. This latter feature explains the absence of the Auspitz sign clinically. The stratum corneum shows parakeratosis, which characteristically alternates in both horizontal and vertical directions.

DIAGNOSIS AND DIFFERENTIAL

- There are no specific lab tests to confirm the diagnosis of PRP. The diagnosis is usually made based on a correlation between clinical and histologic findings.
- A biopsy can be useful to rule out other possible papulosquamous and erythrodermic disorders.
- Erythroderma is a reaction pattern of the skin that can occur in the setting of several different skin disorders, most commonly psoriasis, eczema, cutaneous T-cell lymphoma, and drug reactions.

TREATMENT

- Topical care with hydration and emollients reduces fissuring and dryness, providing some patient comfort. Petroleum jelly or equivalent emollients may be used.
- Topical steroids are not helpful.
- The treatment of choice is oral retinoids. The majority of patients experience a significant benefit from the use of oral retinoids. Clinical improvement can be expected within 4 to 6 months. High doses of vitamin A were used before synthetic retinoids became available.
- Immunosuppressive drugs such as methotrexate and cyclosporine have been used in retinoid-resistant cases.

REFERENCES

Clayton BD, Jorizzo JL, Hitchcock MG, et al. Adult pityriasis rubra pilaris: A 10-year case series. *J Am Acad Dermatol.* 1997;36:959.

Sorensen KB, Thestrup-Pedersen K. Pityriasis rubra pilaris: A retrospective analysis of 43 patients. *Acta Derm Venereol.* 1999;79:405.

PARAPSORIASIS

PITYRIASIS LICHENOIDES ET VARIOLIFORMIS ACUTA (PLEVA, ACUTE PARAPSORIASIS, MUCHA–HABERMANN DISEASE)

PITYRIASIS LICHENOIDES CHRONICA (CHRONIC PARAPSORIASIS)

EPIDEMIOLOGY

- The nomenclature of parapsoriasis, pityriasis lichenoides et varioliformis acuta (PLEVA), and pityriasis lichenoides chronica (PLC) has been complicated and confusing. The different forms of parapsoriasis have been classified as large-plaque parapsoriasis, small-plaque parapsoriasis, and pityriasis lichenoides. Of these, only pityriasis lichenoides is discussed further in this chapter. Pityriasis lichenoides can be viewed as a single entity with a spectrum of clinical disease, with PLEVA at one end of the spectrum and PLC at the other end.
- No accurate statistics on the incidence and frequency of pityriasis lichenoides (PLEVA or PLC) exist.
- These dermatoses occur in both children and adults.

PATHOPHYSIOLOGY

- The etiology of pityriasis lichenoides (PLEVA or PLC) is unknown.
- Various infections have been proposed as causative agents. Based on the current state of knowledge, no known infectious agents have been conclusively associated with PLEVA or PLC.

CLINICAL FEATURES

- PLEVA begins with the appearance of numerous erythematous, edematous papules that may vesiculate. Some lesions develop central necrosis and heal with varioliform scars. At any point in time, the lesions are in multiple stages.
- The papules are predominantly present on the trunk, arms, and legs, sparing the palms and soles. The face is usually spared.
- Lesions are often pruritic.
- PLC is characterized by erythematous, tan or red-brown, scaly papules. Lesions are typically about 3 to 4 mm in diameter, although lesions up to 1 cm in

diameter may be observed. Vesiculo-necrotic lesions are characteristic of PLEVA but not PLC. Scarring does not usually occur, but the scaly papules may resolve with dyspigmentation.

- The papules of PLC are predominantly present on the trunk and proximal extremities but spare the palms, soles, and face.
- PLC lesions are often asymptomatic. PLC may last a few months or persist for years.

HISTOPATHOLOGY

- Biopsy of PLEVA shows hyperkeratosis, parakeratosis, and epidermal edema. There is invasion of the epidermis by lymphocytes and red blood cells. Often the epidermis shows degeneration, necrosis, or ulceration. The dermis contains a lymphocytic vasculitis with red cell extravasation.
- Biopsy of PLC shows changes similar to a chronic dermatitis and is not diagnostic. The dermis contains a superficial inflammatory infiltrate consisting predominantly of lymphocytes. The epidermis may show atrophy and exocytosis.

DIAGNOSIS AND DIFFERENTIAL

- In children, the differential diagnosis of PLEVA-like lesions may include varicella, insect bites, and Gianotti–Crosti syndrome. In adults, the differential may include bites, dermatitis herpetiformis, lymphomatoid papulosis, and vasculitis. A biopsy can be helpful.
- PLC can be confused with PR, guttate psoriasis, small-plaque parapsoriasis, and secondary syphilis. A biopsy can be helpful.

TREATMENT

- Treatment includes topical steroids and antihistamines for symptomatic relief.
- Tetracycline and erythromycin have each been used for PLEVA, although their efficacy has not been demonstrated conclusively.
- Several investigators report a satisfactory response of PLEVA and PLC to ultraviolet radiation treatment (UVB or PUVA). Regular sun exposure if UVB or PUVA is unavailable may help speed the disappearance of the eruption.

REFERENCES

Fox BJ, Odom RB. Papulosquamous diseases: A review. *J Am Acad Dermatol.* 1985;12:597.

Romani J, Puig L, Fernandez-Figueras MT, de Moragas JM. Pityriasis lichenoides in children: Clinicopathologic review of 22 patients. *Pediatr Dermatol.* 1998;15:1.

2 KERATINIZING DISORDERS

Anna Drosou
Robert S. Kirsner

ICHTHYOSES

- Ichthyosis (from the Greek word for fish, "ichthys") is a term used to describe a wide range of acquired or genotypically distinct diseases whose main phenotypic characteristic is that of excessive scaling. In this group of diseases there is an abnormal differentiation of the epidermis caused by either an increase of the rate of epidermal proliferation or prolonged retention of the keratinocytes, resulting in the clinical appearance of scales. This is often caused by genetic defects leading to abnormal protein production of enzymes critical to differentiation. The terms disorders of cornification and ichthysiform dermatoses have also been used.
- Ichthyosis in the neonatal period is usually inherited. Ichthyosis occurring in older groups may be either inherited or acquired. The most common diseases among the ichthyoses are ichthyosis vulgaris, X-linked ichthyosis, lamellar ichthyosis, congenital ichthyosiform erythroderma, and bullous ichthyosiform erythroderma. Several rare inherited syndromes may also include ichthyosis among their features.

ICHTHYOSIS VULGARIS

EPIDEMIOLOGY

- Ichthyosis vulgaris is the most common of the ichthyoses (vulgaris is Latin for "common"). It presents in 1 in 250 to 500 live births.
- It is transmitted as an autosomal dominant trait.
- Ichthyosis vulgaris is not present at birth, but occurs usually in infancy, most commonly between 3 and 12 months of age. More rarely, it occurs in early childhood.

PATHOPHYSIOLOGY

- Ichthyosis vulgaris is a retention hyperkeratosis, that is, scales are not shed in the normal fashion. The rate of epidermal turnover is normal.

- The exact abnormality is unknown; however, filagrin is absent in involved skin, and the m-RNA for pro-filaggrin is unstable. Filagrin is a protein found in the keratohyalin granules. These structures are essential for the aggregation of keratin, which contributes to the structural integrity of keratinocytes. The absence or reduction of filagrin leads to abnormal keratinocyte differentiation.
- As a result, the barrier function of the involved skin is compromised.

CLINICAL FEATURES

- Ichthyosis vulgaris is characterized by fine white scales covering the entire body and pronounced skin dryness. The scale can be centrally attached with superficial fissuring at the edges.
- The scales are more prominent and coarser at the lower extremities and at the extensor surfaces. The axillary and gluteal folds are usually not involved, and the elbow and knee flexures as well as the diaper area (in children) are most often spared. Hyperkeratosis of the palms and soles usually coexists. Hypohidrosis (decreased sweating) may occur, because of the involvement of the adnexal structures of the skin, with subsequent heat intolerance.
- The scales increase in severity and extent with cold and dry weather and ameliorate in warm, humid climates.
- Several conditions, including keratosis pilaris and atopic dermatitis, are more frequent in patients with ichthyosis vulgaris.

DIAGNOSIS AND DIFFERENTIAL

- Usually the diagnosis is made based on the clinical findings. The existence of associated conditions such as hyperlinear palms and soles associated with atopy, or keratosis pilaris, strongly suggest ichthyosis vulgaris.
- Family history and family pedigree point to a dominant mode of inheritance.
- Biopsies from involved areas show moderate hyperkeratosis with a markedly reduced or absent granular

layer. The thickness of the spinous layer is normal. The findings are distinctive but not pathognomonic. Examination with electron microscopy reveals irregular (fragmented or spongy) keratohyalin granules.

- Mild forms can be confused with xerosis (dry skin), while severe forms in males are difficult to distinguish from X-linked ichthyosis. Other inherited forms of ichthyosis as well as acquired ichthyosis are also included in the differential diagnosis.

TREATMENT

- Lubricating and emollient creams can be efficient in the mild forms.
- Hydration can improve the clinical findings. Salt-water baths followed by application of lubricants are often helpful. Propylene glycol (40 to 60%) in water applied under occlusion for several nights also increases the removal of scales.
- Keratolytic agents, such as 10% urea cream, 3 to 6% salicylic acid preparations, and alpha hydroxy acid formulations, are also used.
- Care must be given when treating widespread areas on infants and pediatric patients. Systemic absorption of the topical medications can be substantial because of the compromised barrier function and the greater body-surface-to-weight ratio. Increased incidence of adverse effects may occur in this group of patients.

X-LINKED ICHTHYOSIS

EPIDEMIOLOGY

- X-linked ichthyosis presents in 1 in every 2000 to 6000 live births of males. It has no ethnic or racial predominance.
- It is transmitted as an X-linked recessive trait.
- X-linked ichthyosis can present at birth, and occurs usually before 3 months of age.

PATHOPHYSIOLOGY

- X-linked ichthyosis is a retention hyperkeratosis with decreased desquamation and normal rate of epidermal turnover.
- Mutations in the gene encoding the enzyme steroid sulfatase (aryl sulfatase c), most commonly deletions at the Xp22 chromosome, have been found. This enzyme catalyses the hydrolysis of cholesterol sulfate

in the epidermis. Cholesterol sulfate accumulates and causes the abnormal cornification.
- The barrier function of the involved skin is compromised.

CLINICAL FEATURES

- X-linked ichthyosis is characterized by fine to large yellow brown scales.
- The scales are more prominent on the anterior and sides of the neck giving a dirty, unwashed appearance to the patient. The involvement of the trunk, primarily the abdomen, and the extensor surfaces of the extremities is also pronounced. The antecubital and popliteal fossae can have mild abnormalities. The scalp and face are relatively spared as are the palms and soles.
- Ophthalmologic slit-lamp examination reveals corneal opacities on the posterior capsule in about 50% of the patients. The opacities do not affect vision. Similar abnormalities may be found in female carriers.
- Cryptorchidism may exist in 12 to 15% of patients with X-linked ichthyosis, increasing the risk for testicular cancer if it is not discovered and treated early.
- Conditions, such as keratosis pilaris and atopy, that usually coexist with ichthyosis vulgaris, do not have increased incidence in patients with X-linked ichthyosis.
- Difficulty in initiating labor during the birth of these patients frequently occurs. This failure of spontaneous parturition is caused by deficiency of placental sulfatase.

DIAGNOSIS AND DIFFERENTIAL

- Clinical findings are very helpful for the diagnosis. The quality and distribution of the scales, existence of cryptorchidism, and corneal opacities are of importance.
- Family history and family pedigree suggest an X-linked mode of inheritance. Ophthalmologic examination of the mother may reveal corneal opacities.
- Histology is nonspecific, with hyperkeratosis and mild hypergranulosis.
- Lipoprotein electrophoresis can strongly indicate the diagnosis since the increase of cholesterol sulfate causes low-density lipoproteins to migrate more rapidly in affected individuals.
- Increased serum cholesterol sulfate confirms the diagnosis. Decreased enzyme activity can also be found in fibroblasts, keratinocytes, and leukocytes.
- Other ichthyosiform dermatoses are included in the differential diagnosis.

- Prenatal diagnosis can be made by finding reduced steroid sulfatase activity in fibroblasts obtained from amniotic fluid. Noninvasive techniques, such as the detection of nonhydrolyzed, sulphated steroids in the urine of pregnant women, may be helpful.

TREATMENT

- Lubricating, emollient creams, keratolytics, and increased hydration are helpful.
- 10% cholesterol cream and calcipotriol ointment has been used.
- In severe cases oral acitretin can reduce scaling and ameliorate the clinical appearance.

LAMELLAR ICHTHYOSIS

EPIDEMIOLOGY

- Lamellar ichthyosis occurs in about 1 in every 300,000 live births.
- It is transmitted as an autosomal recessive trait. Autosomal dominant inheritance has also been reported.
- Lamellar ichthyosis is usually present at birth, or soon after birth. Collodion baby presentation may occur.

PATHOPHYSIOLOGY

- In lamellar ichthyosis there is a normal or slightly increased rate of epidermal proliferation.
- Mutations in the gene encoding the enzyme trans-glutaminase-1 (TGM-1) have been found. Reduced or absent TGM-1 activity is found in about half of the patients. This enzyme catalyses the cross-linking of epidermal proteins, such as involucrin, that are normally deposited on the membrane of keratinocytes. Without cross-linking an abnormal cornified cell envelope develops.
- Genetic heterogeneity exists as cases of lamellar ichthyosis have been found with normal TGM-1 activity and the reason for an increased rate of epidermal proliferation is not completely understood.
- The barrier function of the involved skin is compromised.

CLINICAL FEATURES

- Patients with lamellar ichthyosis are usually enclosed in a collodion-like membrane at birth. This membrane desquamates after 1 to 2 weeks, revealing underlying red skin. Large, platelike, dark, brown scales in a mosaic pattern appear later. The scales are free at the edges and adherent in the center. The hair follicles may have a crateriform appearance. Adult patients are not erythrodermic.
- The scales cover almost the entire body. They are more prominent on the lower extremities resembling a dry riverbed. The face and flexures are involved. The lips and mucous membranes are spared. Palms and soles have hyperkeratosis, which may vary from mild hyperlinearity to keratoderma.
- Ectropion and eclabium are common in patients with lamellar ichthyosis. Exposure keratitis may develop. Scarring alopecia is also a frequent finding. Nails can be thickened and dystrophic. The patients also suffer from heat intolerance as a result of hypo-hidrosis.

DIAGNOSIS AND DIFFERENTIAL

- Among the clinical findings, the existence of ectropion, eclabium, and alopecia as well as the quality and distribution of the scales are most helpful.
- Family history and family pedigree suggest an autosomal recessive mode of inheritance.
- Histology is nonspecific and hyperkeratosis with acanthosis is found.
- Other ichthyosiform dermatoses are included in the differential diagnosis. The findings of lamellar ichthyosis may overlap with congenital ichthyosiform erythroderma, rendering the diagnosis difficult.

TREATMENT

- Lubricating, emollient creams, keratolytics, and increased hydration are helpful.
- Topical retinoids and topical vitamin D derivatives can ameliorate the scaling.
- Oral retinoids, such as acitretin (soriatane) or isotretinoin (accutane), may improve the condition, but the risk/benefit ratio should be considered if long-term treatment is indicated.
- Eye care with liquid tears and lubricants is important in patients with ectropion.
- In the neonatal period the patients presenting as collodion babies are at risk for temperature imbalance, hyponatremia, dehydration, and infections, especially pneumonia. These possible complications should be addressed, as well as the requirement for increased protein and caloric intake.

Nonbullous Congenital Ichthyosiform Erythroderma (CIE)

EPIDEMIOLOGY

- CIE occurs in about 1 in every 300,000 live births.
- It is transmitted as an autosomal recessive trait.
- CIE is usually present at birth. A collodion baby presentation often occurs.

PATHOPHYSIOLOGY

- In CIE, in contrast to lamellar ichthyosis, there is marked increase of the rate of epidermal turnover.
- The etiology of CIE is unknown.
- The barrier function of the involved skin is compromised.

CLINICAL FEATURES

- Patients with CIE are usually enclosed in a collodion-like membrane at birth. Fissuring and desquamation of the membrane usually begins within 1 day and is complete after 1 to 2 weeks, revealing underlying red skin with scaling.
- Generalized involvement with large scales on the lower extremities and finer on the trunk, face, and scalp is typical. Palms and soles are almost always affected and palmoplantar hyperkeratosis is frequent. The mucous membranes are spared.
- In contrast to lamellar ichthyosis, ectropion and eclabium are not common in patients with CIE. Cicatricial alopecia may be seen.
- The patients may suffer from severe heat intolerance as a result of decreased sweating. Nail dystrophy may exist, and fungal infections of the nails are common.

DIAGNOSIS AND DIFFERENTIAL

- Clinical findings and family pedigree are very helpful for the diagnosis.
- Histology is nonspecific as it shows hyperkeratosis, acanthosis, and parakeratosis.
- CIE is the most common cause of collodion baby. However, lamellar ichthyosis, other forms of ichthyosis, and normal infants (lamellar exfoliation of the newborn or self-healing collodion baby) should be included in the differential diagnosis.

TREATMENT

- Lubricating, emollient creams, and increased hydration are helpful. Keratolytics should be avoided. Oral retinoids can be particularly helpful.
- Special care to avoid infection in fissured areas is of importance.

Epidermolytic Hyperkeratosis or Bullous Congenital Ichthyosiform Erythroderma (EHK)

EPIDEMIOLOGY

- EHK occurs in about 1 in every 200,000 to 300,000 live births. It affects all races and both genders.
- It is transmitted as an autosomal dominant trait. However, in many cases there is no family history and the disease is the result of a new spontaneous mutation.
- EHK is usually present at birth or shortly after birth.

PATHOPHYSIOLOGY

- EHK is a hyperproliferative hyperkeratosis.
- Mutations in the genes encoding for one of the suprabasal keratins (keratins 1 and 10) result in keratin clumping and the formation of abnormal keratohyalin granules. These defects lead to abnormal cytoskeleton, mechanical fragility, and easy formation of intraepidermal blisters. The mechanism by which increased proliferation occurs is not yet clear.

CLINICAL FEATURES

- Patients with EHK usually present, at birth or shortly after, with widespread blisters and erosions on erythrodermic skin. Later, thick, warty scales can cover the entire body. The skin has a characteristic foul odor.
- Secondary cutaneous bacterial infections are common and systemic infection may also occur.
- Generalized involvement is typical with disease more prominent on the flexures and intertriginous areas. Palms and soles may be involved, and digital contractures have been found in some patients. Keratoderma

(palmar/plantar hyperkeratosis) may exist and erythroderma may be lacking.

- There is a marked clinical heterogeneity in regard to the clinical appearance and distribution of the lesions, and several different subtypes of EHK have been described.
- The disorder can also appear in the form of an epidermal nevus caused by a postmitotic mutation.

DIAGNOSIS AND DIFFERENTIAL

- Clinical findings and family pedigree are helpful for the diagnosis. However, in cases of spontaneous mutation there is no family history.
- Histology is very distinctive in EHK, but not pathognomonic. The findings include marked hyperkeratosis and vacuolar degeneration of the epidermal granular layer (epidermolytic hyperkeratosis). The granular layer is thickened and contains irregular keratohyaline granules. The histologic picture is very useful in establishing the diagnosis.
- In the neonatal period EHK must be differentiated from epidermolysis bullosa or staphylococcal scalded skin syndrome.
- Prenatal diagnosis can be made by finding the characteristic histologic picture after fetal skin biopsy.

TREATMENT

- Lubricants, keratolytics, hydration, and topical retinoids are helpful in thickened areas with scale. Systemic retinoids can be helpful in cases of extensive involvement, but they may increase the blistering and should be used carefully. Antibacterial soaps are helpful in reducing the foul odor of the skin lesions.
- In newborns, fluid and electrolyte imbalance and sepsis are serious problems and should be addressed.

ACQUIRED ICHTHYOSIS

- Acquired ichthyosis can present in patients of any age with systemic disease. The clinical and histologic appearance resembles, in most cases, one of ichthyosis vulgaris. Some of the most common causes of acquired ichthyosis are described next.
- *Malignancies.* Hodgkin's disease is the most common malignancy causing acquired ichthyosis. The ichthyosis can precede the manifestations of the lymphoma,

although it often presents in already diagnosed patients. The scaling is more prominent on the lower extremities. Other malignancies, mainly lymphoreticular, such as non-Hodgkin's lymphoma, as well as solid tumors, such as bronchogenic carcinomas, have also been associated with ichthyosis.
- *Infections.* Ichthyosis and xerotic skin is commonly observed in patients with AIDS. Ichthyosis usually occurs after profound T-cell decrease. Leprosy can also be associated with ichthyosis.
- *Medications.* Several medications, especially cholesterol-lowering drugs, have been associated with ichthyosis. Nicotinic acid, triparanol, butyrophenone, phenothiazine, cimetidine, and isoniazid are among the most frequent offenders.
- *Autoimmune or diseases of unknown etiology.* Ichthyosis in patients with systemic lupus erythematosus, dermatomyositis, sarcoidosis, and mixed connective tissue disease has been reported.
- *Nutritional deficiencies.* Nutritional deficiencies, including essential fatty acid deficiency, malabsorption, Kwashiorkor, and hypo and hypervitaminosis, may be associated with acquired ichthyosis.
- *Endocrine and metabolic diseases.* Patients with hypothyroidism may present ichthyosiform skin with scaling mainly on the trunk and extremities. Chronic renal failure can also cause acquired ichthyosis.

TREATMENT

- Treatment is symptomatic. In many cases treatment of the underlying disorder causes improvement of the skin lesions. Previously healthy adults with sudden onset of ichthyosis should be screened for an underlying cause of the ichthyosis. Screening and evaluation for malignancy may be appropriate.

SYNDROMES ASSOCIATED WITH ICHTHYOSIS

- Several rare inherited syndromes can present with ichthyosis. Usually extracutaneous manifestations coexist. Among the most well described are the following.
- Sjögren–Larsson syndrome, a rare autosomal recessive disorder, characterized by congenital ichthyosis, neurologic manifestations during early childhood, and mental retardation.

- Erythrokeratoderma variabilis, a rare autosomal recessive disorder, characterized by hyperkeratosis and localized migrating erythema presenting at birth or shortly thereafter.
- Netherton's syndrome, a rare autosomal recessive disorder, characterized by congenital ichthyosis, hair abnormalities ("bamboo hair"), and atopy.
- Refsum's disease, a rare autosomal recessive disorder, characterized by neurologic manifestations, skeletal abnormalities, ichthyosis, and cardiac and renal abnormalities. Defective lipid metabolism and accumulation of phytanic acid due to a deficiency of phytanic acid oxidase has been identified as the cause.

REFERENCES

Akiyama M. The pathogenesis of severe congenital ichthyosis of the neonate. *J Dermatol Sci.* 1999;21:96.

Akiyama M. Severe congenital ichthyosis of the neonate. *Int J Dermatol.* 1998;37:722.

Campell JM, Banta-Wright SA. Neonatal skin disorders: A review of selected dermatologic abnormalities. *J Perinat Neonat Nurs.* 2000;14:63.

Hernadez-Martin A, Gonzalez-Sarmiento R, De Unamuno P. X-linked ichthyosis: an update. *Br J Dermatol.* 1999;141:617.

Ishida-Yamamoto A, Tanaka H, et al. Inherited disorders of epidermal keratinization. *J Dermatol Sci.* 1998;18:139.

Shwayder T. Ichthyosis in a nutshell. *Pediatr Rev.* 1999; 20:1.

KERATOSIS PILARIS (KP)

EPIDEMIOLOGY

- KP is a common disorder with a prevalence of up to 80% in adolescent women and 20% in adult women. Generally it affects about 40% of the population, without any racial predilection. It is usually seen in young women and teenagers.
- It is probably transmitted as an autosomal dominant trait with incomplete penetrance. More than 50% of the patients lack a family history.
- The disease usually starts during childhood, with more than 80% of the cases presenting before the age of 20.

PATHOPHYSIOLOGY

- The pathogenesis of the disease is unknown. Excessive follicular production of keratin leads to the formation of keratin plugs, which subsequently block and dilate the follicular orifice.

CLINICAL FEATURES

- The main clinical characteristics of KP are small follicular papules, which represent keratinous plugging of the follicular orifices. Skin acquires a rough texture and looks like "goose flesh." The sites more frequently affected are the extensor surfaces of the proximal arms, the lateral surface of thighs, and buttocks. The face, especially eyebrows, may be affected.
- Perifollicular erythema may accompany the lesions, in which case it is often referred to as keratosis pilaris rubra. Cases without erythema are called keratosis pilaris alba.
- The disease is usually asymptomatic, painless, and with absent or mild pruritus.
- KP presents seasonal variations. In the majority of the patients the lesions worsen during winter and/or improve during summer.
- The prevalence of KP appears to be higher in patients with dry skin, atopic dermatitis, ichthyosis vulgaris, high body mass index (BMI > 25), and insulin-dependent diabetes mellitus. Conditions that have been associated with KP include vitamin B_2 deficiency and Cushing's disease.

DIAGNOSIS AND DIFFERENTIAL

- The diagnosis is usually based on clinical findings. A family history may reveal other members affected with KP.
- The biopsy is helpful showing an orthokeratotic keratin plug that blocks and dilates the orifice and the upper portion of the follicular infundibulum. Sometimes a twisted hair shaft may be entrapped inside the keratin plug. A mild perivascular cell infiltrate may be present in the upper dermis.
- Lichen spinulosum, phrynoderma, pityriasis rubra pilaris, and keratosis pilaris atrophicans can be included in the differential, but differ clinically and histologically.

THERAPY

- Although no cure for KP exists, several approaches have been found to reduce the intensity of the clinical findings. Some have approached this disease as a follicular disease, while others have treated it as a dermatitis. Prevention of excessive skin dryness by

decreasing the frequency of long hot baths, use of harsh soaps, and by regular use of emollients is helpful.
- Topical medications that have been used with partial success in many cases include tretinoin, glycolic acid, and keratolytic agents such as urea, salicylic acid, and lactic acid. Topical steroids, such as triamcinolone, may also be of help, especially in lesions with associated inflammatory changes.

KERATOSIS PILARIS ATROPHICANS (KPA)

EPIDEMIOLOGY

- KPA is a group of rare inherited diseases. Its precise prevalence is unknown. The most common subtype is keratosis pilaris atrophicans faciei (KPAF), while atrophoderma vermiculatum (AV) and keratosis follicularis spinulosa decalvans (KFSD) are less common. KPAF and KFSD are both characterized by erythematous follicular papules and alopecia starting in infancy; however, their distribution differs. AV starts in childhood and is characterized by scar-like atrophic pits on the cheeks.
- The subtypes of KPA have different modes of inheritance (Table 2–1).

PATHOPHYSIOLOGY

- The etiology of KPA is unknown. The primary event appears to be abnormal production of keratin from the upper part of the hair follicle. A keratin plug is formed that blocks and dilates the follicular orifice. However, in later stages fibrosis and atrophy of the hair bulb develop in some of the affected areas, causing scarring and destruction of the hair.

CLINICAL FEATURES

- The main clinical feature of KPA is follicular hyperkeratosis combined with scarring alopecia. The individual features of the variants of KPA are described next (Table 2–1).

KERATOSIS PILARIS ATROPHICANS FACIEI (KPAF) (ULERYTHEMA OOPHRYOGENES)
- Its onset is usually during infancy or even at birth.
- The main characteristic of KPAF is the appearance of several follicular papules with erythema on the face. During childhood, there is loss of eyebrow hair and scarring.
- The main areas affected are the eyebrows, cheeks, and forehead.
- Keratosis pilaris usually coexists on the extremities or other sites of the body.
- It may be associated with atopy, wooly hair syndrome, Noonan's syndrome, and other congenital abnormalities. In wooly hair syndrome a variable degree of tight curling is present in all hairs throughout the scalp. Noonan's syndrome is a genetic disorder characterized by short stature, webbed neck, skeletal, cardiac, and endocrine abnormalities; and some degree of mental retardation.

ATROPHODERMA VERMICULATUM (AV)
- AV usually presents during childhood, after the age of 5. Presentation at older ages, even during adulthood, has been reported, but is rare.
- AV begins as multiple pinhead follicular plugs surrounded by erythema, which gradually progress to form irregular atrophic pits giving a "worm-eaten" appearance to the skin.

TABLE 2–1 Subtypes of Keratosis Pilaris Atrophicans

	KPAF	AV	KFSD
Mode of Inheritance	Autosomal dominant	Autosomal dominant or recessive	X-linked
Onset	Birth or infancy	Childhood, adulthood (rarely)	Infancy
Main Lesion	Erythematous follicular papules	Small follicular pits, "worm-eaten" skin	Erythematous follicular plugs and milia
Distribution	Face, esp. eyebrows	Face, esp. cheeks. Eyebrows and scalp are spared	Face, scalp, trunk
Other Findings	Loss of eyebrows and scarring		Absent eyelashes, scarring alopecia, xerosis, corneal dystrophy, photophobia
Associated Diseases	Atopy, wooly hair, Noonan's syndrome, other congenital abnormalities	Mongolism	Keratosis pilaris, atopic dermatitis

- Affecting mainly the cheeks, AV can progress to involve the forehead, lips, preauricular areas, and ears. It is usually symmetric. The eyebrows and scalp are typically spared.
- AV in some patients is associated with other abnormalities such as mongolism.

KERATOSIS FOLLICULARIS SPINULOSA DECALVANS (KFSD)

- KFSD usually begins during infancy.
- KFSD starts with multiple follicular plugs and milia on the face (nose, cheeks, eyebrows) and extends to other parts of the body (scalp, neck, and trunk). Erythema commonly accompanies the lesions. It causes patchy scarring alopecia of the scalp and eyebrows. Eyelashes may also be absent.
- Folliculitis spinulosa decalvans (FSD), a subtype of KFSD that occurs in the scalp, is characterized by pronounced inflammation and pustule formation.
- Associated findings include keratosis pilaris of the extremities, ichthyosiform xerosis, hyperkeratosis of palms and soles, photophobia, and atopic dermatitis of the scalp. Corneal dystrophy with opacities of Bowman's membrane may be found during ophthalmologic examination.
- Female carriers may have dry skin, mild hyperkeratosis of the soles, and minimal follicular hyperkeratosis.

DIAGNOSIS AND DIFFERENTIAL

- The diagnosis is based primarily on the clinical findings. A positive family history exists in most cases.
- The histologic findings depend on the stage of the disease. Early lesions show hyperkeratosis of the infudibulum and isthmus of the hair follicle and hypergranulosis. Later lesions show destruction of the hair wall and mixed lymphohistiocyte infiltrate. However, fully developed lesions may lack specific findings with predominant fibrosis. The lower follicle is uninvolved at the early stages and becomes affected only later.
- KPAF should be differentiated from seborrheic dermatitis. Atopic dermatitis may be confused with KFSP. The KID (keratitis, ichthyosis, deafness) syndrome may resemble KFSP as well. KFSD should be considered in the differential diagnosis of scarring alopecia. AV scars may resemble acne scars.

TREATMENT

- No effective cure exists for KPA. However, the symptoms may improve with topical therapy, including emollients, keratolytic agents, corticosteroids, and tretinoin. Oral retinoids have also been effective. Follicular depressions on the face may be treated with dermabrasion, laser abrasion, or deep chemical peels. Pulsed dye laser has been reported to be useful for the reduction of the facial erythema, but not of the associated skin roughness.

REFERENCES

Baden HP, Byers RH. Clinical findings, cutaneous pathology, and response to therapy in 21 patients with keratosis pilaris atrophicans. *Arch Dermatol.* 1994;130:469.

Garwood JD. Keratosis pilaris. *Am Fam Physician.* 1978; 17:151.

Lateef A, Schwartz RA. Keratosis pilaris. *Cutis.* 1999; 63:205.

Potskitt L, Wilkinson JD. Natural history of keratosis pilaris. *Br J Dermatol* 1994;130:711.

Rand R, Baden HP. Keratosis follicularis spinulosa decalvans. *Arch Dermatol.* 1983;119:22.

DARIER'S DISEASE

KERATOSIS FOLLICULARIS, DARIER–WHITE DISEASE

EPIDEMIOLOGY

- Although the exact prevalence of Darier's disease is not known, it has been reported to be between 1:36,000 and 1:100,000 in European countries. There does not appear to be a racial or sexual predilection.
- Darier's disease is an autosomal dominant genodermatosis, with high penetrance. The disease presents great phenotypic heterogeneity between and within each generation. New mutations are common, and there is no family history in many cases.
- The onset of the disease typically is before 20 years old, with presentation prior to the third decade in more than 70% of the cases. Peak incidence occurs during the second decade of life. However, in some patients the disease does not manifest until adulthood and in some (< 5%) the disease manifests after the age of 60.

PATHOPHYSIOLOGY

- Recently, mutations in the ATP2A2 gene, a gene that encodes the sarco/endoplasmic reticulum Ca^{2+}-ATPase isoform 2, have been identified as the cause of Darier's disease.

- Disturbances of the function of T cells have been reported, but various studies have yielded conflicting results.
- The disease is characterized by abnormalities of the cornification process. One of the early events of the disease is the loss of the cohesion between keratinocytes, which results in separation of epidermal cells (acantholysis). The acantholysis can present clinically as bullae, although usually this is not a main characteristic of the disease. Moreover, the desmosome-keratin filament complexes become disorganized and keratin filaments aggregate around the nuclei. The disease process results in hyperkeratosis and dyskeratosis and manifests clinically with characteristic keratotic papules. There is, however, no known primary defect in the keratins or cell adhesion proteins.

CLINICAL FEATURES

- Multiple, rough, keratotic papules are the main clinical findings of the disease. Beginning as skin-colored papules, they are later covered by a brown, rough, scaly crust. If the crust is removed, it often reveals a central umbilicated papule. Inflammation may accompany the lesions. The papules may coalesce and form hypertrophic warty plaques or even tumors. Extensive confluent areas of hyperkeratosis may develop. Localized blistering may occur occasionally.
- Depending on the distribution of the lesions, three main patterns have been recognized. In the vast majority of the patients (> 90%) the disease predominantly affects the so-called seborrheic areas, including the chest, supraclavicular fossae, back, scalp, face (especially the nasolabial folds and the forehead), and ears. Mild flexural involvement may coexist. In a less common pattern, the *flexural* pattern, involvement of the flexures, including axillae, inframammary areas, and groin, predominates. In the *nevoid* pattern, there is only unilateral dermatomal or zosteriform involvement. These unilateral cases are considered by many as a form of a nevus that has a Darier-like histology rather than localized Darier's disease. Others believe that they may represent mosaicism.
- Acral lesions exist in more than 90% of the patients. Palmar pits and keratotic papules on the palms are found. Soles are less frequently affected. Hemorrhagic macules may occur rarely. The dorsum of the hands or feet may have acrokeratosis verruciformis-like lesions (flat wart-like lesions). Rarely, hands may be the only area affected by the disease.

- Nail lesions exist in the majority of the patients and, in some cases, they are the presenting manifestation of the disease. Fingernails are more commonly and more severely affected than toenails. Characteristic lesions include longitudinal red or white lines, ridging, nail fragility, and notches at the free edge of the nail, as well as subungual thickening.
- Oral mucosal involvement, with white cobblestone papules, is common (~15%). Vulval and anal lesions have been reported.
- Foul odor, probably due to bacterial hyperproliferation, accompanies the lesions in as many as half of all patients. This can be particularly socially disabling in some patients. Pruritus is also common (~80%), while pain is unusual in uncomplicated Darier's disease.
- Complications include frequent cutaneous viral infections especially with herpes simplex (14% of the patients), cutaneous bacterial infections, chronic dermatophytosis, and rarely salivary gland obstruction.
- Conditions that cause exacerbation of Darier's disease include exposure to sunlight, probably related to excessive heat, as well as sweating. Stress, and wool clothing, have also been reported as exacerbating the disease, as have general anesthesia and oral treatment with lithium. A small percentage of female patients may have premenstrual worsening of the disease.
- Psychological or neurologic diseases, such as epilepsy, mental retardation, and affective disorders, have been reported associated with Darier's disease.

DIAGNOSIS AND DIFFERENTIAL

- The clinical findings, mainly the quality and distribution of the papules and the existence of nail lesions, are quite suggestive of Darier's disease. The combination of white and red longitudinal lines on the nails is considered pathognomonic. Family history exists in more than half of the patients.
- The histologic picture in combination with the clinical presentation confirms the diagnosis. The skin biopsy shows acantholysis with suprabasal clefts (lacunae), dyskeratosis, hyperkeratosis, and papillary overgrowth of the epidermis. Characteristic dyskeratotic cells exist, called "corps ronds" and "corps grains." "Corps ronds" have a darkly stained central nucleus surrounded by clear cytoplasm and are located in the spinous layer. "Corps grains" are small densely staining cells without nucleus located in the stratum corneum.
- The differential diagnosis includes lesions that may have a similar histologic picture to Darier's disease. Transient acantholytic dermatosis (Grover's disease), warty dyskeratoma, epidermal nevi, and Hailey-Hailey

disease (benign familial pemphigus) may have either dyskeratosis or acantholysis histologically. Seborrheic dermatitis may sometimes be confused with Darier's disease because of the similar distribution. Keratosis pilaris, acneiform eruptions, and histiocytosis may bear clinical resemblance to Darier's disease.

TREATMENT

- There is no cure for Darier's disease. The treatment's objective is to control the symptoms of the disease and limit extent and severity of the lesions.
- Avoidance of the triggers that cause exacerbation of the disease is important. Use of sunscreens is recommended. Cotton clothes are preferable.
- Good personal hygiene, frequent washes with antiseptics, and use of topical or oral antibiotics helps control the malodor of the lesions. Retinoids, however, are more effective in both reducing the odor and decreasing keratin production. Emollients and topical steroids may be helpful. Cyclosporine may control severe flares.
- Surgical approaches for localized areas, including dermabrasion, carbon dioxide laser treatment, and surgical excision and grafting, have been used for hypertrophic lesions. Others have used tissue-engineered skin for the resultant wounds.
- Secondary fungal, viral, or bacterial infections should be identified and treated appropriately.

REFERENCES

Bale SJ, Toro JR. Genetic basis of Darier-White disease: Bad pumps cause bumps. *J Cutan Med Surg.* 2000;4:103.
Burge S. Management of Darier's disease. *Clin Exp Dermatol.* 1999;24:53.
Burge SM, Wilkinson JD. Darier-White disease: A review of the clinical features in 163 patients. *J Am Acad Dermatol.* 1992;27:40.
Kumar S, Sharma RC. Common genodermatoses. *Int J Dermatol.* 1996;35:685.

POROKERATOSIS

- Porokeratosis includes a group of phenotypically distinct disorders of epidermal keratinization, which share the clinical feature of annular or circular plaques with a raised keratotic border of the lesions, and a histologic hallmark, called the cornoid lamella.
- Four common subtypes of porokeratosis exist (Table 2–2): (1) porokeratosis of Mibelli (classic porokeratosis or plaque-type porokeratosis), (2) linear porokeratosis, (3) disseminated superficial actinic porokeratosis, and (4) porokeratosis palmaris et plantaris disseminata.
- In some cases, the lesions have increased risk for malignant transformation and porokeratosis is considered by some authors to be a premalignant condition. Up to 10% of patients with porokeratosis develop a porokeratosis-related skin malignancy. Allelic loss has been hypothesized to explain the increased cancer risk of porokeratosis.

PATHOPHYSIOLOGY

- The pathogenesis of porokeratosis is unknown. The predominant hypothesis is that a mutant clone of keratinocytes hyperproliferates and results in an area of hyperkeratosis and parakeratosis. The close association of porokeratosis with immunosuppression has

TABLE 2–2   Types of Porokeratosis

	POROKERATOSIS OF MIBELLI	LINEAR POROKERATOSIS	DSAP	PPPD
Mode of Inheritance	Autosomal dominant	Unknown	Autosomal dominant	Autosomal dominant
Onset	Childhood	Infancy or childhood	Adulthood	Early adulthood
Main Lesion	Variable-sized hyperkeratotic plaque	Multiple, coalescent, small keratotic lesions	Multiple, annular, small, keratotic lesions with central depression	Multiple, uniform, small, keratotic lesions
Distribution	Localized, esp. hands, feet, face, scalp, and perigenital area	Extremities or trunk, zosteriform or dermatomal pattern	Sun-exposed areas	Palms and soles, generalized
Malignant Transformation Rate	Moderate (~8%)	High (~20%)	Low (<5%)	Moderate (~10%)

also led to the hypothesis that abnormalities of the immune surveillance allow the development of the mutant clone of keratinocytes.

- Other authors believe that the primary defect lies in the dermis, and the epidermal findings are due to a reactive phenomenon.

POROKERATOSIS OF MIBELLI (CLASSIC POROKERATOSIS OR PLAQUE-TYPE POROKERATOSIS)

EPIDEMIOLOGY

- Porokeratosis of Mibelli is a rare disease, found more commonly in males (male to female ratio is 2:1).
- It is inherited as an autosomal dominant trait. However, most cases are sporadic.
- The onset is usually during childhood.

CLINICAL FEATURES

- The characteristic lesion is a variable-sized hyperkeratotic plaque, with central atrophy, surrounded by an elevated keratotic brown edge. A small furrow (linear dell) is found on the border. Usually few lesions are found.
- The affected areas lack hair, although sometimes the follicular orifices may be present as tiny projections. The lesions may affect the nail matrix and cause nail dystrophy.
- The lesions tend to appear usually on the hands, fingers, feet, face, scalp, and perigenital areas. However, they may appear on any area of the body. Palms and soles as well as mucous membranes may be involved.
- Predisposing factors include renal transplantation, chemotherapy, PUVA therapy, chronic exposure to sun, and exposure to certain chemicals.
- The affected areas have increased risk for the development of skin cancer, especially squamous cell carcinoma. The malignant transformation rate has been reported to be up to 10%.

DIAGNOSIS AND DIFFERENTIAL

- The characteristic clinical appearance of the lesions in combination with the histologic findings establishes the diagnosis. Histology reveals hyperkeratosis and parakeratosis of the epidermis. The cornoid lamella, a thickened compact column of parakeratotic cells, is found and corresponds to the keratotic ridge of the clinical lesions. The granular layer is absent beneath the cornoid lamella. Similar changes are found in the other subtypes of porokeratosis.
- Elastosis perforans serpiginosa clinically resembles to porokeratosis of Mibelli, but it lacks the characteristic furrow seen in porokeratosis.

TREATMENT

- Topical fluorouracil (5-FU) under occlusion can cause improvement. Oral retinoids (acitretin and isotretinoin) can be used, but the lesions recur after discontinuance.
- Surgical approaches include CO_2 laser ablation, dermabrasion, cryotherapy, and excision and grafting.
- Because of the increased risk of malignant transformation, the patients should practice sun safety, including avoidance of excessive sun exposure, sunscreen use, and periodic full body examination.

LINEAR POROKERATOSIS

EPIDEMIOLOGY

- Linear porokeratosis is a rare disease that usually presents in childhood, often in infancy.
- It is more common in females.

CLINICAL FEATURES

- Linear porokeratosis presents as multiple, coalescent, small lesions with a raised border in a linear, unilateral and/or occasionally dermatomal or zosteriform distribution. In the neonatal period ulcerations and erosions may complicate the clinical picture.
- The lesions are usually distributed on the extremities, or on the trunk in a zosteriform pattern.
- Linear porokeratosis has a high risk of malignant transformation (malignant transformation rate is as high as 19%). Squamous cell (SCC) and basal cell carcinoma, as well as Bowen's disease (SCC in situ) may develop. Older patients, with large and long-standing lesions, are at increased risk of malignant transformation, as are areas of previous radiation therapy.

DIAGNOSIS AND DIFFERENTIAL

- The clinical appearance and the histologic picture establish the diagnosis. Histologic findings are similar to porokeratosis of Mibelli.

- Linear lichen planus and linear verrucous nevus may present similar findings but the raised border and typical histology can differentiate linear porokeratosis.

TREATMENT

- The therapeutic approaches are similar to the approaches used for porokeratosis of Mibelli.

DISSEMINATED SUPERFICIAL ACTINIC POROKERATOSIS (DSAP)

EPIDEMIOLOGY

- DSAP is not an uncommon disease, and is inherited as an autosomal dominant trait. It is more common in women (male to female ratio is 1:3).
- Its onset is usually during adulthood, especially the third and fourth decades of life. However, a mild form of DSAP may develop in older patients (seventh to ninth decades).

CLINICAL FEATURES

- The characteristic lesions in DSAP are numerous, annular small keratotic plaques, with central depression and a slightly raised border. A furrow is found along the edges. The lesions commonly coalesce.
- DSAP lesions are typically found on the sun-exposed areas (disseminated superficial actinic porokeratosis) in a symmetrical distribution. In many patients the disease is more generalized and involves non-sun-exposed areas as well.
- Exacerbation or induction of the lesions may be caused by immunosuppression (organ transplantation, AIDS), exposure to commercial tanning salons, PUVA therapy, and sun exposure.
- DSAP has a low malignant transformation rate (~3.5%).

DIAGNOSIS AND DIFFERENTIAL

- The clinical and histologic picture establishes the diagnosis.
- Actinic keratosis, seborrheic keratosis, and cutaneous T-cell lymphoma may clinically resemble DSAP.

TREATMENT

- The therapeutic approaches are similar to the approaches used for porokeratosis of Mibelli.

POROKERATOSIS PALMARIS ET PLANTARIS DISSEMINATUM (PPPD)

EPIDEMIOLOGY

- PPPD is a rare autosomal dominant disease.
- Its onset is more common during early adulthood.
- It is more common in males (male to female ratio is 2:1)

CLINICAL FEATURES

- PPPD is characterized by multiple, uniform, small keratotic lesions, with the characteristic surrounding ridge and furrow. Beginning on the palms and soles, they subsequently extend to the rest of the body. Mucous membranes may be affected.
- Pruritus often accompanies the lesions.

DIAGNOSIS

- The clinical and histologic picture establishes the diagnosis.

TREATMENT

- The therapeutic approaches are similar to the approaches used for the other forms of porokeratosis.

REFERENCES

Herranz P, Pizarro A, De Lucas R, et al. High incidence of porokeratosis in renal transplant recipients. *Br J Dermatol.* 1997;136:176.

Patrizi A, D'Acunto C, Passarini B, Neri L. Porokeratosis in the elderly: A new subtype of disseminated superficial actinic porokeratosis. *Acta Derm Venereol.* 2000;80:302.

Sasson M, Krain AD. Porokeratosis and cutaneous malignancy. *Dermatol Surg.* 1996;22:339.

Schamroth JM, Zlotogorski A, Gilead L. Porokeratosis of Mibelli. Overview and review of the literature. *Acta Derm Venereol.* 1997;77:207.

PALMOPLANTAR KERATODERMAS

- Keratodermas (palmar/plantar keratosis or PPK) is a group of several phenotypically and genotypically different diseases that share the common clinical finding of palmar and/or plantar hyperkeratosis. Keratodermas can be either acquired or inherited. Moreover, keratodermas can exist alone, or as a part of a syndrome or cutaneous disease. Because of the clinical overlap between different entities and the rarity of some inherited forms of keratodermas, several classifications have been proposed. We will describe both the commonest inherited PPKs (Table 2–3) and the acquired PPKs.

INHERITED PALMOPLANTAR KERATODERMAS

DIFFUSE PALMOPLANTAR KERATODERMAS

- Diffuse palmoplantar keratodermas (PPKs) are characterized by thick hyperkeratosis in a diffuse pattern over the whole of the palms and soles. They do not involve the rest of the body. Diffuse PPKs include four different diseases: epidermolytic PPK, non-epidermolytic PPK, erythrokeratoderma variabilis, and PPK of Symbert.

EPIDERMOLYTIC PPK (VORNER'S PPK)

- Epidermolytic PPK is an autosomal dominantly inherited genodermatosis, and appears to be the most frequent type of inherited PPK. Defects of the gene encoding keratin 9 exist in some families. Keratin 9 is a suprabasal keratin found in the palms and soles.
- It presents during infancy and is characterized by symmetric thickening over the entire palm and sole.
- The diagnosis is confirmed with the histologic findings, which reveal marked hyperkeratosis and acanthosis with epidermolysis.

NON-EPIDERMOLYTIC PPK (UNNA–THOST DISEASE)

- Non-epidermolytic PPK is inherited in an autosomal dominant fashion and is among the commonest inherited PPKs. It occurs worldwide with equal distribution in both sexes. Mutations in the gene encoding keratin 1 have been found.
- It presents from birth or early infancy, and is characterized by marked well-demarcated symmetric thickening over the entire palm and sole. Initially, the

margin may be erythematous or violaceous. The hyperkeratosis may extend to the dorsum of the hands and to the wrists. Nail abnormalities may coexist. Hyperhidrosis is a frequently reported symptom.
- It is often complicated by dermatophyte infections, which result in painful fissures and scaling.
- Histology helps in distinguishing this disease from epidermolytic PPK by revealing hyperkeratosis and acanthosis without epidermolysis.

ERYTHROKERATODERMA VARIABILIS

- This disease is inherited as an autosomal dominant trait.
- It usually presents during infancy and progresses during childhood, with well-demarcated areas of erythrokeratoderma (hyperkeratotic plaques within areas of erythema) over the body. The lesions are symmetrical. Palms and soles present erythematous desquamation. The keratoderma commonly extends to the dorsum of hands and feet. Nail dystrophy may coexist.
- Histology is non-specific, with hyperkeratosis and acanthosis without parakeratosis. Electron microscopy has shown prominent tonofilament/keratohyaline complexes found within the stratum granulosum.

PPK OF SYMBERT (GREITHER'S PPK)

- PPK of Symbert is a rare autosomal dominant genodermatosis.
- It presents with severe symmetric keratoderma of palms and soles. Keratoderma may involve knees and elbows as well. Rarely, autoamputation of the fingers may occur. It is commonly associated with hyperhidrosis.
- The histology shows accumulation of lipid-laden cells in the stratum corneum, while amyloid deposition may develop in the dermis, especially after treatment with retinoids.

FOCAL PPKS

- Focal PPKs are characterized by focuses of hyperkeratosis at sites of friction or pressure on the palms and soles.

STRIATE PPK

- Striate PPK is a rare autosomal dominant keratoderma.
- Its onset is usually during infancy or childhood.

TABLE 2–3 Inherited Palmoplantar Keratodermas (Excluding Palmoplantar Ectodermal Dysplasias)

	MODE OF INHERITANCE	GENE DEFECT	ONSET	CHARACTERISTIC LESION	ASSOCIATED FINDINGS	HISTOLOGY
A. DIFFUSE PPKS						
Epidermolytic PPK (Vorner's)	Autosomal dominant	Keratin 9	Infancy	Even, thick, symmetric hyperkeratosis of palms and soles	None	Characteristic (hyperkeratosis, acanthosis, and epidermolysis)
Non-epidermolytic PPK (Unna–Thost disease)	Autosomal dominant	Keratin gene cluster (12q and 17q), keratin 1	Birth or infancy	Even, thick, symmetric hyperkeratosis of palms and soles ± violaceous margin	Nail abnormalities, hyperhidrosis, dermatophyte infections	Nonspecific (hyperkeratosis and acanthosis without epidermolysis)
Erythrokeratoderma Variabilis	Autosomal dominant	Rhesus blood group locus (1p36.2-p34)	Infancy	Erythematous desquamation of palms and soles, symmetric areas of erythrokeratoderma over rest of body	Nail dystrophy, neurologic abnormalities (rarely)	Nonspecific (hyperkeratosis and acanthosis)
PPK of Symbert (Greither's PPK)	Autosomal dominant	Rhesus blood group locus (1p36.2-p34)	Infancy	Severe symmetric hyperkeratosis of palms and soles, involvement of knees and elbows	Hyperhidrosis, autoamputation of fingers (rarely)	Hyperkeratosis, lipid-laden cells in stratum corneum
FOCAL PPKS						
Striate PPK	Autosomal dominant	Desmosomal cadherins, desmogleins, and desmocollin gene cluster on 18q12, keratin 16 gene	Infancy, childhood	Hyperkeratosis in sites of friction and calluses on the soles, possible involvement of palms, genitalia, and other places	Skin fragility, hair abnormalities, wooly hair (rarely)	Nonspecific (hyperkeratosis, acanthosis, papillomatosis)
PUNCTATE PPKS						
Keratosis Punctata Palmaris and Plantaris	Autosomal dominant	No linkage to keratin gene clusters	Adolescence, early adulthood	Multiple, tiny punctuate keratoses, coalesce over points of friction, on palms and soles	Nail abnormalities, facial sebaceous hyperplasia, increased risk for non-skin malignancies	Massive hyperkeratosis over a sharply limited area
Spiny Keratoderma	Autosomal dominant	Unknown	Adolescence, early adulthood	Multiple, tiny, horny projections (like music box spines) on palms and soles	Facial sebaceous hyperplasia	Columns of parakeratosis (like cornoid lamella of porokeratoses)
Focal Acral Hyperkeratosis	Autosomal dominant	Unknown	Adulthood	Crateriform keratotic papules on the border of hands, wrists, and feet	None	

- Large masses of keratin develop at sites of recurrent friction. Nummular or linear calluses develop. Follicular, oral, and genital hyperkeratosis are common.
- The sites of predilection are the soles; however, palms and other sites may develop lesions as well.
- Skin fragility, nail and hair abnormalities commonly coexist.
- Histology is nonspecific with prominent hyperkeratosis, acanthosis, and papillomatosis.

PUNCTATE PPKS

TYPE I PUNCTATE PPK (KERATOSIS PUNCTATA PALMARIS ET PLANTARIS)

- This is an autosomal dominant keratoderma.
- It usually develops between the ages of 12 and 30 years.
- It is clinically characterized by multiple tiny punctate keratoses over the palms and soles, which may coalesce over the points of friction of the sole. Physical trauma appears to induce the lesions.
- Nail abnormalities are commonly found.
- It may be associated with increased risk for various noncutaneous malignancies.

TYPE II PUNCTATE PPK (SPINY KERATODERMA)

- This is an autosomal dominant keratoderma.
- Its onset is late and may present in patients in adolescence or adulthood.
- The clinical characteristic lesions are multiple tiny horny projections, resembling the spines of a music box, distributed over the entire surface of palms and soles.
- Histology shows columns of parakeratosis, resembling the cornoid lamella found in porokeratoses.

TYPE III PUNCTATE PPK (FOCAL ACRAL HYPERKERATOSIS)

- This keratoderma is inherited as an autosomal dominant trait.
- It is a late-onset keratoderma, presenting more frequently in blacks.
- It is characterized by oval or polygonal crateriform papules, found on the border of the hand, foot, and wrist. A confluent pattern may exist in the center of

the palms and soles. Elastorrhexis (fragmentation of the elastic fibers of the dermis) is a variable feature.

PALMOPLANTAR ECTODERMAL DYSPLASIAS (PEDs)

- Palmoplantar ectodermal dysplasias include a variety of syndromes that have palmar or plantar keratoderma as a common feature. More than 20 entities have been classified as PEDs. The majority of them are inherited as autosomal dominant or recessive traits.
- Nail and hair lesions coexist in most PEDs. Oral mucosal hyperkeratosis may also develop. In addition to skin, other structures that are derived by the ectoderm, including teeth, inner ear, lens, and central nervous system, may be affected. Deafness, bone abnormalities, and eye and teeth lesions have been described in these conditions, and several syndromes have increased risk for development of malignancies.
- Among the most common PEDs are the following.
- Pachyonychia congenita type I (type I PED), which presents during infancy or childhood and is characterized by the combination of nail abnormalities in addition to plantar keratoderma (mutations in keratins 6,16).
- Pachyonychia congenita type II (type II PED), which resembles pachyonychia congenital type I but is also characterized by the presence of multiple epidermal cysts, steatocytoma, and wooly hair in addition to the palmar keratoderma and nail abnormalities (mutations in keratin 17).
- PPK associated with esophageal cancer (type III PED, Howel–Evans syndrome), which presents during childhood as focal plantar keratoderma. Follicular hyperkeratosis and oral leukokeratosis are common. These patients have a risk up to 90% of developing esophageal cancer by the age of 65.
- Papillon–Lefèvre syndrome (type IV PED), which presents during infancy and is characterized by the combination of palmoplantar keratoderma and severe periodontitis resulting in tooth loss. Other lesions may coexist.
- Oculocutaneous tyrosinemia (type V PED), which has an onset at 2 to 4 years of age. Callosities over the pressure points of the soles as well as photophobia and corneal ulcerations develop. Mental retardation may result. Treatment consists of a low tyrosine and phenylalanine diet.
- Olmsted syndrome (type VI PED), which is characterized by diffuse PPK with flexion deformities of the digits and autoamputation of the digits. Perioral, perianal, and perineal lesions coexist.

- Keratitis–ichthyosis–deafness syndrome (type XV PED), which is present from birth and is characterized by ichthyosiform erythroderma, corneal involvement, deafness, and diffuse keratoderma. It is associated with the development of multiple cutaneous squamous cell carcinomas.

ACQUIRED KERATODERMAS

- Keratoderma (palmar or plantar hyperkeratosis) may be found as a feature of several other diseases including psoriasis, atopic dermatitis, Reiter's syndrome, secondary syphilis, tinea pedis, and Sézary syndrome (mycosis fungoides, cutaneous T-cell lymphoma). Norwegian scabies may cause marked hyperkeratosis. Keratoderma may also develop in patients with AIDS.
- Paraneoplastic keratoderma is usually a diffuse PPK. Spiny keratoderma has also been reported in association with malignancy.
- Arsenic ingestion can cause arsenical keratosis, which is a form of punctate PPK. Increased incidence of angiosarcoma of the liver, basal cell carcinoma, and bronchial adenocarcinoma has been reported in patients with arsenical keratosis.
- Idiopathic filiform porokeratotic PPK is an acquired form of punctate keratoderma, which has been associated with colon, breast, lung, and renal cancer.
- Keratosis punctata of the palmar creases is a common form of punctate keratoderma, predominantly found in Afro-Caribbeans. Small depression and keratotic pits are found on the creases of palms and on the fingers.
- Punctate keratosis of the palms and soles is a type of acquired punctate keratoderma found more commonly in black men. Multiple pruritic keratotic papules are found on the palms. It commonly presents as spiny keratoderma. It has been associated with increased risk of internal malignancies.
- Keratoderma climactericum is a form of focal keratoderma that develops on the soles at sites of pressure in women during menopause. It resembles plantar psoriasis.
- How and why acquired keratodermas develop is not known.

TREATMENT OF KERATODERMAS

- Topical emollients and keratolytic agents, with or without occlusion, have been used with variable results. Topical retinoids, such as tazarotene, may be helpful. Manual paring of hyperkeratosis improves the lesions.
- Podiatric evaluation and occasionally surgery may be beneficial especially in focal PPKs.
- Topical 5-FU may be helpful and occlusion may increase the therapeutic benefit.
- Oral retinoids are effective. Acitretin seems to be more effective than isotretinoin.
- Associated dermatophyte infections are treated with topical or oral antifungal agents.

REFERENCES

Helm TN, Lee J, Helm KF. Spiny keratoderma. *Cutis.* 2000; 66:191.

Ishida-Yamamoto A, Tanaka H, et al. Inherited disorders of epidermal keratinization. *J Dermatol Sci* 1998;18:139.

Lucker GPH, Van De Kerkof PCM, Steijlen PM. The hereditary palmoplantar keratosis: An updated review and classification. *Br J Dermatol.* 1994;131:1.

McGovern TW, Gentry RH. Spiny keratodermas: Case report, classification, and treatment of music box spine dermatoses. *Cutis.* 1994;54:389.

Ratnavel RC, Griffins WAD. The inherited palmoplantar keratodermas. *Br J Dermatol.* 1997;137:485.

Stevens HP, Kelsell DP, Bryant SP, et al. Linkage of an American pedigree with palmoplantar keratoderma and malignancy (palmoplantar ectodermal dysplasia type III) to 17q24. Literature survey and proposed updated classification of the keratodermas. *Arch Dermatol.* 1996;132:640.

3 REACTIVE ERYTHEMAS

Onofre Sanmartín

URTICARIA

- Urticaria is a vascular reaction of the skin marked by the transient appearance of numerous wheals. Wheals can be defined as smooth, slightly elevated, erythematous, pruriginous lesions. While urticaria results from transient extravasation of plasma into the dermis, angioedema is the subcutaneous extension of urticaria that results in deep swelling within subcutaneous sites. Urticarial lesions commonly involve the extremities and trunk but may appear on any part of the body. Angioedema has a predilection to areas of loose connective tissue such as the face, lips, or tongue. If angioedema involves the upper respiratory tract, life-threatening obstruction of the laryngeal airway may occur.
- Urticaria has been arbitrarily divided in two types, acute urticaria, when it lasts less than 6 weeks, and chronic urticaria, when it lasts more than 6 weeks.

EPIDEMIOLOGY

- Urticaria affects 15 to 20% of the population. The mean age of those affected is the second to third decade of life, although it is also frequent in the pediatric population (2 to 3% of children). Females have a slightly higher incidence than males, especially in chronic forms of urticaria. In general, more than 80% of new-onset urticaria resolves in 2 weeks, and more than 95% resolves by 3 months.
- The main known etiologic factors of urticaria are medications, foods, infections, contactants, autoimmune disorders, malignancies, physical factors, and genetics. The etiology of acute urticaria can be determined in up to 50% of new cases. In one recent study, 39.5% of total cases were associated with viral upper respiratory tract infections, 9% with analgesics intake, and 0.9% with food intolerance. However, the majority of cases of new-onset urticaria are idiopathic in nature. The longer the urticaria persists, the more difficult it is to determine a specific etiology.
- Chronic urticarias can be subdivided according to the etiologic agent into three groups: physical urticarias, urticaria secondary to an underlying medical condition, and chronic idiopathic urticaria. Unfortunately, most cases of chronic urticaria belong to the category of idiopathic urticaria. Physical urticarias are the most common, accounting for approximately 20% of cases. Thyroid diseases such as Hashimoto's disease, and less commonly Graves' disease, should be ruled out in patients with chronic urticaria. The percentage of patients with chronic urticaria who have antithyroglobulin antibody, antimicrosomal antibody, or both is 27%, and 19% have abnormal thyroid function. In a substantial fraction of patients with chronic idiopathic urticaria (35 to 40%) circulating IgG antibodies directed against the alpha subunit of the IgE mast cell receptor have been detected. These antibodies activate basophils and mast cells to release histamine.
- A number of drugs such as aspirin, nonsteroidal anti-inflammatory drugs (NSAIDs), and opioids may cause or exacerbate urticaria. Angiotensin-converting enzyme inhibitors can cause chronic angioedema. Penicillin and cephalosporins may induce type I and type III hypersensitivity reactions.
- Some patients report the onset of urticaria associated with the consumption of certain foods, such as shellfish, eggs, nuts, strawberries, or certain baked goods.
- Besides a viral syndrome or an upper respiratory illness, the other infection strongly associated with urticaria is viral hepatitis. The association with other agents such as Streptococcus and Mycoplasma species, *Helicobacter pylori*, *Mycobacterium tuberculosis*, and Herpes Simplex Virus is controversial. Parasitic infections (Ascaris, Ancylostoma, Strongyloides, Echinococcus, Trichinella, Filaria) may cause chronic urticaria.
- Contact urticaria can be divided in two broad categories: nonimmunologic and immunologic. Some of the more commonly reported causes of nonimmune contact urticarias include balsam of Peru, benzoic acid, cinnamic alcohol, sorbic acid, and dimethylsulfoxide. Immune-mediated contact urticaria can be caused by latex (especially in health care workers), plants, insects (caterpillars), medications (penicillin), and food (fish, garlic, onions, tomato). It represents a type I IgE hypersensitivity reaction. Prior immune sensitization is required and sensitization can be at the cutaneous level, but it occurs more frequently via mucous membranes.

- Urticaria has been associated with a number of autoimmune diseases including autoimmune thyroid disease, lupus erythematosus, cryoglobulinemia, and juvenile rheumatoid arthritis.
- Little evidence exists to support the association of urticaria with malignant diseases. Acquired angioedema associated with C1 esterase inhibitor deficiency may be associated with lymphoproliferative disorders. Schnitzler syndrome is a variant of urticarial vasculitis frequently associated with IgM myeloma.
- Heredity may play a role in some variants of urticaria. An autosomal dominant form of angioedema (not urticaria) results from C1-esterase inhibitor deficiency. Specific subcategories of urticaria, including vibratory angioedema, heat urticaria, solar urticaria, and cold urticaria, have inherited forms.

PATHOPHYSIOLOGY

- Urticaria, for the most part, represents the end result of mast cell activation. Mast cell activation results in the release of both preformed (histamine) and newly formed mediators from cytoplasmic granules, which cause wheal formation, vasodilatation, and erythema. Granules of these cells contain histamine and chemotactic factors for eosinophils and neutrophils. Newly formed mediators include prostaglandin D2, platelet-activating factor, and leukotrienes C4, D4, and E4. Mast cells are also rich in numerous cytokines including TNF-α, IL-4, IL-5, IL-6, IL-8, and stem cell factor. Mast cells express high-affinity IgE receptors on their cell surface, to which the Fc portion of IgE antibodies bind.
- Histamine is the ligand for at least two types of receptors, H_1 and H_2, which are present on different cells. Activation of H_1 receptors on smooth muscle cells and endothelial vascular cells leads to smooth muscle cell contraction and increased vascular permeability. Activation of H_2 vascular receptors causes vasodilatation.
- The mechanism of action resulting in the release of the intracellular contents (mediators) of mast cells is varied and can occur through immune-mediated or nonimmune mechanisms. Immune-mediated urticaria may respond to two different hypersensitivity mechanisms: type I allergic IgE response and type III response mediated by immune-complexes. In type I response, specific IgE antibodies that recognize certain antigens bind to Fc IgE receptors on the mast cell surface. The combination of mast cell IgE with the specific antigen induces the release of mast cell mediators. Allergens involved in type I reactions may include certain drugs, foods, and insect venoms. Type III immune-complex disease is associated with urticarial vasculitis, systemic lupus erythematosus (SLE), and other connective tissue disorders that activate urticaria.
- Nonimmune-mediated urticaria responds to direct degranulation of mast cells without immune mechanism. Direct degranulation of mast cells may occur under three different situations: (1) infections, where complement fragments (C3a) may activate mast cells to release histamine; (2) drugs that can directly induce mast cell degranulation, presumably by altering the membrane properties (opiates, antibiotics, curare, radiocontrast media, azo dyes, aspirin, and NSAIDs); and (3) in physical urticaria, where in addition to histamine, neuropeptides and complement products can play a role in the pathogenesis of this urticaria.
- Hereditary angioedema is due to mutations within the C1-inhibitor (C1-INH) gene. The disorder is transmitted as an autosomal dominant trait. There are two variants of hereditary angioedema: type I (85%) and type II (15%). Type I is characterized by low antigenic and functional plasma levels of a normal C1-INH protein. Type II is characterized by the presence of normal or elevated antigenic levels of a dysfunctional mutant protein together with reduced levels of the functional protein. C1-INH deficiency allows autoactivation of the first component of complement with consumption of C4 and C2. The activation of C4 and C2 does not result in the formation of an effective classical pathway C3 convertase (C4b2a), and consequently C3 and all of the later-acting components are present in normal amounts in the serum of these patients. C1-INH is one of the major inhibitors of plasma kallikrein, the contact system protease that cleaves kininogen and releases bradykinin. It is presumed that because of uncontrolled activation of the contact system, kinin-like mediators are episodically released, resulting in edema of the subcutaneous or submucosal tissues. Kinins are potent bioactive molecules that are important in inflammation by mediating pain, vasodilatation, edema, and secondary activation of leukocytes.
- An acquired deficiency of C1-INH has been described. Acquired angioedema (AAE) is a rare disorder that has been categorized into two forms: type I associated with B-lymphoproliferative disorders, and type-II, defined by the presence of an autoantibody directed against the C1-inhibitor molecule.

CLINICAL FEATURES

ACUTE URTICARIA
- Acute urticaria is characterized by the abrupt onset of numerous itchy, short-lived wheals. The wheals consist of edematous, evanescent, erythematous papules, plaques, and polycyclic forms with peripheral

TABLE 3–1   Physical Urticarias

PHYSICAL URTICARIA	PRECIPITATING FACTORS	CLINICAL MANIFESTATIONS	DIAGNOSTIC TEST
Dermatographism	Rubbing the skin	Wheals with linear distribution appearing minutes after stimuli	Stroking uninvolved skin
Pressure urticaria	Pressure	Dermal and subcutaneous swellings appearing 4 to 6 hours after a pressure. Remains for 8 hours to 3 days	Pressure challenge on shoulder (7 kg for 15 minutes)
Solar urticaria	UVB, UVA, or visible rays	Wheals within minutes of sun exposure lasting 30 minutes to 2 hours	Phototest
Cold urticaria	Low temperature	Urticarial plaques can be generalized or confined to the area exposed to the cold	Ice cube test (contact for 20 minutes)
Heat urticaria	High temperature	Well-defined urticarial lesions confined to sites of heat exposure	Warming of the skin (43° C for 5 minutes)
Aquagenic	Contact with water	Small pruritic wheals developing within minutes at the sites of contact with water (regardless water source or temperature)	Water compresses at 36° C (contact for 10 minutes)
Cholinergic	Heat, exercise, or stress	Pinpoint wheals surrounded by an erythematous flare after sweating	Exercise or hot bath provocation
Vibrational	Vibration	Angioedema and urticaria on exposed areas	Vibration with a kitchen mixer on the forearm

blanching. Individual lesions remain less than 24 hours, exhibiting a transitory and migratory behavior. If the location of the wheals remains fixed for longer than 24 hours, the diagnosis of urticaria is doubtful, being more frequently urticarial vasculitis or bullous pemphigoid. Although there are episodes of less than 24 hours of duration, acute urticaria usually clears in 1 to 6 weeks.

CHRONIC URTICARIA

• During the course of chronic urticaria, symptoms may be daily or episodic. It is not possible to predict the duration of chronic urticaria. Spontaneous remissions often occur within 12 months, but without correction of the underlying problem, patients continue to have symptoms at least periodically for years. Angioedema accompanies chronic urticaria in approximately 40% of patients, another 40% of patients have hives alone, and about 20% of patients have angioedema but not urticaria.

PHYSICAL URTICARIA

• In physical urticaria, wheals are induced by a physical stimulus such as heat, rubbing, pressure, cold, sunlight, or vibration. Depending on the precipitating factor, physical urticaria can be classified in several types, and it is not uncommon for a single patient to have more than one type. Table 3–1 summarizes the triggering factors and clinical manifestations of physical urticaria. Dermatographism is the most common form of physical urticaria (up to 9% of the population). It is defined as erythema and whealing seen within minutes after stroking the skin. Other types of physical urticaria, such as aquagenic, cholinergic, and cold urticaria, may be accompanied by systemic symptoms (such as hypotension or wheezing).

CONTACT URTICARIA

• Contact urticaria refers to the onset of urticaria within 30 to 60 minutes of contact with an inciting agent. Nonimmunologic contact urticaria, the most frequent type, appears without prior sensitization, is restricted to the contact area, and no generalized symptoms occur. Immunologic contact urticaria may spread beyond the site of contact and progress to generalized urticaria. The most frequent antigen involved is natural rubber latex. In severe cases, systemic symptoms such as asthma, hypotension, and anaphylactic shock may occur.

HEREDITARY ANGIOEDEMA

• Hereditary angioedema is characterized by recurrent self-limited attacks involving the skin, upper respiratory tract, or gastrointestinal tract. Patients usually develop symptoms within the second decade of life. Family history is usually positive. Patients have local swellings at three predominant sites: subcutaneous tissues (hands, arms, legs, genitals, and buttocks) with

TABLE 3–2   Laboratory Evaluation of Urticaria

LABORATORY EVALUATION	INDICATIONS
Complete blood count with differential	Eosinophilia indicates a parasitic infection or drug reaction
Erythrocyte sedimentation rate	Elevated ESR indicates chronic inflammation (urticarial vasculitis)
Multichemistry panel	Hepatic and renal dysfunction may indicate associated systemic diseases
Throat culture for streptococcal infection	Indicated when positive history
Urinalysis	Evidence of urinary tract infection responsible for urticaria
Stool ova and parasites	Indicated if eosinophilia or positive history
Hepatitis B and C titers	May be positive in chronic urticaria and cryoglobulin associated cold urticaria
Serum cryoglobulins	May be positive in cold urticaria and urticarial vasculitis
Thyroid functions and antithyroid antibodies	Strong association to chronic urticaria
Antinuclear antibody titers	Indicated in urticarial vasculitis
Complement studies	Low C4 in C1 INH deficiency, low C3 in systemic vasculitis
RAST and prick	Needed if suggestive history of food allergy or contact urticaria

low preference for the face; abdominal organs (stomach, intestines, bladder), which can mimic surgical emergencies; and the upper airway, which may result in life-threatening laryngeal edema. A typical feature is the absence of urticarial lesions. Attacks may last from several hours to 2 to 3 days. Local trauma is one of the most important trigger factors. Acquired angioedema presents with symptoms identical to those of hereditary angioedema but with the onset after the fourth decade of life and absence of family history.

URTICARIAL VASCULITIS

- Occasionally, chronic urticaria and angioedema can be manifestations of an underlying connective-tissue disorder or a systemic vasculitis in which the histologic findings of the involved skin may be consistent with a leukocytoclastic vasculitis. This condition is known as urticarial vasculitis. The skin lesions differ from classic urticaria in that they are palpable, purpuric, and persist at least 24 hours. Urticarial vasculitis accounts for less than 1% of all cases of chronic hives.

DIAGNOSIS AND DIFFERENTIAL

- History and examination helps to identify the type of urticaria and eliminate nonurticarial diseases.
- Skin biopsy is only indicated if a particular lesion remains longer than 24 hours. Histology of acute urticaria looks like normal skin. The dermis may show edema between collagen fibers. Dilated vessels can be

seen in the involved skin with a mild perivascular lymphocytic infiltrate. Occasionally isolated eosinophils can be seen. Histology of urticarial vasculitis shows a true leukocytoclastic vasculitis in dermal vessels.

- The selection of laboratory tests must be directed using the information elicited from the history and physical examination. Table 3–2 summarizes the specific laboratory tests. When a connective-tissue disorder is suspected, antinuclear antibodies and other serologic tests may be indicated. Complement determinations are indicated only for patients who have urticarial vasculitis or angioedema. Patients with a hereditary or acquired deficiency of C1 inhibitor do not have hives. Only in patients who present with angioedema alone is measurement of C4 indicated, followed by a determination of the levels and function of C1 inhibitor if C4 levels are below normal. In patients with urticarial vasculitis, C3 levels can be low, due to complement consumption. Thyroid-function tests, including antithyroglobulin and antimicrosomal antibodies, may be helpful, given the association of chronic urticaria with thyroid disease.
- Allergies (to food or food additives) are so rarely a cause of chronic urticaria that routine testing is not recommended unless particular clues are present.

TREATMENT

- The first step of treatment is the identification and avoidance of the inciting agent. Unfortunately, this is not always possible, and recurrences of urticaria are common.

- Acute urticaria is frequently treated in emergency rooms. In these cases, systemic corticosteroids are commonly used to induce rapid remission of wheals. Thereafter, most patients with acute urticaria respond to oral daily doses of prednisone (20 to 40 mg/d) within 4 to 5 days. During this time different combinations of antihistamines can be introduced to maintain remission, allowing withdrawal of corticosteroids. In those cases in which urticaria is part of an anaphylactic reaction, the preservation of the airway and the use of subcutaneous epinephrine (0.2 to 0.4 mL of epinephrine 1:1000) are clearly warranted.

- Nonsedating, long-acting H_1 antihistamines are the first line of treatment of urticaria. They include astemizole, loratadine, desloratadine, fexofenadine, cetirizine, mizolastine, and ebastine. Doses must be sufficient to improve symptoms. If disease remains uncontrolled, the addition of another short-acting sedating H_1 antihistamine is indicated. Traditional H_1 blockers include diphenhydramine, hydroxyzine, chlorpheniramine, and cyproheptadine. In general they are more efficacious than nonsedating antihistamines, but their use is limited by the sedating effects.

- The addition of an H_2-receptor antagonist (cimetidine, ranitidine, or famotidine) to an H_1-receptor antagonist augments the inhibition of a histamine-induced wheal-and-flare reaction. Doxepin, a tricyclic antidepressant, blocks both types of histamine receptors and is a much more potent inhibitor of H_1 receptors than either diphenhydramine or hydroxyzine; however it is also a potent sedating agent.

- Leukotriene antagonists (zafirlukast and montelukast) have been shown to be superior to placebo in the treatment of patients with chronic urticaria, indicating that leukotrienes may also contribute to hives and swelling. Its use is indicated in difficult cases of urticaria.

- Many patients with chronic urticaria and angioedema unresponsive to antihistamines and with disability due to the disease warrant consideration for corticosteroid therapy. In such cases a short intermittent course of corticosteroids may be helpful.

- Patients with urticaria in which the inflammatory infiltrate is predominantly neutrophilic may require the addition of colchicine (0.6 mg b.i.d.) or dapsone (50 to 150 mg/d). Plasmapheresis and cyclosporine have been used as experimental therapies in a small number of patients.

- Dietary modification is only necessary if food allergy or food-additive hypersensitivity has been established. Food additives or preservatives have been reported to cause chronic urticaria in 3 to 4% of cases, but the data is scarce and questionable. In chronic idiopathic urticaria, salicylate dietary restriction can be useful. NSAIDs and other drugs that cause histamine release should be avoided.

- Treatment of recurrent severe attacks of hereditary angioedema revolves around anticipation of trauma. Most severe attacks occur during manipulation of the upper airway. Infusions of 2 units of fresh frozen plasma immediately prior to airway manipulation or surgery is advised. Long-term therapy includes androgens to boost levels of all complement components (danazol 200 mg twice per day, or stanozolol 1 to 2 mg twice per day, are the most commonly used androgens).

REFERENCES

Beltrani VS. Urticaria and angioedema. *Dermatol Clin.* 1996;14:171.

Hide M, Francis DM, Grattan CEH, et al. Autoantibodies against the high-affinity IgE receptor as a cause of histamine release in chronic urticaria. *N Engl J Med.* 1993;328:1599.

Kozel MM, Mekkes JR, Bossuyt PM, Bos JD. Natural course of physical and chronic urticaria and angioedema in 220 patients. *J Am Acad Dermatol.* 2001;45:387.

Leznoff A, Sussman GL. Syndrome of idiopathic chronic urticaria and angioedema with thyroid autoimmunity: A study of 90 patients. *J Allergy Clin Immunol.* 1989;84:66.

Lin RY, Curry A, Pesola GR. Improved outcomes in patients with acute allergic syndromes who are treated with combined H1 and H2 antagonists. *Ann Emerg Med.* 2000;36:462.

Nzeako UC, Frigas E, Tremaine WJ. Hereditary angioedema: A broad review for clinicians. *Arch Intern Med.* 2001; 161:2417.

Shipley D, Ormerod AD. Drug-induced urticaria. Recognition and treatment. *Am J Clin Dermatol.* 2001;2:151.

Spector S, Tan RA. Antileukotrienes in chronic urticaria. *J Allergy Clin Immunol.* 1998;101:572.

Wakelin SH. Contact urticaria. *Clin Exp Dermatol.* 2001; 26:132.

Wanderer AA, Bernstein IL, Goodman DL, et al. The diagnosis and management of urticaria: A practice parameter. *Ann Allergy Asthma Immunol.* 2000;85:521.

ERYTHEMA MULTIFORME

- Erythema multiforme (EM) is an acute, self-limited, inflammatory eruption characterized by symmetric erythematous, edematous, or bullous lesions of the skin and mucous membranes. The distinctive lesion of erythema multiforme is the iris or target lesion. EM may be divided into a minor and major form, according to the severity. Mild cases are referred as EM minor.

TABLE 3–3   Causes of Erythema Multiforme and Stevens–Johnson Syndrome

Post-Infectious	VIRAL
	Most frequent: Herpes simplex I & II
	Other viruses: Adenovirus, coxsackievirus B5, echoviruses, enteroviruses, Epstein-Barr, hepatitis A, hepatitis B, measles, vaccinia, varicella, influenza, mumps, poliovirus
	BACTERIAL
	Most frequent: *Mycoplasma pneumoniae*
	Other bacteria: Proteus sp., Salmonella sp., Mycobaterium sp., Vibrio sp., *Chalmidia psitacci*, *Rochimalea henseale*, Brucella sp., *Francisella tularensis*, *Neisseria gonorrhoeae*, Salmonella sp., Corynebacterium diphteriae, *Yersinia enterocolitica*
	FUNGAL
	Histoplasmosis, Coccidioides sp.
	POSTVACCINATION
	Bacille Calmette-Guérin (BCG), oral polio vaccine, tetanus/diphtheria
Drug-Induced	**Common agents**: Sulfonamides, anticonvulsants (barbiturates, hydantoins, carbamazepine), nonsteroidal anti-inflammatory drugs (piroxicam, pyrazolones), antibiotics (aminopenicillins, quinolones), allopurinol, phenylbutazone, antituberculous agents (pirazinamide, ethambutol)
Other Causes	Malignancy
	Hormonal
	Collagen vascular disease
	Sarcoidosis
	Radiotherapy

Severe cases are referred as EM major or as Stevens–Johnson syndrome (SJS). Toxic epidermal necrolysis (TEN) or Lyell syndrome is the most aggressive and extensive form of SJS.

- There is a clear correlation between clinical severity pattern and etiology. EM is usually postinfectious (generally postherpetic), with good prognosis. Conversely, SJS/TEN is a severe drug-induced disease with high morbidity, and its prognosis may be poor in some patients. These differences allow the separation of infection-induced EM spectrum (EM minor and EM major) from drug-induced EM spectrum (SJS and TEN).

EPIDEMIOLOGY

- The exact incidence of EM minor is unknown. SJS occurs at 1 to 7 cases per million inhabitants per year, while TEN occurs in 0.4 to 1.3 cases per million per year. EM minor shows the highest incidence in the second to fourth decades, with 20% of cases occurring in children and adolescents. SJS is more common in people younger than 30 or older than 65, and TEN has a much higher incidence in the elderly.
- EM minor is induced by herpes simplex virus in nearly 100% of cases. Most cases of idiopathic EM minor are induced by subclinical herpetic infections. EM

major is related to herpes in 55% of cases. Mycoplasma infection appears to be another common cause.

- Drugs are the reported culprits in many documented cases of SJS and EM major (Table 3–3). Sulfonamides and anticonvulsants are the most common triggers. A slow acetylator genotype is a risk factor for sulphonamide-induced SJS.

PATHOPHYSIOLOGY

- In the past, the presence of IgM and C3 around the blood vessels of EM as well as the presence of circulating immune-complexes in the serum of patients with EM suggested that this condition represented a form of vasculitis. However, herpes-associated EM appears to represent the result of a cell-mediated immune reaction associated with herpes simplex virus antigen. The herpes simplex DNA has been identified by polymerase chain reaction amplification primarily within the keratinocytes in almost all cases of EM minor. The immunologic reaction affects herpes virus-expressing keratinocytes. Cytotoxic effector cells (CD8+ T lymphocytes) in epidermis induce apoptosis of scattered keratinocytes and lead to satellite cell necrosis.
- Clearly not all EM is due to herpes simplex, particularly those of EM major. In this setting drugs or

mycoplasma organisms may act in a similar way to the herpes simple virus.

- Apoptosis caused by the interaction of FAS (CD95) and its ligand (CD95L) is believed to play a role in TEN.

CLINICAL FEATURES

ERYTHEMA MULTIFORME MINOR AND ERYTHEMA MULTIFORME MAJOR

- Onset is usually sudden, with erythematous macules, papules, and vesicles appearing mainly on the distal portion of the extremities. In the case of postinfectious EM, the lesions are located initially in acral areas and follow a centripetal spreading. Many affected patients have a history of a preceding herpes labialis or herpes genitalis.
- The skin lesions, known as target or iris lesions, are symmetric in distribution, with concentric rings. Typical target lesions show a small papule or vesicle in the center, a pale edematous intermediate ring, and a violaceous peripheral ring. Some lesions are atypical targets that consist of only two concentric rings. Skin tenderness is absent with an occasional mild burning sensation and itching.
- Mucosal involvement is present in up to 70% of cases. The degree is mild with limitation to one mucosal surface in EM minor, and more prominent in EM major. Hemorrhagic lesions and erosions of the lips and oral mucosa may make eating difficult. Eye involvement may cause lacrimation and photophobia. The genital lesions are painful and may result in urinary retention.
- Fifty percent of patients with EM major have moderate fever, general discomfort, cough, chest pain, or gastrointestinal symptoms. These are usually present for one week preceding the eruption.
- Most cases of EM minor subside completely within 2 to 3 weeks without any complication. The reported mortality rate of EM major is less than 5% and clearing requires 3 to 6 weeks.

STEVENS–JOHNSON SYNDROME AND TOXIC EPIDERMAL NECROLYSIS

- These reactions generally begin with prodromal symptoms including fever, cough, and burning eyes, which are followed in 1 to 3 days by skin and mucous membrane lesions.
- A painful, burning rash rapidly spreads from the face and trunk to the extremities. In a few days (or sometimes even in hours) the lesions are maximally extended, with numerous blisters. Epidermal detachment occurs with lateral pressure (Nikolsky sign). Skin lesions consist of purpuric macules, blisters, and atypical targets (only two concentric rings). It is possible to separate EM major from SJS on the basis

of clinical symptoms. Thus, EM major is defined by mucosal erosions with characteristic skin lesions, typical targets with or without blisters, and a symmetrical and mainly acral distribution. SJS presents with mucosal erosions, widespread purpuric cutaneous macules, atypical targets, and bullous lesions mainly of truncal distribution.

- 90% of patients with SJS or TEN have mucosal lesions. The most commonly affected sites are the oropharynx, eyes, genitalia, and anus. These painful and hemorrhagic lesions cause crusted lips, salivation, photophobia, and painful micturition. Ocular lesions need particular attention due to high risk of sequelae such as synechiae and erosions, which can result in blindness.
- Because the extent of necrolysis is one of the principal prognostic factors, the limit of 10% of the body surface area involved by epidermal detachment is used as an arbitrary boundary between SJS and TEN. SJS includes cases with mucosal erosions plus widespread purpuric macules and epidermal detachment below 10%; overlap SJS–TEN, cases with epidermal detachment between 10% and 30%; and TEN, cases with epidermal detachment above 30%.
- Patients with SJS have a mortality rate of around 5%, while patients with TEN have a much higher rate at 25 to 30%. Complications are similar to those seen in extensively burned patients. There is loss of large areas of skin, fluid loss, electrolyte abnormalities, and multiorgan toxicity including pneumonia, esophageal strictures, hepatitis, and nephritis. Sepsis is the most common cause of death, followed by pulmonary complications.

DIAGNOSIS AND DIFFERENTIAL

- Diagnosis can be made according to clinical features and histopathologic findings. The skin lesions of erythema multiforme must be distinguished from bullous pemphigoid, urticaria, and dermatitis herpetiformis. The oral lesions can resemble aphthous stomatitis, pemphigus, and herpetic stomatitis.
- Histopathology of EM shows a diffuse inflammatory infiltrate at the dermal–epidermal junction composed mainly of lymphocytes. The epidermis shows exocytosis, spongiosis, and isolated necrotic keratinocytes. The dermis shows edema and lymphocytic vasculitis with extravasation of red blood cells. More intense cases show partial to full-thickness epidermal necrosis, intraepidermal vesiculation, and subepidermal blisters.
- Complete blood count, electrolytes, erythrocyte sedimentation rate, liver function tests, and cultures from blood, sputum, and erosive areas are indicated in severe cases of EM major.

TREATMENT

- Mild cases require only symptomatic treatment, including oral antihistamines, analgesics, local skin care, and soothing mouthwashes. Topical steroids may be considered. The use of systemic corticosteroids should be avoided.
- Herpes-induced EM may benefit from oral or IV acyclovir. The goal is to shorten the clinical course, prevent complications, and prevent development of latency and/or subsequent recurrences. In recurrent EM, continued 6-month treatment with low doses of acyclovir is recommended. It must be considered when recurrences are more frequent than 5 per year.
- Patients with EM major, SJS, or TEN should be admitted to the hospital where airway support as well as careful monitoring of electrolytes, fluid imbalance, and secondary infection is undertaken routinely. Local supportive care for eye involvement is important and includes topical lubricants for dry eyes and removal of fresh adhesions. The use of systemic corticosteroids is controversial and some authors consider that it may predispose to complications.
- Intravenous immunoglobulin appears to be efficacious in TEN.

REFERENCES

Assier H, Bastuji-Garin S, Revuz J. Erythema multiforme with mucous membrane involvement and Stevens–Johnson syndrome are clinically different disorders with distinct causes. *Arch Dermatol.* 1995;131:539.

Bastuji-Garin S, Rzany B, Stern RS. Clinical classification of cases of toxic epidermal necrolysis, Stevens–Johnson syndrome, and erythema multiforme. *Arch Dermatol.* 1993; 129:92.

Roujeau JC. The spectrum of Stevens–Johnson syndrome and toxic epidermal necrolysis: A clinical classification. *J Invest Dermatol.* 1994;102:28S.

Schofield JK, Tatnall FM, Leigh IM. Recurrent erythema multiforme: Clinical features and treatment in a large series of patients. *Br J Dermatol.* 1993;128:542.

Tatnall FM, Schofield JK, Leigh IM. A double-blind, placebo-controlled trial of continuous acyclovir therapy in recurrent erythema multiforme. *Br J Dermatol.* 1995; 132:267.

ANNULAR ERYTHEMAS

- A number of chronic annular and figurate eruptions are considered annular erythemas. The etiology and clinical features are sufficiently characteristic to distinguish several entities: erythema annulare centrifugum, erythema chronicum migrans, erythema gyratum repens, erythema marginatum rheumaticum, and necrolytic migratory erythema.

ERYTHEMA ANNULARE CENTRIFUGUM

EPIDEMIOLOGY

- Erythema annulare centrifugum (EAC) has been reported at an incidence of 1 case per 100,000 population per year. The etiology is uncertain. Most cases are idiopathic, but the literature contains numerous case reports associated with a variety of agents including drugs, arthropod bites, infections, or underlying systemic diseases (liver disease, autoimmune diseases, appendicitis).

PATHOPHYSIOLOGY

- The pathogenesis of EAC is unknown, but it is probably due to a hypersensitivity reaction to a variety of agents. Intradermal injections of different antigens (Trichophyton, Candida, tuberculin, and tumor extracts) may reproduce lesions of EAC, supporting a type IV hypersensitivity reaction as one possible mechanism for its development.

CLINICAL FEATURES

- The patient usually presents an asymptomatic or pruritic papular eruption that spread peripherally while clearing centrally. These enlarge at a rate of approximately 2 to 5 mm/d to produce annular or polycyclic plaques. The peripheral margin is indurated and shows a trailing scale on the inner aspect. The diameter of the polycyclic lesions varies from a few to several centimeters, but not exceeding 7 cm. Lesions demonstrate a predilection for the thighs and legs, but they may occur on the upper extremities, trunk or face. The palms and soles are spared.
- Superficial and deep variants of EAC have been recognized. Superficial annular erythema is characterized by a pruritic, annular lesion with trailing scale. Deep annular erythema is characterized by a nonpruritic annular red lesion without scale.
- The mean duration of EAC is 11 months. However, the course has ranged from 4 weeks to 34 years (recurrent attacks).

TABLE 3–4   Differential Diagnosis of Annular Erythemas

DIAGNOSIS	CLINICAL	HISTOLOGIC
Erythema annulare centrifugum	Rate of enlargement: 2 to 5 mm/d Lesions are 4 to 5 cm in diameter	Perivascular lymphocytic infiltrates
Erythema chronicum migrans	Lesions less numerous (solitary) History of tick bite (Ixodes) Slower rate of spread (weeks rather than days) Size > 5 cm Persistence of lesions: 3 weeks	Patchy lymphohistiocytic infiltrate with plasma cells. Spirochetae may be found
Erythema gyratum repens	Rate of spread: days rather than weeks (> 1 cm/d) Bizarre configuration Underlying malignancy	Perivascular lymphocytic infiltrates
Erythema marginatum rheumaticum	Association with rheumatic fever (10 to 18%) Rate of spread is measurable in hours Lesions fade in 2 to 3 hours Lesions may recur intermittently for weeks to months	Neutrophilic infiltrate as opposed to lymphohistiocytic
Necrolytic migratory erythema	Erythema and scaling with flaccid bullae, erosions, and crusting Associated with glucagonoma	Superficial epidermal necrosis

DIAGNOSIS AND DIFFERENTIAL

- A biopsy is helpful in confirming the diagnosis of EAC. In the superficial type, there is a perivascular lymphohistiocytic infiltrate associated with epidermal changes (parakeratosis and spongiosis). In the deep type, there is an intense superficial and deep lymphohistiocytic perivascular infiltrate in a "coat-sleeve" fashion without epidermal changes.
- The differential diagnosis includes other dermatosis with annular configuration such are erythema gyratum repens, granuloma faciale, lupus erythematosus, annular urticaria, erythema chronicum migrans, necrolytic migratory erythema, and erythema marginatum rheumaticum. The differential characteristics of these entities are summarized in Table 3–4.

TREATMENT

- Erythema annulare centrifugum is usually self-limited. Most cases require no treatment and resolve spontaneously. Topical steroids will usually cause involution of the treated lesions. Search for and treatment of the underlying disorder is the primary therapy to prevent recurrences.

ERYTHEMA MARGINATUM RHEUMATICUM

EPIDEMIOLOGY

- This characteristic rash is one of the major diagnostic criteria of rheumatic fever, occurring in 5 to 13% of patients with acute rheumatic fever. It is more frequently seen in children.

CLINICAL FINDINGS

- The eruption consists of rings, (arcuate or polycyclic lesions), pale or dull red in color, flat, or palpably thickened. Erythema marginatum begins as 1 to 3 cm in diameter, pink to red, nonpruritic macules or papules located on the trunk and proximal limbs. The lesions spread outward to form a serpiginous ring with erythematous raised margins and central clearing.
- The rash may fade and reappear within an hour. It is exacerbated by heat and is more intense in the afternoon. The rash occurs early in the course of the disease and remains long past the resolution of other symptoms.

ERYTHEMA CHRONICUM MIGRANS

PATHOPHYSIOLOGY

- Erythema chronicum migrans is one of the dermatological manifestations of Lyme disease. The Ixodes tick is the principal vector for _Borrelia burgdorferi_, the etiologic agent of Lyme disease.
- Lyme disease is characterized by local and general manifestations and can be subdivided in three stages. The first stage is the dispersion and replication of spirochetes in the tick bite. The characteristic erythema chronicum migrans can be seen in roughly half of the patients. The second stage corresponds to the

dissemination of the *B. burgdorferi* through blood and can manifest weeks or months after the contact with the tick. This stage is characterized by neurologic (meningitis), rheumatologic (arthralgia), and cardiac (myocarditis and pericarditis) symptoms. The third stage can appear months or years after infection, and is characterized by cutaneous (lymphadenosis benigna cutis and acrodermatitis chronica atrophicans), nervous system, and musculoskeletal manifestations.

CLINICAL FEATURES

- Erythema chronicum migrans starts as an erythematous papular lesion, clear in the center, with centrifugal ring-shaped extension over several days. The size can vary, but is frequently around 5 cm. It may be asymptomatic or may itch and burn. The eruption appears 1 to 36 (average, 9) days after the bite, and is due to local spread of the spirochete, usually in a ring formation enlarging at a rate of several centimeters per week. It often occurs at or near the site of the tick bite. The most commonly affected sites are the inferior extremities, trunk, and neck; however, the lesions may arise in an area not normally visualized by individuals, such as the axilla, groin, or popliteal areas.
- Untreated, the rash persists for 2 to 3 weeks, but the duration may even last 14 months. Eighty percent of patients have only one episode of erythema migrans, while 20% may have recurrent episodes. Multiple lesions may occur in 40% of patients and may be an important marker of hematogenous dissemination rather than the result of multiple tick bites.

DIAGNOSIS AND DIFFERENTIAL

- The skin biopsy shows a superficial and deep perivascular and interstitial lymphohistiocytic infiltrate containing plasma cells. The Warthin–Starry stain identifies spirochetes in 40% of cases.
- The current recommendation from the Centers for Disease Control (CDC) for the serologic diagnosis is a two-step testing process. The first step, in patients with symptoms consistent with Lyme disease, is to order an antibody titer. This can be either a total Lyme titer or separate immunoglobulin G (IgG) and immunoglobulin M (IgM) titers. The second step is to confirm positive titers with a Western blot. It should be taken into account that antibody testing in patients with erythema migrans can be negative because the rash may develop before the antibodies.

TREATMENT

- Treatment with oral doxycycline (100 mg b.i.d.) or amoxicillin (500 mg t.i.d.) or erythromycin (1 g daily) is indicated in cases of erythema chronicum migrans. A 30-day course also reduces the number of patients who relapse after the shorter regimens.

ERYTHEMA GYRATUM REPENS

EPIDEMIOLOGY

- Erythema gyratum repens (EGR) has been reported in association with an underlying neoplasm in 84% of cases, most commonly lung cancer, followed by tumors of the esophagus and breast. In cases without malignancy it has been reported in association with benign breast hypertrophy, pulmonary tuberculosis, CREST syndrome, and bullous pemphigoid.

CLINICAL FEATURES

- This infrequent dermatosis shows a quite distinctive clinical picture characterized by multiple, scaling, erythematous lesions, which form concentric rings, giving a wood-grain appearance to the skin. The lesions are frequently pruritic and may migrate up to 1 cm each day.
- Complete evaluation for internal malignancy is essential, and dramatic responses have occurred after tumor resection.
- Histologic examination is usually nonspecific and indistinguishable from the changes seen in erythema annulare centrifugum.

NECROLYTIC MIGRATORY ERYTHEMA

EPIDEMIOLOGY

- Necrolytic migratory erythema (NME) is a characteristic eruption usually associated with glucagonoma, although it has been reported also in association with malabsorption disorders and chronic pancreatitis.
- The majority of patients with glucagonoma have symptoms for 1 to 2 years before the diagnosis is made, and 50% of patients already have metastatic disease at the time of diagnosis.

CLINICAL FEATURES

- Patients with NME are usually middle-aged to elderly women. Typical cutaneous manifestations include

multiple erythematous, scaly macules with flaccid bullae, erosions, and crusting. Lesions tend to spread peripherally and are localized primarily on the groin and lower extremities.
- Glucagonoma syndrome initially starts with a non-specific clinical scenario characterized by weight loss, diabetes mellitus, diarrhea, and stomatitis.

DIAGNOSIS AND DIFFERENTIAL

- NME can be mistaken clinically for a blistering disorder, eczema, or psoriasis. The biopsy can be diagnostic, showing a characteristic eosinophilic appearance at the epidermal spinous layer due to keratinocyte necrosis, associated with spongiosis and neutrophils exocytosis.
- High levels of plasma glucagon are found in patients with glucagonoma.

REFERENCES

Bisno AL. Group A streptococcal infections and acute rheumatic fever. *N Engl J Med.* 1991;325:783.

Bressler GS, Jones RE. Erythema annulare centrifugum. *J Am Acad Dermatol.* 1981;4:597.

Masters E, Granter M, Paul Duray P, et al. Physician-diagnosed erythema migrans and erythema migrans-like rashes following lone star tick bites. *Arch Dermatol.* 1998;134:955.

Melski JW. Lyme borreliosis. *Semin Cutan Med Surg.* 2000;19:10.

Tyring SK. Reactive erythemas: Erythema annulare centrifugum and erythema gyratum repens. *Clin Dermatol.* 1993;11:135.

Wermers RA, Fatourechi V, Wynne AG, et al. The glucagonoma syndrome. Clinical and pathologic features in 21 patients. *Medicine.* 1996;75:53.

DRUG ERUPTIONS

- Drug eruptions may be defined as the occurrence of cutaneous lesions as a consequence of adverse effects of drugs. Cutaneous drug eruptions vary in their appearance, time of onset, severity, potential sequelae, and underlying immunopathologic mechanism. For these reasons, drug eruptions have a wide range of different morphologic presentations.

EPIDEMIOLOGY

- The incidence of cutaneous drug reactions is approximately 2 to 5% in hospitalized patients and 1% in the outpatient setting. Persons who are immunocompromised have a 10-fold higher risk of developing a drug eruption than the general population. Women have a 35% higher incidence of adverse cutaneous reactions to drugs than men.
- Categories of drugs most commonly implicated are antimicrobial agents, nonsteroidal anti-inflammatory drugs and anticonvulsants.

PATHOPHYSIOLOGY

- The pathogenesis of drug eruptions can be divided into three groups: non-immunologic, immunologic, and unknown origin. Some of the nonimmunologic reactions are predictable (dose-related) while some are unpredictable (idiosyncratic). They generally have of high incidence and morbidity, but low mortality. Immunologic reactions are less common and unpredictable. Table 3–5 lists the various pathogenetic mechanisms with examples of different drug eruptions.

CLINICAL FEATURES

- Cutaneous drug reactions have a wide range of clinical presentations. Some of the clinical patterns are more frequently associated with certain drugs. Table 3–6 summarizes the different clinical patterns identified in drug reactions along with their most frequent causative agents. Most eruptions are mild and self-limited, resolving after the offending agent is discontinued. However, severe potentially life-threatening eruptions can occur in approximately 1 in 1000 hospitalized patients. Drugs that commonly cause serious reactions include allopurinol, anticonvulsants, NSAIDs, sulphonamides, furosemide, thiazide diuretics, captopril, penicillamine, and piroxicam. In this section we will describe the clinical findings of the most common cutaneous reaction patterns. Drug-induced urticaria, Stevens–Johnson/TEN syndrome, drug-induced leukocytoclastic vasculitis, and drug-induced erythroderma will be discussed in their respective sections.

MORBILLIFORM OR MACULOPAPULAR EXANTHEMS

- Morbilliform rash is the most common cutaneous drug eruption (30 to 50% of cutaneous drug eruptions) and is characterized by a measles-like viral exanthem.
- They usually begin 2 to 10 days after initiation of the drug, with intense pruritus. The lesions are widely distributed, symmetric, often with confluent erythematous

TABLE 3–5   Pathophysiologic Mechanisms of Drug Eruptions

NONIMMUNOLOGIC DRUG REACTIONS		
MECHANISM		EXAMPLE
Expected adverse effects		Chemotherapy-induced alopecia
Ecologic disturbance		Candidiasis and antiobiotics
Overdosage		Coumadin purpura
Drug interreaction		Barbiturates and coumadin (purpura)
Cumulative		Argyria (silver nitrate)
		Antimalarial pigmentantion
Idiosyncratic causes	Altered metabolism	Drug-induced lupus in response to procainamide in slow acetylators of N-acetyltransferase coumadin necrosis and lack of protein C
	Exacerbation of underlying disorder	Lithium and psoriasis
Phototoxic		Increased sensitivity to sun caused by toxic photoproducts of different drugs (tetracyclines)
Direct release of mast cell mediators		Aspirin, NSAID, radiographic contrast material
Jarisch–Herxheimer phenomenon		Penicillin therapy for syphilis, antifungal therapy for dermatophyte

IMMUNOLOGIC TYPE DRUG REACTIONS	
MECHANISM	EXAMPLE
Type I: Classic immediate hypersensitivity	Urticaria, angioedema, anaphylaxis
Type III: Immune complex	Leukocytoclastic vasculitis, serum sickness, urticaria, angioedema
Type IV: Delayed hypersensitivity	Contact dermatitis, exanthematous reactions, photoallergic reactions
Systemic infection impairing immune response	Infectious mononucleosis: Ampicillin-induced rash
	HIV infection: Sulphonamide-induced toxic epidermal necrolysis (TEN)
Unknown immunologic mechanisms	Lichenoid reactions
	Fixed drug eruption

macules and papules that typically spare the palms and soles. Most rashes resolve with some degree of superficial skin desquamation, but continued administration of the offending drug may lead to a generalized eruption and exfoliative erythroderma.

- Morbilliform rash is frequently related to antimicrobial therapy and anticonvulsants.

HYPERSENSITIVITY SYNDROME

- Hypersensitivity syndrome is a potentially life-threatening complex of symptoms including fever, sore throat, skin rash, and internal organ involvement. Lymphadenopathy, hepatitis, nephritis, and leukocytosis with atypical lymphocytes followed by eosinophilia are common clinical findings.
- The reaction usually begins within 1 to 3 weeks after initiating a new drug; however, it may develop as late as 3 months or longer into the course of therapy. The

skin rash is a maculopapular exanthem similar to morbilliform rash.

- The most frequent causative drugs are anticonvulsants. It is estimated to occur as frequently as 1 per 1000 patients treated with phenytoin, carbamazepine, phenobarbital, and lamotrigine. Frequently, cross-reactions occur between these agents. Allopurinol and sulphonamides may induce a similar reaction.

ACUTE GENERALIZED EXANTHEMATOUS PUSTULOSIS

- Acute generalized exanthematous pustulosis (AGEP) is characterized by the acute onset of fever and a generalized scarlatiniform erythema with numerous, small, sterile, nonfollicular pustules. Lesions are mainly distributed on flexural areas. The clinical presentation is similar to pustular psoriasis; however, patients with AGEP show more marked leukocytosis with

TABLE 3–6 Drugs Associated With Specific Morphologic Patterns

Morbiliform exanthems	*Commonly associated drugs:* Amoxicillin, ampicillin, carbamazepine, phenytoin, sulfonamides
	Less commonly associated drugs: ACE inhibitors, allopurinol, other anticonvulsants, barbiturates, isoniazid, NSAIDs, phenothiazine, quinolones, thiazides
Urticaria	*Commonly associated drugs:* Aspirin/NSAIDs, blood products, cephalosporins, dextran, opiates, penicillin
	Less commonly associated drugs: Peptide hormones, polymixin, radiocontrast dye, ranitidine, vaccines, ACE inhibitors
SJS/TEN	*Commonly associated drugs:* Sulfonamides, penicillin, Phenobarbital, phenytoin, NSAIDs
	Less commonly associated drugs: Allopurinol, carbamazepine, barbiturates, cimetidine, codeine, diltiazem, furosemide, griseofulvin, nitrogen mustard, phenothiazine, phenylbutazone, rifampicin, tetracyclines, fansidar, isoniazid
Acute generalized exanthematous pustulosis	*Commonly associated drugs:* Beta-lactam antibiotics, macrolides, mercury
Leucocytoclastic vasculitis	*Commonly associated drugs:* Allopurinol, penicillins, sulfonamides
	Less commonly associated drugs: Aspirin/NSAIDs, cimetidine, gold, hydralazine, phenytoin, propythiouracil, quinolones, tetracycline, and thiazides
Hypersensitivity syndrome	*Commonly associated drugs:* Carbamazepine, phenobarbital and phenytoin
	Less commonly associated drugs: Allopurinol, dapsone, lamotrigine, minocycline, NSAIDs, and sulfonamides
Erythroderma	*Commonly associated drugs:* Gold salts, sulfonamides
	Less commonly associated drugs: Allopurinol, anticonvulsants, barbiturates, captopril, carbamazepine, cefoxitin, chloroquine, chlorpromazine, cimetidine, diltiazem, griseofulvin, lithium, nitrofurantoin
Fixed drug eruptions	Acetaminophen, anticonvulsants, aspirin/nonsteroidal anti-inflammatory drugs (aspirin/NSAIDs), barbiturates, benzodiazepines, butalbital, dapsone, metronidazole, oral contraceptives, penicillins, phenacetin, phenolphthalein, sulfonamides, tetracyclines, tolmetin
Photosensitivity	Amiodarone, chlorpromazine, furosemide, griseofulvin, lovastatin, phenothiazine, piroxicam, quinolones, sulfonamides, tetracycline, thiazide
Lichenoid eruptions	Antimalarials, beta blockers, captopril, diflunisal, furosemide, gold, levamisole, penicillamine, phenothiazine, tetracycline, thiazides
Alopecia	Allopurinol, anticoagulants, hormones, NSAIDs, phenytoin, valproate, cytotoxic agents
Erythema nodosum	Halogens, oral contraceptives, penicillin, sulfonamides, tetracycline
Aceneiform	Amoxapine, corticosteroids, halogens, haloperidol, isoniazid, lithium, phenytoin, dactynomicyn, docetaxel
Linear IgA dermatosis	Captopril, diclofenac, glibenclamide, lithium, vancomycin
Drug-induced SLE	*Most common:* Hydralazine, procainamide, minocycline, hydrochlorothiazide

neutrophilia and eosinophilia. The rash resolves spontaneously and rapidly, with fever and pustules lasting 7 to 10 days, followed by desquamation over a few days.

- Most cases are caused by drugs (primarily beta-lactam antibiotics) with a short time of onset, often within the first few days of drug administration.

FIXED DRUG ERUPTION

- Fixed drug eruptions develop during the first 2 weeks of treatment with agents such as tetracycline, phenolphthalein (laxative), NSAIDs, and sulphonamides.

- They are characterized by the development of a solitary pruritic erythematous macule, which can evolve into a raised plaque or even a blister. In some cases, multiple plaques 2 to 4 cm in diameter may appear. Lesions occur preferentially on the oral or genital mucosa, face, and the extremities.
- After withdrawal of the drug, the lesion resolves, leaving hyperpigmentation. Typically, when the drug is reintroduced the fixed drug eruption will recur at the same location.

PHOTOSENSITIVE DRUG ERUPTIONS

- Depending on the type of photosensitizing drug, either a phototoxic or a photoallergic rash will occur. A phototoxic drug reaction involves absorption of ultraviolet radiation by the causative drug and the release of free radicals causing damage to epidermal cells. A photoallergic drug reaction occurs when ultraviolet energy causes the drug hapten to bind to native protein on epidermal cells, thereby creating a complete antigen. This antigen sensitizes the immune system and a photodistributed eczematous reaction develops.
- Clinically, phototoxic reactions manifest as an exaggerated sunburn, with diffuse erythema, edema, and blisters in severe cases. No previous sensitization is required and the reaction will develop after the first administration of the drug. Lesions are distributed only on sun-exposed areas such as face, neck, dorsum of the hands, and anterior legs. Phototoxic drugs are tetracyclines, sulphamides, amiodarone, nalidixic acid, psoralens, and tolbutamide.
- Photoallergic reactions manifest as a pruritic eczematous eruption involving not only sun-exposed areas but neighboring areas. After cessation of the drug, re-exposure to sunlight may cause a recurrence of the rash in the case of photoallergic but not in phototoxic reactions.

OTHER UNCOMMON PATTERNS OF DRUG ERUPTIONS

- Other patterns of drug eruptions less frequently seen include acneiform eruptions, erythema nodosum, drug-induced lupus erythematosus, exfoliative dermatitis, lichenoid drug reactions, and vesiculobullous eruptions.
- The introduction of cytokines in routine therapy of many diseases has resulted in the appearance of new reaction patterns.

DIAGNOSIS AND DIFFERENTIAL

- Diagnosis of a drug reaction requires a high index of suspicion, a detailed history, careful examination, and a complete laboratory study according to clinical findings.
- Important clinical information that must be obtained with the history includes the names and dosage of the drugs taken, temporal relationship between the intake of the drugs and the onset of skin lesions (allergic drug reactions usually require more than 1 week of treatment), previous history of drug allergy, and similar skin lesions after taking similar drugs.

TREATMENT

- Once the offending drug has been identified, it should be discontinued promptly. If the patient is on multiple medications and it is not possible to isolate the responsible drug, the number of medications must be reduced as much as possible.
- After withdrawal of the offending drug most eruptions are treated with supportive therapy. Oral antihistamines may be used for pruritus, and moisturizing lotions may be helpful during the late desquamative phase of reaction. Topical steroids may be used for mild cases.
- Severe widespread drug eruptions may require a short course of oral prednisone (0.5 to 1 mg/kg per day). Prednisone may be used in the treatment of hypersensitivity syndrome with interstitial nephritis, as well as in the treatment of severe urticaria vasculitis, leukocytoclastic vasculitis, angioedema, erythroderma, and widespread morbilliform exanthem.

REFERENCES

Beylot C, Doutre MS, Beylot-Barry M. Acute generalized exanthematous pustulosis. *Semin Cutan Med Surg.* 1996; 15:244.

Daoud MS, Schanbacher CF, Dicken CH. Recognizing cutaneous drug eruptions. Reaction patterns provide clues to causes. *Postgrad Med.* 1998;104:101.

Gould JW, Mercurio MG, Elmets CA. Cutaneous photosensitivity diseases induced by exogenous agents. *J Am Acad Dermatol.* 1995;33:551.

Hunziker T, Kunzi UP, Braunschweig S, et al. Comprehensive hospital drug monitoring (CHDM): Adverse skin reactions, a 20-year survey. *Allergy.* 1997;52:388.

Knowles SR, Shapiro LE, Shear NH. Anticonvulsant hypersensitivity syndrome: Incidence, prevention and management. *Drug Saf.* 1999;21:489.

Stern RS, Steinberg LA. Epidemiology of adverse cutaneous reactions to drugs. *Dermatol Clin.* 1995;13:681.

TABLE 3–7   Etiology of Erythroderma

Adults

Systemic diseases (10 to 40%)	Lymphoma (CTCL and Hodgkin's) Leukemia Multiple myeloma
	Solid tumors (carcinoma of the lung, prostate, colon, and thyroid)
	Graft versus host disease Immunodeficiency (including HIV) Reiter syndrome
Cutaneous diseases (10 to 40%)	Psoriasis
	Eczematous disorders (seborrheic dermatitis, atopic dermatitis, stasis dermatitis, contact dermatitis)
	Congenital ichthyosis Pityriasis rubra pilaris Pemphigus foliaceus and pemphigoid Sarcoidosis Dermatophytosis Lichen planus Hailey–Hailey disease Lupus erythematosus
Drugs (3 to 10%) **Idiopathic** (15 to 45%)	See Table 3–6
Infants	Congenital ichthyosiform erythroderma
	Congenital bullous epidermolysis
	Leiner's syndrome Atopic dermatitis Seborrheic eczema Psoriasis
	Staphylococcal scalded skin syndrome
	Kawasaki disease Diffuse mastocytosis Chronic candidiasis Congenital immunodeficiency

ERYTHRODERMA

- Erythroderma or exfoliative dermatitis (ED) refers to a scaling erythematous dermatitis involving 90% or more of the cutaneous surface.

EPIDEMIOLOGY

- The annual incidence of ED has been estimated at 1 to 2 per 100,000 inhabitants. It is more frequent in males (male to female ratio of 2:1 to 4:1). The onset usually occurs in persons older than 40 years, except when the condition results from an eczematous disorder or a hereditary ichthyosis.
- This generalized eruption is considered the end-point of different processes like drug eruptions and cutaneous or systemic diseases. The most important causes are summarized in Table 3–7. Approximately 40% of cases are related with preexisting cutaneous diseases, another 40% with an underlying systemic disease, 10% are secondary to drug reactions, and the remaining 10% of cases are of unknown origin (idiopathic). In children, immunodeficiency (30%), congenital ichthyosis (24%), Netherton syndrome (18%), and eczematous or papulosquamous dermatitis (20%) are the most frequent causes.

PATHOPHYSIOLOGY

- Patients with ED develop an increased skin blood perfusion that results in heat loss and possible high-output cardiac failure. The basal metabolic rate rises to compensate for the resultant heat loss. Fluid loss by transpiration is increased. A marked loss of exfoliated scales occurs (20 to 30 g/d), which contributes to the depletion of proteins. Hypoalbuminemia is commonly associated to peripheral edema in most patients. The situation is similar to that observed in patients following burns (negative nitrogen balance characterized by edema, hypoalbuminemia, and loss of muscle mass).

CLINICAL FEATURES

- Patients often present with a generalized erythema, followed by scaling 2 to 6 days after the onset of erythema, usually starting from flexural areas. The entire skin surface becomes red, scaly, thickened, and occasionally crusted. The patient usually feels cold, and pruritus is a very prominent and frequent symptom. In some cases hairs may shed and nails may become ridged and thickened.
- When exfoliative dermatitis persists for weeks, the patient presents with weight loss, hypoproteinemia, hypocalcemia, iron deficiency, or high-output heart failure. Generalized superficial lymphadenopathy is frequent, but biopsy usually shows a benign lymphadenitis (dermatopathic lymphadenopathy).
- ED is a severe clinical situation, with a high mortality rate. Mortality varies according to the disease's cause. A mortality rate of 43% has been observed, but only 18% of deaths are directly related to ED. The typical mean duration of illness is 5 years, with a median of 10 months.

TABLE 3–8   Diagnostic Tests in Erythroderma

TEST	FINDING	DIAGNOSIS
Blood analysis	Increased ESR, anemia, hypoalbuminemia, hyperglobulinemia Increased IgE Peripheral blood smears	Frequent and nonspecific findings May be observed atopic dermatitis Abnormal in leukemia
Skin scraping	Hyphae or scabies mites	Dermatophytosis, Norwegian scabies
Cultures	Bacterial overgrowth, herpes simplex virus	Infectious cause
Skin biopsy	Skin biopsies reveal nonspecific findings of spongiotic dermatitis	Primary disease may be evident
HIV testing	ED has been reported to predict seroconversion in HIV infection	HIV infection
Imaging studies	Computed tomography, magnetic resonance imaging, chest x-ray, mammogram (according to the clinical features)	Solid tumors, lymphoma
Other tests	Bone marrow examination if myeloproliferative disorder is suspected	Leukemia
	Immunophenotyping, flow cytometry, B-cell and T-cell gene rearrangement analysis if lymphoma is suspected	Lymphoma
	Routine cancer screenings appropriate for age and gender (mammogram, stool occult blood test, sigmoidoscopy, prostate examination, serum PSA, cervical smear) if cause of ED is in doubt	Solid tumors
Patch testing	Contact allergens (should be performed only during periods of remission)	Contact dermatitis

DIAGNOSIS AND DIFFERENTIAL

- The intense erythema and scaling frequently obscure any underlying primary dermatitis. Residual signs may include islands of normal-appearing skin and orange palmar keratoderma in pityriasis rubra pilaris, isolated psoriatic plaques in erythrodermic psoriasis, oral lesions in lichen planus, superficial blisters in pemphigus foliaceus, erythematous papular lesions in drug eruptions, and hepatomegaly and splenomegaly in lymphoma.
- The most common histopathologic appearance of ED is a subacute or chronic spongiotic dermatitis. The appearance of ED usually masks the underlying disease's specific histologic features. Detailed histopathologic analysis with clinicopathologic correlation is mandatory for cases in which a specific cause is not apparent. With multiple biopsies, the diagnosis may be confirmed in as many as 45% of patients.
- The laboratory studies that can be undertaken to find out the cause of ED are summarized in Table 3–8. Patients with idiopathic ED should be carefully followed using multiple serial biopsies to exclude cutaneous T-cell lymphoma.

TREATMENT

- Patients with ED often require admission for inpatient management and should be kept in a warm and humid environment. Fluid intake needs to be monitorized, adequate nutrition with emphasis on protein intake should be provided, and body temperature controlled. In cases of known cause, adequate treatment of the underlying disease should be performed.
- The use of wet compresses, warm baths, and lubricants is generally recommended in order to maintain skin moisture and avoid scratching. Oral antihistamines and topical steroids help to reduce pruritus. Systemic steroids may be helpful in some cases but should be avoided in suspected cases of psoriasis. Systemic antibiotics are indicated if signs of secondary infection are observed.
- Weekly methotrexate has been advocated, between reevaluation periods, in patients with idiopathic ED that is unremitting despite the use of topical steroids.

REFERENCES

Botella-Estrada R, Sanmartin O, Oliver V, et al. Erythroderma: A clinicopathological study of 56 cases. *Arch Dermatol.* 1994;130:1503.

Karakayli G, Beckham G, Orengo I, Rosen T. Exfoliative dermatitis. *Am Fam Physician.* 1999;59:625.

Pruszkowski A, Bodemer C, Fraitag S, et al. Neonatal and infantile erythrodermas: A retrospective study of 51 patients. *Arch Dermatol.* 2000;136:875.

Sigurdsson V, Toonstra J, Hezemans-Boer M, Van Vloten WA. Erythroderma: A clinical and follow-up study of 102 patients, with special emphasis on survival. *J Am Acad Dermatol.* 1996;35:53.

Zackheim HS, Kashani-Sabet M, Hwang ST. Low-dose methotrexate to treat erythrodermic cutaneous T-cell lymphoma: Results in twenty-nine patients. *J Am Acad Dermatol.* 1996;34:626.

SWEET'S SYNDROME

- Sweet's syndrome, also termed acute febrile neutrophilic dermatosis (AFND), is an inflammatory condition characterized by the abrupt development of erythematous plaques accompanied by fever and peripheral neutrophilia. Sweet's syndrome is believed to be a reactive phenomenon that occurs in association with certain malignancies, systemic infections, autoimmune conditions, or drug exposure.

EPIDEMIOLOGY

- Sweet's syndrome is uncommon. Its incidence has been estimated to be 2.7 cases/year per one million population. Women are predominantly affected in non-malignancy associated Sweet's syndrome, with a female to male ratio of 2:1 to 3:1. However, in cancer-associated cases, the female to male ratio is 1:1.
- Table 3–9 summarizes the conditions associated with Sweet's syndrome. Most cases (71%) are of unknown origin, occurring 4 to 14 days after a non-specific gastrointestinal or upper respiratory infection or after vaccination. Sweet's syndrome has also been described in patients with chronic inflammatory disorders (16%) such as rheumatoid arthritis or inflammatory bowel diseases, in pregnancy (2%), or as an adverse effect of drug therapy. Sweet's syndrome can be a paraneoplastic phenomenon (11%), associated with a hemoproliferative disorder (especially acute myeloid leukaemia) or a solid carcinoma.

PATHOPHYSIOLOGY

- The pathogenesis is still unknown, but convincing evidence suggests that Sweet's syndrome is a cytokine (IL-8) T-cell mediated disease with secondary activation and participation of neutrophils. Neutrophils are basic in the pathogenesis of Sweet's syndrome, as evidenced by its histopathologic appearance, associated neutrophilia, and increased neutrophil function.

CLINICAL FEATURES

- Abrupt onset of multiple tender, well-demarcated plaques distributed on the face, neck, upper trunk, and extremities is characteristic. Skin lesions start as multiple, isolated erythematous papules that often coalesce into circinate or arcuate plaques. The surface of cutaneous plaques shows a mamillated appearance and intense edema with pseudovesiculation. Skin lesions are characteristically painful but not itchy. Oral lesions (apthae) occur in about 30% of the cases. Sweet's syndrome may be associated with erythema nodosum on the lower legs (12 to 30% of cases).

TABLE 3–9   Conditions Associated with Sweet's Syndrome

Classic (71%)	Focal upper respiratory infections Gastrointestinal infection
Inflammatory (16%)	**Autoimmune diseases** o Behçet's disease o Inflammatory bowel disease o Sjögren's syndrome o Lupus erythematosus/mixed connective tissue disease o Rheumatoid arthritis o Thyroiditis o Sarcoidosis **Systemic infections** o Yersiniosis o Toxoplasmosis, histoplasmosis, ureaplasmosis o Tuberculosis
Paraneoplastic (11%)	**Leukemia and lymphoma** (most frequent) o AML, AMML, ALL o Myelodysplasia, polycythemia, myeloid metaplasia o CML, CLL o Multiple myeloma o Hairy cell leukemia o Non-Hodgkin's lymphomas **Solid tumors** (very rare) o Carcinoma of the breast, prostate, uterus, vagina, colon, stomach, rarely others
Drug-Induced	Vaccination Therapy with growth factors (G- and GM CSF) Sulfonamides, all-*trans* retinoic acid, minocycline

- Each crop of lesions is usually preceded by fever, headache, and malaise. In very rare cases, Sweet's syndrome has the potential to involve other organ systems. Pulmonary manifestations are the most common extracutaneous findings and may manifest as a chronic cough or pulmonary infiltrates on chest x-ray films.
- Clinical lesions may persist for days to weeks without treatment. Outcome depends on the underlying condition, but recurrences may occur in up to 50% of patients and is most likely in cases associated with hematologic malignancy or drug reactions. In isolated cases recurrent crops cause the condition to persist indefinitely, like a chronic disease; this is termed chronic neutrophilic dermatosis.

DIAGNOSIS AND DIFFERENTIAL

- Diagnosis is made according to clinical, histopathologic, and laboratory findings. A number of diagnostic criteria have been proposed (Table 3–10).

TABLE 3–10 Diagnostic Criteria for Sweet's Syndrome[a]

MAJOR CRITERIA

1. Abrupt onset of tender of painful erythematous plaques or nodules occasionally with vesicles, pustules, or bullae

2. Neutrophilic infiltration in the dermis *without* leukocytoclastic vasculitis

MINOR CRITERIA

1. Associations
   o Preceded by an unspecific respiratory or gastrointestinal tract infections or vaccination
   o Associated with inflammatory diseases (autoimmune, infections), cancer (hemoproliferative disorders or solid malignant tumors), or pregnancy

2. Accompanied by periods of general malaise and fever (>38°C)

3. Laboratory values during onset (three out of four necessary):
   o ESR > 20 mm
   o C-reactive protein positive
   o Neutrophils > 70%
   o Leukocytosis > 8.000
   o Excellent response to systemic corticosteroids or potassium iodide

[a]Both major and two minor criteria are needed for diagnosis.

- The classic histopathologic pattern of Sweet's syndrome consists of a dense diffuse neutrophilic infiltrate in the reticular dermis and massive papillary dermal edema. Although leukocytoclastic nuclear debris is typically present, true vasculitic changes are typically absent.
- Leukocytosis and neutrophilia are typically present, but their absence does not rule out Sweet's syndrome. The sedimentation rate, reactive C protein, and other acute reactants are usually elevated.
- Features that suggest a malignant association are the lack of antecedents of upper respiratory infections, heterogeneity of cutaneous lesions with blistering and/or ulceration, tendency to recurrences, and abnormal laboratory results (anemia, thrombocytosis, thrombocytopenia). These cases should enforce thorough diagnostic investigations including a bone marrow aspiration.

TREATMENT

- Standard treatment of Sweet's syndrome is the oral administration of corticosteroids. In most cases, prednisone is extremely and rapidly effective (1.0 mg/kg of body weight).
- A number of non-steroidal drugs, especially potassium iodide, have been used alternatively to prednisone. These treatments are indicated for longer-term management and in recurrent and chronic cases.

REFERENCES

Bourke JF, Keohane S, Long CC, et al. Sweet's syndrome and malignancy in the U.K. *Br J Dermatol.* 1997;137:609.

Su WP, Liu HN. Diagnostic criteria for Sweet's syndrome. *Cutis* 1986;37:167.

Von den Driesch P. Sweet's syndrome (acute febrile neutrophilic dermatosis). *J Am Acad Dermatol.* 1994;31:535.

POLYMORPHOUS LIGHT ERUPTION

- Polymorphous light eruption (PMLE) is an inflammatory, ultraviolet light-induced eruption characterized by itchy, transient, and recurrent lesions on sun-exposed areas.

EPIDEMIOLOGY

- PMLE is a common photodermatosis with a prevalence estimated in 5 to 15%. Onset is usually in young adult life. It can affect all racial skin types, but it is more common in fair-skinned individuals.
- Family history is positive in only about 15% of the affected patients. Actinic prurigo, a hereditary variant of PMLE more frequent in native Americans, appears to be inherited in an autosomal dominant manner (75% of patients reveal disease in a family member).

PATHOPHYSIOLOGY

- The pathogenesis of PMLE is not fully known, but it has been suggested that it might represent a type IV hypersensitivity to a UV-induced neoantigen produced after sun exposure in the involved skin.
- Although UV-A light is currently considered as the causative factor in PMLE eruption, UV-B or even visible light, may be responsible in some individuals.

CLINICAL FEATURES

- As the name implies, clinical lesions are polymorphous. Many different morphologies may appear, but typically only one type of lesion predominates the clinical findings in any one person. Multiple erythematous papules on sun-exposed areas are the most frequent type of lesions, followed by plaques, papulovesicles, and erythema multiforme-like lesions. Upper chest, arms, and upper back are the most frequently involved areas, although generalized involvement or atypical locations may appear. The skin lesions are intensely pruritic.

- Lesions appear following the first days of sun exposure and disappear after several days of sun avoidance. Thirty minutes to several hours of sun exposure are required to trigger the eruption. The eruption of PMLE typically starts in spring and decreases in severity until it disappears as the summer progresses. This adaptation is known as the hardening phenomenon and may explain the progressive reduction in severity of PMLE during the summer. PMLE tends to recur during several years. Each spring or summer the lesions tend to recur in the same locations as in the preceding year.
- A variant of this disease, known as juvenile spring eruption of the ears, is characterized by recurrent UV-induced crops of vesicular lesions on the helix of young males.

DIAGNOSIS AND DIFFERENTIAL

- Diagnosis is usually based on the clinical picture. But in some cases, skin biopsy, photobiologic studies and laboratory analysis are required. Fully developed lesions of PMLE show a dense superficial and deep perivascular lymphocytic infiltrate and intense edema of the papillary dermis. Phototests with UV-A, UV-B, and visible light sources must be performed. The minimal erythema dose (MED) is normal in PMLE. Repeated phototesting on the same area may reproduce lesions of PMLE in up to 60 to 100% of the patients.
- Differential diagnosis includes patients with lupus erythematosus (positive ANA), erythropoietic porphyria (anomalies in porphyrin levels), chronic actinic dermatitis (CAD) and solar urticaria. Under the term of CAD are included patients with chronic photosensitivity, abnormal phototests, and photodermatitis determined by biopsy findings. CAD includes other

diseases previously known as persistent light reactivity, photosensitive eczema, and actinic reticuloid. Clinical presentation consists in chronic erythematous patches, lichenified papules and plaques on sun-exposed areas. Biopsy shows a chronic eczema with a pseudolymphomatous appearance in the infiltrate.

TREATMENT

- Prophylactic therapy—avoiding sunlight, wearing protective clothing, and using sunscreen—is mandatory in the care of these patients. Prophylactic phototherapy (PUVA and UVB) at the beginning of the spring may prevent flare-ups throughout the summer. This therapy is based on the hardening phenomenon of PMLE.
- Topical corticosteroids, antihistamines, or systemic steroids are useful to treat acute flares and control pruritus. Antimalarials at low doses may be helpful. This treatment may induce remission and prevent new relapses of the disease during the summer. Beta-carotene, may be an alternative to antimalarials. Azathioprine may be indicated in severe, resistant cases.

REFERENCES

Boonstra HE, Van Weelden H, Toonstra J, van Vloten WA. Polymorphous light eruption: A clinical, photobiologic, and follow-up study of 110 patients. *J Am Acad Dermatol.* 2000;42:199.

Hasan T, Ranki A, Jansen CT, Karvonen J. Disease associations in polymorphous light eruption. A long-term follow-up study of 94 patients. *Arch Dermatol.* 1998;134:1081.

Lim HW, Epstein J. Photosensitivity diseases. *J Am Acad Dermatol.* 1997;36:84.

Murphy GM, Logan RA, Lovell CR. Prophylactic PUVA and UVB therapy in polymorphous light eruption. *Br J Dermatol.* 1987;116:531.

4 CUTANEOUS VASCULITIDES

Adrienne Rencic
Alfredo C. Rivadeneira
Deborah Cummins
H. Carlos Nousari

- Vasculitic syndromes remain one of the greatest imitators in medicine. Evaluation of cutaneous vasculitis requires a thorough physical examination and careful correlation of immunopathologic and serologic data. This chapter proposes a practical algorithmic approach for the diagnosis and management of patients with cutaneous vasculitis.
- *"Cutaneous vasculitis is an idiopathic, complex, and dynamic inflammatory disorder characterized by a disruption of the architecture of the cutaneous blood vessels by inflammatory cells and by clinical morphologic presentations that correlate with the size of the dominant affected vessel."* The components of this definition will be dissected and discussed throughout this chapter.
- Many systems of classification for systemic vasculitis have been suggested. Among these, the one that renders the most accurate clinicopathologic correlation and thus best diagnostic yield for cutaneous vasculitis is the one based on the size of the predominant affected vessels.
- Cutaneous small-sized vessels include arterioles, capillaries, and postcapillary venules. These vessels lack a fully developed muscular layer, measure less than 50 microns in diameter, and are located predominantly in the upper dermis.
- Cutaneous medium-sized vessels contain a fully developed muscular layer, measure greater than 50 microns in diameter, and are predominantly in the deep dermis, dermal subcutaneous fat, and the fascia.
- Large vessels are rarely found in the skin and the discussion of large vessel vasculitis is beyond the scope of this chapter.

SMALL-SIZED VESSEL VASCULITIS OF THE SKIN

CLINICAL FEATURES

- The most common clinical presentations of small-sized vessel vasculitis (SVV) of the skin are purpuric and/or urticarial lesions.

- The purpuric lesions are nonblanchable and are most prominent in dependent areas, typically the lower extremities. These purpuric lesions can be nonpalpable (e.g., macules) or palpable (e.g., papules). Other clinical presentations of SVV such as vesicular, pustular, or small, superficial ulcerations (usually less than 1 cm in diameter) are not uncommonly observed. These lesions resolve with postinflammatory hyperpigmentation.
- Urticarial vasculitis lesions may be associated with burning or pain sensation, but not with clinically significant pruritus. Individual lesions in urticarial vasculitis last longer than those in classic urticaria. An individual lesion in classic urticaria is traditionally thought to last less than 24 hours, but some otherwise typical urticarial lesions may last longer.
- Lack of pruritus and the presence of purpura, postinflammatory hyperpigmentation, and significant constitutional symptoms are more useful features than the duration of the lesions in the diagnosis of urticarial vasculitis.

HISTOLOGY

- A standard 4 to 6-mm punch lesional biopsy of a nonulcerated lesion less than 48 to 96 hours old should be performed to render the best diagnostic yield. The specimen should be split. Half should be sent for routine histology and half for direct immunofluorescence examination.
- The histologic features of SVV are listed in Table 4–1.
- However, in lymphocyte-predominant vasculitis, most of the classic histologic features of vasculitis are absent and the findings are subtle. Thus, lymphocytic vasculitis is commonly misdiagnosed.
- Table 4–2 lists the differential diagnosis for lymphocytic vasculitis.

TABLE 4–1   Histologic Features of SVV

Fibrinoid necrosis
Perivascular/intravascular inflammatory cell infiltrate
Edema of the vessel wall
Extravasation of red blood cells
Leukocytoclasis
Endothelial cell swelling
Intraluminal thrombi

ESSENTIAL INFORMATION IN THE HISTOLOGIC EVALUATION OF CUTANEOUS VASCULITIS

Confirmation of cutaneous vasculitis and distinction from other perivascular infiltrates

Determination of predominant vessel size involved
Determination of the predominant inflammatory cell

ADDITIONAL RELEVANT COMPONENTS

Location of the vessel that is predominantly affected
Associated palisaded neutrophilic and granulomatous dermatitis
Staining for microorganisms

MEDIUM-SIZED VESSEL VASCULITIS OF THE SKIN

CLINICAL FEATURES

- The clinical presentation of medium-sized vessel vasculitis (MVV) of the skin may consist of nodules, ulcerations, digital infarcts, and livedo reticularis. Papulo-nodular necrotic lesions on extensor surfaces and granulomatous lesions can also be seen in MVV.
- Because of the involvement of deeper vessels, it is necessary to sample sufficient subcutaneous tissue. Wedge biopsies or deep punch biopsies are more appropriate for diagnosis in these cases.
- Yield is highest with biopsy of nodules (95%), and less for ulcers (50%) and livedo Reticularis (25%). Biopsy of digital infarcts should be avoided as diagnostic yield is very low (5%) and the wounds heal poorly.

HISTOLOGY

- Vasculitis of these vessels is commonly referred to as necrotizing vasculitis. This reflects the hyalinization, coagulative necrosis, and degeneration of the vessel muscular layers, where it is readily visible. The infiltrate is mixed, with polymorphonuclear predominance in early stages and mononuclear in late stages.
- Eosinophilic infiltrates may be present in any vasculitis. The diagnosis of Churg–Strauss syndrome (CSS), however, requires eosinophil predominance.

TABLE 4–2   Differential Diagnoses of Lymphocytic Vasculitis

Late or resolving stage of leukocytoclastic vasculitis
Purpuric mycosis fungoides
Angiocentric lymphoma
Intravascular lymphoma (angiotropic lymphoma)
CMV vasculitis
Pityriasis lichenoides
Lymphomatoid papulosis

DIRECT IMMUNOFLUORESCENCE

- Direct immunofluorescence (DIF) is an essential diagnostic tool in the evaluation of cutaneous vasculitis, especially in the small-vessel group. This technique consists of the detection of immunoglobulins and complement deposited within the affected tissues.
- The skin specimens are placed in Michels's transport medium and stored at 4°C prior to processing in a dermatoimmunology laboratory.
- The specimen is then washed, snap frozen, sectioned, and probed with antihuman IgG, IgA, IgM, C3, C5b-9.
- Careful interpretation is necessary; otherwise false-positive and negatives results are commonly encountered. Both C3 in superficial vessels and patchy vascular IgM are frequent artifacts in nonvasculitic lesions.
- Older lesions do not usually show immunoreactants, due to degradation as a result of proteolysis from polymorphonuclear cell degranulation products.
- IgA deposits are usually patchy and subtle, affecting only a few vessels. This is important in the evaluation of a possible IgA vasculitis.

REFERENCES

Callen JP. A clinical approach to the vasculitis patient in the dermatologic office. *Clin Dermatol.* 1999;17:549.

Chu P, Connolly MK, LeBoit PE. The histopathologic spectrum of palisaded neutrophilic and granulomatous dermatitis in patients with collagen vascular disease. *Arch Dermatol.* 1994;130:1278.

Gibson LE, Su WP. Cutaneous vasculitis. *Rheum Dis Clin North Am.* 1995;21:1097.

Gonzalez-Gay MA, Garcia-Porrua C. Epidemiology of the vasculidities. *Rheum Dis Clin North Am.* 2001;27:729.

Jennette JC, Falk RJ, Andrassy K, et al. Nomenclature of systemic vasculitides. Proposal of an international consensus conference. *Arthritis Rheum.* 1994;37:187.

Stone JH, Nousari HC. "Essential" cutaneous vasculitis: What every rheumatologist should know about vasculitis of the skin. *Curr Opin Rheumatol.* 2001;13:23.

CUTANEOUS VASCULITIS SYNDROMES

SMALL-SIZED VESSEL VASCULITIS

CUTANEOUS LEUKOCYTOCLASTIC ANGIITIS (HYPERSENSITIVITY VASCULITIS)

- Cutaneous leukocytoclastic angiitis (CLA) is the term coined by the Chapel Hill Consensus conference to better identify patients with the so-called hypersensitivity vasculitis.

EPIDEMIOLOGY

- In Norwich, England from 1990 to 1994 the incidence was found to be 15.4 per million. In Lugo, Spain, the mean age of onset was 58.7 years.

PATHOPHYSIOLOGY

- This type of vasculitis is commonly triggered by medications, infections, or inflammatory disorders.
- The eruption usually occurs within 5 to 20 days after exposure to these triggers.
- Relapsing episodes of CLA can be caused by chronic infections such as osteomyelitis or AIDS, inflammatory bowel disease, or neoplasms (hematologic malignancies).
- Serum sickness, originally described as a response to injection of heterologous serum into humans, is a variant of CLA. It now occurs most frequently as a reaction to medications, often 7 to 21 days after primary exposure to the offending agent, and after 2 to 4 days on re-exposure.
- The inciting stimulus initiates the production of lymphokines and cytokines, which induce circulating IgM immune complexes that do not strongly activate complement. Consequently, a chemokine-mediated inflammatory cascade in the endothelium of cutaneous small vessels is the final insult leading to the clinical manifestations of CLA.
- Polymorphonuclear dominant vasculitis of small vessels of the upper dermis is most typical. In most instances neutrophils and eosinophils share the dominance of the infiltrate.
- DIF is positive in no more than 50% of the specimens, and typically shows granular IgM with weak or absent C3 in the superficial dermal vessels.

- However, DIF remains a very important tool in the exclusion of IgA vasculitis, since the latter shares similar clinical features and triggers (infections and drugs).
- Relevant laboratory data include ESR, which is elevated in 50% of cases; and complement levels, which are normal, except in serum sickness syndrome.

CLINICAL FEATURES

- The onset is abrupt and characteristically the skin findings are palpable or nonpalpable purpuric and urticarial lesions.
- All the lesions typically occur at one time and appear of similar age. Ulceration of these lesions is rarely seen. The lesions favor the lower extremities.
- Although the cutaneous involvement can be striking, clinically significant systemic involvement is rare with the exception of constitutional symptoms and mild synovitis.
- An exception remains in serum sickness syndrome, where patients by definition have significant systemic disease; fortunately, this variant is rarely seen nowadays.

TREATMENT

- Treatment consists of identification and withdrawal of the responsible medication, and eradication of the infection. In most instances the lesions will resolve even with continuation of the offending drug.
- Systemic immunosuppressive drugs are largely unnecessary. However, systemic corticosteroids, usually at moderate doses of 0.5 mg/kg per day for a few weeks, may play a role in palliative treatment of the constitutional symptoms and synovitis.
- In chronic relapsing cases, a thorough investigation for an underlying chronic inflammatory, infectious, or a neoplastic disease is mandatory. Treatment of these underlying disorders is associated with improvement or eradication of the CLA.
- CLA resolves most often within 3 weeks or less after onset without treatment.

HENOCH–SCHOENLEIN PURPURA (IGA VASCULITIS)

EPIDEMIOLOGY

- In Norwich, England the incidence was 13 per million from 1990 to 1994. In Lugo, Spain the incidence was

14.3 per million from 1988 to 1997. About half of cases occur in children under the age of 5 years. The incidence in Denmark for children under the age of 14 years was 135 to 180 per million, whereas in adults (over age 14) it was 8 per million.

PATHOPHYSIOLOGY

- As in CLA, the most common triggers in HSP are infections and drugs. Upper respiratory infections are the most common; however, gastrointestinal infections and genitourinary infections have also been reported. This may account for some HSP patients with gastrointestinal symptoms and not true intestinal vasculitis.
- These triggers through a cascade of lymphokines and cytokines induce IgA1 immune complexes. An inflammatory cascade in the endothelium of cutaneous small vessels in the skin, mesenteric vessels, and renal vessels leads to the clinical manifestations of HSP.
- Patients with fibronectin rich IgA1 immune complexes tend to have higher incidence of renal disease, as well as patients with an abnormality in glycosylation of the hinge region of IgA1.
- Routine histologic features show neutrophil dominant perivascular and intravascular infiltrates, disrupting the architecture of the small vessels in the upper dermis. These findings are indistinguishable from other pure SVV such as CLA and urticarial vasculitis.
- The gold standard diagnostic tool is DIF; virtually all patients should have IgA deposits in superficial blood vessels. False-negative results are not uncommon and are usually a consequence of the patchy and occasionally subtle granular nature of the deposits or due to evaluation of old lesions.
- Weaker IgG, IgM, and C3 in conjunction with stronger IgA deposits can also be seen in HSP lesions, especially in HIV patients.
- More extensive IgA deposits in deeper blood vessels can be observed in cases of HSP associated with monoclonal gammopathy.
- 60% of patients may have an IgA polyclonal gammopathy, but no other serologic abnormalities.

CLINICAL FEATURES

- HSP is a syndrome typically characterized by purpura, abdominal pain, arthralgias, and hematuria.
- The skin lesions have been reported as either typical palpable purpura or urticaria rapidly turning into purpura with annular configuration.
- HSP predominantly affects the lower extremities and characteristically the buttocks.

- Gastrointestinal involvement is thought to be the result of vasculitic involvement in the gut.
- Renal involvement (glomerulonephritis) can produce irreversible renal damage.
- Recently, the prevalence of this vasculitis in adults has come with the recognition of DIF findings and the more extensive use of DIF in evaluation of cutaneous vasculitis.
- The skin lesions are present in all patients. The most common lesions are purpuric (palpable and nonpalpable), preceded or not by an urticarial component. Some of the patients may have only urticarial lesions.
- The lower extremities are always affected; more extensive disease may have lesions on the buttocks, trunk, or upper extremities.
- Ulcerative lesions are uncommonly observed; however, this presentation seems to be more common in patients with HIV-associated HSP.
- The Koebner phenomenon (appearance of a lesion after trauma) occurs frequently in these patients due to involvement of the superficial plexus of small vessels in the papillary dermal tips.
- Growing evidence suggests that acute hemorrhagic edema of childhood is a clinical variant of HSP. These children have purpuric lesions, acral edema, low incidence of systemic involvement, such as fever and a possible infectious trigger. Skin lesions are urticarial, purpuric, and annular with a stockade configuration that involves extremities, and typically, face and ears.
- Gastrointestinal involvement in HSP ranges from pain due to edema to frank bleeding.
- Synovitis is usually mild and affects the ankles, but other joints may be affected.
- The renal involvement ranges from 0 to 40%. It has been shown that the renal involvement in the pediatric population has been underestimated; some children will have higher incidence of hypertension and chronic renal failure as adults.
- Adults seem to have a higher incidence of renal disease. Interestingly, in these patients the skin lesions may be observed above the waistline; preceding infections and elevated acute phase reactants seem to be factors associated with higher incidence of renal involvement.
- IgA monoclonal gammopathy and HIV have been recently recognized associations, in adults. In addition, HSP is recognized as one of the most common causes of chronic relapsing cutaneous SVV in this age group.
- Patients with extensive cutaneous involvement and persistent or recurrent disease require further tests including HIV testing, serum protein electrophoresis, random urine electrophoresis, and total immunoglobulin quantitation; and immunofixation should be performed to rule out IgA monoclonal gammopathy.

TREATMENT

- Treatment of the cutaneous disease is largely unnecessary, unless significant ulceration is present.
- The constitutional symptoms (synovitis, gastrointestinal edema, and inflammation) are quite responsive to systemic corticosteroids at moderate doses. Systemic corticosteroids are associated with initial response, but tapering is associated with rapid relapse.
- There is no gold standard treatment for glomerulonephritis; often a combination of systemic corticosteroids with immunosuppressants such as azathioprine or mycophenolate mofetil can be effective. Alkylating agents may be employed in more severe cases.
- Several experimental studies have shown up-regulation of TNF. Recent trials using anti-TNF drugs have been initiated, but definite data about the effectiveness of these drugs in HSP is pending.
- The cutaneous disease is refractory for treatment, especially in patients with monoclonal gammopathy and HIV.
- The complication of HSP that is of greatest concern is renal failure due to glomerulonephritis. About 5% of patients develop chronic renal disease, and 15% of children on hemodialysis have renal failure due to HSP.
- Renal involvement is most likely to occur within the first 3 months of disease. The best screening test for renal involvement is a urinalysis. Hematuria is the most sensitive parameter for measuring disease activity.
- Adult patients with HSP appear to have a higher incidence of renal disease.
- Other internal organs can be affected, such as the lungs, with pulmonary hemorrhage, although some cases are difficult to distinguish from a potential respiratory infection triggering the disease. Liver, testicular, pancreatic, and CNS involvement are uncommon.

REFERENCES

Besbas N, Duzova A, Topaloglu R, et al. Pulmonary haemorrhage in a 6-year-old boy with purpura. *Clin Rheumatol.* 2001;20:293.

Birchmore D, Sweeney C, Choudhury D, et al. IgA multiple myeloma presenting as Henoch-Schonlein purpura/polyarteritis nodosa overlap syndrome. *Arthritis Rheum.* 1996;39:698.

Garcia-Porrua C, Gonzalez-Louzao C, Llorca J, et al. Predictive factors for renal sequelae in adults with Henoch-Schonlein purpura. *J Rheumatol.* 2001;28:1019.

Paradisi M, Annessi G, Corrado A. Infantile acute hemorrhagic edema of the skin. *Cutis.* 2001;68:127.

Saulsbury FT. Henoch-Schonlein purpura. *Curr Opin Rheumatol.* 2001;13:35.

URTICARIAL VASCULITIS

EPIDEMIOLOGY

- Because urticarial vasculitis is a morphologic finding and is composed of several distinct entities including normocomplementemic urticarial vasculitis, hypocomplementemic urticarial vasculitis, and urticarial HSP, it is difficult to estimate the incidence of urticarial vasculitis.

NORMOCOMPLEMENTEMIC URTICARIAL VASCULITIS

CLINICAL FEATURES

- Normocomplementemic urticarial vasculitis (NMV) is the most common variant, which is a subset of CLA and has a similar prognosis and pathogenesis. Infections and medications trigger 90% of these cases. The eruption is self-limited, lasting 4 weeks or less with no evidence of systemic involvement.

HYPOCOMPLEMENTEMIC URTICARIAL VASCULITIS SYNDROME

- Hypocomplementemic urticarial vasculitis syndrome (HUVS) is a chronic relapsing condition. All patients have constitutional symptoms such as fever, myalgias, and arthralgias, resembling symptoms and signs seen in systemic lupus erythematosus (SLE).
- The lesions favor the trunk and proximal extremities in both NUV and HUVS.
- Lesions are typically pruritic, but some concomitant symptoms like burning sensation, pain, and mild constitutional symptoms are not uncommon.
- As opposed to the lesions in NUV, careful examination of the urticarial lesions of HUVS would show a purpuric component in most if not in all of these lesions. This may be facilitated by using diascopy (viewing after pressure with a glass slide).
- The most common associated systemic involvement includes synovitis, glomerulonephritis, gastrointestinal involvement, and scleritis, as well as other ocular symptoms.
- Also, an association with chronic obstructive pulmonary disease has been suggested, but this appears to be a coincidental finding.
- A group of patients with more overt SLE symptoms and HUVS may have associated angioedema.

PATHOPHYSIOLOGY

- The two forms of urticarial vasculitis: normocomplementemic (NUV) and hypocomplementemic (HUVS) are distinguished by complement consumption as evidenced by decreased levels of C3, C4, and CH50.
- NUV is very likely a subset of cutaneous leukocytoclastic angiitis, and the hypocomplementemic variant is a subset of SLE.
- When more sensitive assays for the investigation of complement activation such as levels of C3a, C5a, and C3bi are used, a number of patients formerly classified as normocomplementemic would be switched into the category of hypocomplementemic. These tests are not widely commercially available and are performed only in research laboratories.
- Patients with associated angioedema have an acquired deficiency of C1 esterase, believed to be the result of a high rate of consumption caused by antibodies to C1q.
- In both NUV and HUVS lesions, histologic examination reveals a dense neutrophilic predominant perivascular and intravascular infiltrate disrupting the architecture of small vessels of the superficial dermis with frequent spillage into the interstitium. These lesions have the heaviest neutrophilic infiltrate among all cutaneous vasculitides.
- In HUVS the neutrophilic infiltrate may extend to the dermal–epidermal junction, inducing vacuolar changes in the epidermis, along with significant upper dermal edema resulting in a histologic cleft of the basement membrane zone.
- HUVS lesions, in virtually all patients, show a typical DIF finding: IgG and significant C3 deposits around and within the superficial papillary small vessels and at the basement membrane zone. The latter finding resembles the lupus band test, supporting the notion of HUVS as a subset of SLE.
- In NUV lesions as in CLA, 50% of patients have positive DIF showing predominantly IgM and less IgG within the blood vessel walls. If C3 is observed, it is patchy and weak.
- In NUV the only serologic marker is an elevated ESR, which is present in up to 70% of patients.
- Virtually all HUVS patients have an elevated ESR and have or will develop an ANA titer of 1:320 or more.
- CH50 is a more sensitive predictor of hypocomplementemia since C3 and C4 are acute-phase reactants and may be normal in mild disease or early-stage disease.

DIAGNOSIS AND DIFFERENTIAL

- Neutrophilic urticaria, also known as polymorphonuclear predominant urticaria (PPU), is an under-recognized variant of chronic urticaria and is the most common misdiagnosis of NUV. The chronicity of the lesion without a trigger or underlying disease (e.g. inflammatory bowel disease) speak against the diagnosis of NUV and should prompt to the exclusion of PPU even in the setting of a histology report that overall favors vasculitis. DIF is consistently negative.
- Neutrophilic dermatoses with or without the association of periodic fever syndromes are also in the clinical and immunopathologic differential of NUV. Schnitzler syndrome, which is characterized by urticaria, periodic fever, lymphadenopathy, hepatosplenomegaly, bone pain, and sensorimotor neuropathy, should also be considered in the differential.

TREATMENT

- NUV as in CLA does not usually require treatment.
- In HUVS, early and effective systemic immunosuppressive therapy is required.
- In milder cases, leflunomide, antimetabolites, and anti-inflammatory agents may be effective.
- Corticosteroids and antimetabolite immunosuppressives such as azathioprine (3 to 4 mg/kg per day) or mycophenylate mofetil (40 to 50 mg/kg per day) are effective.
- In severe cases, alkylating agents such as cyclophosphamide may be needed.
- Pure anti-inflammatory drugs such as dapsone, colchicine, calcineurin inhibitors, and methotrexate, may block a secondary inflammatory process; however, these have no effect on the production of immune complexes or anti-C1q antibody synthesis. Thus they are not very effective in the management of these patients.
- NUV resolves without treatment and does not tend to recur.
- HUVS is a chronic relapsing condition. It is associated with systemic symptoms and can often be associated with SLE and angioedema. It can be refractory to treatment.

REFERENCES

Davis MD, Daoud MS, Kirby B, et al. Clinicopathologic correlation of hypocomplementemic and normocomplementemic urticarial vasculitis. *J Am Acad Dermatol.* 1998; 38:899.

Mehregan DR, Hall MJ, Gibson LE. Urticarial vasculitis: A histopathologic and clinical review of 72 cases. *J Am Acad Dermatol.* 1992;26:441.

VASCULITIS AFFECTING SMALL AND MEDIUM-SIZED VESSELS

CRYOGLOBULINEMIA

- Cryoglobulins are immunoglobulins that precipitate in cold temperatures.
- There are three types of cryoglobulinemia.
- Type I most commonly presents with hyperviscosity and thrombotic phenomena and occurs in the context of myeloproliferative disorders.
- Types II and III commonly occur with infections and connective tissue diseases and present as small and medium-sized vessel vasculitis.

EPIDEMIOLOGY

- The incidence of essential mixed cryoglobulinemia in Lugo, Spain for 1988 to 1997 was 4.8 per million. Hepatitis C (HCV) has been associated in 40% of cases of essential mixed cryoglobulinemia. The presence of HLA-DRB1*11 has been associated with patients with HCV who develop cryoglobulinemia.

PATHOPHYSIOLOGY

- Type I cryoglobulinemia results from a pure monoclonal gammopathy.
- Type II cryoglobulinemia is composed of mixed cryoglobulins with a monoclonal component, usually an IgM rheumatoid factor in conjunction with polyclonal gammopathy. Type III consists of polyclonal cryoglobulins.
- Types II and III cryoglobulins are present at lower titers than type I and avidly form immune complexes; thus, as opposed to the thrombotic vasculopathy seen in type I, types II and III cause vasculitis.
- Type II cryoglobulinemia is commonly caused by subacute and chronic infections such as viral hepatitis, HIV, and endocarditis. Hepatitis C is by far the most common cause, and represents most if not all cases previously labeled as essential mixed cryoglobulinemia.
- Autoimmune disorders including connective tissue diseases and neoplasms such as lymphoproliferative and myeloproliferative disorders can also be associated with cryoglobulinemia type II or type III.
- Pathology can show either small or medium-sized vessel vasculitis, or both. The routine histologic features of small or medium-sized vessels affected are identical to those seen in any SVV and MVV. Some dermatopathologists claim that the presence of homogeneous intravascular material is typical for cryoglobulinemic vasculitis. In most instances, those cases are associated with cryoglobulinemia type I, which histologically shows a thrombotic vasculopathy with mild perivascular infiltrates and not a true vasculitis.
- DIF in cryoglobulinemia type II often shows significant granular IgM and C3 in and around small and medium-sized blood vessels.
- Cryoglobulinemia type III has both IgM and IgG along with C3 in and around primarily small vessels. However, in most cases it is almost impossible to make the distinction between cryoglobulinemia types II and III based on IF findings. The complexes frequently consist of monoclonal IgM rheumatoid factor (RF) and polyclonal IgG.
- More than 90% of cases can have decreased C4 and relatively normal C3. 100% have a rheumatoid factor titer greater than 1:320.
- A negative cryoglobulin assay in the absence of RF activity and low C4 virtually excludes cryoglobulin II. This is very important, because, as previously mentioned, false-negative results in testing for cryoglobulins are very common.
- A positive cryoglobulin at low titer, without any clinical signs of a vasculitic syndrome, is common after infections. Therefore a positive cryoglobulin assay in the setting of normal complement levels and in the absence of RF activity usually represents an "innocent bystander" cryoglobulin.
- Type III cryoglobulinemia presents with pure polyclonal gammopathy and low complement, usually both C4 and C3. The high avidity for fixing complement and forming immune complexes at low levels in cryoglobulinemia type II explains why clinical syndromes of type II are far more common than type III.

CLINICAL FEATURES

- Cryoglobulinemia affects both small and medium-sized skin blood vessels. The skin lesions in types II and III are clinically indistinguishable.
- As in all SVV, palpable and nonpalpable purpura and urticarial lesions are the most frequent clinical presentation. The lesions typically occur on the distal lower extremities. The palpable purpura lesions are indistinguishable from those seen in any SVV.
- MVV lesions are not uncommon, and when they are present there is almost always underlying SVV as well. However, SVV lesions can, and often do, present without MVV lesions. The presence of ulcer-ations with urticarial lesions suggests the diagnosis of cryoglobulinemia rather than urticarial vasculitis, since the latter rarely affect medium-sized blood vessels.

Arthralgias and renal, gastrointestinal, and neurologic symptoms are often observed in these patients. The systemic involvement in cryoglobulinemia parallels the extent of the cutaneous eruption due to SVV and the presence of MVV. Virtually all the patients with significant cutaneous MVV lesions, especially those with extensive ulceration, have an associated clinical or subclinical peripheral neuropathy.

DIAGNOSIS AND DIFFERENTIAL

- Schamberg's disease-like pigmented purpuric eruption is a common presentation for the nonpalpable purpuric lesions in cryoglobulinemia.
- Some clinical features helpful in differentiating cryoglobulinemic vasculitis from Schamberg's disease in patients presenting with a pigmented purpuric eruption are outlined in Table 4–3.
- Classic urticarial vasculitis typically favors trunk and proximal extremities. A predilection for the lower extremities helps clinically in the distinction of urticarial cryoglobulinemia from classic urticarial vasculitis.
- Lymphocytic vasculitis (benign hypergammaglobulinemic purpura of Waldenström), can also present with Schamberg's-like eruption clinically, thus indistinguishable from the lesions in cryoglobulinemia.
- Platelet disorders typically present with dependent nonpalpable purpura.
- Pigmented purpura-like mycosis fungoides may mimic cryoglobulinemia

TREATMENT

- Although on clinical and immunopathologic grounds cryoglobulinemia types II and III are indistinguishable, in terms of therapy, making the distinction is crucial. This is because the therapy should be directed toward both the underlying condition and treatment of the vasculitis.

TABLE 4–3 Clinical Features that Favor Cryoglobulinemia Vasculitis over Schamberg's Disease in Patients Presenting With a Pigmented Purpura Eruption

Extensive pigmented purpuric eruption with lesions above waistline
Pigmented purpuric eruption with lesions at different stages of evolution
Pigmented purpuric eruption with ulcerative lesions
Pigmented purpuric eruption with lesions involving the soles of the feet
Pigmented purpuric eruption associated with constitutional symptoms

- One common situation in which this is illustrated is in the setting of hepatitis C-induced cryoglobulinemia. In the presence of extensive vasculitis and high titers of cryoglobulins, antiviral treatment with interferon should be initiated cautiously, as this may promote massive release and precipitation of immune complexes and rapid exacerbation of cutaneous vasculitis and renal failure.
- These patients should be treated with corticosteroids and immunosuppressive medications with low incidence of liver toxicity, such as mycophenolate mofetil or alkylating agents, for at least 3 to 6 months before starting interferon therapy. The vasculitis therapy is not different from other regimens that aim to reduce immunoglobulin and immune complexes.
- One of the main differences in the management between cryoglobulinemia types II and III is the effectiveness of plasmapheresis in removing the IgM RF in type II.
- IgM RF in type II as well as in rheumatoid vasculitis is the main pathogenetic immunoglobulin and is largely present in the intravascular compartment. Thus few plasma exchanges are usually effective. Immunosuppressants (prednisone and cyclophosphamide) are necessary to prevent the rebound effect in the synthesis of IgM.
- Because the cryoglobulins in type III are polyclonal and are located both intravascularly and extravascularly (in the tissues), the extravascular component is not affected by plasmapheresis. Therefore, plasmapheresis in cryoglobulinemia type III is less effective and requires more plasma exchanges to achieve a significant effect.

REFERENCES

Karlsberg PL, Lee WM, Casey DL, et al. Cutaneous vasculitis and rheumatoid factor positivity as presenting signs of hepatitis C virus-induced mixed cryoglobulinemia. *Arch Dermatol.* 1995;131:1119.

Mendez P, Saeian K, Reddy KR, et al. Hepatitis C, cryoglobulinemia, and cutaneous vasculitis associated with unusual and serious manifestations. *Am J Gastroenterol.* 2001;96: 2489.

Pawlotsky JM, Dhumeaux D, Bagot M. Hepatitis C virus in dermatology. A review. *Arch Dermatol.* 1995;131:1185.

Scelsa SN, Herskovitz S, Reichler B. Treatment of mononeuropathy multiplex in hepatitis C virus and cryoglobulinemia. *Muscle Nerve.* 1998;21:1526.

CONNECTIVE TISSUE DISEASE-ASSOCIATED VASCULITIS

- Several vasculitic syndromes can occur in the setting of connective tissue disease (CTD).

- CTD patients are more susceptible to infections and drug exposure and as a result, have higher risks of developing either CLA or IgA-mediated vasculitis.
- Also, cryoglobulinemia types II and III can be associated with CTDs.
- However, there are three vasculitic syndromes that are primarily related to CTD: CTD-associated vasculitis, HUVS, and lymphocytic vasculitis (LV).

EPIDEMIOLOGY

- The annual incidence of vasculitis in SLE in Lugo, Spain between 1988 and 1997 was 5.3 per million, and was four times more prevalent in women than in men. In one study of 75 patients with dermatomyositis/polymyositis in Singapore, 18.7% exhibited cutaneous vasculitis.

PATHOPHYSIOLOGY

- Histologically CTD-associated vasculitis shows SVV and MVV indistinguishable from any SVV and/or MVV. High titers of ANA and low complement are relatively constant features in CTD associated vasculitis.
- Several combinations of ANA are commonly seen in these patients. The most common ANA combinations present are positive dsDNA and RNP, positive RNP and Ro, or positive Sm and RNP.
- Any combination of the dsDNA, Sm, and RNP increases the patient's risk of developing vasculitis. LV is commonly associated with Anti-Ro, RF, polyclonal gammopathy, and cryoglobulins.
- LV, although rare, is more commonly seen in SS and SLE; however it can occur in association with other CTDs.
  - LV is also known as benign hypergammaglobulinemic purpura of Waldenström (BHP). Most experts believe that both LV and BHP of Waldenström are cryoglobulinemia type III associated with CTDs.
  - DIF, as opposed to cryoglobulinemia, shows IgG as the predominant immunoglobulin in and around small and medium-sized vessels. C3 is usually very strongly deposited. A positive ANA is very commonly present.
  - Hypocomplementemia is found in virtually all of these patients.
  - Lymphocytic vasculitis is often misdiagnosed. The most frequent false-positive diagnosis is when a specimen of leukocytoclastic vasculitis is taken from an old lesion. On the other hand, the most common false-negative diagnosis is pigmented purpura.
  - Less than 50% of the specimens show granular IgG, IgM, and C3 in the vessels. Thus, a clinical

immunopathologic correlation is required for the diagnosis of this form of vasculitis.

CLINICAL FEATURES

- CTD-associated vasculitis is most commonly seen in SLE, but can be seen in other connective tissue diseases, such as dermatomyositis, systemic sclerosis, mixed connective tissue disease, and Sjögren's syndrome. This typically presents in patients with advanced and overt disease and with internal organ involvement.
- CTD-associated vasculitis commonly presents as SVV, with purpuric lesions of the lower extremities.
- MVV lesions (nodules, ulcers, livedo reticularis, and digital infarcts) are also common. Most patients with MVV lesions also have clinical evidence of SVV.
- However, unlike cryoglobulinemia, several cases of CTD may present with pure MVV indistinguishable from PAN. Otherwise the lesions are clinically indistinguishable from cryoglobulinemia.
- Virtually all of these patients have systemic involvement. Renal failure and glomerulonephritis are the most common problems. Also, central and peripheral nervous system, gastrointestinal, and cardiac involvement are not uncommon.
- Lymphocytic vasculitis (LV) is rare. The most common clinical presentation of LV is self-limited nonpalpable purpura Schamberg's-like eruption (Table 4–3). Peripheral and central nervous system involvement is not uncommon in these patients, especially those with Sjögren's syndrome.

DIAGNOSIS AND DIFFERENTIAL

- The differential for CTD is other forms of small vessel vasculitis. The differential for lymphocytic vasculitis includes late or resolving stage of leukocytoclastic vasculitis, purpuric mycosis fungoides, angiocentric lymphoma, intravascular lymphoma (angiotropic lymphoma), pityriasis lichenoides, and lymphomatoid papulosis.

TREATMENT

- Usually a combination of corticosteroids, with high doses of antimetabolites or more commonly alkylating agents and even plasmapheresis, is necessary to control the progression of CTD-associated vasculitis.
- In CTD-associated vasculitis, the presence of high titers of circulating immunocomplexes, and a positive

ANA, are the rule. Thus, aggressive treatment of the underlying CTD is mandatory, since this complication in CTDs is often associated with an ominous prognosis.

- LV is typically very responsive to a short course of immunosuppressive therapy.

REFERENCE

Tsokos M, Lazarou SA, Moutsopoulos HM. Vasculitis in primary Sjögren's syndrome. Histologic classification and clinical presentation. *Am J Clin Pathol.* 1987;88:26.

RHEUMATOID VASCULITIS

- This variant is a rare but severe complication in patients with advanced, usually otherwise quiescent seropositive RA.

EPIDEMIOLOGY

- In Norwich, England the incidence was 12.5 per million between 1988 and 1994. In Lugo, Spain the average annual incidence was 6.4 per million.

PATHOPHYSIOLOGY

- Histologically RV lesions are indistinguishable from SVV and/or MVV.
- DIF is indistinguishable from cryoglobulinemia type II, with heavy granular IgM and variable degrees of C3 in small and medium-sized vessels. A high titer of RF, often with low complement levels of both C3 and C4, is characteristic of RV. This often helps in distinguishing RV from cryoglobulinemia II, since in both RF is elevated and even in RA patients with a higher titer of RF, a low titer of cryoglobulinemia type II antibodies is not uncommon.
- Thorough evaluation is mandatory to exclude other causes of MVV, including hepatitis C, hepatitis B, HIV, and lymphomas in RA patients with cryoglobulins. The RF in RV as a rule is present at very high titers (>1: 320).
- The most common RF is IgM; however, in exceptional cases, IgG RF is encountered. A typical RV syndrome in the setting of a negative standard RF serology (nephelometry or latex agglutination), often directed to detect IgM RF, should prompt to the exclusion of IgG RF by other methods such as ELISA.

CLINICAL FEATURES

- Rheumatoid vasculitis (RV) can affect all sized vessels from small to the largest. This serious vasculitis typically complicates end-stage, seropositive RA patients whose arthritis is quiescent.
- The most common presentation is purpura. Isolated fluctuating periungual splinter hemorrhages, known as Bywater's lesions, are caused by digital SVV, and are not uncommon.
- Concomitant MVV is present in 30% of cases. Consequently, clinical manifestations can include purpura, with variable degrees of ulcerations, livedo reticularis, digital infarcts, or cutaneous nodules.
- MVV in RV often presents as deep geographic ulcers at the malleoli. These patients frequently have accompanying mononeuritis multiplex.

TREATMENT

- The aim of the therapy is to reduce IgM RF immunocomplexes through using combinations of corticosteroids with antimetabolites and or alkylating agents.
- Methotrexate is effective for the synovitis and more T-cell mediated symptoms in RA, but is not effective in RV.
- Because of the IgM RF, plasmapheresis, in combination with steroids and alkylating agents as in cryoglobulinemia type II, is a good choice in patients with life-threatening disease.
- Bywaters lesions alone do not necessitate aggressive systemic therapy.
- Generally, RV is extremely difficult to treat, and these patients have a poor prognosis with an associated high mortality.

REFERENCES

Nousari HC, Kimyai-Asadi A, Stebbing J, Stone JH. Purple toes in a patient with end-stage rheumatoid arthritis. *Arch Dermatol.* 1999;135:648.

Schneider HA, Yonker RA, Katz P, et al. Rheumatoid vasculitis: experience with 13 patients and review of the literature. *Semin Arthritis Rheum.* 1985;14:280.

Winkelstein A, Starz TW, Agarwal A. Efficacy of combined therapy with plasmapheresis and immunosuppressants in rheumatoid vasculitis. *J Rheumatol.* 1984;11:162.

ANCA-ASSOCIATED VASCULITIS

- ANCAs are antineutrophilic cytoplasmic antibodies. These antibodies are found in numerous autoimmune disorders. However, they have become the serologic hallmark for three vasculitic syndromes: Wegener's granulomatosis (WG), microscopic polyangiitis (MPA), and Churg–Strauss syndrome (CSS).

- WG is a vasculitis (SVV and/or MVV) associated with significant systemic involvement, including upper and lower respiratory tracts, kidneys, and nervous system. Virtually all of these patients are C-ANCA positive.
- MPA is a SVV, separated from the PAN group, often associated with systemic involvement. MPA is the most common vasculitis syndrome causing pulmonary-renal syndrome. Most, if not all, of these patients are P-ANCA positive.
- CSS is virtually indistinguishable from WG, with the exception of significant eosinophilia in both tissue and peripheral blood, higher prevalence of P-ANCA, and atopy (asthma, allergic rhinitis).

EPIDEMIOLOGY

- The overall annual incidence of the ANCA-mediated (pauci-immune) vasculitides in Norwich, England between 1988 and 1997 was 19.8 per million. These disorders are more common in men (23.5 per million) than in women (16.4 per million).
- The incidence of MPA ranges from a low of 0.5 per million from 1980 to 1986 in Leicester, England to a high of 24 per million in Kuwait from 1993 to 1996.
- The incidence of Wegener's granulomatosis has been reported to range from 0.5 per million to 15 per million. The only incidence data from the United States is from Olmsted County, Minnesota for 1976 to 1979, which was 0.7 per million.
- The incidence of Churg–Strauss syndrome was 4.0 per million from Olmsted County, Minnesota for 1976 to 1979, 2.7 per million in Norwich, England from 1988 to 1997, and 1.1 per million in Lugo, Spain from 1988 to 1997.

PATHOPHYSIOLOGY

- There are two histologic patterns in ANCA-mediated vasculitides: medium and/or small-sized vessel vasculitis and palisaded neutrophilic and granulomatous dermatitis (cutaneous necrotizing extravascular granulomas, Churg–Strauss granuloma).
- It is noteworthy that cutaneous necrotizing extravascular granulomas and Churg–Strauss granuloma are misnomers, since very frequently the blood vessels in the infiltrates show clear evidence of vasculitis and can be found in vasculitides other than CSS. Therefore, we prefer the term palisaded neutrophilic and granulomatous dermatitis (PNGD).

- Erythema nodosum-like nodules, geographic deep ulcers, livedo reticularis and digital infarcts represent MVV, whereas the palpable and nonpalpable purpuric lesions represent SVV histologically.
- In CSS the eosinophilic infiltrate in the vasculitic lesion or in palisaded neutrophilic and granulomatous dermatitis is striking, usually accounting for more than 60% of the inflammatory cells in the infiltrates.
- DIF is positive in 80% of the lesions and is often IgG and IgM without significant C3.
- IF evaluation of ANCA is a good screening test, since this technique will determine the C (cytoplasmic) or P (perinuclear) pattern. Nevertheless, experience is required in performing and interpreting the results.
- Nearly all patients with WG and MPA will be positive for C-ANCA and P-ANCA respectively, especially those with significant systemic involvement. On the other hand, in CSS only 60% will be positive for P-ANCA. Some serologic overlap results are not uncommon.
- C-ANCA is represented by only one antigen, proteinase-3. Thus, an ELISA for proteinase-3 is definitely more sensitive and even more specific.
- In contrast, since several antigens are responsible for the P-ANCA pattern including myeloperoxidase and elastase, as well as other antigens, IF remains as the main tool for the diagnosis of P-ANCA vasculitides.

CLINICAL FEATURES

- All cases with WG, MPA, and CSS will develop skin disease in the setting of systemic involvement. The clinical features of WG and CSS are those of SVV and/or MVV.
- SVV lesions including palpable purpura are the most common.
- Interestingly, some of the CSS patients report pruritus as a preceding symptom of SVV purpuric lesions. It is thought that this is due to the eosinophilic infiltration.
- Any of the lesions of MVV including nodules, ulcers, livedo reticularis, or digital infarcts can be observed in WG or CSS, with or without SVV lesions.
- Miscellaneous presentations in WG and CSS are papules and nodules often ulcero-necrotic on extensor surfaces, and ulcers with violaceous overhanging borders that mimic pyoderma gangrenosum.
- Essential or primary cutaneous disease in these three syndromes is extremely rare. However, some cases of WG may present with cutaneous disease, the so-called "pyoderma maligna," often in preauricular areas and dorsa of the hands.
- These lesions clinically mimic pyoderma gangrenosum and may be associated with just limited systemic disease including ocular, ear, and/or upper respiratory tract.

- Another unusual presentation of WG is so-called strawberry-like gingivitis.
- Cutaneous lesions in MPA are uncommon, and when present, are primarily manifested by purpuric lesions of SVV.

TREATMENT

- The cutaneous involvement of ANCA-mediated vasculitides virtually always occurs in the setting of overt or smoldering systemic disease. The treatment of the primary vasculitis will treat the cutaneous disease. In general, a combination of corticosteroids at high doses, associated with antimetabolites or alkylating agents, is the standard management.

REFERENCES

Daoud MS, Gibson LE, DeRemee RA, et al. Cutaneous Wegener's granulomatosis: Clinical, histopathologic, and immunopathologic features of thirty patients. *J Am Acad Dermatol*. 1994;31:605.

Gibson LE, Daoud MS, Muller SA, Perry HO. Malignant pyodermas revisited. *Mayo Clin Proc*. 1997;72:734.

Guillevin L, Cohen P, Gayraud M, et al. Churg–Strauss syndrome. Clinical study and long-term follow-up of 96 patients. *Medicine* (Baltimore). 1999;78:26.

Lauque D, Cadranel J, Lazor R, et al. Microscopic polyangiitis with alveolar hemorrhage. A study of 29 cases and review of the literature. Groupe d'études et de recherché sur les maladies "orphelines" pulmonaires (GERM"O"P). *Medicine* (Baltimore). 2000;79:222.

Mangold MC, Callen JP. Cutaneous leukocytoclastic vasculitis associated with active Wegener's granulomatosis. *J Am Acad Dermatol*. 1992;26:579.

Raustia AM, Autio-Harmainen HI, Knuuttila ML, Raustia JM. Ultrastructural findings and clinical follow-up of "strawberry gums" in Wegener's granulomatosis. *J Oral Pathol*. 1985;14:581.

PURE MEDIUM-SIZED VESSEL VASCULITIS

POLYARTERITIS NODOSA

- Polyarteritis nodosa (PAN), the prototype of a pure MVV, often presents as a systemic illness with multiorgan involvement. PAN is a diagnosis of exclusion.

EPIDEMIOLOGY

- The annual incidence of polyarteritis nodosa ranges from a low of 2.0 per million in Michigan from 1957 to 1971 to a high of 77.0 per million in Alaska from 1974 to 1985.

PATHOPHYSIOLOGY

- The diagnostic yield for MVV in PAN is the following: nodules (90 to 100%), ulcer (50 to 80%), livedo reticularis (0 to 20%), and digital infarcts (0 to 5%).
- Papulonecrotic lesions present on extensor surfaces show PNGD histologically.
- Nerve conduction studies with nerve and muscle biopsies or angiogram are useful diagnostic tools for MVV in patients in whom definitive histologic diagnosis cannot be achieved by skin biopsies.
- DIF in 60% of biopsies will show granular IgM in medium-sized vessel and weak C3 deposition.
- Serologic testing may but will not always show an elevated ESR with hypocomplementemia. ANCA, ANA, and RF are typically negative, but may be present at insignificant titers.
- Many patients have antibodies against hepatitis B surface antigens.

CLINICAL FEATURES

- Since PAN is a pure MVV, the clinical presentation encompasses nodules, deep ulcers, livedo reticularis, and digital infarcts, and less frequently papulonecrotic lesions on extensor surfaces.
- The most common presentation is with painful cutaneous nodules and ulcerations with a predilection for the malleoli. These ulcerations heal with stellate atrophic ivory-colored scars or alternatively with hyperpigmentation.
- Ulcerations are often accompanied by neuropathic pain resulting from involvement of the vasa nervorum.
- Focal synovitis and subsequent arthralgias may be present in the joints close to areas of cutaneous involvement. This is particularly common in the ankle joint. This is in contradistinction to erythema nodosum, in which generalized arthralgias may be present.
- Systemic disease is present in almost all of the patients with extensive nodulo-ulcerative disease.

DIAGNOSIS AND DIFFERENTIAL

- Differential diagnosis for nodular lesions includes erythema nodosum, nodular vasculitis, and erythema induratum. The latter two are most likely variants of PAN with a prominent component of panniculitis.
- Infectious causes of ulceration, pyoderma gangrenosum, calciphylaxis, lymphomas, and other causes of

medium-sized vessel vasculitis must be included in the differential.

TREATMENT

- Corticosteroids alone may be sufficient for mild nodular disease.
- Ulcerative disease without significant systemic involvement may respond to prednisone and azathioprine.
- Severe cutaneous disease with digital infarcts and systemic disease should be treated with corticosteroids and alkylating agents.
- Plasmapheresis is not effective in PAN since IgM immune complexes and RF do not play a prominent role in this disease, in contrast to the high titers of these seen in RV and cryoglobulinemia.
- With adequate treatment, patients with purely cutaneous PAN do well.
- Even patients with nodules limited to the ankles require close and long-term follow-up for progression to systemic disease.
- Without adequate treatment many will develop signs and symptoms of peripheral neuropathy.

TABLE 4–4   Miscellaneous Causes of Vasculitis

Infectious (bacterial endocarditis, *Rickettsia, Zygomycetes*, CMV)
Behçet's disease
Kawasaki's disease
Erythema elevatum diutinum
Bowel-associated dermatosis arthritis

Mycobacterial-associated vasculitides (erythema nodosum leprosum and erythema induratum of Bazin)

Paraneoplastic
Buerger's disease

REFERENCES

Daoud MS, Hutton KP, Gibson LE. Cutaneous periarteritis nodosa: A clinicopathological study of 79 cases. *Br J Dermatol.* 1997;136:706.

Kumar L, Thapa BR, Sarkar B, et al. Benign cutaneous polyarteritis nodosa in children below 10 years of age—a clinical experience. *Ann Rheum Dis.* 1995;54:134.

Maillard H, Szczesniak S, Martin L, et al. Cutaneous periarteritis nodosa: Diagnostic and therapeutic aspects of 9 cases. *Ann Dermatol Venereol.* 1999;126:125.

Siberry GK, Cohen BA, Johnson B. Cutaneous polyarteritis nodosa. Reports of two cases in children and review of the literature. *Arch Dermatol.* 1994;130:884.

MISCELLANEOUS FORMS OF VASCULITIS

- Table 4–4 summarizes miscellaneous causes of vasculitis. Figures 4–1 and 4–2 illustrate practical diagnostic algorithms for SVV and MVV, respectively. A comprehensive and accurate clinical and immunopathologic correlation is required for a correct diagnosis and classification of cutaneous vasculitides.

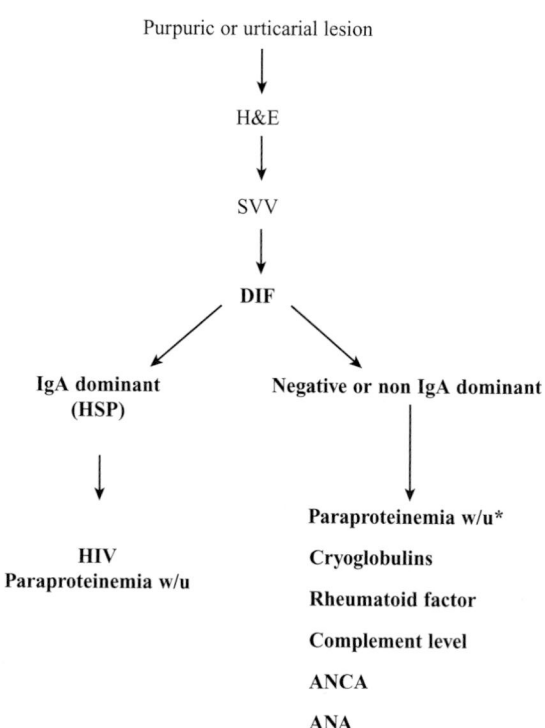

*Paraproteinemia work-up includes serum protein electrophoresis, serum protein immunofixation, urine protein immunofixation, total immunoglobulins

FIGURE 4–1. Diagnostic algorithm in cutaneous SVV.

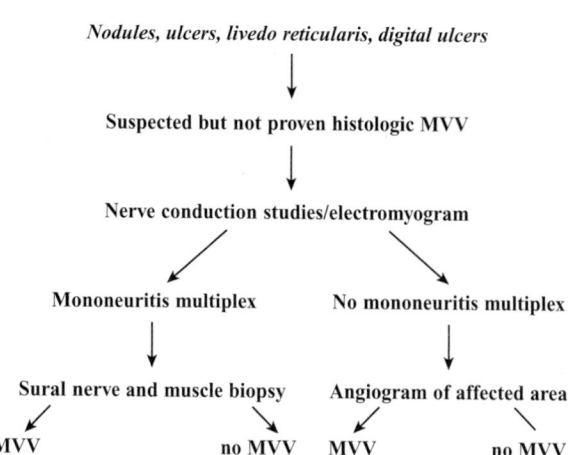

FIGURE 4–2. Diagnostic algorithm in cutaneous MVV.

5 PILOSEBACEOUS AND SWEAT GLAND DISORDERS

Marianne N. O'Donoghue

ACNE

EPIDEMIOLOGY

- Acne vulgaris is common.
- Can be seen at birth, but most often develops at puberty.

PATHOPHYSIOLOGY

- Acne vulgaris results from the obstruction of the sebaceous follicles located primarily on the face, back, and chest. There is excessive production of sebum and excessive numbers of desquamated epithelial cells from the walls of the sebaceous follicles. "The obstruction causes the formation of a microcomedo that may evolve into either a comedo or an inflammatory lesion. A resident anaerobic organism, *Propionibacterium acnes,* proliferates in the environment created by the mixture of excessive sebum and follicular cells and produces chemotactic factors and produces chemotactic factors and proinflammatory mediators that may lead to inflammation." In summary, the four factors causing acne are (1) follicular keratinization, (2) excessive sebum, (3) bacterial proliferation, and (4) inflammation.

FOLLICULAR KERATINIZATION
- The origin of acne is in the sebaceous follicle. Normally the sebaceous follicle contains keratinous material, which is loosely organized. At the lowermost part of the follicle, the layer is very thin.
- In acne, the follicular epithelium becomes thicker (hyperkeratotic) with increased adhesion of the keratin instead of loose shedding. This increased adherence is the beginning of a microcomedone.

SEBUM PRODUCTION
- Acne patients have been demonstrated to possess increased sebum production, and the areas that have acne are areas where there are more sebaceous glands (face, back, chest).

- Androgens stimulate sebum production, which increases at puberty correlating with acne onset. The sebum produced has less linoleic acid, and this linoleic acid reduction causes an increased desquamation of follicular epithelial cells, causing a "traffic jam" at the exit of the follicles.
- The success of many therapeutic agents (isotretinoin, estrogens, and anti-androgens) is based on the decrease of sebum production.

BACTERIAL PROLIFERATION
- *Propionibacterium acnes* is an anaerobic diphtheroid that contains a lipase, which splits triglycerides into glycerol and comedogenic free fatty acids. Glycerol is a major nutrient for *P. acnes.*
- Other bacteria are present in the sebaceous follicle and include *Staphylococcal epidermidis* and *Pityrosporum ovale.* Control of these bacteria helps control the acne.

INFLAMMATION
- Inflammation may be caused by an overly vigorous immune response to *P. acnes,* but it also may be caused as a reaction to the rupture of the intact comedones.
- Neutrophils and lymphocytes are present in acne lesions, although reactive oxygen species, collagenase, and other elements are also responsible for the chronic inflammation.
- Antibacterial agents with inflammatory properties such as tetracyclines and erythromycin have a dual beneficial action in acne by inhibiting the production of *P. acnes* chemotactic factor, neutrophil migration, reactive oxygen species, and collagenase levels.

CLINICAL FEATURES

- Acne lesions consist of closed and open comedones (noninflammatory lesions), papules, pustules, and nodules. These latter lesions are erythematous, may be tender, and may leave marks of prolonged discoloration or even scarring.
- The distribution of acne is most commonly on the face, chest, and back. There may also be involvement of the neck and upper arms.

DIAGNOSIS AND DIFFERENTIAL

- For most patients the diagnosis is fairly straight-forward. Exceptions to this are women who may have hirsutism, abnormal menses, or excessive weight gain. These patients may need a further work-up for endocrine abnormalities, such as Stein–Levenson syndrome.
- There is also a form of newborn acne because of the stimulation of the baby's sebaceous glands by the mother's hormones. This usually resolves spontaneously without need of treatment.

TREATMENT

- Therapy can be divided into topical and systemic. Most physicians would probably combine the two.

TOPICAL THERAPY

- Comedolytic agents: For patients with noninflammatory acne, retinoids such as tretinoin and adapalene are the treatments of choice. They slow the desquamative process of follicular epithelium in sebaceous follicles. They also increase penetration of other topical medications.
- Other excellent products for keratolytics are the sulfur and sodium sulfacetamide topical medications. There may be less irritating to patients with sensitive skin. Salicylic acid, alpha-hydroxy acids, and azelaic acids are also helpful.
- Antibacterial agents: Benzoyl peroxide products are lipophilic (accumulate in the sebaceous gland), reduce the population of *P. acnes* by generating reactive oxygen species in the sebaceous follicle, and decrease the free fatty acid content. These products are available in 2.5 to 10% concentration, and are particularly helpful in papular, pustular, and nodular acne. They may be drying, and they occasionally cause contact dermatitis.
- Topical clindamycin and erythromycin act by decreasing the population of *P. acnes* but also have their anti-inflammatory characteristics.
- A combination of benzoyl peroxide and either clindamycin or erythromycin can synergize and work better than either ingredient alone.

SYSTEMIC THERAPY

ORAL ANTIBIOTICS
- Tetracycline: Tetracycline is lipophilic, anti-inflammatory, and antibacterial. In doses from 250 mg daily to 500 mg b.i.d., this medication is safe and inexpensive.
- Tetracycline cannot be used in children before the second teeth are set, and may not be used in pregnant women. Rarely, a secondary *Candida albicans* vaginitis can occur. There is a risk of mild photosensitivity.
- Most patients with inflammatory acne require treatment orally during the fall and winter seasons.
- Erythromycin: Erythromycin is lipophilic, anti-inflammatory, and antibacterial. The dose ranges from 250 to 1000 mg per day in divided doses.
- Erythromycin is safe for children because it does not affect the dentition. It is also inexpensive and has no photosensitivity. There may be greater GI toxicity than with tetracycline.
- Minocycline: Minocycline has the same advantages as tetracycline. In addition it is more easily absorbed from the GI tract, is more lipophilic, can be taken with food, and does not produce photosensitivity.
- The dose for minocycline ranges from 50 mg/d to 100 mg b.i.d. and it is one of the most effective medications for nodular-cystic acne.
- The major disadvantage of minocycline is that it can cause vertigo. In addition, a very small number of patients who have been taking 100 mg b.i.d. for an extended period can develop a lupus-like syndrome as well as hepatitis.
- Doxycyline: Doxycline is similar to minocycline in that it has superior absorption from the GI tract, is very lipophilic, can be taken with food, and is very effective in moderately severe acne.
- The major drawback of doxycyline is that there is marked photosensitivity while taking this drug. The dose is 50 mg/d to 100 mg b.i.d. Both minocycline and doxycycline are relatively expensive.

RETINOIDS
- For patients who have failed all other medical therapy with the above regimens and who have severe papulonodular acne, isotretinoin has been an excellent medication.
- Because of the severe birth defects caused while taking this medication, it is currently being monitored very closely. Pregnancy tests before and during treatments, two methods of birth control, and careful dispensing of the medication for 4 weeks at a time are necessary.
- The advantages of this medication are that it is anti-inflammatory, decreases the size of the sebaceous glands, and decreases sebum production, so *P. acnes* cannot thrive; causes a prolonged remission of acne (especially if the dose is 1 mg/kg for 20 weeks); and appears to decrease scarring.
- Side effects are common and include dryness of the mucous membranes, arthralgias, stiffness, tendonitis,

increased serum lipids, increased liver enzymes (requiring the absence of alcohol during therapy), rare headaches and depression, and cost.

- Patients need to be monitored with a monthly CBC and comprehensive chemistry tests, including liver function studies, triglyceride and cholesterol levels, and pregnancy tests in women.

HORMONES

- In women who have mild hirsutism, a male escutcheon, abnormal menses, and distribution of the acne lesions on the lower face, jaw line, and chin, birth control pills may be helpful. If these problems are severe, testing of the patient's dehydroepiandrosterone and free testosterone levels may be needed.

REFERENCES

Cunliffe WJ. Acne. In: *Year Book*, 1989:178.

Harris HH, Downing DT, Stewart ME, Strauss JS. Sustainable rates of sebum secretion of acne patients and matched normal control subjects. *J Am Acad Dermatol.* 1983;8:200.

Karvonen SL. Acne fulminans. *J Am Acad Dermatol.* 1993;28:572.

Leyden JJ. Therapy for acne vulgaris. *N Engl J Med.* 1997;336:16:1156.

Lookingbill DP, Chalke DK, Lindholm JS, et al. Treatment of acne with a combination clindamycin/benzoyl peroxide gel compared with clindamycin gel, benzoyl peroxide gel, and vehicle gel. Combined results of two double-blind investigations. *J Am Acad Dermatol.* 1997;37:590.

Webster GF. Inflammation in acne vulgaris. *J Am Acad Dermatol.* 1995;33:247.

OTHER ACNE SYNDROMES

ACNE CONGLOBATA

- This highly inflammatory acne usually starts in adult life. It consists of comedones, nodules, abscesses, and draining sinus tracts.
- It may be associated with hidradenitis suppurtiva and folliculitis decalvans. The lesions themselves may scar and persist for many years.
- Isotretinoin has been helpful in the management of these patients.

ACNE FULMINANS

- This is a form of acne that occurs acutely in teenage boys. The lesions are explosive with inflammatory nodules and cysts especially on the face and the back.
- Fever and leukocytosis are common. Often the only therapy that will stop this progression is systemic steroids.
- Dapsone in relatively high doses (100 to 300 mg/d) has also been used.

DIAGNOSIS AND DIFFERENTIAL

- The mixture of papules, pustules, comedones, and cysts together with the age and sex of the patient help with the differential. Folliculitis, rosacea, and other acneiform eruptions due to drugs or environment must be excluded.

ROSACEA

EPIDEMIOLOGY

- Common disorder of high prevalence in people of Celtic or Northern European Heritage, rare in dark-skinned individuals.

PATHOPHYSIOLOGY

- Rosacea is an erythematous disorder that occurs primarily on the central face, often as the result of too much sun as a child and oily skin as an adult.
- Vasomotor lability secondary to caffeine, heat, and highly spiced foods may contribute to this problem.
- It may be associated with excessive seborrhea, seborrheic dermatitis, and perioral dermatitis. There is also an inflammatory reaction from the breakdown products of sebum to free fatty acids.
- *Demodex folliculorum* mites as well as *Propionibacterium acnes* may influence the severity of rosacea.
- Dyspepsia with gastric hypochlorhydria and infestation with the microaerophilic gram-negative bacterium *helicobacter pylori* has also been associated with this condition. This association is not universally accepted. There is improvement of rosacea in the patients who have this bacteria successfully treated.

CLINICAL FEATURES

- Rosacea consists of diffuse redness, papules, and telangiectasias on the central face. The nose and cheeks

are most commonly affected. Occasionally eyelids and the conjunctivae may also be involved.
• In some long-standing rosacea patients, especially men, a thickness of the skin on the nose may result in a bulbous, greasy, hypertrophic skin called rhynophyma.

TREATMENT

• Avoiding stimulants that cause facial erythema, such as sunburn, spicy foods, hot drinks, and alcohol, can be very effective in controlling rosacea.
• Topical therapy: Sulfur and sodium sulfacetamide cleansers and lotions decrease bacteria and reduce erythema and oiliness. These products rarely cross-react with patients who are allergic to systemic sulfur medication. They are usually inexpensive if generic products are used.
• Topical metronidazole gels, lotions, and creams have been useful to decrease the Demodex mite. Once a day application of these products appears to be sufficient to improve the erythema and pustules.
• If there is an element of seborrheic dermatitis of the face, sudsing with a zinc pyrithione or a ketoconazole shampoo may be effective.
• Oral antibiotics such as tetracycline, minocycline, or doxycycline may be required to control severe rosacea. The doses needed appear to be less than that required for acne vulgaris.
• Some tinted sulfur preparations or green-tinted sunblocks may be used to camouflage the violaceous or red appearance of the nose and cheeks. If rhynophyma develops, cosmetic surgery with lasers, electrocautery, or cold steel blade can be very effective.

DIAGNOSIS AND DIFFERENTIAL

• Rosacea must be distinguished from acne vulgaris, perioral dermatitis, seborrheic dermatitis, and lupus miliaris disseminatus faciei. The use of topical steroids on the face can also contribute to a clinical appearance of rosacea. Classical presentation of centro facial papules, pustules, vivid erythema, telangiectasias, and flushing, without comedones should be very convincing of this diagnosis.

REFERENCES

Dahl MV, Jarratt M, Kaplan D, et al. Once-daily topical metronidazole cream formulations in the treatment of the papules and pustules of rosacea. *J Am Acad Dermatol.* 2001; 45:723.

Serap U, Ozbakir O, Turasan H, Cengiz U. *Helicobacter pylori* eradication treatment reduces severity of rosacea. *J Am Acad Dermatol.* 1999;40:433.

HIDRADENITIS SUPPURATIVA (HS)

EPIDEMIOLOGY

• HS occurs in both sexes but more common in women (up to 4% of women).
• Rare before puberty.

CLINICAL FEATURES

• This disease is acne but of the apocrine glands.
• It consists of multiple nodules, abscesses, draining sinuses, undermining cysts, and fistulas. They involve the axillae, groins, perirectal skin, and occasionally the suprapubic and submammary areas.
• Related diseases are dissecting cellulitis of the scalp, and a severe type of acne called acne conglobata.
• This disease lasts for many years and needs constant therapy.
• A helpful sign to distinguish between furunculosis and hidradenitis is the presence of comedones in hidradenitis.
• The pustules and nodules may rupture and cause dissecting tunnels between the lesions. Incision and drainage of these lesions should be discouraged, because this contributes to more tunneling.
• The usual age of patients is between 20 and 40 years, but it can occur as young as puberty and into old age.
• Women have more disease in the axillae, while men have more involvement in the groin and perianal area. Women will often suffer flares during their menstrual periods and they often improve after menopause.
• Squamous cell carcinoma can occur secondary to the chronic inflammation. This complication most commonly occurs in the anogenital region and may be related to infection with the human papillomavirus.

TREATMENT

• Treatment consists of broad-spectrum antibiotics such as tetracycline, minocycline, and doxycline. These antibiotics are used for their antibacterial and anti-inflammatory characteristics as outlined in the acne section earlier in the chapter. Topical clindamycin in mild cases has proved to be as effective as oral tetracycline.

- Incision and drainage of the cystic lesions should be avoided because it may contribute to the greater formation of tunneling and fistulas.
- Isotretinoin has been used with effectiveness in hidradenitis suppurativa.
- The definitive treatment of choice is to surgically excise the affected skin that contains these glands.
- The best results were obtained when wide surgical excision was performed. This type of surgery, however, is often complicated and can produce an extensive defect.

DIAGNOSIS AND DIFFERENTIAL

- Patients with one abscess may have a furuncle. Multiple abscesses in the apocrine area are most likely hidradenitis suppurativa. Histopathology reveals follicular plugging and poral occlusion. Fibrosis is often seen in the dermis and may extend into the subcutaneous tissue. Folliculitis and perifolliculitis are common. Abscesses, neutrophils, lymphocytes, plasma cells, and eosinophils are seen.

REFERENCES

Boer J, vanTenmert MJP. Long-term results of isotretinoin in the treatment of 68 patients with hidradenitis suppurativa. *J Am Acad Dermatol.* 1999;40:73.

Cosman BC, O'Grady TC, Pekarske S. Verrucous carcinoma arising in hidradenitis suppurativa. *Int J Colorectal Dis.* 2000;15:342.

Daoud MS, Dicken CH. Hidradenitis suppurativa. In: Freedberg IM, Eisen AZ, Wolff K, et al., eds. *Fitzpatrick's Dermatology in General Medicine,* ed 5. New York:McGraw-Hill, 1999:815.

Jemef GB, Wendelboe P. Topical clindamycin versus systemic tetracycline in the treatment of hidradenitis suppurativa. *J Am Acad Dermatol.* 1998;39:971.

Rompel R, Petres J. Long-term results of wide surgical excision in 106 patients with hidradenitis suppurativa. *Dermatol Surg.* 2000;26:638.

MILIARIA

PATHOPHYSIOLOGY/CLINICAL FEATURES

- Miliaria or heat rash is the obstruction of the sweat ducts. Most commonly this disease occurs because of excess sweating due to heat and high humidity.

- The three types of miliaria depending upon the level of obstruction of the sweat duct are miliaria crystallina, miliaria rubra, and miliaria profunda.
- Miliaria crystallina occurs when the obstruction is in the subcorneal layer with easily ruptured vesicles. There is no erythema present. This condition occurs most frequently when the patient has a high fever.
- Miliaria rubra occurs when the obstruction is in the epidermis and upper dermis. There is erythema present. The lesions are usually very pruritic and are often referred to as "prickly heat." Infants are subject to this condition when they are dressed too warmly. Adults may develop this when they are subjected to a hot, humid environment. Occasionally there is a temporary anhidrosis (lack of sweating) following a severe episode of miliaria rubra that may last as long as two weeks.
- Miliaria profunda occurs when the obstruction is deeper in the dermis. Sweat may occasionally leak into the dermis in this condition. Nonpruritic flesh-colored, deep-seated white papules are found with this disease. This usually occurs in the tropics or following a severe case of miliaria rubra. Anhidrosis and heat retention may occur.

DIAGNOSIS AND DIFFERENTIAL

- In neonatal patients, toxic erythema neonatorum, bacterial sepsis, transient neonatal pustular melanosis, and acne neonatorum may easily be excluded with a Gram stain, culture, or biopsy.
- In adults, steroid-induced acne is excluded by history. The types of miliaria are distinguished by the clinical appearance and biopsy.

TREATMENT

- Removing the patient from the excessive heat and humidity is the first therapy. Zinc shake lotion may help to cool the patient down.
- Keeping the patient in air conditioning is also very successful.
- It is important to establish the function of the sweat glands before the individual is subjected to a warm climate to avoid heat stroke.

REFERENCE

Wenzel FG, Horn TD. Non-neoplastic disorders of the eccrine glands. *J Am Acad Dermatol.* 1998;38:1.

FOX-FORDYCE DISEASE

EPIDEMIOLOGY

• Incidence is unknown, it occurs mainly in women between the ages of 15 and 35 years.

PATHOPHYSIOLOGY

• It is thought that obstruction of the excretory duct of the apocrine gland by a keratin plug provokes dilation of the sweat gland.
• The pressure of the secretion of the apocrine gland induces spongiotic vesicles.
• An inflammatory infiltrate around the glands is also present.

CLINICAL FEAUTRES

• Fox-Fordyce disease is a chronic, pruritic, papular eruption, strictly localized to areas that have apocrine glands. It occurs mainly in women.
• The lesions are noninflammatory and occur after puberty in women between the ages of 15 and 35.
• It is worse in hot weather and occasionally improves with pregnancy or with oral contraceptives.

DIAGNOSIS AND DIFFERENTIAL

• The diagnosis is usually made on clinical assessment of conical papules in the apocrine areas.

• There may be a decrease of hair and sweat in those areas.
• Pruritus is usually the chief complaint.
• Other papular diseases such as lichen planus, lichen nititis, syringomas, miliaria, and chronic dermatitis should be easily excluded with a skin biopsy.

TREATMENT

• Oral contraceptives have been used in many patients. Topical clindamycin has been used successfully in some patients. The most exciting new therapy has been the successful use of liposuction of the axillae to remove the apocrine glands.

REFERENCES

Chae KM, Marshall MA, Marshall SF. Fox-Fordyce disease treated with liposuction-assisted curettage. *Arch Dermatol.* In press.

Daoud MS, Dicken CH. Apocrine glands. In: Freedberg IM, Eisen AZ, Wolff K, et al., eds. *Dermatology in General Medicine*, ed 5. New York McGraw-Hill, 1999:812.

Feldmann R, Masouye I, Chavaz P, Saurat JH. Fox-Fordyce disease: Successful treatment with topical clindamycin in alcoholic propylene glycol solution. *Dermatology.* 1992; 184:310.

Ghislain PD, van Der Endt JD, Delescluse J. Itchy papules of the axillae. *Arch Dermatol.* 2002;138:259.

Miller ML, Harford RR, Yeager JK. Fox-Fordyce disease treated with topical clindamycin solution. *Arch Dermatol.* 1995;131:1112.

Stashower ME, Krivda SJ, Turiansky GW. Fox-Fordyce disease: Diagnosis with transverse histologic section. *J Am Acad Dermatol.* 2000;42:89.

6 DERMATITIS

Esperanza C. Welsh
Francisco A. Kerdel

ATOPIC DERMATITIS

- Atopic dermatitis (AD) is a chronic skin disease that generally starts in childhood. It is commonly associated with asthma and allergic rhinitis.

EPIDEMIOLOGY

- Affects 10 to 15% of the population.
- Onset of AD within the first year of life is approximately 60%, and by age 5 the incidence increases to 85%.
- 40% of affected children outgrow the disease by adulthood.
- When both parents are affected, there is an 81% chance that the child will be affected, 59% if only one parent had AD and the other a respiratory atopy, and 56% if only one parent is affected.
- 75 to 80% of patients with AD have history of atopy.
- It is thought that inheritance of this trait is autosomal dominant, but polygenic inheritance influenced strongly by environmental factors is also possible.
- Mast cell chymase gene located on chromosome 14q11.2 has been linked to atopic dermatitis.
- A mutation of the gene encoding for the IL-4 receptor located on chromosome 16p11.2-12 leading to increased receptor activity has also been reported.

PATHOPHYSIOLOGY

- There is an increase of the lymphocyte TH2 response producing cytokines such as IL-4, IL-5, IL-10, and IL-13, which promote IgE immunoglobulin production through B-cell proliferation.
- There is a suppression of lymphocyte T_H1 cell-mediated response in which interferon-γ, interleukin-2, and tumor necrosis factor are the active cytokines.
- In AD there is increased phosphodiesterase activity of monocytes, which leads to increased postoglandin E_2, which has been shown to increase the IL-4 production of T_H2 cells and to inhibit T_H1 response.
- Increased mast cells are seen in chronic AD, which also produce IL-4.
- Abnormal epidermal Langerhans cells with hyperstimulatory antigen-presenting activity have been found in the affected and normal skin of atopic patients.
- AD patients are frequently colonized with *Staphylococcus aureus*, and many of the strains that colonize AD patients produce superantigens, which exacerbate the inflammatory response in these patients.
- IgE antibodies to resident staphylococcal superantigens have been identified from the serum of some patients with atopic dermatitis.
- In chronic AD there is an increase in IL-12 mRNA. It has been proposed that there could be a biphasic model in AD with expression of T_H2 cytokines in acute disease and T_H1 cytokines in the chronic phase.
- Decrease in ceramide concentrations as well as of sphingomyelin acyclase has been described. This enzyme is needed for epidermal-cell function.
- Certain foods have been associated with the exacerbation of atopic dermatitis, among them eggs, milk, wheat, peanuts, soy, fish, and chicken. This appears to be important in childhood disease.
- In the early phase of AD there is mild spongiosis in the epidermis, parakeratosis, and a perivascular lymphohystiocytic infiltrate. In long-standing lesions, the rete ridges are elongated and the spongiosis is decreased. Eosinophils can be present, but less numerous than in allergic contact or nummular dermatitis. There is an increase in mast cells.

CLINICAL FEATURES

- Pruritus is a cardinal feature in AD.
- Infants: Face and extensor surfaces of the skin are affected with sparing of the diaper area.
- Older children and adults: Flexural surfaces commonly affected.
- The lesions can be morphologically varied, but they mainly include red, scaly patches and plaques, hypopigmented patches, excoriations, lichenified plaques, and yellow crusting when infected.

TABLE 6–1 Other Findings in Atopic Dermatitis

Anterior neck folds
Cataracts
Cheilitis
Conjunctivitis
Dennie–Morgan fold (infraorbital fold)
Dermographism
Early age of onset
Facial pallor or erythema
Food intolerance
Ichthyosis
Immediate skin test reactivity
Increased IgE levels
Keratoconus
Keratosis pilaris
Nipple eczema
Orbital darkening
Perifollicular accentuation
Periorbital darkening
Pityriasis alba
Postauricular fissures
Scalp scaling
Tendency towards cutaneous infections, especially *S. aureus* and
    herpes simplex
Wool intolerance
Worsens with environmental emotional factors
Xerosis

- There are other findings associated with atopic dermatitis (Table 6–1).
- A personal or family history of atopy such as asthma, allergic rhinitis, or AD are important clues in making a diagnosis.
- Dry skin especially in winter is a common finding.
- Wool will exacerbate the dermatitis due to mechanical irritation.
- The diagnostic criteria recommended by Hanifin and Rajka are the most widely used. To make the diagnosis, the patient should have three or more of the following plus three or more of the associated findings in Table 6–1:
  - Pruritus
  - Typical morphology and distribution of the skin lesions (described above)
  - Chronic relapsing dermatitis
  - Personal or family history of atopy

DIAGNOSIS AND DIFFERENTIAL

- Ichthyosis vulgaris, contact dermatitis, lichen simplex chronicus, scabies, dermatophytosis, cutaneous T-cell lymphoma, zinc deficiency, and certain immunodeficiencies.

TREATMENT

- General recommendations: Use an antibacterial or a hypoallergenic soap, avoid the use of irritating fabrics such as wool, keep the skin well lubricated at all times with ointments, avoid heat, and perspiration.
- Topical steroids are the mainstay of the therapy. Ointments should be used whenever possible. A low-potency steroid should be used for the face and intertriginous areas while a mid-potency steroid can be used on the body.
- If steroids are used for a long period of time without interruption, a cortisol level needs to be checked.
- Antihistamines such as hydroxizine and cetirizine play an important role in decreasing the itching.
- Atopic patients have a higher tendency to develop bacterial infections. These are often associated with flares of the disease. A course of oral antibiotics should be considered.
- Nasal application of mupirocin (topical antibiotic) for 5 days is recommended to prevent carriage of *S. aureus*.
- Light therapy with UVA and UVB (including UVB narrowband) as well as PUVA (UVA plus psoralens) has been reported to be a good therapeutic option.
- The combination of UVA and UVB light is 90% effective in clearing lesions, while either alone is 70% effective.
- Daily UVA1 (340 to 400 nm) therapy has also been shown to be more effective than combined UVA and UVB after 10 days. This could be because high-dose UVA1 penetrates deeper.
- Psoralens plus UVA was shown in a study to clear AD lesions in 10 to 25 weeks.
- When the disease is severe and does not respond to first-line therapy, other agents can be considered. Among these are the macrolides: cyclosporine, tacrolimus, and pimecrolimus. These agents inhibit the transcription of genes for cytokines such as IL-2.
- Cyclosporine is given orally, and has been used successfully in the pediatric population. It is important to note that cyclosporine has important side effects such as nephrotoxicity, and can also increase the blood pressure. These need to be monitored carefully. The initial dosage is 5 mg/kg with an effective and rapid clearance. This is subsequently tapered gradually. There is a risk that the AD will relapse after stopping the therapy if no other ancillary treatment is started before cyclosporine is discontinued.
- Tacrolimus (FK 506) has similar effects to cyclosporine. Even though it can be used systemically, the topical form has been shown to be very efficacious in the treatment of moderate to severe atopic dermatitis. This topical agent penetrates inflamed skin but not normal skin, making it very safe. Tacrolimus is available in a 0.1 and 0.03% ointment. The lower concentration is preferred for children under two years of age.

- Pimecrolimus is a new ascomycin derivative that has also been shown to be effective in mild to moderate atopic dermatitis. It is less irritating and comes in a 0.1% concentration. Pimecrolimus has been shown to inhibit IL-2 cytokine production and mast cell activation.
- Interferon-γ, which inhibits IL-4 production, has been used to treat AD. Recombinant interferon is given at a dose of 50 μg/m² by subcutaneous injection.
- Recently, mycophenolate mofetil (MMF) was reported to be a successful treatment of severe AD. MMF is given orally at doses that range from 1 to 2 g daily.
- Azathioprine has also been used in AD patients and has been shown to be effective in both relieving the symptoms and having fewer hospitalizations. The recommended dose is 100 mg/d. Blood counts need to be monitored. Before therapy is started, thiopurine S-methyltransferase (TMPT) may be evaluated. One in 300 patients have deficient TMPT and can develop toxicity due to the medication.
- Zafirlukast is a leukotriene inhibitor. It is given daily at a dose of 20 mg PO b.i.d. It has been shown to inhibit LTD4 and histamine-mediated cutaneous vascular permeability.
- Other agents that have been used to treat atopic dermatitis include methotrexate and IVIG (intravenous immunoglobulin).

REFERENCES

Hanifin JM, Ling MR, Langley R, et al. Tacrolimus ointment for the treatment of atopic dermatitis in adult patients. Part I, efficacy. *J Am Acad Dermatol.* 2001;44:S28.

Odom B, James WD, Berger TG. *Diseases of the Skin.* New York:Saunders, 2000.

Rudikoff D, Lebwohl M. Atopic dermatitis. *Lancet.* 1998; 351:1715.

Tofte S, Hanifin J. Current management and therapy of atopic dermatitis. *J Am Acad Dermatol.* 2001;44:S13.

CONTACT DERMATITIS

- Contact dermatitis is subdivided into allergic contact dermatitis and irritant contact dermatitis.
- Allergic contact dermatitis (ACD) is the result of a sensitization to a specific substance.
- Irritant contact dermatitis (ICD) is an irritation of the skin by a particular substance but there is no sensitization. ICD potentially can affect all those who are exposed to the substance.

- Allergic contact dermatitis accounts for 20% of contact dermatitis, whereas irritant contact dermatitis represents 80%.

PATHOPHYSIOLOGY

- Allergic contact dermatitis is a delayed hypersensitivity reaction (cell-mediated immunity).
- The allergen is processed by antigen-presenting cells (APCs), which in the skin are the Langerhans cells. The antigen is then transported to the lymph nodes where it is presented to T cells
- Clone expansion of T cells occurs, and these cells act as memory cells ready to react upon further exposure to the allergen.
- Persons may be exposed for years to an allergen before hypersensitivity develops.
- In ICD the irritant chemical damages the skin barrier and causes inflammation. This depends on the nature of the irritant chemical, its concentration, and the duration of the contact with the skin. Broad categories of irritants include soaps, detergents, acids, alkalis, metal salts, and solvents.

CLINICAL FEATURES

- The clinical findings include red patches, papules and plaques, vesicles, and bullae.
- The area of the body affected helps determine the most common allergen:
  - Eyes (cosmetics and nail polish)
  - Lips (cosmetics, toothpaste, mango)
  - Ears (nickel, neomycin), neck (perfumes)
  - Axilla plus axillary vault (deodorant), sparing the vault (particularly formaldehyde used in clothing)
  - Trunk: fabrics, nickel on wires (brasierre, corsettes)
  - Abdomen: nickel (belts), rubber (elastic band)
  - Genital area (poison ivy, latex)
  - Feet: shoe dermatitis secondary to chrome-tanned leather, rubber, adhesives.

COMMON ALLERGENS

- The most common causes of contact dermatitis are toxicodendron (poison ivy, oak, or sumac), nickel (most common metal allergen), fragrance, thimerosal, quartenium 15, neomycin, formaldehyde, bacitracin, and rubber compounds (Table 6–2).
- The allergen in toxicodendron (*Rhus*) is urushiol, a catechol. This allergen is found in poison ivy, poison sumac, poison oak, the Japanese lacquer tree, cashew nut tree (nutshell), mango (rind, leaves, or sap), rengas tree, and the Indian marking nut tree. The ginko tree

TABLE 6–2   Common Occupational Contact Allergens

Artists	Acrylic, vinyl acrylic resins, epoxy and polyester resins, benzene, toluene, acetone, turpentine, azo dyes, nickel, chromium pigments, clay, plaster
Barbers	Quinine, resorcin, mercury, nickel, paraphenylendiamine, capsicum, arsenic, sulfur
Carpenters	Teak, mahogany, rosewood, glues, nickel, rubber, polishes, turpentine, plastics
Cooks	Soap, detergents, vegetables (garlic, carrots, onions, artichokes, potatoes)
Dentists	Benzalconium chloride, soaps, detergents, acrylic monomers, anesthetics (procaine), eucalyptol, menthol, formaldehyde
Gardeners	Plants, arsenic, insecticides, lime dust, fertilizers, formaldehyde, chrysanthemum, tulip, narcissus, primula, manure
Hairdressers	Paraphenylendiamine, soaps, peroxide, ammonium, thioglycolate, rubber, nickel, perfumes, acrylic plastics
Jewelers	Cyanide, nickel, metal polish
Painters	Turpentine, varnish remover, arsenic, linseed oil, aniline dyes, paints, benzene, paint thinners, formaldehyde, polyester resins
Surgeons	Antiseptics, iodine, mercurials, hexachlorophene, latex, procaine, formaldehyde, acrylic polymers
Tanners	Dichromate, hydrochloric acid, vegetable tanning agents, glutaraldehyde, anti-mildew chemicals

(fruit), silver oak, and Brazilian pepper tree have nearly identical allergens.

- The characteristic rash is a linear dermatitis that can be vesicular, bullous, or plaque like.
- Other causes of plant dermatitis include tuliposidase A (tulips, alstroemeria), colophony (pine trees), and serqueterpene lactone (chrysanthemums, daisies, dandelions, sunflowers, artichokes, endevies, feverfew, and liverwort).
- Among the cosmetic contact allergens, fragrance accounts for 30%. Preservatives, parapenylenediamine (PPD), lanolin, toluene sulphonamide formaldehyde resin (TSF resin), cyanoacrylates, and sunscreens are also frequent offenders.
- The most common contact allergen in hair-coloring products is PPD.
- Persons allergic to PPD in hair dyes can use henna, lead oxide, and temporary hair coloring that uses food-coloring agents.
- Ammonium persulfate used for hair bleaching causes mainly an irritant dermatitis.
- Among the fragrances the most common allergens are cinnamic aldehyde, cinnamic alcohol, geraniol, eugenol, isoeugenol, oak moss absolute, hydroxycitronella, alpha-amyl cinnamic alcohol, and balsam of Peru.
- The preservatives commonly used include quaternium 15, DMDM hydantoin, imidazolidinyl urea, diazonidyl urea, and bronopol. Also parabens, kathon CG, Euxyl K400, iodopropynyl butylcarbamate (IPBC), and thimerosal (found in contact lens products).
- Colophony is an extract from pine that is found in eye shadow, mascara, blusher, nail products, and ethnic hair products.

- Glyceryl thioglycolate in permanent wave products.
- TSF resins are found in nail polish, and methyl methacrylate is found in artificial nails. Nail glues contain cyanoacrylates.
- Lanolin is derived from fleece of sheep and is used as a moisturizer.
- Sunscreens that contain PABA, and oxybenzone, can cause contact allergy.
- Other common allergens include the local anesthetics. Among them benzocaine, monocaine, novocaine, and tetracaine are the most common offending agents. These cross-react with PABA.
- Hexavalent chromate is an allergen found in cement that commonly predisposes to ACD in construction workers.

COMMON IRRITANTS

- Irritants can be subdivided into seven major categories: soaps and detergents, acids, alkalis, solvents, metal salts, fabrics, and plant irritants.
- The soaps and detergents that cause irritant dermatitis are mainly the ones used as industrial skin cleansers. Some of these also have abrasive substances such as sand or pumice, which worsen the irritation.
- Among the most common acids are sulfuric, hydrochloric, hydrofluoric, chromic, nitric, and phosphoric acids. These are strong acids that can cause not only dermatitis but ulceration. Hydrofluoric acid can penetrate even bone on exposed terminal phalanges.
- Sulfuric acid is used in fertilizers, pigments, paper, and explosives. It is also used in the jewelry industry and for electroplating.

- Hydrochloric acid is used in fertilizers, paints, electroplating, and leather tanning.
- Hydrofluoric acid is used in the semiconductor industry.
- The most common alkalis causing ICD include sodium hydroxide, potassium hydroxide, calcium oxide, calcium hydroxide, and sodium and potassium carbonate. Alkalis are used in bleaches, soaps, detergents, dyes, paper, plastics, and in the cement industry.
- Sodium and potassium hydroxides are used as hair relaxers mainly in ethnic hair products. Guanidine carbamate has less irritation potential and can be used as an alternative.
- Metal salts most commonly include arsenic, beryllium, and dichromates.
- Many solvents cause ICD, including benzene, toluene, gasoline, kerosene, carbon tetrachloride, alcohol solvents, and dimethyl sulphoxide (DMSO).
- Fibrous glass particles can penetrate the clothing and cause severe skin irritation.
- Wool and several irritating synthetic fibers can cause ICD or exacerbate AD.
- Phototoxic plant dermatitis is caused by plant psoralens such as furocoumarins plus UVA (320 to 400 nm). These chemicals can be found in celery, fig tree, hogweed, parsley, parsnip, rue, and lime.
- ICD can be caused by plants; due to a chemical burn by the plant, or by mechanical irritation such as that caused by spines. Plant extracts are commonly used in alternative medicine as well as in cosmetics.

CONTACT URTICARIA

- Contact urticaria can occur after direct contact with a variety of substances. This can be immunologic (IgE mediated) or nonimmunologic. The nonimmunologic variety is the most common, and it is caused by direct release of vasoactive substances from mast cells. Examples of nonimmunologic causes are nettle rash (plants), dimethyl sulfoxide (DMSO), sorbic acid, benzoic acid, cinnamic aldehyde, and cobalt chloride. Some allergens causing immunologic urticaria include apple, bacitracin, henna, latex rubber, and mechlorethamine.

DIAGNOSIS AND DIFFERENTIAL

- The most important factor in establishing the diagnosis of contact dermatitis due to a specific agent is the history, but when this is unclear, patch testing can help.
- Patch testing consists of the application of the most common allergens onto the skin. The most common patch test is the one that is left for 48 hours and then reread 48 hours later. But for contact urticaria, an open patch test is done, where the waiting time is only 30 minutes.

- If a photocontactant is suspected, photopatch testing can be performed. This consists of applying a patch test, exposing the site 24 hours later to UVA ($10\,J/cm^2$), and read the test 48 hours later. A duplicate patch test is applied at the same time but without exposing it to the light. Common photocontactants include phenothiazines and sulphonamides.

TREATMENT

- Avoid the allergen or irritant.
- Use moisturizing agents and gloves.
- Mid to high-potency topical steroids play an important role in mild to moderate cases.
- Systemic steroids are often needed in severe cases.
- Barrier creams and protective clothing can be used for those patients who cannot avoid exposure.

REFERENCES

Bolduc C, Shapiro J. Hair care products: Waving, straightening, conditioning, and coloring. *Clin Dermatol*. 2001;19:431.

De Leo VA, et al. Allergic contact dermatitis. *Arch Dermatol*. 1992;128:1513.

Wolf R, Wolf D. Contact dermatitis. *Clin Dermatol*. 2000;18:661.

DIAPER DERMATITIS

- Diaper dermatitis or napkin rash is an erythematous papular and or vesicular rash that affects the buttocks, lower abdomen, genitalia, and thighs, sparing the folds.

EPIDEMIOLOGY

- It is frequently seen in children between 6 and 12 months of age, but also in incontinent patients.
- There is no predilation for age or sex.
- The prevalence ranges from 7 to 35% in infants.
- It is the most common cutaneous disorder of infancy.

PATHOPHYSIOLOGY

- Several factors play a role in diaper dermatitis. Ammonia increases the irritation on already damaged skin. Change in skin pH, maceration, friction, proteolytic, and lipolytic digestive enzymes disrupt the epidermal barrier, which can be secondarily colonized by *Candida* and other bacteria.

DIAGNOSIS AND DIFFERENTIAL

- Differential diagnosis includes contact dermatitis, atopic dermatitis, seborrheic dermatitis, Langerhans cell histiocytoses, tinea cruris, zinc and biotin deficiency, scabies, and candidiasis.

TREATMENT

- Change diapers more frequently, in neonates every hour and throughout infancy every 3 to 4 hours.
- Use a mild soap not more than twice a day, and zinc-oxide pastes to protect the epidermal barrier.
- Baby wipes are not recommended due to allergens present in the wipes.
- Low-potency topical steroids and topical antifungals help with the inflammation and secondary yeast infection, respectively.
- Use of superabsorbent diapers is recommended, but taking into account that they should not be left in place longer just because they are more absorbent.

REFERENCES

Odio M, Fallon-Friedlander S. Diaper dermatitis and advances in diaper technology. *Curr Op Pediatr.* 2000;12:342.

Wolfe R, Wolf D, Tuzun B, Tuzun Y. Diaper dermatitis. *Clin Dermatol.* 2000;18:657.

PERIORAL DERMATITIS

- Perioral dermatitis consists of grouped, erythematous papules, vesicles, or pustules around the mouth. Generally there is a space of unaffected skin between the vermilion border and the eruption.

EPIDEMIOLOGY

- Primarily affects women between 16 and 45 years of age.
- It has also been reported to occur in children.

PATHOPHYSIOLOGY

- It has been associated with overuse of potent topical steroids.
- Allergens, bacteria, and *Demodex folliculorum* have also been suggested as possible triggers of this condition.
- Mild perivascular and perifollicular lymphohistio-cytic infiltrate with spongiosis is found on biopsy.
- A granulomatous perioral dermatitis has been described in children.

DIAGNOSIS AND DIFFERENTIAL

- Differential diagnosis includes rosacea, seborrheic dermatitis, contact dermatitis, acne, and papular sarcoid.

TREATMENT

- The mainstay of treatment is to stop any topical corticosteroid and to start oral tetracycline.
- Other antibiotics that have been successfully used are doxycycline, minocycline, and erythromycin. Tetracycline is contraindicated in children younger than 8 years of age due to teeth pigmentation.
- Topical metronidazole, erythromycin, clindamycin, sulfacetamide, and benzoyl peroxide can also be used.
- For granulomatous perioral dermatitis, dapsone and isotretinoin have been tried successfully.

REFERENCES

Katsambas AD, Nicolaidou E. Acne, perioral dermatitis, flushing + rosacea: unapproved treatments or indications. *Clin Dermatol.* 2000;18:171.

Manders SM, Lucky AW. Perioral dermatitis in childhood. *J Am Acad Dermatol.* 1992;27:688.

NUMMULAR DERMATITIS

- Nummular dermatitis is derived from the Latin term "nummulus," meaning coin shaped. It is a localized inflammation of the skin.

PATHOPHYSIOLOGY

- The etiology is unknown; however in the past it has been associated with *Staphylococcus aureus*.

CLINICAL FEATURES

- It presents as coin-shaped plaques that can be erythematous, vesicular, or crusted. The size can vary from 0.5 to 5 cm in diameter.
- Itching is a common finding.
- It commonly starts on the legs and spreads to the trunk and arms.

TREATMENT

- Treatment consists of mid and high-potency topical steroids. Short courses of antibiotics have been reported to be beneficial. If this is ineffective, intralesional steroids or PO steroids can be used in severe cases.
- Moisturizers and antihistamines for itching are warranted.
- The disease has a variable course, but it tends to resolve in 1 to 2 years.

LICHEN SIMPLEX CHRONICUS (LSC)

- Also known as neurodermatitis circumscripta, LSC is localized cutaneous inflammation with prominent skin thickening.

PATHOPHYSIOLOGY

- Lichen simplex chronicus is the result of constant scratching or rubbing of the skin.

CLINICAL FEATURES

- There is lichenification, which is the thickening of the skin with pronounced skin lines.
- LSC is mostly seen on the neck, wrist, ankles, scrotum, anal area, and shins.

TREATMENT

- High-potency topical steroids. These work better under occlusion.
- Antihistamines for itching.
- Topical capsaicin (chili extract) cream has been reported to be effective.
- In severe cases, intralesional steroids can be used.
- Covering the extremity with an occlusive dressing may suppress the urge to scratch.
- Ultraviolet light therapy may be used as an adjuvant.

REFERENCES

Jones RO. Lichen simplex chronicus. *Clin Pediatr Med Surg.* 1996;13:47.

Kantor GR, et al. Treatment of lichen simplex chronicus with topical capsaicin cream. *Acta Derm Venereol.* 1992; 76:161.

VENOUS DERMATITIS

- Venous dermatitis comprises all the dermatitic changes of the skin secondary to venous insufficiency.

EPIDEMIOLOGY

- Venous ulcers are very common. 80% of leg ulcers are caused by venous insufficiency, and 10 to 25% are due to arterial disease. The prevalence of venous ulceration ranges from 0.06 to 2% of the population, it is more common in females (1.6:1), and it peaks between 60 and 80 years of age.
- Obesity is an important factor.

PATHOPHYSIOLOGY

- Loss or dysfunction of the valves of the superficial and/or the communicating veins.
- Loss or lack of function of the valves of the deep vein.
- Mechanical obstruction of the deep venous system.
- Dysfunction of the calf muscle pump
- These factors produce venous hypertension with the subsequent extravasation of red blood cells and fibrinogen into the interstitial fluid. This causes hemosiderin deposition on the skin, which gives the brown pigmentation. The precipitation of fibrin produces

fibrin cuffs around the vessels and prevents oxygen and/or nutrients from reaching the tissues.

- Other hypotheses suggest that trapping growth factors in the dermis inhibits the healing process.
- It has also been suggested that venous hypertension leads to trapping of white cells, which in turn causes localized hypoxia and promotes inflammation through the secretion of cytokines. This then leads to tissue damage.

CLINICAL FEATURES

- Brown pigmentation or mottling of the ankles and inner calves. Scaling with classic dermatitic changes can be present.
- Atrophic white stellate lesions (atrophie blanche) are found in 38% of patients with chronic venous insufficiency.
- Lipodermatosclerosis: Thickening and tender induration of the skin of the ankles resembling an "inverted champagne bottle" is also a change of chronic venous insufficiency.
- Varicose veins are commonly found in these patients.
- Ulcerations on the medial ankle (above the medial maleolus).

DIAGNOSIS AND DIFFERENTIAL

- If there are ulcers, the "gold standard" study is color duplex ultrasound scanning. This to check for valve patency and to rule out deep vein thrombosis.
- Invasive phlebography is recommended if surgery is advised.
- If there is a longstanding ulcer, an osteomyelitis workup can be considered.
- The ankle-to-brachial index measured by Doppler ultrasonography is an important tool to assess for arterial circulation. This is done because part of the mainstay of therapy for venous ulcers is compression, and the ulcers can be of mixed arterial and venous etiology. Arterial ulcers should not be treated with compression.

TREATMENT

- Leg elevation, avoid standing for long hours.
- If venous dermatitis without ulceration is the only finding, a mid-potency steroid can help the inflammation.
- Compression with stockings is recommended with a pressure of 35 to 40 mm Hg.
- If an ulcer is present, compression with multilayered bandage systems has been shown to be effective.

- Mechanical or autolytic debridement can be done if there is an ulceration with necrotic tissue.
- Systemic therapy with stanozolol, an androgenic steroid with fibrinolytic properties, has been reported to help in lipodermatosclerosis.
- Pentoxyfylline at a dose of 800 mg PO t.i.d. has also been shown to be effective for venous ulcerations.
- Other therapies include surgery and tissue-engineered skin equivalents.

REFERENCES

Falanga V, Eaglstein WH. The trap hypothesis of venous ulceration. *Lancet.* 1993;341:1006.

Kirsner RS, Pardes JB, Eaglstein WH, Falanga V. The clinical spectrum of lipodermatosclerosis. *J Am Acad Dermatol.* 1993;28:623.

Phillips TJ, Dover JS. Leg ulcers. *J Am Acad Dermatol.* 1991;25:965.

Valencia IC, Falabella A, Kirsner RS, Eaglstein WH. Chronic venous insufficiency and venous leg ulceration. *J Am Acad Dermatol.* 2001;44:401.

DYSHYDROTIC ECZEMA

- Dyshydrosis or pompholyx, which means "bubble," is a vesicular eruption of the palms and soles frequently accompanied by intense itch.

PATHOPHYSIOLOGY

- The cause is unknown, but it as been found to be worsened by stress and exposure to allergens, and is associated with atopy.
- On histology the sweat glands are not involved, and the vesicles are found superficially in the epidermis. There is spongiosis (edema of epidermis).

CLINICAL FEATURES

- Clinically there are crops of clear deep-seated vesicles on the palms and the sides of the fingers. These have been described as "tapioca" vesicles.

DIAGNOSIS AND DIFFERENTIAL

- Among the differential diagnosis the most common conditions are dermatophyte infections, pustular psoriasis, and contact dermatitis.

TREATMENT

- Burrow's solution soaks (aluminum subacetate) as a drying agent or drysol (aluminum chloride).
- High-potency topical steroids, which can be applied under occlusion.
- Light therapy, in particular PUVA (UVA plus psoralens).
- Other agents that have been tried to treat this condition are keratolytics and topical calcipotriol.
- Oral retinoids have been used for this condition with good results.
- In severe cases, oral steroids or other immunosuppressants have been effective.

REFERENCES

Lodi A, et al. Epidemiological, clinical, and allergological observations on pompholyx. *Contact Dermatitis.* 1992; 26:17.

Pickenacker A, et al. Dyshydrotic eczema treated with mycophenolate mofetil. *Arch Dermatol.* 1998;134:378.

AUTOECZEMATIZATION SYNDROME

- This refers to the development of a distant dermatitis from a primary inflammatory focus. This is also referred to as an "id" reaction.

PATHOPHYSIOLOGY

- Common causes for autoeczematization include contact dermatitis and dermatophyte infection.

CLINICAL FEATURES

- The classic presentation is seen in patients with venous dermatitis. One to two weeks after the onset of the dermatitis, symmetric, pruritic, papular, or vesicular plaques appear on the body in a sudden fashion.

DIAGNOSIS AND DIFFERENTIAL

- The diagnosis is made by exclusion.

TREATMENT

- Eliminate the cause of the inflammation of the original focus.
- Apply topical steroids to affected area
- Antihistamines for itching.

STEATOTIC ECZEMA

- Also called eczema craquele, this is a dermatitis caused by low humidity of the skin.

EPIDEMIOLOGY

- It is most common in the elderly population.

CLINICAL FEATURES

- It is more severe on the shins and arms.
- The skin is dry and there are flakes on the skin making it look "cracked."
- Commonly worsens over the winter.

TREATMENT

- Emollients and moisturizing creams.
- When bathing, wash only the axillae and groin area with soap and use bath oils.

7 BACTERIAL INFECTIONS

Justin J. Vujevich
Francisco A. Kerdel

IMPETIGO (IMPETIGO OF BOCKHART, BULLOUS IMPETIGO, IMPETIGO CONTAGIOSA)

EPIDEMIOLOGY

- *Staphylococcus aureus* is the most common pathogen in impetigo of Bockhart and impetigo contagiosa. The remainder of infections are caused by *Streptococcus pyogenes*, with or without *S. aureus*. Impetigo is frequently seen in children.
- Bullous impetigo, most of which is caused by phage 71 type coagulase-positive *S. aureus*, or related group 2 phage type, occurs primarily in newborn infants (age 4 to 10 days old). It is highly contagious in nurseries, but occurs in adults in warmer climates.
- Impetigo can occur as a primary infection or as a secondary event. Common sources of primary infection include pets, fingernails, children in close confinement, swimming pools, hair cutteries, and infected children. Secondary infection occurs commonly in scabies, herpes simplex, insect bites, dermatitis, and poison ivy.

PATHOPHYSIOLOGY

- Infection arises as the result of superficial breaks in the skin, which allow bacteria to invade.
- Histologically, there is a vesicopustule containing few cocci, neutrophils, and epidermal debris. A mild inflammatory reaction is seen in the dermis.
- In bullous impetigo, *S. aureus* produces a toxin capable of producing a split in the superficial epidermis, resulting in bullae formation.

CLINICAL FEATURES

- Impetigo generally begins as a superficial vesicle or pustule, which ruptures, turning into a crusted erosion. The lesions are typically found on the nose, cheek, lips, and chin.
- In impetigo contagiosa, superficial erythematous macules develop into vesicles or bullae. These lesions rupture, releasing a straw-colored discharge, which dries and gives a honey-colored crust. These extremely friable crusts are easily removed, leaving a residual moist red surface. The infection spreads peripherally, forming larger gyrating circles of erythema and crusting. There may be local lymphadenopathy.
- Impetigo contagiosa occurs primarily on exposed parts of body, usually on the face and hands.
- In bullous impetigo, vesicles and bullae arise with surrounding erythema. These easily rupture, forming an erosion. Lesions most commonly occur on the face and hands of children.

DIAGNOSIS AND DIFFERENTIAL

- Impetigo is predominantly a clinical diagnosis. Lesions may be cultured for isolation and sensitivities.
- Circular patches, especially in children, may resemble tinea; however, tinea usually has more scale and erythema at the edges of the plaque.
- Differential diagnosis also includes ecthyma, varicella, contact dermatitis, and herpes simplex.
- Bullous impetigo lesions may also resemble pemphigus vulgaris and bullous pemphigoid.

TREATMENT

- Topical mupirocin combined with oral antibiotics if needed. A semisynthetic penicillin or first-generation cephalosporin is usually given for 7 to 10 days.
- Soak with warm compresses/Burrows solution.
- Recurrent impetigo patients may be harboring *S. aureus* in their nares and may benefit from application of nasal mupriocin to the anterior nares b.i.d. or rifampin 600 mg PO q.d. × 5 days.
- Most cases respond quickly to therapy without scarring.

REFERENCES

Barton LL. Impetigo. *Pediatr Dermatol.* 1987;4:185.
Dillon HC. Treatment of staphylococcal skin infections. *J Am Acad Dermatol.* 1983;8:177.
Shriner DL, Schwartz RA, Janniger CK. Impetigo. *Dermatol Clin.* 1999;17:561.

ECTHYMA

EPIDEMIOLOGY

- Caused by *Streptococcus pyogenes, Staphylococcus aureus*, or a combination of both.
- Ecthyma is usually seen in patients with preceding trauma, poor hygiene, and malnutrition. Also seen in HIV and drug-abusing patient populations.

PATHOPHYSIOLOGY

- A deeper infection than impetigo. Histology demonstrates a dermal perivascular infiltrate of lymphocytes and neutrophils.
- A defect in the stratum corneum allows bacteria to invade.

CLINICAL FEATURES

- Pustules/papules coalesce, forming an ulceration covered with thick crusts. When the crust is removed, it leaves a saucer-shaped, well-circumscribed ulceration with a slightly raised border and surrounding erythema.
- It is usually seen in the lower extremities, on the shins or the dorsal feet.
- Looks like a deep form of impetigo. Heals with scarring.

DIAGNOSIS AND DIFFERENTIAL

- Generally a clinical diagnosis. The pathogen may be identified in a Gram stain or culture of the lesion.
- Differential diagnosis includes herpetic ulceration, herpes zoster, and insect bites. Venous or arterial ulcers may have a similar appearance, though medical history should help differentiate.

TREATMENT

- Cleanse with soap/water, apply topical antimicrobial ointment b.i.d. (mupirocin) and oral antibiotics covering the pathogens indicated. A semisynthetic penicillin or first-generation cephalosporin is commonly used.
- Encourage proper hygiene/wound checks in patients prone to trauma or in an immunocompromised host.
- Lesions heal after few weeks, frequently leaving scars.

REFERENCES

James WD. Cutaneous group B streptococcal infection. *Arch Dermatol.* 1984;120:85.
Kelly C, Taplin D, Allen AM. Streptococcal ecthyma. *Arch Dermatol.* 1971;103:306.

FOLLICULITIS (SUPERFICIAL)

EPIDEMIOLOGY

- Folliculitis may be bacterial, fungal, or viral in origin. The most common bacterial pathogen is *Staphylococcus aureus*. Other bacterial pathogens include *Pseudomonas aeruginosa.*
- Predisposing factors include living in warm climates, chronic use of topical steroids, systemic antibiotic therapy, and immunocompromised hosts.

PATHOPHYSIOLOGY

- Folliculitis is an infection of the hair follicle.

CLINICAL FEATURES

- *S. aureus* folliculitis presents as erythematous papules or pustules surrounding hair, occurring singly or in crops. These may rupture and form erosions. Lesions may also progress to furuncle or abscess formation. Commonly seen in scalp, trunk, and extremities.
- *P. aeruginosa* folliculitis presents as multiple follicular papules and pustules on the trunk and is frequently seen in individuals after exposure to hot tubs (Jacuzzi).
- Gram-negative folliculitis is characterized by small follicular erythematous pustules on cheeks and upper trunk. Typically occurs in individuals treated for acne with oral antibiotics.

DIAGNOSIS AND DIFFERENTIAL

- Diagnosis is made by the clinical picture, and confirmed Gram stain or lesion culture.

- Differential diagnosis includes any other follicular inflammatory disease such as acne vulgaris, rosacea, and perioral dermatitis. Also included are chemical-induced acne (chloracne), eosinophillic folliculitis, drug reactions, atopic dermatitis, and keratosis pilaris.

TREATMENT

- Cleanse area with antibacterial soap/water t.i.d. Mupirocin ointment topically.
- If required, oral antibiotics covering the pathogens indicated. A semisynthetic penicillin or a first-generation cephalosporin is commonly used.
- *P. aeruginosa* folliculitis may require the use of an oral quinolone.

REFERENCES

Dillon HC. Treatment of staphylococcal skin infections. *J Am Acad Dermatol.* 1983;30:319.

Kovacs A, et al. Bacterial infections. *Med Clin Noth Am.* 1997;81:319.

Smith KJ, et al. *S. aureus* carriage and HIV disease. *Arch Dermatol.* 1994;130:521.

SYCOSIS BARBAE (BARBER'S ITCH)

EPIDEMIOLOGY

- Staphylococcal infection of the bearded region associated with frequent washing and shaving.

PATHOPHYSIOLOGY

- Chronic perifollicular, pustular staphylococcal infection of the beard. When these lesions are ruptured with repeated shaving, the infection spreads.

CLINICAL FEATURES

- Starts off as erythema associated with burning and itching, especially on the upper lip region. The erythema progresses to small pustules with small out-shooting of hairs.
- As the patient's shaving regimen continues, these pustules rupture, reinfecting the local bearded area.
- In children, it can be seen in the scalp or extremities.

DIAGNOSIS AND DIFFERENTIAL

- Diagnosis is made by the clinical picture and ruling out other differential diagnoses.
- Tinea barbae, which is typically seen in the submaxillary region and not on the upper lip, may be ruled out by KOH scraping. Acne vulgaris may be hard to distinguish in the bearded region; however, papules/pustules are also seen in unbearded regions. Pseudofolliculitis barbae (ingrown hair) is typically manifested by larger papules at the site of an outgrowing hair. Herpes simplex occurs with vesicular outbreaks lasting a few days.

TREATMENT

- Cessation of close razor shaving for a period of time until infection resolves. Stringent cleansing regimen with antibacterial soap and water t.i.d. Mupirocin ointment may be used topically.
- If required, oral antibiotic, such as a first-generation cephalosporin/penicillinase-resistant penicillin.

REFERENCE

Feingold DS, et al. Bacterial infections of the skin. *J Am Acad Dermatol.* 1989;20:469.

FURUNCULOSIS (BOIL)

EPIDEMIOLOGY

- Furuncles are commonly found on areas of the skin exposed to irritation, pressure, moisture, dermatitis, and shaving. These factors provide *Staphylococcus aureus* with a portal of entry.
- Entry of *Staphylococcus* is either from contagion, or autoinoculation in chronic carriers of *S. aureus*. Autoinoculation originates from the nose, intriginous areas, or axillae. Atopic dermatitis also predisposes to a carrier state.
- Certain medical illnesses can predispose patients to furuncles, including alcoholism, malnutrition, neutrophilic function disorders, diabetes, and HIV.

PATHOPHYSIOLOGY

- A furuncle is an infection of the hair follicle that becomes deeper than folliculitis. The inflammation extends into the dermis.

- Histologically, a deep abscess is seen with both lymphocytes and neutrophils.

CLINICAL FEATURES

- Clinically presents as an acute, tender, round, inflammatory nodule, sometimes topped by a pustule through which a hair emerges. Furuncles are commonly found on the legs and face.
- Two or more furuncles may become confluent and form a carbuncle, in which each nodule has a separate head.

DIAGNOSIS AND DIFFERENTIAL

- Diagnosis is made by clinical presentation.
- Differential diagnosis includes a ruptured epidermoid or pilar cyst, though the latter two are not infected. Folliculitis is generally more superficial without resulting in deeper nodules. Hidradenitis suppurativa is generally found in the axillae, groin, and vulva. Herpes simplex generally exhibits vesicles on erythematous base.

TREATMENT

- Initial care may include warm saline solution compresses and topical antimicrobials.
- Generally, oral antibiotics are needed, which include a penicillinase-resistant penicillin or first-generation cephalosporin (1 to 2 g/d). For those cases that do not respond to conventional antibiotics, sensitivities should be checked. In hospital settings, *S. aureus* can be methicillin-resistant.
- When lesions are acutely inflamed, avoid surgical manipulation unless there is definite fluctuation. In these cases, incision and drainage (with culture of fluid) is indicated.
- Hospital outbreaks may be prevented through meticulous hand washing.
- Patients who suffer from chronic furuncles may be carriers of *S. aureus*. Antibacterial soap, frequent laundering of bedding and clothing, and meticulous hand-washing are recommended. In addition, Bactroban ointment applied to the anterior nares b.i.d. every fourth week may break the carrier state. Rifampin 600 mg PO q.d. +/− cloxacillin 500 mg PO q.i.d. for 10 days, or clindamycin 150 mg PO q.d. for 3 months, may eradicate the nasal carrier state.

REFERENCES

Mertz PM, et al. Topical mupirocin treatment of impetigo is equal to oral erythromycin therapy. *Arch Dermatol.* 1989; 125:1069.

Reagan DR, et al. Elimination of coincident *S. aureus* nasal and hand carriage with intranasal application of mupirocin calcium ointment. *Ann Intern Med.* 1991;114:101.

Sadick NS. Current aspects of bacterial infections of the skin. *Dermatol Clin.* 1997;15:341.

ANTHRAX

EPIDEMIOLOGY

- Uncommon bacterial disease of wild domestic animals caused by *Bacillus anthracis* (gram positive, spore-forming rod) transmitted to humans by inoculation, inhalation, or ingestion.
- Sources of infection include the hides, bristles, meat, and bones of diseased herbivores. These animals shed the bacilli via the blood at death. On exposure to air, the bacteria sproulates and the spores remain in the soil for long periods of time, resistant to adverse environmental conditions.
- Bioterrorism remains a potential threat of delivering spores via mail, aerosolization, or other means.
- There are two forms of the acute bacterial disease: cutaneous anthrax and inhalation anthrax.

PATHOPHYSIOLOGY

- Spores from the environment are introduced into the skin via abrasion of the skin, scratching, or even arthropod bite. Transmission from human to human has not been documented.
- The disease has an inoculation period of 1 to 7 days. Once inside the host, spores germinate, multiply, and produce a complex toxin. The toxin causes hemorrhagic necrosis of the epidermis and dermis, resulting in ulceration with neutrophil dermal infiltration.

CLINICAL FEATURES

- In cutaneous anthrax, itching of exposed skin surface occurs first. A papular lesion develops, becoming vesicular, then forming a depressed black eschar surrounded by severe edema. The lesion is painful and is most commonly found on the head, forearms, and hands within 2 to 6 days. Untreated, it may spread to regional lymph nodes and bloodstream, leading to septicemia.

- In inhalation anthrax, the patient presents with non-specific fever, malaise, cough, and chest pain. There may be mediastinal widening on chest x-ray. Subsequently, the patients develop septicemia, shock, and frequently die in a short period of time (3 to 5 days after onset of symptoms).

DIAGNOSIS AND DIFFERENTIAL

- The clinical picture of an ulcer that does not respond to conventional therapy is suggestive. Gram stain demonstrates gram-positive rods and culture eventually confirms the diagnosis.
- Early specific diagnosis is achievable with a direct immunofluorescence antibody test. Other diagnostic tests include an ELISA, which detects anticapsule antibodies, and electrophoretic immunotransblot (EITB), which detects lethal factor and protective antibodies.
- Differential diagnosis includes disease processes that produce vesicles that eventually form ulcerations and scar: leishmaniasis, orf, and other bacterial abcesses.

TREATMENT

- Antibiotic therapy may sterilize the skin lesion within 24 hours, but does not alter its cycle of ulceration, sloughing, and resolution.
- For cutaneous anthrax, oral penicillin V (30 mg/kg per day) divided in q.i.d. doses for 5 to 7 days. Tetracyclines, erythromycin, and chloramphenicol are also effective. For inhalation anthrax, ciprofloxacin or doxycycline may be given orally for up to 60 days. For systemic disease, penicillin G (20 to 30 mg/kg per day) IM in two equal doses for 5 to 7 days.
- Persons who may have been exposed should be advised to await laboratory results and may not need to be placed on chemoprophylaxis. However, if threat or exposure to aerosolized anthrax is credible or confirmed, individuals at risk should begin postexposure prophylaxis with appropriate antibiotic.
- Postexposure immunization with an inactivated, cell-free anthrax vaccine is indicated in conjunction with chemoprophylaxis following proven biologic incident, because of uncertainty of when or if inhaled spores may germinate. Immunization consists of three injections—one as soon as possible postexposure, and then at 2 and 4 weeks postexposure.

- Untreated cutaneous anthrax has a case-fatality rate between 5 and 20%. With antibiotic therapy, however, it is rarely fatal.
- Untreated inhalation anthrax is almost always fatal.

REFERENCES

Chin J. Anthrax. In: Chin J, ed. *Control of Communicable Diseases Manual*, ed 17. Washington: American Public Health Association, 2000.

King P. Recognition and management of anthrax. *N Engl J Med.* 2002;346:943.

ERYSIPELAS/CELLULITIS

EPIDEMIOLOGY

- Most frequently caused by *Staphylcoccus aureus* and group A beta-hemolytic *Streptococcus pyogenes* (GAS).
- Compromised skin such as underlying dermatoses, trauma, surgical wounds, and mucosal infection provides portal of entry for bacterial pathogens.

PATHOPHYSIOLOGY

- Infection of the dermal and subcutaneous tissues.

CLINICAL FEATURES

- Erysipelas is a superficial cellulitis involving the lymphatics. Margins of the lesions are raised, sharply demarcated from the adjacent normal skin. The lesions are typically seen on the face, lower legs, and areas of preexisting lymphedema.
- Cellulitis is an acute, spreading infection with erythematous, warm, tender skin. An apparent portal of entry is usually evident.
- Patients may present with fever, chills, and malaise.

DIAGNOSIS AND DIFFERENTIAL

- Usually a clinical diagnosis. Culture rarely helpful.
- On the lower extremities, it may be difficult to distinguish cellulitis from deep venous thrombosis. Deep venous thrombosis, however, does not respond to antimicrobial therapy.
- The differential diagnosis also includes stasis dermatitis and contact dermatitis.

TREATMENT

- Oral antibiotic therapy if immunocompetent and if cellulitis or erysipelas is limited. Otherwise, would require IV antibiotic therapy.
- It is also important to treat medical condition predisposing patient to developing cellulitis or erysipelas, such as controlling blood sugar and monitoring trauma in diabetics.

REFERENCES

Chartier C, et al. Erysipelas. *Int J Dermatol.* 1990;29:459.
Hook EW III. Acute cellulitis. *Arch Dermatol.* 1987;123:460.
Sachs MK. Cutaneous cellulites. *Arch Dermatol.* 1991; 127:481.

NECROTIZING FASCIITIS

EPIDEMIOLOGY

- Necrotizing fasciitis is categorized into two types of infections.
- Type I necrotizing fasciitis is caused by at least one anaerobic species (most commonly Bacteroides and Peptostreptococcus spp.) in combination with one or more facultative anaerobic species such as streptococci (other than group A) and members of the Enterobacteriaceae family (*E. coli*, Enterobacter, Klebsiella, Proteus).
- Type II necrotizing fasciitis is caused by group A streptococci, isolated either alone or in combination with other species (*S. aureus* most commonly).
- May occur de novo or follow surgery or perforating trauma.

PATHOPHYSIOLOGY

- Aggressive soft-tissue infection, which has centered itself in the superficial fascia and subcutaneous tissue. Infection may involve muscle in severe cases.

CLINICAL FEATURES

- May present only as mild erythema, particularly in the lower extremities. However, the pain may be out of proportion to the other clinical findings. Associated with fever and systemic toxicity.
- Within 24 to 48 hours, the infection extends through the fascial planes. Because nerves and blood vessels that penetrate the fascia are often damaged, edema and erythema quickly progress to patches of dusky blue discoloration and anesthesia.
- Blisters with hemorrhagic fluid commonly present, and by fourth or fifth day, these areas become gangrenous.

DIAGNOSIS AND DIFFERENTIAL

- Early surgical exploration is needed for both diagnosis and therapy. Fascial necrosis is seen through surgical exploration and histopathologic examination.
- MRI may aid in demonstrating the extent of bacterial involvement.
- Suspected cellulitis that does not respond or worsens to antimicrobial treatment alone should be suspected of being necrotizing faciitis. The presence of hemorrhagic blisters or excessive pain should prompt early intervention. An elevated WBC and CPK herald a worse prognosis.

TREATMENT

- Early surgical debridement is essential. Both aerobic and anaerobic cultures should be taken immediately prior to commencing antimicrobial therapy.
- Antibiotic therapy directed at the offending pathogen is indicated. Group A *Streptococcus* and clostridia can be treated with IV clindamycin (600 to 900 mg IV q 8 hr). With suspected polymicrobial infection, utilize drug combination of metronidazole 750 mg IV q 6 hr, ampicillin 2 to 3 g IV q 6 hr, plus gentamicin 1 to 1.5 mg/kg q 8 hr. Hyperbaric oxygen therapy can also be used in clostridial infection.
- Even with appropriate therapy, the mortality rate may reach 50%. Poor prognostic factors include increased age, underlying diabetes, myositis, high white blood cell count, delay of more than 7 days in diagnosis and surgical debridement, use of nonsteroidal anti-inflammatory medication (masks inflammation of a serious infection), and infection on the trunk or head and neck rather than the more commonly involved extremities.

REFERENCES

Banerjee AK. Necrotizing faciitis. *Br J Surg.* 1991;78:1402.
Kaul R, et al. Population-based surveillance for group A streptococcal necrotizing faciitis. *Am J Med.* 1997;103:18.
Majeski JA. Necrotizing faciitis. *Am Fam Physician.* 1984;4:221.

ERYSIPELOID

EPIDEMIOLOGY

- Occupational disease often seen in individuals who handle dead animal matter. Widespread among commercial fisherman, veterinarians, and meat packers.
- *Erysipelothrix rhusiopathiae*, a gram-positive rod, is the causative organism. It is found on dead matter of animal origin, particularly pig and turkey. Also found in saltwater fish, crabs, and other shellfish.

PATHOPHYSIOLOGY

- *E. rhusiopathiae* infection contaminates a wound sustained while handling material containing this organism.

CLINICAL FEATURES

- The lesions are painful, swollen, violaceous plaques with well-defined, irregularly raised borders occurring at site of inoculation. Vesicles frequently occur. Typically seen on the fingers or the hands.
- Lesions may be migratory in nature.

DIAGNOSIS AND DIFFERENTIAL

- Clinical diagnosis is made by history of exposure. Lesional biopsy may lead to isolation of *E. rhusiopathiae*.
- May resemble other bacterial cellulitis or contact dermatitis.

TREATMENT

- Mild cases run a self-limited course, usually clearing after about 3 weeks.
- For localized disease which requires antimicrobial therapy, penicillin 1 g/d for 5 to 10 days or erythromycin 250 mg PO q 6 hr × 7 to 10 days should be effective. IV penicillin may be necessary for severe forms of the disease.

REFERENCES

Barnett JH. Erysipeloid. *J Am Acad Dermatol.* 1983;9:116.
Razsi L, et al. Progressively enlarging painful annular plaque on the hand: Erysipeloid. *Arch Dermatol.* 1994; 130:1311.

ERYTHRASMA

EPIDEMIOLOGY

- Chronic bacterial infection caused by Corynebacterium minutissimum, a gram-positive rod.
- Advancing age, diabetes, obesity, living in warm, humid climates, and prolonged occlusion of the skin predisposes patients to this disease.

PATHOPHYSIOLOGY

- Infection occurs in intertriginous areas with high moisture content. Friction and maceration of the stratum corneum play a role.

CLINICAL FEATURES

- Sharply demarcated, brown, scaly patches and plaques in intertriginous areas.
- May cause burning and itching. Commonly found in the axillae, groin, and webs of toes (particularly between the fourth and fifth interspace). In toe web spaces, erythrasma presents as maceration.

DIAGNOSIS AND DIFFERENTIAL

- Lesions examined with Wood's lamp show a coral red fluorescence (bacteria produces porphyrins). Cultures usually do not yield the organism.
- Tinea cruris and Candida can be excluded with negative KOH preparation. Seborrheic dermatitis usually has predilection for seborrheic areas of face, scalp, and chest. Inverse psoriasis has other features of psoriasis such as nail pitting, scalp lesions, and response to topical steroids.

TREATMENT

- Erythromycin 250 mg PO q.i.d. for 1 week. Also effective is tolnaftate cream or erythromycin solution applied b.i.d. for 2 to 3 weeks.
- Preventative measures include daily use of benzoyl peroxide wash.

REFERENCES

Shelly WB, et al. Coexistent erythrasma, trichomycosis axillaris, and pitted keratolysis. *J Am Acad Dermatol.* 1982;7:752.
Sindhuphak W, et al. Erythrasma. *Int J Dermatol.* 1985;24:95.

TRICHOMYCOSIS AXILLARIS

EPIDEMIOLOGY

- The causative agent is not a fungus, but a variety of aerobic Corynebacterium species.
- Predilection in patients with poor personal hygiene, excessive sweating, and those who do not wear deodorant.

PATHOPHYSIOLOGY

- Large colonies of coryneform bacteria coating the hairs of affected regions.

CLINICAL FEATURES

- Yellow, red, or black waxy nodules forming on the hair in the axillary or pubic areas. There may be associated hyperhidrosis in affected regions.

DIAGNOSIS AND DIFFERENTIAL

- Clinical diagnosis. Affected regions may fluoresce various colors under Wood's lamp.
- Differential diagnosis includes primary or secondary axillary hyperhidrosis.

TREATMENT

- Shaving hairs in the area is usually effective. Encourage use of deodorant.
- May treat with topical antibiotic preparations such as topical clindamycin or erythromycin.

REFERENCES

Shelley WB, et al. Electronmicroscopy, histochemistry, and microbiology of bacterial adhesion in trichomycosis axillaris. *J Am Acad Dermatol.* 1984;10:1005.

Shelly WB, et al. Coexistent erythrasma, trichomycosis axillaris, and pitted keratolysis. *J Am Acad Dermatol.* 1982;7:752.

PITTED KERATOLYSIS

EPIDEMIOLOGY

- Excessive sweating, warm climates, and damp occlusion are predisposing factors.
- Several bacterial agents have been implicated as the causative organism, including *Dermatophilus congolensis* and *Micrococcus sedentarius*.

PATHOPHYSIOLOGY

- Causative bacteria produces enzymes that digest keratin to create pitting in the stratum corneum.

CLINICAL FEATURES

- Weight-bearing portions of the soles covered with shallow, asymptomatic discrete round 1 to 3-mm pits. Some pits become confluent, forming furrows. Less commonly occurs on palms.
- Usually asymptomatic, but may be associated with pruritus, burning, pain, tenderness, and malodor.

DIAGNOSIS AND DIFFERENTIAL

- Clinical diagnosis, given unique appearance.
- Rule out tinea pedis with a KOH preparation.

TREATMENT

- Topical azoles such as miconazole and clotimazole are usually effective. Topical erythromycin and clarithromycin also appear to be effective.
- Benzoyl peroxide gel and aluminum chloride solution may decrease sweating.

REFERENCES

Nordstom KM, et al. Pitted keratolysis. *Arch Dermatol.* 1987;123:1320.

Takama H, et al. Pitted keratolysis. *Br J Dermatol.* 1997; 137:282.

SCARLET FEVER

EPIDEMIOLOGY

- Occurs during outbreak of pharyngitis, with the causative organism being group A beta-hemolytic *Streptococcus pyogenes* (GAS). Uncommonly caused by exotoxin-producing *Staphylococcus aureus*.
- Scarlet fever primarily affects children.

PATHOPHYSIOLOGY

- The incubation period is about 1 to 3 days. The upper respiratory tract is the usual portal of entry.
- The exanthem is produced by erythrogenic, exotoxin-producing group A streptococci. There are three antigenically unrelated types of the toxin: A, B, and C. Type B is the most frequent toxin responsible for cases in the United States, Germany, and England.

CLINICAL FEATURES

- Fever and pharyngitis is followed shortly by nausea, vomiting, headache, and abdominal pain. A diffuse erythematous exanthem develops 24 to 48 hours after onset of pharyngeal symptoms.
- The exanthem features small erythematous papules (with "sandpaper feel") starting on the neck and spreading to the trunk and extremities. The palms and soles are usually spared. Linear petechiae occur over the body folds (Pastia's sign). The exanthem fades within 4 to 5 days and is followed by desquamation of the trunk and extremities, and a sheet-like exfoliation of the palms by 2 weeks.
- The tonsils are red, edematous, and covered with hemorrhages. The tongue is bright red with prominent papillae and white coating ("strawberry tongue"). A transverse groove may be produced on all of the nails (Beau's lines).

DIAGNOSIS AND DIFFERENTIAL

- Diagnosis is based on clinical features and confirmation of streptococcal antigen on rapid strep test and/or throat swab cultures. Serology may show an elevated antistreptolysin O titer if cultures are not taken early.
- Other processes that manifest by generalized exanthem include enteroviral exanthems, drug eruption, Kawasaki's syndrome, and staphylococcal or streptococcal toxic shock syndrome.

TREATMENT

- Treat pain and fever with aspirin or acetaminophen.
- Penicillin is the antibiotic of choice because of its effectiveness in preventing rheumatic fever. Given as penicillin G 1.2 million units IM in adults and 600,000 units IM in children, or by penicillin V 250 mg PO q.i.d. for 10 days. Erythromycin, azithromycin, or cephalosporin may also be used.

- Streptococcal infection may result in acute rheumatic fever, acute glomerulonephritis, and erythema nodosum.

REFERENCES

Del Castillo LD, et al. Group A streptococcal pharyngitis and scarlatiniform rash in an 8-week-old infant. *Am J Emerg Med.* 2000;18:233.

Golledge C. Sore throat and a rash. *Aust Fam Physician.* 1999;28:379.

Weisse ME. The fourth disease, 1900–2000. *Lancet.* 2001;357:299.

STAPHYLOCOCCAL SCALDED SKIN SYNDROME

EPIDEMIOLOGY

- Most commonly affects neonates during the first 3 months of life, and young children. Occurs rarely in adults, with immunosupression and renal failure being predisposing factors.
- Age distribution thought to be secondary to reduced renal clearance of toxin in neonates and lack of neutralizing antibodies to the toxin.

PATHOPHYSIOLOGY

- Colonizing or localized infection of *Staphylococcus aureus* from distant focus on the body produces exotoxin (ET-A and ET-B) that reaches other areas of the skin. Toxin causes acanthosis and intraepidermal cleavage just below the stratum granulosum. This results in exfoliation of the skin. The toxin binds to desmoglein 1.

CLINICAL FEATURES

- Patients present with fever, skin tenderness, and erythema primarily in flexural and periorificial areas. There is sparing of the palms, soles, and axillae.
- Blisters and generalized exfoliation develop within 24 to 48 hours. Firm rubbing of the skin produces disruption of the skin (positive Nikolsky's sign).

DIAGNOSIS AND DIFFERENTIAL

- Clinical findings with cultures from mucous membranes or other infected foci helps confirm the

diagnosis. Frozen sections of the blister roof show mainly stratum corneum.
- Differential diagnosis includes toxic epidermal necrolysis, which demonstrates full thickness cleavage and necrotic epidermis on frozen section. Staph/strep toxic shock syndrome typically have more systemic organ involvement. Others in differential include Kawasaki's syndrome, erythema multiforme, Rocky Mountain spotted fever, rubeola, and enteroviral exanthems.

TREATMENT

- Hospitalization is recommended for neonates and young children. Antibiotic therapy is necessary with a penicillinase-resistant penicillin. Oxacillin or dicloxacillin are commonly used. Volume status and electrolytes should be maintained due to loss of fluids through exfoliation.
- Topical antimicrobial therapy may be applied to impetiginized foci.
- The prognosis is good.

REFERENCES

Cribier B, et al. Staphylococcal scaled skin syndrome in adults. *J Am Acad Dermatol.* 1994;30:319.

Pollak S. Staphylococcal scaled skin syndrome. *Pediatr Rev.* 1996;17:18.

Sahn EE. Vesiculopustular diseases of neonates and infants. *Curr Opin Pediatr.* 1994;6:442.

STAPHYLOCOCCAL TOXIC SHOCK SYNDROME

EPIDEMIOLOGY

- Caused by toxin-producing strains of *Staphylococcus aureus*.
- Original cases described in young women who developed illness during first and sixth days of the menstrual period. The majority of these women were using superabsorbent tampons.
- Other cases have been associated in women using sponges for contraception, patients with nasal packing after rhinoplasty, and patients with other local staphylococcal infections.

PATHOPHYSIOLOGY

- Toxic shock syndrome toxin-1 (TSST-1), which is produced by certain staphylococcal species, is responsible for the disease.
- Histopathology shows spongiosis, scattered neutrophils in the epidermis, necrotic keratinocytes, and perivascular and interstitial lymphocytic and neutophillic infiltrates.

CLINICAL FEATURES

- Sudden onset of fever associated with vomiting, diarrhea, headache, pharyngitis, myalgia, and hypotension.
- A diffuse, erythematous, macular exanthemous eruption develops on the trunk, which eventually spreads to the arms and legs. The rash favors flexural regions of body. Palms and soles become erythematous and edematous. Mucous membranes, including conjunctivae, become intensely erythematous.
- Generalized desquamation with prominent sheet-like peeling of the hands and feet occurs around 10 to 21 days after presentation.

DIAGNOSIS AND DIFFERENTIAL

- Diagnosed by clinical features exhibiting the following criteria: temperature over 38.9°C, an erythematous rash, desquamation of the palms and soles 1 to 2 weeks after onset of rash, hypotension, and involvement of three or more other systems (gastrointestinal, muscular, mucous membrane, renal, central nervous system).
- Differential diagnosis includes other processes that produce exanthemous rash such as enteroviral exanthems, Rocky Mountain spotted fever, Kawasaki's disease, scarlet fever, and drug eruptions.

TREATMENT

- Must first manage multisystem organ involvement of illness. Volume status must be maintained due to massive extravascular fluid loss, desquamation, and fever. Cardiovascular pressor agents may be required. Remove offending foreign body, if found, or drain the focus of infection, if present.
- Systemic antibiotics are needed to cover staphylococcal species, such as nafcillin (1 to 1.5 g) IV q 4 hr.

REFERENCES

Bach MC. Dermatologic signs of toxic shock syndrome. *J Am Acad Dermatol.* 1983;8:343.

Eykyn SJ. Staphylococcal sepsis. *Lancet.* 1988;1:100.

Kain KC, et al. Clinical spectrum of nonmenstrual TSS. *Clin Infect Dis.* 1993;16:100.

STREPTOCOCCAL TOXIC SHOCK SYNDROME

EPIDEMIOLOGY

- Caused by type A streptococci. Eighty percent of the isolates produce pyrogenic exotoxin A.
- Increasing age, diabetes, alcoholism, trauma, and prevalence of invasive strains in the community are predisposing risk factors.

PATHOPHYSIOLOGY

- The portals of entry for streptococci are the pharynx, skin, and vagina in 50% of cases.
- The streptococci produce pyrogenic exotoxins that have the ability to cause fever, enhance susceptibility to endotoxin, suppress IgM-antibody synthesis, and act as superantigens. This leads to the induction of cytokine synthesis, which plays an important role in the production of shock and organ failure.

CLINICAL FEATURES

- Patients present with hypotension and multiorgan failure, similar to the systemic involvement in staphylococcal TSS. Most of the patients have a diffuse exanthemous rash at the time of presentation. This leads to generalized erythroderma with desquamation and localized cellulitis with vesiculation or bulla formation.
- Unlike in staphylococcal TSS, however, a focus of pyogenic inflammation is usually present, such as necrotizing fasciitis. A large proportion of the patients develop bacteremia. This infection is usually rapidly progressive, and destructive soft-tissue injury from infection is common.

DIAGNOSIS AND DIFFERENTIAL

- Shock and multiorgan failure with associated necrotizing infection should prompt attention to this diagnosis. Laboratory findings include rising BUN/creatinine and creatine phosphokinase levels.
- Differential diagnosis includes staphylococcal TSS, enteroviral exanthems, Rocky Mountain spotted fever, Kawasaki's disease, scarlet fever, and drug eruptions.

TREATMENT

- Presentation may require patient stabilization with IV fluids and pressors.
- Prompt and aggressive surgical exploration and debridement of suspected deep-seated streptococcal infection are mandatory. Once necrosis is determined, debridement is necessary. Amputation is not an uncommon sequelae.
- Prompt antimicrobial therapy with empiric broad-spectrum coverage for septic shock should be instituted. Once the streptococcal cause is confirmed, high-dose penicillin and clindamycin should be given. In addition, several reports have described the successful use of intravenous gammaglobulin in patients with streptococcal TSS.
- Streptococcal TSS has a case fatality rate of 30 to 40%. The rapidity with which shock and multiorgan failure can progress is impressive, and many patients die within 24 to 48 hours of hospitalization.

REFERENCES

Cone LA, et al. Clinical and bacteriologic observations of a toxic shock-like syndrome due to *S. pyogenes. N Engl J Med.* 1987;317:146.

Hoge CW, et al. The changing epidemiology of invasive group A streptococcal infections and the emergence of streptococcal toxic shock-like syndrome. *JAMA.* 1993;269:384.

Taub DD. Superantigens and microbial pathogenesis. *Ann Intern Med.* 1993;119:89.

CUTANEOUS TUBERCULOSIS

EPIDEMIOLOGY

- Caused by *Mycobacterium tuberculosis*, a non-spore-forming anaerobic rod demonstrating acid-fastness by the Ziehl–Neelsen method.
- More commonly found in infants and immunodeficient adults. Predisposing factors include close contact, poverty, intravenous drug use, and immunodeficient states. Seen more commonly in Third-World countries.

PATHOPHYSIOLOGY

- Cutaneous tuberculosis is transmitted by three routes. The patient may be exogenously infected via percutaneous inoculation in an immunocompromised host (primary inoculation tuberculosis or tuberculosis verrucosa cutis). Cutaneous tuberculosis may also be contiguously spread through an endogenous source with breakdown of the overlying skin (scrofuloderma), or spread via lymphatics (lupus vulgaris). Cutaneous tuberculosis may by hematogenously disseminated (lupus vulgaris and miliary tuberculosis). Finally, cutaneous tuberculosis may be autoinoculated from extensive internal organ involvement.
- Tuberculoid granulomas containing epithelioid cells, Langhans' giant cells, lymphocytes, and caseation necrosis are seen on histopathology.

CLINICAL FEATURES

- Cutaneous tuberculosis manifests clinically depending on the route of infection, virulence of the organism, and immune status of the patient.
- *Primary inoculation tuberculosis*: Initial papule at the inoculation site, which enlarges to a painless indurated ulceration. It is associated with lymphadenopathy. Commonly found on exposed skin at site of minor injury. The patient has no prior exposure to tuberculosis.
- *Tuberculosis verrucosa cutis*: Initial erythematous papule with violaceous halo at inoculation site, enlarging to become an irregular, crusty keratoic plaque. There is no associated lymphadenopathy. Primary site on dorsolateral hands and fingers. This occurs in patients previously sensitized to the organism.
- *Lupus vulgaris*: Initial erythematous papule at infected site that develops into reddish-brown plaque. Diascopy (pressing glass slide against the skin) reveals an "apple-jelly" color. Typically located on head and neck, and gradually spreads. May involve mucous membranes. Occurs in previously sensitized individuals.
- *Scrofuloderma*: Hard subcutaneous nodule that becomes soft and evolves into an irregular plaque. This liquefies and becomes a large violaceous abscess, and invariably is contiguous with involved adenopathy. It is more common in children.
- *Acute miliary tuberculosis*: Erythematous macules and papules disseminated on all parts of the body, but often favoring the trunk. Occurs in immunosuppressed adults or children. Focus of infection is typically pulmonary or meningeal.
- *Oroficial tuberculosis*: Rare condition involving tuberculosis of the mucous membranes and skin surrounding orifices caused by autoinoculation into these areas. Generally, these patients have tuberculosis of the internal organs. The mouth is the most common site. Presents as a painful red nodule that forms a punched-out ulceration.

DIAGNOSIS AND DIFFERENTIAL

- Need high index of clinical suspicion. May show positive tuberculin skin test. However, may not be helpful in immunocompromized individuals, or those with miliary TB.
- To confirm with certainty, need to demonstrate acid-fast bacilli in the lesion via microscopy (acid-fast staining), culture (up to 8 weeks), or polymerase chain reaction.
- Differential diagnosis depends on the subtype of cutaneous tuberculosis. Primary inoculation tuberculosis can be similar to cat-scratch fever, primary chancre (syphilis), tularemia, sporotrichosis, and actinomycosis. Verruca vulgaris, seborrheic keratosis, and blastomycosis may be mistaken for tuberculosis verrucosa cutis. Lupus vulgaris may mimic discoid lupus, sarcoidosis, or other mycoses. Scrofuloderma resembles tertiary syphilis, actinomycosis.

TREATMENT

- Therapy for cutaneous tuberculosis consists of 6 months of antibiotic chemotherapy. This includes 4 months of isoniazid, rifampin, pyrazinamide, and ethambutol for 2 months, followed by rifampin and isoniazid for an additional 4 months. A cure rate of around 95% can be expected in patients undergoing a strict regimen.

REFERENCES

Barnes PF, et al. Tuberculosis in the 1990s. *Ann Intern Med.* 1993;119:400.

MacGregor RR. Cutaneous tuberculosis. *Clin Dermatol.* 1995;13:245.

Pozniak A. Multi-drug resistant tuberculosis and HIV infection. *Ann NY Acad Sci.* 2001;953:192.

ATYPICAL MYCOBACTERIAL INFECTIONS

EPIDEMIOLOGY

- Atypical mycobacteria are a heterogeneous group of pathogens grouped by their rate of growth and ability to produce pigment. Atypical mycobacteria are classified into slow-growing photochromogens (*Mycobacterium marinum*, *M. kanasii*) and nonchromogens (*M. avium* and *M. kansasii*), and fast-growing mycobacteria (*M. fortuitum* and *M. chelonae*).

- Most cutaneous lesions caused by atypical mycobacteria are caused by *M. marinum* and *M. ulcerans.* These pathogens are commonly found in water and soil.
- *M. marinum* infection, which is commonly referred to as "swimming pool" granuloma or "fish tank" granuloma, occurs in individuals with aquatic occupations, who are continuously around water, or who maintain fish tanks, and are at increased risk for inoculation.
- *M. ulcerans*, an environmental saprophyte, is generally found in individuals living in subequatorial regions.
- *M. kansasii* is found particularly in temperate zones of the world, and is most often associated with pulmonary disease in middle-aged men.
- *M. avium* complex lesions occur after traumatic inoculation or as the result of disseminated infection. Infection is frequently seen in immunocompromised patients.
- *M. fortuitum* and *M. chelonae* are commonly found in water or soil, and inoculate into the skin via trauma.

PATHOPHYSIOLOGY

- In general, these organisms have low-grade pathogenicity. The mycobacterium is inoculated into the skin during an environmental exposure (*M. marinum*, *M. ulcerans*, *M. fortuitum*) or hematogenous spread (*M. kansasii*, *M. avium* complex). Following exposure, incubation period typically lasts a few weeks to months.
- Histologic features range from acute and chronic inflammation to well-formed tuberculoid granuloma.

CLINICAL FEATURES

- *M. marinum* infection: At the site of inoculation, there are verrucous, violaceous papules/plaques/nodules with central clearing. Sporotrichoid spread is commonly seen. Usually found at skin sites prone to trauma, such as hands, feet, elbow, or knee. Heals with scarring.
- *M. ulcerans* infection: Patients present with a solitary nodule that ulcerates with undermined edges. Lesions are typically found on the arms and legs.
- *M. kansasii* infection: Patients present with verrucous nodules, papules, pustules, and crusted ulcerations.
- *M. avium* complex infection: While this infection affects the lungs and lymph nodes, cutaneous lesions may occur after hematogenous spread. Lesions consist of papules and ulcers.

- *M. fortuitum* and *M. chelonae* infections: Patients present with red, painful lesions at the site of trauma (e.g., infection or surgery). These lesions may develop into an abscess.

DIAGNOSIS AND DIFFERENTIAL

- Diagnosis is confirmed by histopathology or by isolating the mycobacterium from a lesion culture.
- Differential diagnosis includes fungal infections such as sporotrichosis, blastomycosis, histoplasmosis, and coccidiomycosis. *M. tuberculosis* (tuberculosis verrucosa cutis), nocardiosis, leichmaniasis, and syphilis should also be considered.

TREATMENT

- Lesions are typically benign and occasionally, self-limited (except *M. ulcerans*).
- A consensus for ideal therapeutic antibiotic regimens has yet to be established. Initially treat with doxycycline, minocycline, or clarithromycin until sensitivities from cultures become available.
- For *M. ulcerans* infection, the treatment of choice is surgery aimed at removing the lesion.

REFERENCES

French AL, et al. Nontuberculosis mycobacterial infections. *Med Clin North Am.* 1997;81:361.

Gluckman SJ. Mycobacterium marinum. *Clin Dermatol.* 1995;13:273.

Street ML, et al. Nontuberculosis mycobacterial infections of the skin. *J Am Acad Dermatol.* 1991;24:208.

HANSEN'S DISEASE (LEPROSY)

EPIDEMIOLOGY

- Leprosy is caused by *Mycobacterium leprae*, an acid-fast bacillus.
- There are five variants of Hansen's disease, representing a clinical, histologic, and immunologic spectrum: tuberculoid tuberculoid (TT), borderline tuberculoid (BT), borderline borderline (BB), borderline lepromatous (BL), and lepromatous lepromatous (LL). In India and Africa, 60% of cases are of the tuberculoid type, whereas in Mexico, 90% of cases are of the lepromatous variant.

- Children and young adults are most susceptible to developing Hansen's disease.
- Leprosy is common throughout the tropics. In the United States, Southern Texas and Louisiana are considered endemic regions. Infected wild armadillos have been found in Louisiana.
- Prevalent in hot and humid climates. Predisposing factors include residence in an endemic area, having a blood relative with leprosy, close contact, poverty, and contact with infected armadillos.

PATHOPHYSIOLOGY

- *M. leprae* is most likely transmitted via the nasorespiratory route. The incubation period is 3 to 5 years. The bacilli have a predilection for neural tissue. The bacilli grow best at low temperatures; therefore the cooler areas of the body, such as the ear lobes, are usually affected.
- Patients with tuberculoid leprosy have a high degree of immunity against *M. leprae*. Therefore, the infection is limited to a few skin sites and peripheral nerves. Histology shows tuberculoid granulomas around nerves and skin appendages with a dense lymphocytic infiltrate.
- Patients with lepromatous leprosy have low immunity against *M. leprae* and have numerous skin lesions. The bacilli spread via the bloodstream to cool areas of body and skin, and to peripheral nerves. Histology shows a thin epidermis and flat rete ridges, with the dermis containing enormous numbers of acid-fast bacilli.

CLINICAL FEATURES

- Hansen's disease affects the skin, peripheral nerves, anterior part of the eyes, and nasal area. The major clinical features recognized are the visible skin lesions or areas of cutaneous anesthesia.
- *Tuberculoid leprosy* (*TT*): Lesions are few in number, and consist of asymmetrically distributed, sharply demarcated, erythematous scaly plaques. The lesions may be hypopigmented are usually dry and hairless. They are commonly located on the face, limbs, or trunk. The scalp, axillae, groin, and perineum are not involved. Sensation may be lost within the center of the skin lesion. Cutaneous anesthesia occurs early and is prominent and well defined. Nerve enlargement is marked, especially in the superficial peroneal nerve and the greater auricular nerve. There may be atrophy and wasting of the muscles of the hands and fingers. Mucosal and systemic involvement is absent.

- *Lepromatous leprosy* (*LL*): Lesions are numerous, and consist of symmetrically distributed, poorly demarcated, hypopigmented macules. Lesions may occur anywhere on the body, but are commonly seen on the face, arms, legs, and buttocks. There is little or no loss of sensation over the lesions. Cutaneous anesthesia occurs late, initially as slight and ill-defined, but becoming extensive. The longest peripheral nerves are the first to be affected. A slow progressive loss of hair occurs on the outer portion of the eyebrows, eyelashes, and finally, the whole body. The face may become diffusely infiltrated, with loss of eyebrows and the development of a waxy, shiny appearance. Nodules may develop, called lepromas, and occur on the acral parts of the body. The nasal mucosa may be infiltrated with organisms, and if untreated, may cause chronic nasal congestion and epistaxis, leading to a "saddle nose" deformity.
- *Borderline lepromatous leprosy* (*BL*): Lesions have varying morphology. Annular, poorly demarcated lesions are characteristic. Loss of sensation present.
- *Borderline tuberculoid leprosy* (*BT*): Lesions are smaller and more numerous than TT leprosy.
- *Borderline leprosy* (*BB*): Borderline leprosy is unstable, and the disease progresses toward the lepromatous spectum if untreated, and toward the tuberculoid variant if treated.
- *Indeterminate leprosy*: This classification is assigned to an early lesion that appears before the host makes an immunologic response. Clinically, the lesion is a hypopigmented macule with or without a sensory deficit.

DIAGNOSIS AND DIFFERENTIAL

- Diagnosed primarily by demonstrating cutaneous anesthesia, enlarged peripheral nerves, and histopathology demonstrating leprosy bacilli. *M. leprae* may be demonstrated by a slit skin smear (ear lobes commonly used) or skin biopsy.
- Differential diagnosis depends on lesion type at presentation and includes atopic dermatitis, vitiligo, pityriasis versicolor, and tinea corporis for macular presentation. Plaque lesions have a differential including sarcoidosis and cutaneous tuberculosis. Finally, nodular presentation (including leonine facies) includes leishmania and scleromyxedema.

TREATMENT

- The evolution of lesions is slow in tuberculoid leprosy, and there can be spontaneous remission of the lesions within 3 years. The National Hansen's Disease Program and World Health Organization have standard treatment regimens. Antibacillary therapy regimens are based on whether smears or tissue sections are multibacillary (bacilli detectable) or paucibacillary (no bacilli detectable).

- *National Hansen's Disease Program*: For multibacillary leprosy, the regimen is rifampin 600 mg daily, dapsone 100 mg daily, and clofazimine 50 mg daily for 2 years. For paucibacillary leprosy, the regimen is rifampin 600 mg daily and dapsone 100 mg daily for 1 year.
- *World Health Organization*: For multibacillary leprosy, the regimen is rifampicin 600 mg once a month, dapsone 100 mg daily, and clofazimine 300 mg monthly and 50 mg daily for 1 year. For paucibacillary leprosy, the regimen is rifampicin 600 mg monthly and dapsone 100 mg daily for 6 months.
- Approximately one-half of all Hansen's patients experience one of two acute inflammatory episodes, once therapy has been initiated. *Reversal reaction* (type I reaction) is seen in borderline leprosy, representing an upgrade or downgrade in cell-mediated immunity towards *M. leprae*. The patient's existing lesions become acutely inflamed and edematous. There is no systemic involvement. A major complication of this cell-mediated inflammation is an acute neuritis. In this setting, nerves may become enlarged, tender, and lose function, making this type I reaction a medical emergency. Treatment with prednisone may be required. *Erythema nodosum leprosum* (*ENL*) (type II reaction) is seen in lepromatous leprosy, representing precipitation of *M. leprae* immune complexes in blood vessels (vasculitis) as the result of antibiotic therapy. Systemic involvement is present, represented by fever, myalgias, and anorexia. Skin lesions are erythematous, painful nodules on the extremities, not occurring at sites of previous skin lesions. In diffuse leprosy (Lepra Bonita), a severe type II reaction can occur (Lucio's Phenomenon). Treatment may consist of conventional anti-inflammatory therapy and thalidomide.

REFERENCES

Marlowe SN, et al. Update on leprosy. *Hosp Med.* 2001; 62:471.
Myers WM. Leprosy. *Dermatol Clin.* 1992;10:73.
Sehgal VN. Leprosy. *Dermatol Clin.* 1994;12:629.

8 VIRAL INFECTIONS

Jeffrey J. Meffert
Jay L. Viernes
Sandra P. Osswald
Chetan Maingi

HERPES SIMPLEX VIRUS (HSV)

EPIDEMIOLOGY

- Exists as two closely related DNA virus types, HSV 1 and HSV 2. Each has affinities for different body sites. Approximately 90% of infections caused by HSV 1 are oral-labial, and 90% caused by HSV 2 are genital. However, either viral type can cause disease in both areas. They are clinically indistinguishable.
- Oral labial HSV affects about one-third of the both the world and U.S. populations. Worldwide, more than 85% of adults show serologic evidence of prior HSV 1 exposure.
- Genital lesions due to HSV 2 affect about 23% of the U.S. population and are increasing.

PATHOPHYSIOLOGY

- Primary infection is the first viral exposure in a seronegative individual. The virus initially enters the host through abraded skin or intact mucous membranes. Epithelial cells are the initial targets. After infection, these injured epithelial cells die, with the resulting inflammation causing vesicle or blister formation, and merge with other cells to create multinucleated giant cells.
- After a primary infection, the virus establishes latency in the sensory nerve ganglia innervating that site. Retrograde transport through adjacent neural tissue to sensory ganglia leads to life-long latency. Various stimuli, such as fever, stress, menses, immunodeficiency, trauma, and ultraviolet light, can provoke virus reactivation.
- Once reactivated, the virus is transported by the neuron back to the epithelium, where more replication occurs, and another outbreak begins. Although recurrences are generally less severe than the initial/primary infection, it is through asymptomatic recurrences that most disease is transmitted.

CLINICAL FEATURES

OROLABIAL HERPES
- Primary orolabial infection manifests after about 5 to 10 days from exposure.
- Most common in children and young adults.
- May present with spectrum of subclinical to severe—typically with painful vesicles and/or ulcerative erosions on the lips, gingiva, buccal mucosa, tongue, and palate. Edema, halitosis, and drooling may be present, along with tender submandibular and cervical lymphadenopathy. Systemic symptoms are often present, including fever, malaise, and myalgia.
- Duration of primary illness is about 2 to 3 weeks and oral shedding of virus may continue for as long as 23 days.
- Recurrence 3 to 4 times/year, usually shorter and less discomforting than the primary infection. Lesions are often single and more localized, often at the border of the lip and heal in 8 to 10 days. Pain is present for about 4 to 5 days.

GENITAL HERPES
- Primary genital infection has an incubation period of 2 to 12 days (mean 4 days), followed with a prodrome of itching, burning, and erythema.
- The prodrome is followed by multiple, grouped painful vesicles that appear on the penis, perineum, vulva, vagina, or cervix, along with tender inguinal lymphadenopathy. The vesicles progress to ulcers in a few days. Accompanying symptoms can include dysuria and urinary retention. Systemic symptoms are common in primary disease and include fever, headache, malaise, abdominal pain, and myalgia.
- Duration of primary illness in immunocompetent patients is 7 to 10 days, with complete resolution of lesions in 3 weeks. Shedding of viable viral particles occur frequently. Of concern is that up to 90% of infected individuals are asymptomatically shedding viable virus.
- Recurrences typically occur within 1 year of the primary infection and recur about 3 to 4 times a year.

Outbreaks are heralded by a prodrome of burning or tingling at the site of the outbreak. Symptoms are usually less severe and shorter in duration than the initial outbreak.

OTHER

- Neonatal herpes occurs upon exposure of neonate to infected maternal vaginal secretions during delivery, and if left untreated, is associated with a high mortality rate.
- Herpes gladiatorum is a cutaneous or ocular HSV 1 infection acquired in wrestlers or other athletes through sports contact due to direct skin to skin contact.
- Herpetic whitlow is herpes infection of the fingers or hands.
- Erythema multiforme can follow recurrent herpes infections.

DIAGNOSIS AND DIFFERENTIAL

- Diagnosis can often be made by clinical presentation that shows grouped vesicles and/or erosions on an erythematous base on mucocutaneous surfaces.
- Diagnosis can be confirmed by performing any of the following tests:
  1. Tzanck smear (find presence of multinucleated keratinocytic giant cells, which signifies presence of a herpes virus family infection)
  2. Direct fluorescent antibody (DFA) test/polymerase chain reaction (PCR)
  3. Tissue biopsy
  4. Viral culture (gold standard) of vesicular fluid or skin biopsy material
  5. Serologic studies are not helpful, since positivity merely indicates prior exposure.
- Differential diagnoses for primary orolabial HSV infection include: aphthous ulcers, candidiasis, pemphigus, erythema multiforme, bacterial pharyngitis, enterovirus infections (such as hand-foot-mouth and herpangina), and primary HIV infection. Recurrent orolabial infections include impetigo, aphthous stomatitis, and erythema multiforme. Primary and recurrent genital HSV infections include: syphilis, lymphogranuloma venereum, chancroid, gonorrhea, candidiasis, granuloma inguinale, and trauma.

TREATMENT

PRIMARY OROLABIAL HERPES

- Acyclovir 200 mg five times daily for 5 days (older children and adults) or 15 mg/kg five times daily for 7 days (children up to age 6 years).

- Standard analgesic therapy with acetaminophen or ibuprofen, careful monitoring of hydration status, and aggressive early rehydration are usually sufficient to prevent inpatient admission for most children.
- Topical medication is not significantly effective.

PRIMARY GENITAL HERPES

To reduce or shorten length of time with symptoms:
- Acyclovir (Zovirax) 200 mg five times daily for 10 days *or*
- Famciclovir (Famvir) 250 mg three times daily for 10 days *or*
- Valacyclovir (Valtrex) 1 g twice daily for 10 days

RECURRENT GENITAL OR ORAL HERPES

For "suppressive therapy" to reduce frequency of recurrences and amount of viral shedding:
- Acyclovir 400 mg twice daily *or*
- Famciclovir 250 mg twice daily *or*
- Valacyclovir 1 g once daily (or 500 mg once daily for <10 outbreaks/year)

EPISODIC TREATMENTS

To reduce symptoms and infectivity during recurrences:
- Acyclovir 200 mg five times daily or 800 mg twice daily for 5 days *or*
- Famciclovir 125 mg twice daily for 5 days *or*
- Valacyclovir 500 mg twice daily for 5 days

  The above treatments do NOT influence the frequency or number of recurrences and cannot eradicate latent virus nor affect the long-term natural history of the infection.

INFECTION IN PREGNANT WOMEN

- Consult high-risk obstetrics physician.
- High risk for TORCH syndrome for infections acquired in first trimester.
- High risk for neonatal herpes for infections acquired late in pregnancy and without completed seroconversion before labor and/or active lesions at time of delivery. Antiviral therapy at week 36 and cesarean section to minimize neonatal exposure to virus.

TREATMENT

- Abstention from sexual activity or limiting life-time number of sexual partners to prevent exposure and transmission of virus.
- Use of condoms to limit exposure.
- Education about transmission and shedding to avoid high-risk exposure.
- Education about autoinoculation to prevent spread to nongenital areas of body.

- There are currently no effective vaccines to prevent transmission.

REFERENCES

Amir J, Hare L, Semtana Z, Varsan I. Treatment of herpes simplex gingivostomatitis with acyclovir in children: A randomized double blind placebo controlled study. *Br Med J.* 1997; 314:1800.

Corey L, Holmes KK. Genital herpes simplex virus infections: Clinical manifestations, course, and complications. *Ann Intern Med.* 1992;116:197.

Johnson RE, Nahmias AJ, Magder LS. A seroepidemiologic survey of the prevalence of herpes simplex virus type 2 infection in the United States. N Engl J Med. 1990;321:7.

Mertz GJ. Epidemiology of genital herpes infections. *Infect Dis Clin North Am.* 1993;7:825.

Su SJ, Wu HH, Lin YH, Lin HY. Comparative studies of types 1 and 2 herpes simplex virus infection of cultured normal keratinocytes. *J Clin Pathol.* 1995;48:75.

Wald A. Virologic characteristics of subclinical and symptomatic genital herpes infections. *N Engl J Med.* 1995;333:770.

Whitley RJ, Kimberlin DW, Roizman B. Herpes simplex viruses. *Clin Infect Dis.* 1998;26:541.

VARICELLA ZOSTER VIRUS (VZV)

EPIDEMIOLOGY

- A member of the human herpes virus family. It is a double-stranded DNA virus that is unique in that it can produce two different syndromes: varicella (chickenpox) and herpes zoster (shingles).
- VZV infections occur worldwide, and both genders are affected equally. In the absence of vaccination, almost all persons acquire varicella over the course of their lifetime; an estimated 4 million cases occur annually in the United States, with the highest incidence occurring in children ages 5 to 9 years. By age 11 years, less than 10% of all children remain susceptible.
- The prevalence of herpes zoster increases dramatically among individuals over 50 years old to approximately 1010 per 100,000 people per year among people 80 to 90 years old (from 74 per 100,000 among children less than 10 years old).

PATHOPHYSIOLOGY

PRIMARY VARICELLA

- Acquired by inhalation of respiratory secretions or contact with skin lesions, varicella typically infects the mucosa in the upper respiratory tract or the conjunctiva.
- Followed by the first cycle of viral replication in the regional lymph nodes on days 2 to 4, and a primary viremia between days 4 and 6.
- The second replication cycle follows in the liver, spleen, and other organs, and a secondary viremia, which distributes viral particles which invade first the capillary endothelial cells, then the capillaries, and ultimately, the epidermis on about days 14 to 16.

HERPES ZOSTER

- It is believed that during the course of primary varicella, the VZV spreads from the skin and mucosal lesions into the sensory nerve endings.
- From there, it travels centripetally along these nerve fibers until it reaches the dorsal ganglion cells where it enters a "latent" state.
- The virus, probably due to a decline in cell-mediated immunity, it is reactivated. The CMI decline is seen in persons with increased incidence of shingles, including the elderly and persons with HIV infection or other immunocompromising conditions, such as organ transplantation (with immunosuppression), malignancy requiring chemotherapy or radiation therapy, or long-term corticosteroid use.
- After reactivation, the VZV undergoes an initial phase of replication within the affected sensory ganglion and produces active ganglionitis. The inflammatory response and neuronal necrosis that result cause a severe neuralgia. The pain intensifies as the virus moves down the sensory nerve, producing a radiculoneuritis.

CLINICAL FEATURES

PRIMARY VARICELLA

- Prodrome of headache, myalgia, nausea, anorexia, and vomiting in older children and adults a few days before skin lesions.
- In young children, prodrome may not occur; simultaneous onset of rash, low-grade fever, and malaise.
- Small, red macules appear on the face and trunk and progress rapidly over 12 to 14 hours to papules, vesicles, pustules, and finally crusts. Lesions are typically more abundant centrally and on the proximal upper extremities (including palms and soles) and are present in all stages of development. The characteristic vesicle is often characterized as a "dewdrop on a rose petal." Pruritus is usually present. Crusted lesions ultimately resolve over 1 to 2 weeks.
- In immunocompetent children, the disease is often benign and self-limiting, lasting about 1 week or less. The most common complication is secondary bacterial

infection (with strep or staph) with subsequent scarring. In adult varicella, varicella pneumonia is a frequent complication occurring in 1/400 cases. The mortality rate in adult varicella pneumonia is high, with death occurring in 10% of immunocompetent and 30% of immunocompromised patients.

- In immunocompromised hosts, the disease may be more severe with greater number of lesions, prolonged healing time, visceral complications, and resulting increased mortality.
- Reye's syndrome has been linked with varicella infection and aspirin use.
- Neonatal varicella occurs when maternal varicella occurs from 5 days before to 2 days after delivery and is associated with increased infant mortality. Maternal varicella occurring between 8 and 20 weeks of gestation causes fetal varicella syndrome (prematurity, low birth weight, hypoplasia, and ocular/neurologic abnormalities).

HERPES ZOSTER

- Intense pain (hyperesthesia, paresthesias, burning dysesthesias) and/or pruritus in the involved dermatome typically precedes the rash of herpes zoster by 1 to 3 days in more than 90% of patients. The thoracic dermatome is most frequently involved, followed by the lumbar, trigeminal, cervical, and sacral dermatomes. The pain is subject to a wide variety of misdiagnoses depending on the location including myocardial infarction, pleurisy, cholecystitis, appendicitis, ulcer, herniated disks, thrombophlebitis, or biliary or renal colic. Some patients may have symptoms without developing the characteristic rash (known as "zoster sine herpete").
- About 5% of patients have a prodrome of fever, malaise, and headache.
- A unilateral dermatomal rash appears as erythematous macules and papules, which progress to vesicles (within 12 to 24 hours), then to pustules (3 to 4 days), and finally to crusts (7 to 10 days). Scarring can result, especially in dark skinned patients. There can be regionally lymphadenopathy. Pain can be severe requiring narcotic analgesics.
- Like chickenpox, the pain and rash of zoster are usually more severe in immunocompromised patients.
- Ophthalmic zoster is zoster localized to the ophthalmic branch of the trigeminal nerve (VI). Presence of lesions on the tip or side of the nose (Hutchinson's sign) reflects VI distribution and may indicate ocular involvement. Scarring of the cornea can occur.
- Herpes zoster oticus is zoster localized to the geniculate ganglion. This syndrome, called "Ramsay Hunt syndrome," is characterized by a polycranial neuropathy involving cranial nerves VI and VII. Patients may have ear pain, ipsilateral facial nerve palsy, tinnitus, vertigo, deafness, and loss of taste. Lesions may occur on the external ear, tympanic membrane, and anterior two thirds of the tongue.
- Postherpetic neuralgia (PHN) exists when pain persists either after a certain period or after all crusts have fallen off. PHN is relatively common; affecting 10 to 15% of all patients with zoster and at least 50% of patients older than 60 years. Pain usually significantly reduces after about 6 months. Other symptoms that may persist in addition to pain include pruritus, paresthesia, dysesthesia, and anesthesia. Patients may require referral for pain management.

DIAGNOSIS AND DIFFERENTIAL

- Both varicella and zoster are typically diagnosed clinically with a compatible history and physical examination.
- To confirm the diagnosis, a Tzanck smear may be performed. It will show multinucleated epithelial giant cells. The Tzanck smear, however, cannot differentiate VZV from HSV.
- To differentiate VZV from HSV, a culture of vesicular fluid or tissue may be performed. In addition, cellular material may be submitted for direct immunofluorescence or PCR.
- The differential diagnosis for primary varicella includes other viral exanthems, insect bites, scabies, erythema multiforme, papular urticaria, drug eruptions, and other vesicular dermatoses such as dermatitis herpetiformis.
- The differential for herpes zoster includes dermatomal HSV infection, cellulitis, or erysipelas.

TREATMENT

PREVENTION OF PRIMARY VARICELLA (CHICKENPOX)

- Varicella-zoster vaccine is recommended for all children between the ages of 12 and 18 months, and older children and most adults who have not had chickenpox. If patient is unsure, antibody titers to varicella may be checked prior to administering vaccine.

PRIMARY VARICELLA

- In healthy children, symptomatic treatment is typically sufficient (bathing, cutting fingernails short to prevent excoriation, antipruritics, antipyretics).
- No aspirin use (to prevent Reye's syndrome).
- In children, may consider acyclovir 20 mg/kg four times daily for 5 days; shown to decrease duration and severity of infection; may allow children to return to school sooner increasing cost effectiveness by allowing parents to return to work sooner.

- Adults may be treated with acyclovir 800 mg five times daily for 7 days.
- In immunocompromised, acyclovir 10 mg/kg IV every 8 hours for 7 to 10 days.

Acute Herpes Zoster (Shingles)

- No antiviral treatment can prevent PHN; however, early treatment (within 48 to 72 hours of the first vesicle) can reduce its severity and duration:
  1. Valacyclovir (Valtrex) 1 g three times daily for 7 days *or*
  2. Famciclovir (Famvir) 500 mg three times daily for 7 days *or*
  3. Acyclovir (Zovirax) 800 mg five times daily for 7 days
  4. Prednisone alone or with antiviral agents does NOT decrease risk or severity of PHN. For acyclovir-resistant strains in AIDS patients, foscarnet found effective.

Postherpetic Neuralgia

- Analgesics, narcotics, cutaneous stimulation, tricyclic antidepressants, capsaicin, biofeedback, and nerve blocks have been reported to be effective in relieving the pain in some patients.

REFERENCES

Alkalay AL, Pomerance JJ, Rimoin DL. Fetal varicella syndrome. *J Pediatr.* 1987;111:320.

Dunkel LM, Arvin AM, Whitley RJ, et al. A controlled trial of acyclovir for chickenpox in normal children. *N Engl J Med.* 1983;309:133.

Grose C. The pathogenesis of chickenpox. *Pediatrics.* 1981;68:735.

Hope-Simpson RE. The nature of herpes zoster: A long-term study and a new hypothesis. *Proc R Soc Med.* 1965;58:9.

Kanski JJ. *Clinical Ophthalmology,* ed 2. London: Butterworth-Heineman, 1989:101.

Krugman S, Goodrich CH, Ward R. Primary varicella pneumonia. *N Engl J Med.* 1957;257:843.

Lewis GW. Zoster sine herpete. *Br Med J.* 1958;2:418.

Perronne C, Lazanas M, Leport C, et al. Varicella in patients infected with the human immunodeficiency virus. *Arch Dermatol.* 1990;126:1033.

VanLoon F, Markowitz L, McQuillan G, et al. Varicella seroprevalence in U.S. population. In: Program and Abstracts of the 33rd Interscience Conference on Antimicrobial Agents and Chemotherapy. New Orleans, 1993.

Weber DM, Pellecchia JA. Varicella pneumonia: Study of prevalence in adult men. *JAMA.* 1965;192:572.

Whitley RJ. Therapeutic approaches to varicella-zoster virus infection. *J Infect Dis.* 1992;166(suppl 1):S51.

Whitley RJ, Weiss H, Gnann JW, et al. Acyclovir with and without prednisone for the treatment of herpes zoster. *Ann Intern Med.* 1996;125:376.

Whitney RJ. Varicella-zoster virus infections. In: Galasso GJ, Whitley RJ, Merigan TC, eds. *Antiviral Agents and Viral Diseases in Man.* New York:Raven Press, 1990:235.

Wood MJ, Johnson RW, McKendrick MW, et al. A randomized trial of acyclovir for 7 days or 21 days with and without prednisolone for treatment of acute herpes zoster. *N Engl J Med.* 1994;330:896.

Human Papilloma Virus

EPIDEMIOLOGY

- Human papilloma virus (HPV) is a large family of double-stranded DNA viruses. PV affects many animal species but the host specificity prevents contagion from one species to another. It spreads from person to person through casual contact and they may survive on surfaces, such as floors, for an unknown period of time.
- Modern antigen identification and amplification techniques have shown that the virus may be carried and shed by asymptomatic individuals from infected, but normal appearing, skin. Susceptibility will depend on the host's native immune status, acquired immune defects by way of disease or medication, method and intensity of exposure, and prior exposure of the host to that particular viral epitope.
- Neutralizing antibodies to a given HPV may block reinfection with that particular epitope.

PATHOPHYSIOLOGY

- There are more than 80 HPV types (and counting) and, while there will always be exceptions, a given epitope will usually cause infection of a certain type in a certain body location (see Table 8–1).
- Maceration (such as a swimmer's foot) or abrasion (as in sexual transmission) of the skin may provide a portal of infection. Clinical infection usually will not be apparent for 1 to 12 months after infection and some people never show a wart although the skin is infected and shedding live virions.
- While most warts are benign nuisances, several are oncogenic for squamous cell carcinoma (SCCA). In some people, this is related to the increased susceptibility of epidermodysplasia verruciformis patients to HPV in general and specific HPV types in particular. In the general population, the oncogenic HPVs may be a significant proponent of genital SCCA and have recently been linked with other cutaneous malignancies.

TABLE 8–1   Common Wart Types and Associated Serotypes

WART TYPE	DESCRIPTION	HPV TYPE (COMMON REPORTS)
Verruca vulgaris	Rough, flesh-colored papules	2, 4, 7, 27, 29
Verruca plana	Flat-topped papules	3, 10, 28, 49
Verruca plantaris/palmaris	Thick lesions on soles or palms	1
Condyloma acuminata	Anogenital papules and plaques (lower risk for malignancy)	6, 11, 43
Condyloma acuminata: oncogenic	Bowenoid papulosis and SCCA	16 (primary), 18, 31, 32, 34, 35, 39, 42, 48, 51–54
Epidermodysplasia verruciformis	Flat, hypopigmented macules (variable malignancy risk, especially 5, 8, 9)	5, 8 (primary), 9, 12, 14, 15, 17, 19–26, 36, 46, 47, 50

CLINICAL FEATURES

- Verruca vulgaris (common warts) are scaly, rough or mamillated surface papules, nodules, and, occasionally, small plaques that may occur singly or in confluent groups. The extremities are the most common location, although single or grouped long, thin, finger-like projections ("digitate" or "filiform") will often occur on the face of older patients. Usually, they are the color of the skin. They may be red if irritated or traumatized.
- Verruca plana (flat warts) are 1- to 4-mm flat topped, slightly scaly papules. They are especially common on the face and extremities. They may be hyperpigmented and resemble small seborrheic keratoses or hypopigmented and resemble idiopathic guttate hypomelanosis or lichen nitidus. They also may be associated with filiform warts described above and, in this setting, may occur at cutaneous/mucosal junctures, such as the vermilion of the lip, eyelid margin, or nostril.
- Verruca plantaris/palmaris (plantar and palmar warts) are referred to by most patients as "planter's warts," although even non-gardeners will get these thick, hyperkeratotic papules, nodules, and plaques. They are often painful when they are over bony prominences and weight-bearing areas. Occasionally, the small vessels within the wart will be thrombosed and appear to be a number of tiny black dots. On the soles, such warts will occasionally reach heroic sizes ("mosaic wart") with large plaques made up of a confluence of smaller papules.
- Condyloma acuminata (anogenital warts, venereal warts, and genital warts) are variably sized, mamillated papules that occasionally coalesce into large cauliflower-like excrescences, especially in perineal and crural folds. They may extend into the vagina, the urethra, or rectum. A variation, usually caused by an oncogenic HPV, is bowenoid papulosis, in which the early papule, which is often smoother and darker than the average condyloma, will, in time, develop histologic features of a superficial squamous cell carcinoma.
- Giant condyloma acuminatum (Buschke–Lowenstein tumor) is a low-grade genital malignancy caused by oncogenic HPV. Epithelioma cuniculatum is a similar smoldering malignancy on the sole of foot that arises from a plantar wart.
- Extracutaneous presentations of HPV include oral mucosal lesions, cervical dysplasia with its attendant cancer risk, and laryngeal papillomatosis. The latter may be acquired by the infant in transit through an infected birth canal but is also a concern when laser treatment vaporizes a verruca. Infectious material has been recovered from the laser plume in such cases.

DIAGNOSIS AND DIFFERENTIAL

- The diagnosis of HPV infections can usually be made clinically, both by clinical appearance and history of the lesion. When in doubt, histologic examination of a biopsy specimen can confirm the diagnosis and exclude some of the entities discussed as follows.
- SCCA is the most concerning entity in the differential diagnosis of warts. The reason for this is twofold; first that a superficial SCCA may also be hyperkeratotic and rough surfaced. The second reason is because of oncogenic HPV types, malignant transformation of a clinically benign verruca may occur. A verruca that does not respond to therapy or seems to be growing larger or faster than the "average" wart should be biopsied. An isolated subungual verruca in a patient with sun damage but without other warts should prompt biopsy to exclude a subungual SCCA.
- While melanoma would seem to be easy to distinguish from a wart, there are many cases in which amelanotic or minimally pigmented acral melanomas were subjected to repeated cryotherapy before the correct diagnosis is finally made.
- Calluses and clavi (corns) are often misdiagnosed as verruca, especially on the soles. Punctate keratoderma (punctate porokeratosis) may also resemble plantar warts but careful paring of the surface will reveal a translucent keratin build up rather than evidence of the

tiny thrombosed capillaries. These conditions may initially appear to respond to keratolytic therapies but at some point, will usually become irritated enough for the patient to seek medical attention.

- Flat seborrheic keratoses, especially the stucco keratoses found on the extremities, may closely resemble verruca plana. They will often respond to the same treatments used for verruca.
- Hypertrophic actinic keratoses may closely resemble verruca and do have the potential to become a superficial or invasive SCCA. Consider performing a biopsy on a wart occurring on sun-damaged skin that is not responding to therapy.

TREATMENT

- HPV infections will often "resolve" spontaneously, although this may take years, a time period unacceptable to most patients, especially if the wart is uncomfortable or in a socially embarrassing location (nose, fingers, genital). Even after clinical resolution of the infection, with or without treatment, viral genome may still be recovered from the original or remote sites. The tendency for warts to clear suddenly after variable times and treatments must be remembered when considering the scientific literature suggesting the efficacy of a new treatment.
- An effective treatment of warts depends less on "killing the virus" than on reducing the amount of infected tissue and generating an immune response.
- Salicylic acid preparations are usually the first treatment tried. More effective, but more irritating under occlusion, these products are most effective when applied after gentle debridement of the wart with an emery board or sandpaper. When used on mucosal or genital surfaces, severe inflammation may occur. Consideration of systemic adsorption when applied to large and/or macerated areas is appropriate in children.
- Mechanical destruction is the mainstay of treatment in the physician's office. Cryotherapy may be performed with liquid nitrogen, carbon dioxide probe, and other cooling devices. Freeze time varies with the method used and the size and location of the wart. The goal is to destroy the infected tissue and, hopefully, generate an immune response in that area. The patient should be advised that blister formation is frequent and that if the wart appears to be at the top of the blister, the blister should be trimmed away. Refreezing after allowing the lesion to thaw potentiates the injury. Excessive freeze times or secondary infection of a cryotherapy site may lead to scarring. Laser treatments may include vaporization by carbon dioxide laser or treatment with a vascular laser. The former leaves the patient with a burn; the latter usually requires multiple treatments and does not have a high success rate. Curettage and electrofulguration may also remove a wart but, like the carbon dioxide laser or aggressive cryotherapy, may scar. Occlusion of a plantar wart with occlusive tape, such as duct tape for several days, with treatment repeated after removing dead wart material is effective in some patients. The maceration caused by this treatment encourages the recognition of the HPV by the immune system.

- More direct stimulation of the immune system is reported to work in a variety of HPV infections. Treatments range from injection of interferon directly into the wart, application of topical imiquomod (indicated for condyloma acuminata, but frequently used off label under occlusion for warts in other areas), systemic cimetidine in high doses (contradicting studies regarding efficacy), application of topical sensitizing agents, and injection of substances such as Candida antigen. All have been reported to work but inconvenience, discomfort, side effects, and expense limits their use.
- Other treatments reported to work include topical podofilox (indicated for condyloma acuminata), application of cantherone (a blistering agent used most often in children), 5-fluorouracil (especially for periungual warts), topical tretinoin (especially for verruca plana), chemical peel agents, and direct injection with antineoplastic agents such as bleomycin. Except for the podofilox for genital warts, all these uses are "off-label" and the practitioner should be familiar with the literature describing the treatment and possible side effects before attempting such therapies.
- Psychologic therapies have included hypnosis, visualization exercises, and "buying the warts" from children (promise a certain incentive if warts are gone in a reasonable time, usually 2 months). There is literature and clinical experience supporting the use of these noninvasive therapies. In the book *Tom Sawyer*, Mark Twain documented the efficacy of spunk water.

REFERENCES

Connant MA. Immunomodulatory therapy in the management of viral infections in patients with HIV infection. *J Am Acad Dermatol.* 2000;43:S27.

Edwards L. Imiquimod in clinical practice. *J Am Acad Dermatol.* 2000;43:S12.

Guidelines of care for warts. *J Am Acad Dermatol.* 1995;32:98.

Tyring SK. Human papillomavirus infections: Epidemiology pathogenesis, and host immune response. *J Am Acad Dermatol.* 2000;43:S18.

Vogel LN. Epidemiology of human papilloma virus infection. *Semin Dermatol.* 1992;11:226.

MOLLUSCUM CONTAGIOSUM

EPIDEMIOLOGY

- Molluscum contagiosum (MC) is caused by a molluscipox DNA poxvirus. Except for very rare veterinary reports, humans are the only species known infected.
- MC occurs by skin-to-skin transmission and is most common in children, as a sexually transmitted disease in adults, and in patients with altered immune status.

PATHOPHYSIOLOGY

- After an incubation of a week to several months, the characteristic papules will appear. Autoinoculation is frequent in children, especially those with skin conditions such as atopic dermatitis.
- Unlike other poxviruses, MC does not grow easily in cell cultures. Unlike the human papilloma virus, there is no malignant potential. Only two epitopes have been identified.

CLINICAL FEATURES

- Characteristic lesions are 1- to 3-mm umbilicated papules that usually start out in a cluster but over time may become generalized, especially in children. Most children with a primary infection will have 20 or more individual lesions. At times, the umbilication is not apparent and the lesions may actually appear vesicular until attempts are made to open a lesion for a procedure, such as a Tzanck smear.
- Occasionally, single MC papules may attain great size, reaching 1 cm or more in diameter.
- Adult MC usually presents with genital lesions only, the majority of lesions being found in the infra-umbilical and pubic region.
- Immune-suppressed patients, especially those with untreated or under-managed HIV disease, may present with large plaques of MC, occasionally covering most of the beard area. Unlike the small childhood papules that create a superficial papule, these nodules and plaques may be very deep seated.

DIAGNOSIS AND DIFFERENTIAL

- Clinical appearance and history are usually enough to make the diagnosis of MC. In questionable cases, a shave biopsy of a papule or plaque will confirm the diagnosis, as the histopathology is unmistakable. This may be especially important in immune-suppressed individuals who may have MC-like presentations of deep fungal infections. Alternatively, the core of the papule may be expressed, smeared on a slide and stained as a Tzanck smear to identify the lozenge-shaped molluscum bodies.
- A variety of benign adnexal tumors or inflammatory conditions, such as perforating granuloma annulare, may resemble small MC papules. Especially if slightly irritated, the papules may look vesicular and be mistaken for varicella or herpes simplex. Some HPV infections, especially condyloma acuminata, may resemble MC, although care should be taken to ensure that the patient is not infected with both agents. Some patients with inflamed MC have been misdiagnosed as having folliculitis.
- Single, large lesions may be mistaken for basal cell carcinoma or small infundibular cysts.
- In the immune-suppressed patient, the cutaneous manifestation of a number of systemic fungal infections may create lesions that are indistinguishable from or coexistent with MC. Cryptococcus, Histoplasmosis, and Coccidiomycosis are especially notorious for this masquerade.

TREATMENT

- Many of the same treatments for HPV are effective in MC. Like HPV, molluscum contagiosum will usually spontaneously involute. This is especially true in children but may take 2 months to 2 years.
- Cryotherapy, podophyllin, podofilox, salicylic acid, chemical peel agents, laser therapies, and other destructive methods are reported to be effective.
- Curettage of the lesions, especially after the application of a topical anesthetic, is a rapid way to clear genital lesions in adults and may be used in cooperative children. Treatments unique to MC include tape stripping and forceps squeezing and extraction of the infectious core.
- Immune system modulation through the use of oral cimetidine or intralesional injection with interferon has been reported to benefit some patients. The plaque-like lesions of immune-suppressed patients have proven particularly difficult to treat, although recent reports of the use of topical imiquomod has shown benefit in both immune-competent and HIV patients. Cidofovir (topical and systemic) was also reported to be of benefit.

REFERENCES

Beutner KR. Cutaneous viral infections. *Ann Pediatr.* 1993; 24:247.

Diven DG. An overview of poxviruses. *J Am Acad Dermatol.* 2001;44:1.

Edwards L. Imiquimod in clinical practice. *J Am Acad Dermatol.* 2000;43:S12.

Epstein WL. Molluscum contagiosum. *Semin Dermatol.* 1992;11:184.

Schwartz JJ, Myskowski PL. Molluscum contagiosum in patients with human immunodeficiency virus infection. *J Am Acad Dermatol.* 1992;27:583.

ORF

EPIDEMIOLOGY

- Orf, or ecthyma contagiosum, is a self-limited viral disease caused by the orf virus, which is a double-stranded DNA virus of the Poxviridae family that is transmitted from sheep and goats to humans via direct contact with an infected animal or through contaminated farming equipment. Orf is commonly seen in farming communities, veterinarians, and those who work in the meat industry.

CLINICAL FEATURES

- Orf usually develops as a single, erythematous papule on the dorsum of the hand 1 week after exposure to an infected animal and may be associated with a low-grade fever and regional lymphadenopathy.
- Lesions are usually solitary and typically located on the fingers and hands. In a course of 6 weeks, the papule develops a white halo, giving it a target-like appearance before becoming more weeping, nodular, and, sometimes, hemorrhagic until it begins to dry with a papillomatous surface before finally regressing with a thick crust.
- The lesions are usually 1 to 3 cm in diameter, although cases of "giant orf" up to 6 cm have been reported in immunosuppressed patients and those with atopic dermatitis.
- Orf has rarely been associated with erythema multiforme.

DIAGNOSIS

- The diagnosis of orf can often be made clinically; confirmatory tests include skin biopsy, tissue culture, or complement fixation.
- Establishing a proper diagnosis is important to prevent aggressive surgical or radiation therapy on the assumption that the lesion is a rapidly growing malignancy.

- The differential diagnosis includes milker's nodule, which is clinically identical except that it is seen with exposure to cows, hence, the term "farmyard pox" to cover both entities.
- Other entities to consider are cowpox, herpetic whitlow, anthrax, tuberculosis, atypical mycobacterial infection, syphilitic chancre, sporotrichosis, tularemia, pyogenic granuloma, squamous cell carcinoma, and keratoacanthoma. The characteristic histologic appearance of orf on a skin biopsy is usually sufficient to make the diagnosis.

TREATMENT

- Typically, the natural history of orf is that of a self-limited disease with complete resolution without scarring in about 6 weeks.
- Local wound care and treatment of secondary bacterial infections may be necessary.
- For larger or recalcitrant lesions, surgical therapy (shave excision, cryotherapy with liquid nitrogen, or curettage and electrodesiccation) can be effective.
- Vaccination and isolation of infected animals can prevent the spread of disease; human to human spread does not occur under natural conditions so isolation of infected patients is not indicated.

REFERENCES

Diven DG. An overview of poxviruses. *J Amer Acad Dermatol.* 2001;44:1.

Groves RW. Poxviruses. In: Arndt KA, Leboit PE, Wintoub BU, et al, eds. *Cutaneous Medicine and Surgery: An Integrated Program in Dermatology.* Philadelphia:WB Saunders, 1996: 1097.

Hawayek LH, Rubriz N. Orf. *E Med J.* 2001;2:1.

HAND, FOOT, AND MOUTH DISEASE

EPIDEMIOLOGY

- Hand, foot, and mouth disease (HFMD) typically occurs in young children, but adults are also at risk.
- Individual cases and outbreaks of HFMD occur worldwide. Recently, major outbreaks have occurred in Southeast Asian countries such as Singapore, Malaysia, and Taiwan.

- The disease usually occurs in the warmer months of summer and early autumn in temperate climates.

PATHOPHYSIOLOGY

- HFMD is caused by enteroviruses. The most common cause is coxsackievirus A16, although sporadic cases have been associated with other strains of this group (coxsackievirus A5, A9, A10, B2, and B5) and with enterovirus 71.
- The disease is spread from person to person by the oral-oral, fecal-oral, and respiratory routes via contact with nose and throat discharges, respiratory droplets, blister fluid, and/or stool. It is moderately to highly contagious. A person is most contagious during the first week of illness, although a person may shed virus even when asymptomatic.
- HFMD is not transmitted to or from pets or other animals. HFMD is not related to the foot and mouth disease of cattle, sheep, or swine.

CLINICAL FEATURES

- A patient may present with a brief prodrome for several days consisting of a low-grade fever, malaise, vomiting, loss of appetite, abdominal pain, or respiratory symptoms. Individuals usually present with the combination of oral and cutaneous findings, but may have one without the other.
- Oral lesions are most frequent and usually occur on the gingiva, buccal mucosa, tongue, and hard palate. Lesions begin as small, painful, 3- to 7-mm erythematous macules and papules that progress to form gray, thin-walled vesicles that then ulcerate. The average number of oral lesions ranges from 5 to 10. Smaller lesions may coalesce into larger ones.
- Cutaneous lesions appear concomitant with or shortly after the mucosal lesions. The hands are more commonly involved than the feet. The lesions begin as erythematous macules or papules that then form gray, round to oval vesicles with a red halo. There can be several to over 100 lesions that may be painful, not pruritic. Occasionally, erythematous macules, papules, and vesicles may occur on the buttock or as a generalized eruption.
- Usually, infection is mild with most lesions resolving without treatment and without complication in 7 to 10 days. However, some epidemics, particularly those associated with enterovirus 71, have been associated with more severe symptoms including headache, tremor, ataxia, CNS pleocytosis, aseptic meningitis, meningoencephalitis, a poliomyelitis-like flaccid paralysis, and/or pulmonary edema.

DIAGNOSIS AND DIFFERENTIAL

- Diagnosis is usually made clinically with the findings of fever, oral ulcerations, and a hand and foot exanthem. Viral cultures of the throat, secretions, blister fluid, stool, and blood may be performed. Serum enzyme-linked immunosorbent assay for viral IgM titers may also be performed for acute and convalescent titers, but it is not usually necessary due to the short course of illness. If necessary, a skin biopsy can be performed, which may show intraepidermal or subepidermal vesicles with reticular and ballooning degeneration.
- The differential diagnoses may include aphthous stomatitis, herpangina, herpes viral infection, varicella, group A streptococcal infection, erythema multiforme, and other viral exanthems. Aphthous stomatitis does not usually have associated systemic symptoms and a cutaneous eruption. Herpangina usually produces ulcerations of the posterior pharynx, including the anterior faucial pillars, the soft palate, tonsils, or the uvula. Herpangina does not commonly involve the tongue, gingiva, or buccal mucosa. A Tzanck smear showing viral cytopathic change, viral cultures, and perioral involvement may help diagnose and differentiate herpetic infection. A typical varicella eruption is usually more generalized on the face and trunk. A Tzanck smear and viral cultures again could be beneficial. Although a streptococcal infection may present with similar symptoms and oral ulcerations, it is not usually associated with a hand and foot vesicular eruption. A throat culture and serologies would be helpful. Lesions of erythema multiforme are usually more targetoid and persistent. Although arthropod assault, acropustulosis of infancy, and tinea may mimic acral lesions, the presence of oral lesions would not usually be found in those conditions.

TREATMENT

- HFMD usually resolves spontaneously in approximately 1 week with supportive symptomatic care. Topical oral viscous lidocaine or aphthous ulcer mixes may provide symptomatic relief. Oral acyclovir has been reported to be helpful.
- General preventive practice measures should be explained to families and childcare settings. All children and adults should conduct good hand-washing techniques, particularly after diaper changes, and soiled clothing laundered. Contaminated surfaces should be cleansed with household cleansers such as diluted bleach. Children with significant blistering may need to be removed from childcare programs or schools during the initial symptomatic period.

REFERENCES

Chan LG, Parashar UD, Lye MS, et al. Deaths of children during an outbreak of hand, foot, and mouth disease in Sarawak, Malaysia: Clinical and pathological characteristics of the disease. *Clin Infect Dis.* 2000;31:678.

Chang LY, Lin TY, Hsu KH, et al. Clinical features and risk factors of pulmonary oedema after enterovirus-71-related hand, foot, and mouth disease. *Lancet.* 1999;354:1682.

Chang LY, Lin TY, Huang YC, et al. Comparison of enterovirus 71 and coxsackievirus A16 clinical illnesses during the Taiwan enterovirus epidemic, 1998. *Pediatr Infect Dis J.* 1999;18:1092.

Dolin R. Enterovirus 71—emerging infections and emerging questions. *N Engl J Med.* 1999;341:984.

Haley JC, Hood, AF. Hand-foot-and-mouth disease. In: Freedberg IM, Eisen AZ, Wolff K, et al, eds. *Fitzpatrick's Dermatology in General Medicine,* ed 5. New York: McGraw-Hill, 1999:2403.

Ho M, Chen ER, Hsu KH, et al. An epidemic of enterovirus 71 infection in Taiwan. *N Engl J Med.* 1999;341:929.

Huang CC, Liu CC, Chang YC, et al. Neurologic complication in children with enterovirus 71 infection. *N Engl J Med.* 1999;341:936.

VIRAL EXANTHEMS

MEASLES (RUBEOLA)

EPIDEMIOLOGY

- The etiologic agent is a paramyxovirus in the genus Morbillivirus and is characterized by rash mimicked by many other conditions. Called "morbilli" to distinguish from "morbus" (plague) the term "morbilliform" is now firmly in the dermatologic lexicon, although measles itself is now quite rare in the United States. It is spread by direct contact with infectious droplets or by airborne spread. Winter and spring are the most likely times of year to see measles.
- In the traditional numbering of the "six exanthematous diseases," measles is "first disease."

PATHOPHYSIOLOGY

- Incubation of this single-stranded RNA virus from exposure to onset of symptoms is 8 to 12 days.
- There is conflicting information as to whether the rash is the result of antigen-antibody complex deposition or direct invasion of local tissues by the virus.

CLINICAL FEATURES

- During the incubation period, virus may be cultured from the mucosa of asymptomatic individuals.
- A symptomatic prodrome phase (about 4 days) ensues with fever, malaise, cough, conjunctivitis, and coryza (the last three being the "three Cs" of rubeola). During this time but usually prior to the rash, the characteristic Koplik's spots, white to bluish spots on an erythematous base, may be found on the buccal mucosa. Usually, they are fading or absent by the time of apparent cutaneous eruption.
- The rash begins on the head and neck and moves downward. The rash forms over 3 days, during which time the patient is the sickest. The rash fades in the same order it appears, often appearing brownish or coppery. While the leg lesions usually stay individual and discrete, the facial lesions will usually become confluent.
- Atypical measles occurs in those who received the killed vaccine (pre 1963) and are later infected with the live virus. This usually has a more abrupt onset and a rash that starts on the extremities and spreads centrally. It may also be hemorrhagic or papulovesicular.
- Complications of measles includes pneumonia (either primary viral or secondary bacterial), encephalitis, exacerbation of tuberculosis, and the late complication of subacute sclerosing panencephalopathy.

DIAGNOSIS AND DIFFERENTIAL

- Most diagnoses will be suspected clinically, especially if pathognomonic findings such as Koplik's spots are seen.
- Culture, from blood, urine, or pharynx, is possible but difficult. Complement fixation, hemagglutination-inhibition, direct immunofluorescence, or ELISA techniques may make a more conclusive diagnosis.
- Acute and convalescent titers may be necessary.

TREATMENT

- Treatment is generally supportive.
- Vitamin A (200,000 IU for 3 doses) may be useful, especially in vitamin-deficient populations.
- Measles specific immune globulin may be recommended for household contacts of measles patients, especially for infants under the age of 1 year, immunocompromised patients, and pregnant women.
- Secondary infection should be watched for and treated as appropriate. (Prophylactic antibiotics are NOT recommended.)

- The most effective treatment is prevention through appropriate childhood immunizations. The World Health Organization has targeted measles as a disease capable of eradication. Currently, it is a significant problem in refugee populations.

RUBELLA (GERMAN MEASLES)

EPIDEMIOLOGY

- Infective from the end of the incubation period until clearance of the rash. Rubella is the only member of the Rubivirus genus and humans are the only known hosts. Epidemics usually occur in the spring and generally in urban population centers and in unimmunized victims.
- In the traditional numbering of the "six exanthematous diseases," rubella is "third disease." (Scarlet fever is "second disease.")

PATHOPHYSIOLOGY

- Rubella, an RNA virus, has a 14- to 21-day incubation period.
- The virus is shed in respiratory secretions.
- The first trimester of pregnancy is the most vulnerable time for intrauterine infection and development of neonatal rubella syndrome.

CLINICAL FEATURES

- The prodrome is characterized by symptoms of a mild URI.
- Low-grade fever, headache, conjunctivitis, and lymphadenopathy may also occur during the prodrome.
- Flushing, macules, and papules begin on the face and rapidly migrate. As it appears on the trunk on the second day, it may already be clearing from the face. This helps distinguish rubella from rubeola, which runs a longer course.
- The lymphadenopathy may be severe and cervical, occipital, and postauricular nodes are most involved.
- Pruritus and mild desquamation may follow.
- Except for occasional thrombocytopenia, complications are rare.

DIAGNOSIS AND DIFFERENTIAL

- Cell culture is possible but tedious and variable in accuracy.

- Hemagglutination-inhibition for antirubella antibodies is the standard screening test, although indirect ELISA tests are the most popular. IgM is used to diagnose intrauterine infections.
- IF and other antibody/antigen assays may also be employed.
- Most cases will be diagnosed on clinical grounds.
- Neonatal rubella has a variety of malformations including cardiac, ocular, auditory, orthopedic, central nervous system, and hematologic.

TREATMENT

- Like measles, the best treatment is prevention through appropriate childhood immunizations.
- Treatment is supportive otherwise.

ROSEOLA (EXANTHEM SUBITUM, SIXTH DISEASE)

EPIDEMIOLOGY

- Seropositivity is fairly universal in the adult population and most infants are born with maternal antibodies. Active infection usually occurs between the ages of 6 months and 2 years of life, corresponding no doubt to waning of the natal protection and the constant exposure.
- The virus likely remains a latent infection indefinitely.

PATHOPHYSIOLOGY

- This is caused by human herpes virus 6 and has an incubation of 5 to 15 days.
- The virus is shed in all secretions and likely spread by respiratory route.

CLINICAL FEATURES

- The rash is preceded by a characteristic prodrome of 3 to 4 days of very high fever in a child who is otherwise doing well. The fever onset may be quite abrupt and is a significant etiology of febrile seizures.
- Nonpruritic, pink macules occur on the fourth day, at which time the fever usually resolves suddenly. The macules blanch with pressure and often have a white halo surrounding them.
- Complications, such as thrombocytopenia, are rare. Atypical monocytes and a transient neutropenia may occur, which are generally of no consequence.

DIAGNOSIS AND DIFFERENTIAL

- Diagnosis is made on clinical grounds of the characteristic febrile prodrome followed by defervescence and onset of rash.

TREATMENT

- As the rash is usually asymptomatic and the fever resolves with rash onset; no treatment other than reassurance to the parents is necessary.

FIFTH DISEASE (ERYTHEMA INFECTIOUSUM)

EPIDEMIOLOGY

- Occurring worldwide, it can affect all ages although school age children (5 to 15 years old) are those most likely affected.
- The incubation period is usually 1 to 2 weeks, during which time the virus is being actively shed in respiratory secretions.
- Blood transmission can occur and is a factor in fetal infection.

PATHOPHYSIOLOGY

- Parvovirus B19 is the cause of erythema infectiosum. This is not a veterinary disease and the parvovirus for which dogs are immunized is not infectious to humans.
- The blood group P-antigen is the viral receptor and those without this antigen cannot be infected.

CLINICAL FEATURES

- Usually, the first presentation is a macular eruption on face giving the characteristic "slapped cheek" appearance.
- A macular eruption over the extremities follows over the next week, usually most noticeable on the extensor surface.
- A reticulated erythema follows in the areas of prior involvement (cheeks, arms), which will fade only to dramatically worsen with heat, sunlight, or embarrassment. This is especially distressing to adolescents who may suddenly appear to erupt in a lace-like pattern on their cheeks weeks or even months after initial infection.

- Papular-purpuric gloves and socks syndrome has recently been associated with parvovirus B19. Presentation is, as described by the name of the syndrome, a purpuric eruption of the distal extremities with a very sharp cut-off of the eruption just proximal to the wrists and ankles.
- Those with blood cell dyscrasias and other hematologic abnormalities are more susceptible to the unusual but severe complications of EI, aplastic crisis and hemolytic anemia. This is also the concern in intrauterine infections. A serious, prolonged anemia may also occur in immune-compromised patients.

DIAGNOSIS AND DIFFERENTIAL

- Diagnosis is usually made clinically. Culture is not generally available and antibody testing is only performed in a few research laboratories.

TREATMENT

- Treatment is supportive.
- Pregnant women who may have been exposed may have serologic testing (usually arranged through local health departments) and serial sonography.
- There is no available vaccine at this time.
- Immune-suppressed patients and those with aplastic crisis generally have higher viral shedding and should be placed in respiratory and contact isolation if hospitalized.

GIANOTTI–CROSTI DISEASE

- Originally described as a papulovesicular eruption associated with hepatitis B infection, it is now recognized that there are a number of different presentations of Gianotti–Crosti disease (GCD) and that it is associated with many different viral infections. It is also known by the descriptive terms of "papular acrodermatitis of childhood" and "papulovesicular acrolocated syndrome."

EPIDEMIOLOGY

- It occurs worldwide, with seasonal or clustered appearances coinciding to the underlying viral etiology.
- Children between the ages of 1 and 6 years are most often affected.

PATHOPHYSIOLOGY

An immune response to a variety of viral antigens, GCD has been associated with:
- Human herpes viruses, such as Epstein–Barr virus, cytomegalovirus, and HHV-6
- Enteroviruses, including coxsackie virus
- Respiratory syncytial virus, parainfluenza virus, parvovirus B19
- Hepatitis B
- Immunizations to MMR (measles, mumps, rubella), polio, and influenza vaccines
- Group A beta-hemolytic streptococcus has also been associated with this eruption.

CLINICAL FEATURES

- A viral prodrome occurs in many, followed by a pruritic eruption, which may be associated with malaise and lymphadenopathy.
- Symmetrical pink papules or papules the color of the skin occur suddenly over the extremities, buttocks, and face. Initially, they may have a vesicular or eczematous appearance.
- Over time, several weeks, they will become more lichenoid.
- Symptoms following an uncomplicated viral infection will resolve in 2 to 8 weeks.

DIAGNOSIS AND DIFFERENTIAL

- Unilateral thoracic exanthem (asymmetric periflexural exanthem of childhood) may appear similar but is mostly confined to one side of the body. Other physicians argue that this eruption is better considered a variation of GCD. Usually, GCD spares the trunk.
- Early in the course and depending upon the presentation, contact dermatitis and drug eruptions might be considered.
- Diagnosis of GCD is made clinically. There are no specific laboratory findings. In the right clinical setting CBC, throat culture, monospot, liver function tests, or tests for hepatitis might be indicated.

TREATMENT

- Unless specific treatment is indicated because of an etiology such as streptococcus, treatment is supportive with consideration of topical antipruritics and oral antihistamines.
- Topical steroids are generally not effective.

HIV DISEASE

EPIDEMIOLOGY

- HIV is transmitted by sexual contact, intravenous drug use with contaminated instruments, transplacentally, needle stick injuries, and other methods of mucosal contamination.
- The majority of cases in the United States are still associated with illicit drug use and homosexual practices, particularly that of receptive anal intercourse. Worldwide, however, heterosexual contact with multiple partners has become the primary means of transmission and spread so that now HIV is epidemic in many countries in sub-Saharan Africa.
- Most pediatric cases are associated with transplacental transmission from an infected mother.
- The inoculum necessary to transmit HIV through accidental needle-stick injury is much greater than that needed to transmit hepatitis B.

PATHOPHYSIOLOGY

- Untreated, HIV infection causes a depletion of CD4+ lymphocytes, leading to impaired immunity and the primary or reactivated infection with a variety of agents normally held in check.
- The viral exanthem associated with newly acquired HIV disease may be a nonspecific immune response to the antigen, as is seen in many other viral infections. It may also be an antibiotic related exanthem, such as is seen in Epstein–Barr virus infections, as many of these patients experience malaise and a febrile illness at this time and often receive antibiotics for a presumptive infection.

CLINICAL FEATURES

- The cutaneous manifestations of HIV disease are the result of a long period of suppressed host immune ability and are not seen as often in the United States as they once were due to the success of multidrug, HAART (highly active antiretroviral therapy).
- The "exanthem of HIV" occurs 2 to 6 weeks after exposure and inoculation to the virus and affects up to half of those infected.
- Symptoms may be relatively abrupt in onset and may be associated with fever, malaise, myalgias, sore throat, and lymphadenopathy.
- A truncal macular or macular-papular erythematous eruption is described, although, at other times, the eruption has been described as morbilliform, affecting the

face and upper body and roseola-like on the face, neck, shoulders, and trunk. Other physicians have reported an occasional vesicular component.

- An aphthous stomatitis, as might be seen in coxsackie infections, may occur.
- The eruption usually resolves within 2 weeks.

DIAGNOSIS AND DIFFERENTIAL

- Enteroviruses (coxsackie and echovirus) may present similarly and with variety of exanthematous presentations as described above.
- EBV, especially with concomitant ampicillin use, may also appear similar.
- Diagnosis is by confirmation of seroconversion to the HIV virus. Even modern ELISA techniques may not detect the virus for 1 to 3 months after infection, although examination for p-24 antigen (the core antigen of the HIV virus), PCR, or other HIV RNA assays may detect infection within the first month.

TREATMENT

- Treatment of HIV disease is beyond the scope of this section. In advanced disease, HIV-related diseases require treatments specific to those infections.

Maintaining a high index of suspicion in susceptible and high-risk individuals who have nonspecific viral exanthems may identify victims early and allow for aggressive HAART before clinical evidence of immune suppression occurs.

REFERENCES

Boyd AS. Laboratory testing patients with morbilliform viral eruptions. *Dermatol Clin.* 1994;12:69.

Caputo R, Gelmetti C, Ermacora E, et al. Gianotti–Crosti syndrome: A retrospective analysis of 308 cases. *J Am Acad Dermatol.* 1992;26:207.

Gable EK, Liu G, Morrell DS. Pediatric exanthems. *Primary Care.* 2000;27:353.

Geusau A, Mooseder G. A maculopapular rash in a patient with severe diarrhea. *Arch Dermatol.* 2002;138:117.

McKinnon HD, Thomas H. Evaluating the febrile patient with a rash. *Am Fam Physician.* 2000;62:804.

Murphy ME, Montemarano A. Papulovesicles and fever in a 41-year-old woman. *Arch Dermatol.* 2002;138:117.

Nelson, JS, Stone MS. Update on selected viral exanthems. *Curr Opin Pediatr.* 2000;12:359.

Penneys NS. *Skin Manifestations of AIDS.* Philadelphia: J.B. Lippincott Company, 1990.

Smith KJ, Skelton HG, Yeager J, et al. Cutaneous findings in HIV-1 positive patients: A 42-month prospective study. *J Am Acad Dermatol.* 1994;31:746.

9 FUNGAL INFECTIONS

Boni E. Elewski
Georgette Rodriguez

CANDIDA

EPIDEMIOLOGY

- Cutaneous candidiasis is caused predominantly by the yeast *Candida albicans*, and less often by other species. Candida species are part of the normal flora of the digestive tract and the vagina.
- *C. albicans* is an oval yeast varying in size (2 to 6 μm by 3 to 9 μm). In tissues it may appear as yeasts or as pseudohyphae.
- During certain favorable conditions such as warm, humid weather or when an individual's immune system is impaired, the yeast can cause disease on the skin. Other risk factors predisposing individuals to Candida infections include diabetes mellitus, obesity, systemic antibiotic therapy, history of vaginal candidiasis, use of oral contraceptives, use of spermicides, and excessive sweating.
- Although mucous membranes in the mouth and vagina are commonly infected, Candida can invade blood and deeper tissues, causing life-threatening infection in patients with primary or secondary immunodeficiencies.

CLINICAL FEATURES

- Cutaneous candidiasis is a superficial infection occurring on moist, occluded sites such as the intertriginous regions of the axilla, under the breast, the panniculus, and in the crural fold. The skin is typically bright red, edematous, moist, and has satellite pustules. Differential diagnosis includes psoriasis, erythrasma, dermatophytosis, and pityriasis versicolor.
- Oropharyngeal candidiasis (thrush) occurs with overgrowth of the resident flora in the oral mucosa including the tongue, lips, gingiva, palate, buccal areas, and pharynx. Infection may present as pseudomembranous candidiasis with white, adherent, cottage-cheese-like plaques that vary in size. Erythematous candidiasis presents with smooth, red, atrophic

plaques. Candidal leukoplakia presents as white patches that cannot be wiped off. Differential diagnosis includes condyloma acuminatum, oral hairy leukoplakia, lichen planus, and trauma.
- Genital candidiasis is an infection of the vaginal mucous membranes (Candida vulvitis), glans penis, prepuce and scrotum (Candida balanoposthitis). Like oral candidiasis, infection likely represents overgrowth of resident flora. The presentation usually includes pruritus, erythema, edema, and a creamy white discharge. White plaques and occasionally pustules may occur.
- Differential diagnosis includes lichen planus, trichomoniasis, bacterial vaginosis, psoriasis, and eczema.
- Candidiasis of the nail unit occurs on the proximal nailfold and nail plate. The infection is characterized by erythema, edema, and a painful or purulent discharge. Nail plate and subungal hyperkeratosis may result in onychodystrophy. Differential diagnosis includes tinea unguium, herpetic whitlow, eczematous dermatitis, allergic contact dermatitis, lichen planus, trauma, and psoriasis.
- Chronic mucocutaneous candidiasis (CMC) is a heterogeneous group of disorders consisting of chronic Candida infections, usually *C. albicans*, associated with underlying immunocompromised state and/or onset in infancy or early childhood. Presentations include oropharyngeal candidiasis refractory to conventional treatments resulting in hypertrophic candidiasis, widespread intertrigo, and/or infection of the nail unit. CMC in an immunocompromised infant or child may present with erosions covered with scales and crusts or as hyperkeratoses.

DIAGNOSIS AND DIFFERENTIAL

- Diagnosis can usually be made after patient history and physical examination. Laboratory test may confirm diagnosis. Direct microscopy with potassium hydroxide preparation (KOH) can be used to visualize pseudohyphae and yeast forms to confirm infection.

TREATMENT

- A variety of treatment modalities are available for candidiasis. First, it is important to identify underlying risk factors such as recent systemic antibiotic use, immunocompromised state, and diabetes mellitus.
- Next, alteration or improvement of the cutaneous environment, such as avoiding occlusion and promoting dryness, helps heal and prevent lesions. Using a hair dryer to dry hard-to-reach areas after bathing may help keep the area dry.
- Topical treatment with drying agents, antifungal powders, or Castellani paint may relieve symptoms.
- Topical antifungal agents are sufficient treatment in simple cutaneous candidiasis. These include nystatin, azole antifungals (ketoconazole, econazole, oxiconazole, and so forth), or imidazole cream twice a day.
- Topical corticosteroids may be used sparingly for short periods in conjunction with topical and/or systemic antifungals to relieve symptoms.
- Oral antifungal treatment includes fluconazole, 150 to 200 mg once weekly for 2 to 4 consecutive weeks for skin involvement and up to 6 to 9 months for Candida nail involvement; or itraconazole, 200 mg per day for up to 7 days. Nystatin tablets may be used for treatment of gastrointestinal tract colonization and may be helpful in preventing recurrences or as adjunct to other treatment.
- Systemic antifungal therapy is indicated in widespread disease, recalcitrant disease, and in immunocompromised patients.

REFERENCES

Elewski BE, ed. *Cutaneous Fungal Infections*, ed 2. Oxford: Blackwell Science, 1998.

Richardson MD, Elewski BE. *Superficial Fungal Infections.* Oxford:Health Press, 2000.

Richardson MD, Warnock DW. *Fungal Infection: Diagnosis and Management*, ed 2. Oxford:Blackwell Science, 1997.

PITYRIASIS VERSICOLOR

EPIDEMIOLOGY

- Pityriasis (tinea) versicolor is a superficial infection caused by the mycelial form of the commensal yeast *Pityrosporum orbiculare* (also known as *Malassezia furfur*).
- Pityriasis versicolor is more common in tropical or subtropical areas with high temperatures and a relatively high humidity.
- Young adults are affected most often, but the disease may occur in childhood and old age.
- Risk factors for widespread disease include immunodeficiency states and living in tropical climates.

CLINICAL FEATURES

- Pityriasis versicolor is characterized by well-demarcated white, pink, or brownish patches, and may become confluent over large areas. The color varies according to the normal pigmentation of the patient, exposure of the area to sunlight, and the severity of the disease. Generally the rash is confined to the chest, back, and upper extremities, but occasionally can involve the lower extremities. On sun-protected pale skin the patches are often salmon colored or pale brown, but after sun exposure and in darker races they are hypopigmented. Lesions may be scaly and pruritic.

DIAGNOSIS AND DIFFERENTIAL

- The clinical diagnosis is usually readily confirmed by observation of hyphae and budding cells ("spaghetti and meatballs") in KOH preparations of scales scraped from lesions. These microscopic features are diagnostic for *Malassezia furfur* and culture preparations are usually not necessary. Pityriasis versicolor may fluoresce a pale greenish color under Wood's ultra-violet light. Differential diagnosis: vitiligo, pityriasis alba, postinflammatory hypopigmentation, tuberculoid leprosy, tinea corporis, guttate psoriasis, and nummular eczema.

TREATMENT

- There are quite a number of topical and oral treatments available for pityriasis versicolor. Fortunately, most of these are very effective; however, there can be a tendency for the disease to recur.
- Effective therapies include 1 to 2% ketoconazole shampoo. The shampoo should be generously applied to affected area for 10 to 15 minutes, then washed off well. This should be repeated on a twice-weekly basis for 2 to 4 weeks. Selenium sulfide 2.5% lotion applied for 15 minutes, and then washed off well, every day for 3 days, or one or two overnight applications, may be affective.

- Topical azole antifungals (such as ketoconazole, econazole, or oxiconazole) or allylamines applied twice daily for 2 weeks are also effective.
- For extensive or recurrent lesions, oral therapy is preferred: ketoconazole 200 mg daily for 5 to 7 days, itraconazole dosed at 200 mg daily for 3 to 5 consecutive days, or single doses of fluconazole 400 mg, continued once weekly for 2 to 3 weeks, have been effective. Oral griseofulvin and terbinafine are not effective treatments.
- To help prevent relapse, particularly in the warmer spring, summer, and fall months, use of ketoconazole shampoo as a medicated soap, applied at least once per week, may help prevent infection.
- Patients also need to be warned that it may take many months for their skin pigmentation to return to normal, even after the infection has been successfully treated. Relapse is a regular occurrence and prophylactic treatment with a topical agent once or twice a week is often necessary to avoid recurrence.

REFERENCE

Elewski BE, ed. *Cutaneous Fungal Infections*, ed 2. Oxford:Blackwell Science, 1998.

DERMATOPHYTE INFECTIONS

EPIDEMIOLOGY

- Dermatophytoses are very common and occur worldwide.
- Dermatophytes are part of a group of fungi that are capable of infecting the stratum corneum of the skin and keratinized structures, such as hair and nails, with minimal immune response from the host.
- Dermatophytes belong to three genera: Trichophyton, Microsporum, and Epidermophyton.
- Fungal growth in keratinized tissue is restricted to the production of hyphae, which branch and segment into chains of spores called arthrospores or arthroconidia. These arthrospores are the main mechanism of dissemination and propagation of the fungus, and can remain viable and infective for months to several years.
- Dermatophytes are transmitted from three sources: from another person by direct or indirect contact, from animals such as puppies or kittens, and least commonly from soil.

- Predisposing factors that may facilitate infection are immunosuppression, icthyosis, collagen vascular disease, sweating, occlusion, obesity, geographic location, and occupational exposure.
- The clinical presentation depends on the site of infection, species of fungus, and immune response of host.
- Dermatophytoses are classified using the term "tinea" followed by the Latin designation of the anatomic location of infection.

TINEA CAPITIS

CLINICAL FEATURES

- Tinea capitis is dermatophytosis of the scalp and hair with resultant scale and alopecia caused by various species in the genera Microsporum and Trichophyton. It most commonly affects prepubertal children, but may occur in adults. There are three patterns of in vivo hair invasion: ectothrix, endothrix, and favus. Ectothrix infection occurs when hyphae and arthrospores form a sheath around the outside of hair shaft and endothrix occurs when certain species of dermatophytes remain within the hair shaft. Four types of clinical presentation are likely:
  - Noninflammatory "gray patch." Presents as a round or oval, sharply delineated dry, scaly patch of partial alopecia on the scalp. Lesion is covered by short stubble and there is persistent scale and mild inflammation. This type is most commonly caused by *M. audouinii*, *M. canis*, and *M. ferrugineum*.
  - Black dot (endothrix). Presents as small, multiple, scattered, angular or polygonal patches with poorly defined margins. There is a dotted appearance caused by weakened hairs that break off at or below the surface of the scalp. There is little or no scaling. This type is more commonly caused by *T. tonsurans* and *T. violaceum*; however, *T. tonsurans* may cause more inflammatory lesions described below.
  - Inflammatory. Presentation may range from a mild pustular folliculitis to a kerion (characterized by pustules and abscesses) which is usually tender. The lesion may become sharply delineated, inflammatory, indurated, and is often described as a "boggy mass." Systemic symptoms such as cervical adenopathy, fever, and malaise may be present. Any dermatophyte may cause this reaction, but *T. tonsurans* and *T. verrucosum* are most common.
  - Favus. Presents as a chronic inflammatory reaction of the scalp characterized by formation of scutula and yellow cup-shaped crusts composed of hyphae, neutrophils, epidermal cells, and intertwined hair.

This disfiguring infection is caused by *T. schoenleinii*. Significant scarring and permanent alopecia may result.

DIAGNOSIS AND DIFFERENTIAL

- Diagnosis is made based on physical examination and history. As with other dermatophytoses, fungal culture using Sabouraud's glucose medium, direct microscopy with KOH preparation, and hair fluorescence under a Wood's light will confirm diagnosis. Differential diagnosis: alopecia areata, trichotillomania, seborrhoeic dermatitis, psoriasis, sebo-psoriasis, bacterial infection or abscess, folliculitis, lichen planus, discoid lupus erythematosus, and syphilis.

TREATMENT

- Topical treatment is not effective.
- Oral antifungal agents must be used. The gold standard of treatment is griseofulvin, 15 mg/kg per day of the ultamicrosize preparation or 20 to 25 mg/kg per day of microsize suspension, continued for a minimum of 8 weeks or longer until hair starts regrowing and fungal culture is negative.
- Terbinafine may be used. Dose varies according to body weight, and it is usually administered for 1 to 6 weeks depending on causative pathogen.
- Itraconazole and fluconazole have been shown to be effective in clinical trials. Itraconazole is dosed at 5 mg/kg for 4 to 6 weeks and fluconazole is dosed at 6 mg/kg for 3 to 6 weeks.
- Adjunctive therapy includes intermittent use of 1 to 2% ketoconazole or selenium sulphide shampoo on a daily basis.
- Tinea capitis is highly contagious, so it is important to check all family members and treat accordingly. It is recommended that all family members use the antifungal shampoo until the patient who is being treated is cured.
- Prevention of recurrence can be achieved by discarding inanimate objects, such as hair brushes, combs, barrettes, and other hair accessories. Boiling the brushes and combs in water for 5 minutes may be helpful, but it is better to discard these objects since spores are difficult to destroy.

TINEA CORPORIS

- Tinea corporis is dermatophytosis of the skin of the trunk, limbs, and face, excluding the hair and nails. All dermatophytes can produce lesions on the skin. The clinical presentation is diverse, but usually involves oval, annular, or circinate lesions. The lesions may be pustular, vesicular, eczematous, and at times granulomatous. Most rashes are scaly unless topical corticosteroids have been used. Symptoms usually consist of pruritus, burning, and/or pain. A typical lesion has an active border that progresses outward, with central clearing, less scale, and discoloration.

DIAGNOSIS AND DIFFERENTIAL

- The clinical diagnosis can be confirmed with direct microscopy with potassium hydroxide preparation (KOH). A scale is scraped from the border of the lesion and placed on a slide. KOH dissolves the keratin of the skin. Visualization of branching hyphae confirms the diagnosis. To identify the specific organism, a culture is necessary using Sabouraud's glucose medium. Differential diagnosis: granuloma annulare, eczematous dermatoses, pityriasis rosea, psoriasis, parapsoriasis, discoid lupus erythematosus, and bacterial pyoderma.

TREATMENT

- Most patients are effectively treated with topical antimycotics including imidazoles, allylamines, substituted pyridone derivative, and others. The patient should be instructed to apply the agent once to twice daily, as recommended by the manufacturer, to the affected skin and at least 2.5 cm around the advancing edge.
- Oral antimycotics such as griseofulvin 500 to 750 mg/d for 2 to 4 weeks, fluconazole 150 mg one a week for 2 to 4 weeks, itraconazole 200 mg/d for 2 to 4 weeks, and terbinafine 250 mg/d for 1 week may be used for extensive disease, recalcitrant infection, and in immunocompromised patients.
- Topical steroids are generally not used although their anti-inflammatory effect may reduce symptoms of itching. Their use may inhibit the cellular response to infection.
- Treatment should include search for source of infection to prevent re-exposure and reinfection. A cool, dry environment and avoidance of infected persons prevents infection. The use of antifungal shampoo (1 to 2% ketoconazole) and soap after exposure to damp, moist environments such as locker rooms and gymnasiums may prevent infection.

TINEA IMBRICATA

- Tinea imbricata is a dermatophyte infection caused by *T. concentricum*. Clinical presentation is a classic appearance of numerous concentric rings with pronounced peripheral scaling facing the center of the ring. The rings become confluent, and a bizarre pattern eventually covers most body surfaces. The axillae, palms, soles, and hair are usually spared. It is a tropical disease seen only in Asia, the Pacific Islands, and South and Central America.

DIAGNOSIS AND DIFFERENTIAL

- Same as for tinea corporis. Differential diagnosis: chronic eczematous eruption, erythema annulare centrifugum, annulare form of subacute cutaneous lupus, and atypical granuloma annulare.

TINEA CRURIS

- Tinea cruris is dermatophytosis of the inguinal area, including the proximal thighs, crural folds, and extending to the buttocks. It occurs predominantly in men, but can occasionally develop in women. The intertriginous fold near the scrotum is usually the first site involved, without involvement of the scrotal skin. The lesions are described as large, scaling, well-demarcated red plaques, which may have a central clearing. Papules and pustules may be present at the margins. Chronic infection can lead to lichenification of area involved.

DIAGNOSIS AND DIFFERENTIAL

- Clinical examination, supported with direct microscopy with KOH and fungal culture confirms diagnosis. Differential diagnosis: seborrheic dermatitis, psoriasis vulgaris, erythrasma, nonspecific intertrigo, and candidiasis.

TREATMENT

- Most cases can be treated with topical anti-fungals; however, extensive infection or immunocompromised patients may benefit from systemic therapy.
- To prevent recurrence, patient should be instructed to wear loose clothing and keep area dry. The use of medicated absorbent powders containing antimycotic, such as Micatin or Tinactin, may be helpful in preventing infection.
- Good hygiene as well as using a hair dryer to dry difficult-to-reach areas may be beneficial.
- Patient should be checked for tinea pedis since it may be a risk factor for developing tinea cruris.

TINEA UNGUIUM

- Tinea unguium (onychomycosis) is a dermatophyte infection of nails. It is a common cutaneous fungal infection in adults. Although generally caused by dermatophytes, Candida and some non-dermatophyte molds can also infect the nail unit. There are four recognized patterns of dermatophyte onychomycosis:
  - Distal lateral subungal onychomycosis. Most common presentation. The disease initially affects the distal nail bed and progresses proximally. Subungal hyperkeratosis develops leading to significant onycholysis (nail separation), eventually involving the whole nail bed. Invasion of the nail plate then occurs, making the nail thick and friable and likely to break off secondary to trauma.
  - Superficial white onychomycosis. Much less common and affects the surface of the nail plate. The pathogen is *T. mentagrophytes*. Several non-dermatophyte molds can occasionally infect the nail plate.
  - Proximal subungal onychomycosis. Rare. The disease begins at the proximal edge of the nail bed and is most likely seen with concomitant disease such as AIDS or local peripheral vascular disease.
  - Total dystrophic onychomycosis. The whole nail bed and plate are involved. The above patterns may lead to this. A dense, creamy white area may be seen beneath the nail, which represents pockets of hyphae.

DIAGNOSIS AND DIFFERENTIAL

- Clinical diagnosis can be confirmed with direct microscopy. Nail debris is obtained and placed on a glass slide. It is suspended in a solution of 10 to 15% KOH and gently heated. Observation of fungal elements confirms diagnosis and fungal culture identifies the pathogen. Differential diagnosis: Candida paronychia, psoriasis, pityriasis rubra pilaris, eczematous dermatitis, allergic contact dermatitis, lichen planus.

TREATMENT

- Effective treatment generally includes an oral antimycotic. A number of agents may be used: fluconazole 150 to 200 mg once weekly for about 6 months in toenail infection or about 3 months for fingernail infection, itraconazole 400 mg/d for 1 week/month for 3 to 4 consecutive months for toenail infection or 1 week/month for 2 consecutive months for fingernail infection, and terbinafine 250 mg/d for 12 weeks continuously in toenail disease and 6 weeks for fingernail disease.

• Prevention includes always wearing protective footwear to avoid exposure found in hotel rooms, carpeting, gymnasiums, and public facilities. Regular application of absorbent powder or antifungal powders may also prevent recurrence. Wearing cotton socks and avoiding sharing nail clippers is also recommended. Finally, discarding old, moldy footwear or spraying terbinafine solution or other antifungals on shoes on a periodic basis may minimize recurrence.

TINEA PEDIS

• Tinea pedis refers to dermatophytosis of the foot, including the plantar surface and toe web space. It is probably the most common dermatophytosis worldwide. There are four presentations:
  • Interdigital or chronic intertriginous type is most common and consists of dry, red, scaly toe webs. Most common site between fourth and fifth toes.
  • Differential diagnosis: impetigo, Candida intertrigo, *P. aeruginosa* infection, erythrasma, and soft corn.
  • Moccasin or chronic hyperkeratotic variety is the most recalcitrant to therapy. Most patients have chronic disease and nail infection. *T. rubrum* is the most common pathogen. The entire plantar surface is dry, scaly, and red.
  • Differential diagnosis: eczematous and atopic dermatitis, pitted keratolysis, psoriasis vulgaris, keratodermas.
  • Inflammatory variety includes vesicles and bullous lesions on the medial foot (caused by *T. mentagrophytes*). These are usually painful and pruritic. Differential diagnosis: bullous impetigo, allergic contact dermatitis, bullous disease, and dyshidrotic eczema.
  • Ulcerative or vesiculopustular presentation of toe web is rare and is generally the consequence of a secondary bacterial infection in patients who have other medical problems such as diabetes mellitus, peripheral vascular disease, or are immunocompromised.

DIAGNOSIS AND DIFFERENTIAL

• Clinical diagnosis as well as confirmation with direct microscopy and KOH and culture confirms diagnosis.

TREATMENT

• Treatment is with topical antifungal agents and oral antifungal agents may be given as adjunctive therapy.

In some patients with extensive and hyperkeratotic moccasin tinea pedis, the addition of an exfoliant containing urea, lactic acid, or salicylic acid may help reduce scale for better penetration of antifungal agent. Oral antifungal agents are recommended for moccasin type and inflammatory tinea pedis. Oral agents include terbinafine 250 mg/d for 1 to 2 weeks and itraconazole 400 mg/d for 1 to 2 weeks. Griseofulvin is less effective. Use of fluconazole is also effective but more data are required to determine dosage and duration.
• Some measures may be helpful to prevent reinfection: use of antimicrobial soaps, drying feet thoroughly after bathing, applying antifungal powders to feet after bathing, wearing cotton socks, and wearing protective footwear in hotels, locker rooms, gymnasiums, and other public facilities.

TINEA MANUM

• Tinea manum is a dermatophytosis of the palmar surfaces and interdigital spaces of the hand. It is a much less common infection than tinea pedis. The clinical presentation is similar to that of moccasin type tinea pedis. Usually only one palm is involved. A dry, scaling eruption particularly heavy in the skin creases is usually seen. Vesicular or bullous lesions are unlikely. Fingernail involvement may be present.

DIAGNOSIS AND DIFFERENTIAL

• Clinical diagnosis as well as confirmation with direct microscopy and KOH and culture confirms diagnosis. Differential diagnosis: chronic contact dermatitis, psoriasis, dyshidrotic eczema, bacterial infection, and secondary syphilis.

TREATMENT

• Treatment is similar to tinea corporis.
• Prevention measures similar to tinea pedis.

REFERENCES

Elewski BE, ed. *Cutaneous Fungal Infections*, ed 2. Oxford:Blackwell Science, 1998.
Richardson MD, Elewski BE. *Superficial Fungal Infections*. Oxford:Health Press, 2000.
Richardson MD, Warnock DW. *Fungal Infection: Diagnosis and Management*, ed 2. Oxford:Blackwell Science, 1997.

DEEP MYCOSIS

SPOROTRICHOSIS

EPIDEMIOLOGY

- Sporotrichosis is a ubiquitous fungal infection caused by the dimorphic organism *Sporothrix schenckii*. It usually infects the skin by inoculation from contaminated plants or soil.
- *Sporothrix schenckii* has a worldwide distribution, particularly in tropical and temperate regions. It is commonly found in soil and on decaying vegetation and is a well-known pathogen of humans and animals.
- The tissue form is an oval, cigar-shaped yeast.
- Infections are caused by the traumatic implantation of the fungus into the skin, or very rarely, by inhalation into the lungs. Secondary spread to articular surfaces, bone, and muscle is not infrequent, and the infection may also occasionally involve the central nervous system, lungs, or genitourinary tract.
- Predisposing factors for localized disease include diabetes mellitus and alcoholism. For disseminated disease, immunosuppresion, cancer, and HIV infection may predispose to infection.

CLINICAL FEATURES

- Sporotrichosis is primarily a chronic mycotic infection of the cutaneous or subcutaneous tissues and adjacent lymphatics characterized by nodular lesions, which may suppurate and ulcerate. However, five presentations may be described: lymphocutaneous sporotrichosis, fixed cutaneous sporotrichosis, pulmonary sporotrichosis, osteoarticular sporotrichosis, and rare forms of sporotrichosis.

LYMPHOCUTANEOUS SPOROTRICHOSIS

- This is the most common presentation. Primary lesions start out as painless nodules, which soon become palpable and ulcerate at the site of implantation of the fungus, and subcutaneous secondary nodules are distributed along lymphatic vessels, which follow the same indolent course as the primary lesion. No systemic symptoms are present.

FIXED CUTANEOUS SPOROTRICHOSIS

- The first symptom is usually a small painless papule or nodule resembling an insect bite, which is pink or purple in color. The nodule usually appears on the finger, hand, or arm where the fungus first enters through a traumatic break on the skin. Satellite lesions and lymphadenopathy do not occur in this form of sporotrichosis.

PULMONARY SPOROTRICHOSIS

- This is a rare opportunistic fungal infection usually caused by the inhalation of conidia but cases of hematogenous dissemination from a primary cutaneous site have been reported. Symptoms are nonspecific and include cough, sputum production, fever, weight loss and an upper-lobe lesion. Hemoptysis may occur and it can be massive and fatal. The natural course of the lung lesion is gradual progression to death.

OSTEOARTICULAR SPOROTRICHOSIS

- Most patients have cutaneous lesions as well as stiffness and pain in a large joint, usually the knee, elbow, ankle or wrist.

OTHER RARE FORMS OF SPOROTRICHOSIS

- These include endophthalmitis, chorioretinitis, and meningitis.

DIAGNOSIS AND DIFFERENTIAL

- Diagnosis is made by clinical suspicion and isolation of organism on culture. Histology of tissue sections stained using PAS digest, Grocott's methenamine silver (GMS), or Gram stain show small narrow-base budding yeast cells. Differential diagnosis: atypical mycobacterial infection, tularemia, cutaneous tuberculosis, cat-scratch disease, foreign body granuloma, blastomycosis, and leishmaniasis, and other infective agents such as *Nocardia brasiliensis*, *Francisella tularensis*, and *Mycobacterium marinum*.

TREATMENT

- SSKI drops.
- Itraconazole 400 mg/d and terbinafine 250 mg twice daily have both proved to be effective, although treatment times may be prolonged. Ideally, treatment needs to be maintained for at least a month after clinical cure is achieved.
- Intravenous amphotericin B may be used for disseminated infection.
- Local heat has also been shown to improve cutaneous lesions. Extracutaneous forms of sporotrichosis may need a combination of antifungal treatment with amphotericin B or itraconazole together with surgical debridement.
- Pulmonary sporotrichosis in patients infected with HIV continues to be a difficult therapeutic problem, but itraconazole appears to be at least as effective as amphotericin B as treatment for this form of sporotrichosis.
- Infection can be avoided by careful gardening, so as not to get pricked with a rose bush thorn, especially in immunosuppressed persons.

REFERENCES

Davis BA. Sporotrichosis. *Dermatol Clin.* 1996;14:69.

Elewski BE, ed. *Cutaneous Fungal Infections*, ed 2. Oxford:Blackwell Science, 1998.

MYCETOMA

EPIDEMIOLOGY

- Mycetoma is a chronic, granulomatous disease of the skin and subcutaneous tissue, which sometimes involves muscle, bones, and neighboring organs.
- Mycetoma predominates in farm workers but can also be seen in the general population. Males are predominantly affected.
- The disease was first described by Gill in the Madura district of India in 1842, hence "Madura foot." In 1860 Carter named the condition "mycetoma," describing its fungal etiology. In 1813, Pinoy described the mycetoma produced by aerobic bacteria that belong to the actinomycete group and classified mycetomas as those produced by true fungi (eumycetoma) versus those due to aerobic bacteria (actinomycetoma). Both types have similar clinical findings.
- Risk factors include poor hygiene, poor nutrition, and injured tissue.

- Worldwide, approximately 60% of mycetomas are of actinomycotic origin.
- The most common fungal agents isolated in African countries are *Madurella mycetomatis.* In Central and South America, 98% of the mycetoma is caused by actinomycetes, mainly *Nocardia brasiliensis.*

CLINICAL FEATURES

- Mycetoma is produced by the introduction of microorganisms (bacteria or fungi) via localized trauma of the skin with thorns, wood splinters, or implantation with solid objects. The term eumycetoma refers to disease of fungal origin and actinomycetoma is due to bacteria.
- Clinically, the disease begins as small, painless, firm nodules that can persist (mini-mycetomas) or evolve to form extensive suppurative plaques measuring up to 20 cm in diameter. It usually presents as a clinical syndrome characterized by tumefaction, draining sinuses, and sclerotia (granules, grains).
- Mycetomas are localized infections that involve cutaneous and subcutaneous tissue, fascia, and bone. Sclerotia or grains are present in pus and in tissue around the draining sinus tracts. Granules of the microorganisms may occasionally be seen with the naked eye, as in the case of mycetoma caused by *A. madurae* and *M. mycetomatis,* among others. The granules vary in size, color, and degree of hardness, depending on the etiologic species are the hallmark of mycetoma. It typically affects the lower extremities but can occur in almost any region of the body. Rarely, the disease can spread by hematogenous dissemination.

DIAGNOSIS AND DIFFERENTIAL

- Diagnosis can be made by clinical suspicion and by direct microscopy of serosanguinous fluid containing the granules with 10% KOH and Parker ink. Tissue sections should be stained using H&E, PAS digest, and Grocott's methenamine silver (GMS). Differential diagnosis: botryomycosis and actinomycetoma (produced by bacteria of four genera: Nocardia, Actinomadura, Streptomyces, and Nocardiopsis).

TREATMENT

- Treatment involves surgical excision and systemic antimicrobial therapy. Some cases respond to ketoconazole, itraconazole, amphotericin B, and terbinafine.

- Protective footwear and good hygiene are recommended for prevention.

REFERENCES

Poncio-Mendes R, Negroni R, Bonifaz A, Pappagianis D. New aspects of some endemic mycoses. *Med Mycol.* 2000; 38(suppl 1):237.

Restrepo A. Treatment of tropical mycoses. *J Am Acad Dermatol.* 1994;31:S91.

Welsh O, Salinas MC, Rodriguez MA. Treatment of eumycetoma and actinomycetoma. *Curr Top Med Mycol.* 1995;6:47.

CHROMOBLASTOMYCOSIS

EPIDEMIOLOGY

- Chromoblastomycosis is a cutaneous infection affecting normal, immunocompetent persons mostly in tropical or subtropical areas.
- Five fungal species account for most infections: *Fonsecaea pedrosoi, Phialophora verrucosa, Fonsecaea compactum, Wangiella dermatitidis,* and *Cladosporium carrionii.*
- Agricultural workers, miners, and those exposed to soil barefoot are at risk.

CLINICAL FEATURES

- Chromoblastomycosis presents as a chronic cutaneous and subcutaneous infection characterized by formation of papillomatous nodules that tend to ulcerate. Initial infection may be present for years with minimal discomfort.
- Most infections begin on the foot or leg, but other exposed body parts may be infected, especially where the skin is broken. Early small, itchy, enlarging papules develop and extend to form dull red or violaceous, sharply demarcated patches with indurated bases.

- Several weeks or months later, new lesions, projecting 1 to 2 mm above the skin, may appear along paths of lymphatic drainage. Hard, dull red or grayish verrucous projections may develop in the center of patches, gradually extending to cover extremities over periods as long as 4 to 15 years.
- Lymphatic obstruction resulting in elephantiasis-like edema of the extremity may occur, itching may persist, and secondary bacterial superinfections may cause ulcerations and, occasionally, septicemia.

DIAGNOSIS AND DIFFERENTIAL

- Diagnosis is made with direct microscopy and KOH from scrapings. Differential diagnosis: blastomycosis, lobomycosis, mycetoma, sporotrichosis, foreign body granuloma, pyoderma gangrenosum, squamous cell carcinoma, yaws, and tertiary syphilis.

TREATMENT

- In general, medical therapy for chromoblastomycosis has been disappointing. The combination of newer, more potent antifungal agents plus surgical excision or cryosurgery looks more promising.
- Topical antifungals, potassium iodide, amphotericin B, thiabendazole, vitamin D_2, 5-fluorocytosine (5-FC), ketoconazole, fluconazole, itraconazole, and local heat, have all been reported to have varying degrees of success.
- Currently, itraconazole appears the most promising as medical therapy.
- Prevention includes good hygiene and protective footwear for agricultural workers.

REFERENCES

Bonifaz A, Martinez-Soto E, Carrasco-Gerard E, Peniche J. Treatment of chromoblastomycosis with itraconazole, cryosurgery, and a combination of both. *Int J Dermatol.* 1997;36:542.

McGinnis MR. Chromoblastomycosis and phaeohyphomycosis: New concepts, diagnosis, and mycology. *J Am Acad Dermatol.* 1983;8:1.

10 INFESTATIONS AND PARASITES

Cheryl L. Lonergan
Joseph C. English III

SCABIES

EPIDEMIOLOGY

- *Sarcoptes scabiei var. hominis*, is the ectoparasitic mite that causes the human infestation called scabies. Infestations are acquired through direct cutaneous contact with another infested person.
- It is estimated that approximately 300 million persons worldwide are affected by the scabies mite, and those most commonly affected are children.
- Day care centers, nursing homes, prisons, and military barracks commonly experience outbreaks of scabies infestations due to factors such as a reliance on others for personal care and crowded living conditions. Epidemics have occurred in times of war and famine.
- Patients who are immunocompromised may have heavier infestations or atypical presentations that may be confused with other dermatologic diseases.

PATHOPHYSIOLOGY

- The scabies mite is a rounded, eight-legged arthropod. The adult female is twice the size of the male, and is the only one able to burrow into the epidermis.
- The female mite burrows inside the epidermis creating a tunnel. The male mite follows and dies after mating. A total of 2 to 3 eggs/day are produced. The eggs hatch within 4 days releasing larvae, which molt to adults in up to 14 days. The female adult mite has a lifespan of approximately 30 days.
- The mite can live up to 36 hours away from the human host.
- Scabies mites feed on intercellular fluid for nutrition and hydration.

CLINICAL FEATURES

- Intense pruritus, particularly at night, occurs from a delayed hypersensitivity response to antigens found in the saliva, feces, and eggs of the mites. This symptom

occurs 2 to 6 weeks after initial infestation. If the individual has been previously exposed to scabies, however, symptoms may appear as early as 24 to 48 hours after infestation. In the immunocompromised itching may be absent. The lack of an immune response may also result in a heavier infestation, which is more contagious due to the high concentration of mites in the epidermis. This is referred to as crusted scabies (previously known as Norwegian scabies). This presentation causes grey, hyperkeratotic patches and plaques. Persistent or recurrent scabies may be a clue to the initial diagnosis of an immunodeficiency state.
- Mites are typically found in adults in intertriginous areas, such as the web spaces of fingers and toes, groin, axillae, wrists, genitalia, and intergluteal cleft. In children, however, scabies often have a more widespread distribution affecting the palms, soles, and the scalp.
- Skin lesions include burrows, erythematous papules, pustules, vesiculopustules, and nodules. The intense itching often leads to scratching, which may produce excoriated skin and eventually lead to scaling, crusting, and hyperpigmentation. The classic burrow lesion is not always found, but when existent, it is a strong clue to the diagnosis. The burrow typically presents as a short, zigzag line with a small black dot at the end. The line is the tunnel that has been created by the mite, and the black dot at the end is the mite itself. A pathognomic clinical sign of scabies in men is erythematous papules or nodules on the glans penis. Secondary bacterial infections with *Staphylococcus aureus* and *Streptococcus pyogenes* may occur with long-term infestations.

DIAGNOSIS AND DIFFERENTIAL

- Diagnosis of scabies is accomplished through clinical history and visualization of the mites, eggs, or fecal pellets (scybala).
- An ectoparasite prep is performed by applying a "dab" of immersion oil on the suspected skin lesion, scraping the lesion with a #15 scalpel blade (ensuring the epidermis is removed by noting bleeding in the skin after the scrape), placing the scrapings in

immersion oil on a glass slide, and viewing via light microscopy.

- The differential for a scabies infestation is large and may include: atopic dermatitis, contact dermatitis, dermatitis herpetiformis, folliculitis, HIV-related eosinophilic folliculitis, impetigo, infantile acropustulosis, insect bites, and xerosis.

TREATMENT

- Application of the topical scabicide permethrin 5% cream is the treatment of choice.
- The cream is spread over the skin and under nails of the individual from head to toe, avoiding the eyes and mouth, before bed and is rinsed off in after an 8- to 14-hour duration. This is then repeated in 1 week. Once a diagnosis of scabies is made in an individual, it should be recommended that all close contacts be examined and treated, if necessary, to prevent reinfestation.
- Single dose of oral ivermectin at 200 µg/kg, repeated in 1 week is effective in adults, including the immunocompromised.
- Pruritus can be treated with adjunctive therapy, such as oral antihistamines, topical corticosteroids, mentholated lotion, or moisturizing agents. In cases of severe itching refractory to other treatments, a short course of oral corticosteroids may be appropriate.
- It is important to inform patients that pruritus may continue for up to 4 weeks after effective treatment of a scabies infestation.
- Follow-up examination to ensure free of infestation is recommended after 4 weeks.
- Laundering of all clothing and bedding should be recommended, although it should be emphasized that person-to-person contact is the primary means of transmission. The exception to this rule is crusted scabies, which can be easily spread through environmental contact.

REFERENCES

Hoke AW, Maibach HI. Scabies management: A current perspective. *Cutis.* 1999;64:2.

Meinking TL. Infestations. *Curr Probl Dermatol.* 1999; 11:73.

Meinking TL, Taplin D, Hermida JL, et al. The treatment of scabies with ivermectin. *N Eng J Med.* 1995;333:26.

Vaidhyanathan U. Review of ivermectin in scabies. *J Cutan Med Surg.* 2001;5:496.

Vaidhyanathan U, Gopalakrishnan Nair TV. A comparative study of oral ivermectin and topical permethrin cream in the treatment of scabies. *J Am Acad Dermatol.* 2000;42:236.

Walker GJA, Johnstone PW. A systematic review of the treatment of scabies: Interventions for treating scabies. *Arch Dermatol.* 2000;136:387.

LICE

EPIDEMIOLOGY

- Lice are six-legged, wingless, blood-sucking arthropods that infest humans.
- There are three species of lice that cause infestations in humans: *Pediculus humanus capitis* (head louse), *Pediculus humanus corporis* (body louse), and *Phthirus pubis* (pubic or crab louse).

HEAD LICE
- Head lice can infest the scalp of any individual, at all levels of social class, and the most commonly affected population is children aged 3 to 11 years. It is estimated that to a quarter of school-aged children are infested with head lice. African Americans have the lowest rates of head lice infestations, largely due to differences in the shape of the hair shaft, which may prevent egg attachment to the hair shaft.

BODY LICE
- Body lice are commonly found on the clothing of homeless individuals, refugees, and those forced to live in crowded, unsanitary conditions.

PUBIC LICE
- Pubic lice infestation is considered to be a sexually transmitted disease. Pubic lice are indiscriminant in terms of their target population, and infest individuals of all races and backgrounds in equal numbers.

PATHOPHYSIOLOGY

- Transmission can occur as a result of direct contact between individuals or even as a result of exposure to contaminated items, such as bedding and towels. The sharing of items, such as combs, brushes, hats and sports equipment, promotes transmission.
- Lice cannot be transmitted to or from other animals or household pets.
- Mature lice live for approximately 30 days and up to 3 days without a human host.
- After mating the adult female louse produces up to 120 eggs or nits (30 eggs for the pubic louse). These

are "glued" (amino acid derivative) to the hair shaft (head/pubic lice) or to clothing (body louse). The eggs hatch within 9 days.

- After infestation has occurred, the lice begin taking blood meals from their hosts, generally every 3 to 6 hours.
- The transmission of several serious infections are related to infestations with the human body louse.

BODY LICE
- Epidemic louse-borne typhus fever: *Rickettsia prowazekii.*
- Trench fever: *Bartonella quintana.*
- Louse-borne relapsing fever: *Borrelia recurrentis.*

HEAD LICE
- Scalp pyoderma: *Staphylococcus aureus* and group A *Streptococcus pyogenes.*

CLINICAL FEATURES

- Pruritus is the most common symptom that develops as a result of a lice infestation and is likely due to a host reaction to the lice feces, body parts, and lice saliva when the lice feed. It may take weeks to months for the pruritus to develop; however, if the patient has had a previous infestation, the pruritus may begin within 24 to 48 hours.
- The cutaneous immune response where the lice have taken blood meals produces erythematous macules, papules, or wheals.
- Secondary bacterial infections may develop as a result of skin excoriation due to scratching. If chronic, these infections may lead to lichenification and hyperpigmentation of the skin.
- In some cases, an individual may experience systemic symptoms, such as a low-grade fever, lymphadenopathy, and anemia.
- Chronic pubic lice or body lice infestations can cause a bluish macular discoloration of the skin on the abdomen and thighs referred to as maculae ceruleae.

DIAGNOSIS AND DIFFERENTIAL

- Diagnosis is best accomplished by direct examination and observation of adult lice or nits on skin, clothing, or in hair.
- Head lice can often be found in the retroauricular and nape of the neck areas.
- Pubic lice can infest the eyelashes and is called phthiriasis palpebrarum.

- The differential diagnosis for lice infestation is fairly broad and includes: scalp folliculitis, seborrheic dermatitis, atopic dermatitis, psoriasis, and insect bites.
- The nits found in head lice may be mistaken for hair casts (desquamated epithelial cells), dandruff, and dried hair spray.
- Crab lice can be mistaken for scabs or nevi.

TREATMENT

- Permethrin is the recommended first-line agent and is the most well studied pediculicide. Topical agents are used most commonly and include 1% permethrin cream rinse or 5% permethrin cream.
- Two treatments 1 week apart are required.
- Alternatively, a single, oral dose of the anthelminthic agent ivermectin at 200 μg/kg repeated in 10 days appears to be effective in the eradication of lice.
- With all lice infestations, it is important to thoroughly clean the environment and the individual's personal belongings.
- Commercial environmental pesticides should not be used.
- With all lice infestations, secondary bacterial infections of the skin may require appropriate oral antibiotics.

HEAD LICE

- 1% permethrin cream rinse to a damp scalp for 10 minutes repeated in 1 week.
- In resistant cases, increase the duration of 1% permethrin cream rinse to 30 minutes prior to rinsing, use 5% permethrin cream to the scalp overnight under occlusion with a shower cap, or consider topical malathion 0.5% solution to scalp hair for 12 hours or oral ivermectin.
- All should be repeated in 1 week. In addition, investigating the source of infection may prevent recurrent reinfestations.
- Nits can be removed with the use of metal nit combs in combination with nit remover (i.e., 8% formic acid).
- An alternative, which is usually not cosmetically acceptable, is to shave the head.

BODY LICE

- The main focus in the eradication of body lice is related to the disinfestation of clothing and bedding. Items should be machine washed in hot water, dry

cleaned, fumigated with methyl bromide, or inciner-
ated. This is followed by an 8- to 14-hour application
of 5% permethrin with reapplication 1 week later.

PUBIC LICE

- The key is to treat all hairy parts of the body, as pubic
  lice are not necessarily confined to the pubic and perineal region, and the lice can easily move from one
  location to another if treatment is isolated. Topical
  agents such as 1% permethrin cream rinse, or 5% permethrin cream are recommended.
- Pthiriasis palpebrarum can be treated with a 10-day
  course of trimethoprim-sulfamethoxazole or tetracycline. Another safe and effective way of treating
  this type of infestation is the application of petroleum
  jelly to the eyelashes five times a day for a total of
  10 days.

REFERENCES

Burkhart CG, Burkhart CN, Burkhart KM. An assessment of
topical and oral prescription and over-the-counter treatments
for head lice. *J Am Acad Dermatol.* 1998;38:979.

Goddard J. *Physician's Guide to Arthropods of Medical
Importance*, ed 2. Boca Raton:CRC Press, 1996:189.

Maguire JH, Spielman A. Ectoparasite infestations and arthropod bites and stings. In: Braunwald E, Fauci AS, Isselbacher
KJ, et al, eds. *Harrison's Principles of Internal Medicine,* ed
14. New York:McGraw-Hill, 1998:2548.

Meinking TL. Infestations. *Curr Probl Dermatol.* 1999;11:73.

SPIDER BITES

EPIDEMIOLOGY

- Most spiders use venomous bites to immobilize or kill
  prey.
- North American spiders that cause necrotic skin
  lesions include: brown recluse, hobo, wolf, fishing,
  green lynx, sac and jumping spiders.
- Medically significant necrotic arachnidism is due to
  the brown recluse (*Loxosceles reclusa*) and hobo
  (*Tegenaria agretis*) spiders. Up to 10,000 cases are
  reported annually.

BROWN RECLUSE
- The brown recluse spider is found most commonly in
  the Midwest and south central region of the country.

They are medium-sized (6 to 10 mm body length) and
have a uniform brown appearance with a darkened
violin pattern often seen on the dorsum of the first
body segment. These spiders generally bite victims
only when they are trapped next to the victim's skin.

HOBO SPIDER
- The hobo spider is found mainly in the U.S. Pacific
  Northwest and is 7 to 14 mm in body length, brown in
  color, and often has a herringbone pattern on the dorsal
  abdomen. These spiders can bite without provocation.

BLACK WIDOW SPIDER
- The black widow spider, *Latrodectus mactans*, is
  present in all 48 contiguous states but is found primarily in areas with warmer climates. This spider
  ranges in size from 8 to 15 mm and is black with red
  ventral abdominal markings that often have an hour-
  glass design. These spiders can produce medically
  significant symptoms but the bite site does not
  become necrotic.

TARANTULAS
- The large, mygalomorph spiders bites are generally
  innocuous.
- Other venomous species not found in the United States
  include banana spiders, Australian funnel-web spiders,
  white-tailed spiders, and six-eyed crab spiders. The
  most deadly spider is the Australian funnel-web.

PATHOPHYSIOLOGY

- The pharmacology of the spider bite toxins is quite
  varied between the species, which makes identification of the spider important for medical management.

BROWN RECLUSE
- The venom of the brown recluse spider contains alka-
  line phosphatase, hyaluronidase, lipase, and its major
  component, sphingomyelinase D.
- Sphingomyelinase D activates complement, arachi-
  donic acid metabolites, and neutrophilic chemoattrac-
  tants and causes hemolysis as well as enzymatic
  destruction of myelin.
- The degree of skin necrosis appears to be related to
  neutrophil activity.

HOBO SPIDER
- The components of the venom are unknown.

BLACK WIDOW SPIDER
- The venom component, alpha-latrotoxin, is the neuro-
  toxic agent that leads to release of neurotransmitters.

TARANTULAS
- Although the bites are not symptomatic, the "flicking" of urticating barbed hairs from posterior abdomen in the response to danger can become airborne and lodge in skin, eyes, and nasal passages.

CLINICAL FEATURES

BROWN RECLUSE
- Localized symptoms of the bite appear in 2 to 6 hours and can include: edema, erythema, pain at the site, pruritus, and fever. The edema and erythema may resolve without intervention. Alternatively, a more serious "bull's-eye" type wound can form that may become violaceous, hemorrhagic, bullous, ulcerate, and progress to necrosis. Healing can take weeks to months.
- Systemic symptoms can occur in bites of all severity. These occur within 2 to 3 days and may include hemolysis, thrombocytopenia, and DIC. Although rare, death may result from hemolysis, renal failure, pulmonary edema, and DIC, especially in children.

HOBO SPIDER
- The hobo spider can cause a cutaneous necrosis similar to that of the brown recluse spider but the tissue destruction is less severe.
- Systemic symptoms may include headaches with visual and auditory hallucinations, malaise, vomiting, and diarrhea. The headache can be severe and last up to 1 week in duration.

BLACK WIDOW SPIDER
- Localized symptoms of the black widow bite include erythema, fang marks, and petechiae at the site. Other symptoms are systemic, appear within 1 to 3 hours and include abdominal rigidity with a nontender abdomen, muscle cramping, malaise, sweating, nausea, vomiting, oliguria, hypertension, priapism, and tachycardia or bradycardia. These symptoms can last 3 to 5 days if untreated.

DIAGNOSIS AND DIFFERENTIAL

- Diagnosis is generally made based on history and clinical findings.
- Identification of the spider is ideal for appropriate management.
- The differential diagnosis for necrotic arachnidism includes: arthropod assault, vasculitis, pyoderma gangrenosum, ecthyma gangrenosum, purpura fulminans, and warfarin necrosis.

- Black widow envenomation can be confused with an acute abdomen from appendicitis.

TREATMENT

- All insect bites alter skin integrity, predisposing patients to secondary bacterial infections, which should be treated with appropriate antibiotics.

BROWN RECLUSE SPIDER
- Rest, ice compression, and elevation. Avoid heat, which can worsen lesions.
- Tetanus booster vaccination and analgesics.
- Dapsone in moderate to severe cases; however, controlled trials are lacking.
- Supportive care for systemic symptoms.

HOBO SPIDER
- Same as brown recluse.
- No indication for dapsone.

BLACK WIDOW SPIDER
- Intravenous calcium gluconate and/or antivenom.
- Tetanus booster vaccination.

REFERENCES

Goddard J. *Physician's Guide to Arthropods of Medical Importance*, ed 2. Boca Raton:CRC Press, 1996:271.

Kemp ED. Bites and stings of the arthropod kind: Treating reactions that can range from annoying to menacing. *Postgrad Med.* 1998;130:88.

Sams HH, Dunnick CA, Smith ML, et al. Necrotic arachnidism. *J Am Acad Dermatol.* 2001;44:561.

Vetter RS, Visscher PK. Bites and stings of medically important venomous arthropods. *Int J Dermatol.* 1998;37:481.

LYME DISEASE

EPIDEMIOLOGY

- Lyme disease is the most common vector-borne disease in the United States, with more than 15,000 cases per year reported.
- Lyme disease is a zoonotic, tick-borne illness caused by the spirochete, *Borrelia burgdorferi*, which is transmitted to humans by *Ixodes* ticks.
- *Borrelia burgdorferi* is endemic in over 15 states as well as Europe and Asia. In the United States, the

spirochete is primarily found in the Northeast from Maine to Maryland, in the Midwest in Wisconsin and Minnesota, and in the West in Northern California and Oregon.

- In the NE and Central United States, the transmission of the spirochete moves from nymphal *I. scapularis* tick from its reservoir in the white-footed mouse. Deer serve only as the maintenance host of the adult form of the tick. In the Northwest, the woodrat is reservoir of infection and transmission occurs through *I. pacificus.*

PATHOPHYSIOLOGY

- Transmission of the spirochete occurs when the infected nymphal ticks bite humans to obtain a blood meal.
- *B. burgdorferi* is rarely transmitted when the infected tick has been attached to the human host for less than 48 hours.
- Upon injection of the spirochete by the tick into a human host, the organism migrates to the skin and is subsequently disseminated through the blood and/or lymphatics to other skin sites, organs, or musculoskeletal tissues.
- The key virulence factors of *B. burgdorferi* are surface proteins (Osp A, B, and C) that enable the spirochete to attach to mammalian cells.
- Antibody mediated defense via the classic complement pathway is required for destruction of the organism.

STAGE 1: EARLY LOCALIZED INFECTION
- The rash of Lyme disease, erythema migrans begins 2 to 12 days after the tick bite as a red macule or papule, which is later accompanied by a surrounding area of redness. The area of redness must expand to 5 cm or more with central clearing to be diagnostic of Lyme disease. The center of the rash may become indurated, erythematous, vesicular, or necrotic at the point of tick attachment.
- Erythema migrans can occur in approximately 75% of infected patients.
- Patients often also experience influenza-like symptoms, such as malaise, fatigue, headaches, arthralgias, myalgias, fever, and lymphadenopathy.

STAGE 2: EARLY DISSEMINATED INFECTION
- Within days or weeks disseminated infection can develop involving the nervous system, heart, or joints. Up to 25% of patients will not have a history of erythema migrans.
- Patients may develop symptoms of acute neuroborreliosis. This is characterized by a lymphocytic meningitis

that presents with headaches, meningismus, and mental status changes. In addition, patients may experience facial nerve palsies, motor or sensory radiculoneuritis, mononeuritis multiplex, cerebellar ataxia, or blindness due to optic nerve involvement.
- Patients may have cardiac involvement, which may include AV block, myopericarditis, mild left ventricular dysfunction or, rarely, cardiomegaly.
- Migratory musculoskeletal pain is common in joints, tendons, muscles, and bursae.
- Cutaneous manifestations include a borrelial lymphocytoma, which is a B-lymphocytic infiltrate, manifesting as a blue-red nodule on the ear lobe, nipple, or scrotum. It occurs commonly in Europe and Asia but is rare in the United States.
- Other nonspecific cutaneous reactions include: generalized erythema and urticarial or annular lesions.

STAGE 3: LATE PERSISTENT INFECTION
- After months or years, a persistent infection characterized by subjective symptoms of musculoskeletal pain, neurocognitive difficulties, and fatigue may develop.
- Patients can develop intermittent joint pain and swelling, particularly in the knees.
- A late cutaneous manifestation is acrodermatitis chronica atrophicans, which is characterized by atrophic induration of extremity skin with superficial vein accentuation. This occurs more commonly in cases of European and Asian acquired disease and is rare in the United States.

DIAGNOSIS AND DIFFERENTIAL

- The diagnosis of Lyme disease is based on the above clinical characteristics in an endemic area.
- Serologic testing can not be used primarily for diagnosing Lyme disease.
- Serologic testing will take 4 to 6 weeks for antibodies to be detectable. Enzyme linked immunosorbent assay (ELISA) and immunofluorescent antibodies (IFA) can be performed. Western blot can be used for confirmation of a positive result. False positive results can occur in the setting of relapsing fever, ehrlichiosis, syphilis, and autoimmune disease.
- Serologic testing is useful in patients with arthritis and tick exposure but with no history of erythema migrans.
- Serologic testing does not distinguish between an active infection versus prior infection.
- Tissue/fluid cultures have low yield but PCR testing of synovial fluid is positive in most patients.
- The differential of erythema migrans may include: insect bite, cellulitis, tinea corporis, contact dermatitis,

fixed drug eruption, granuloma annulare, and erythema annulare centrifugum.
- Coinfection with ehrlichiosis and babesiosis can complicate Lyme disease since *I. scapularis* tick is the vector for these diseases as well.
- Connective tissue diseases may manifest with similar symptoms to stage 2 and 3 Lyme disease.

TREATMENT

ANTIBIOTICS
Treatment of early or localized disease includes:
- Doxycycline (100 mg PO b.i.d.) for 21 days in patients > 8 years of age (except for pregnant women).
- Amoxicillin orally (500 mg t.i.d.) for 21 days can be used for pregnant women and children.
- Cefuroxime axetil (500 mg orally b.i.d.) for 21 days.

Treatment of neurologic or cardiac abnormalities includes:
- Ceftriaxone IV for 14- to 21-day course.
- Penicillin G or cefotaxime IV and doxycycline or amoxicillin orally are alternatives.
- A temporary pacemaker may be required for severe AV block.

Treatment of Lyme arthritis includes:
- Doxycycline orally (100 mg b.i.d.) or amoxicillin orally (500 mg t.i.d.) for 28 days.
- Ceftriaxone or penicillin G intravenously for 14 to 28 days.

VACCINATION
- Since infection with *B. burgdorferi* does not confer long-term immunity, the FDA approved a vaccine (LYMErix). The vaccine is a recombinant Osp A protein that induce anti-Osp A antibodies with an efficacy of 76% after a series of three injections. It is recommended for patients 15 to 70 years of age, who live in endemic regions of the country, and have frequent exposure to *I. scapularis* ticks.

PREVENTION
- Protective clothing, topical repellents containing DEET (diethyltoluamide), and vector control.

REFERENCES

Abramowitz M, ed. Treatment of Lyme disease. *Med Lett.* 2000;42:37.

Brown SL, Hansen SL, Langone JJ. Role of serology in the diagnosis of Lyme disease. *JAMA.* 1999;282:62.

Gilbert DN, Moellering Jr RC, Sande MA. *The Sanford Guide to Antimicrobial Therapy 2001*, ed 31. Hyde Park: Antimicrobial Therapy Inc., 2001:87.

Steere AC. Lyme disease. *N Engl J Med.* 2001;345:115.

Steere AC. *Borrelia burgdorferi* (Lyme disease, Lyme borreliosis). In: Mandell GL, Bennett JE, Dolin R, eds. *Principles and Practice of Infectious Diseases*, ed 5. Philadelphia: Churchill Livingstone, 2000:2504.

The Centers for Disease Control. Lyme disease — United States, 1999. *MMWR.* 2001;50:181.

The Centers for Disease Control. Recommendations for the use of Lyme disease vaccine. *MMWR.* 1999;48:11.

Wormser GP, Nadelman RB, Dattwyler RJ, et al. Guidelines from the Infectious Diseases Society of America: Practice guidelines for the treatment of Lyme disease. *Clin Infect Dis.* 2000;31:S1.

LEISHMANIASIS

EPIDEMIOLOGY

- There are three major types of leishmaniasis: cutaneous, mucocutaneous, and visceral (kala azar).
- It is estimated to infect 12,000,000 people worldwide, with 1 to 2 million new cases per year.
- All three types of leishmaniasis are caused by infection with a flagellated, protozoan, obligate intracellular parasite transmitted by the Phlebotomus and Lutzomyia species of sandflies.
- Different species of the protozoa and their resulting form of leishmaniasis include:
  1. *L. aethiopica, L. tropica, L. major*—Old World cutaneous
  2. *L. mexicana, L. panamensis, L. braziliensis*—New World cutaneous
  3. *L. braziliensis*—mucocutaneous
  4. *L. donovani, L. chagasi, L. infantum*—visceral
- Leishmania organisms are widely distributed on every continent except Australia and Antarctica.
- In the Unites States, Leishmania have been found in the state of Texas.

PATHOPHYSIOLOGY

- Transmission of the unflagellated amastigotes occurs from the reservoir (humans, rodents, and mammals) to the vector female sandfly via a blood meal. In the sandfly, the amastigotes are converted to a flagellated, extracellular, metacyclic promastigotes. These are injected via the sandfly bite to the new host and parasitize tissue macrophages of the reticuloendothelial system in the mammalian host and revert to the unflagellated amastigote form causing tissue destruction.

- The incubation period of leishmaniasis can range from weeks to months.
- Cell-mediated immune mechanisms are the primary means of controlling the infection.
- As is true in leprosy, the manifestation of leishmaniasis depends on the immunologic host response to the infection.

CLINICAL FEATURES

- Leishmania organisms can overlap in their clinical presentation and can be geographically specific.

LOCALIZED CUTANEOUS LEISHMANIASIS
- A papule at the site of inoculation that later ulcerates. The lesion is typically circular and erythematous with raised borders and is covered by yellowish exudate. The ulcer generally heals slowly over weeks to months, with resultant hypopigmented scar, and may require treatment for complete resolution.
- In Mexico, earlobe ulcerations are referred to as "Chiclero's" ulcers.
- Lesions can be accompanied by a sporotrichoid-like lymphadenopathy.

DIFFUSE CUTANEOUS LEISHMANIASIS
- Multiple, cutaneous papular to nodular lesions due to dissemination of amastigotes in patients with a minimal cell-mediated immune response.

LEISHMANIASIS RECIDIVANS
- Recurrent psoriasiform cutaneous lesions at sites of previously healed scars.

POST-KALA AZAR DERMAL LEISHMANIASIS
- Cutaneous papules and nodules that develop after apparent cure of visceral leishmaniasis. It is characterized by macules and papules that first appear around the mouth, become more dense and spread downward to cover the entire body. Nodules, vegetations, and ulcerations may develop as well.

MUCOCUTANEOUS
- The mucocutaneous form of the disease may or may not be preceded by a cutaneous lesion.
- If preceded by cutaneous disease, mucocutaneous lesions may develop months to years after cutaneous lesions have healed. This form of the disease is characterized by painful, destructive lesions of the mucosal membranes of the nasopharynx, oropharynx, larynx, and perineum. This is often referred to as espundia in Central/South America.
- Mucocutaneous leishmaniasis evolves slowly over time, is often disfiguring, and is difficult to treat.

VISCERAL (KALA AZAR)
- Visceral leishmaniasis is the most severe and life-threatening form of the disease.
- It behaves like an opportunistic infection in the immunocompromised, particularly HIV-infected individuals and transplant recipients.
- This form of the disease may be characterized by fever, hepatosplenomegaly, and pancytopenia and, if untreated, is often fatal.

DIAGNOSIS AND DIFFERENTIAL

- Clinical symptoms and geographic location.
- Detection of organisms (amastigotes referred to as Leishman–Donovan bodies) by tissue histopathologic microscopic (H&E and Giemsa stained tissue specimens).
- Culture of tissue using specialized culture medium (Novy–MacNeal–Nicolle) to isolate promastigotes. May take weeks to months.
- ELISA and indirect immunofluorescent antibody tests are only supportive of the diagnosis. False positives occur due to cross-reactivity with Chagas' disease, malaria, leprosy, and schistosomiasis.
- Leishmanin skin test (Montenegro test) can be used when the microscopic examination is not helpful. This test is generally positive in the cutaneous and mucosal forms of the disease and negative in the visceral form of the disease. This test is not approved in the United States.

The differential diagnosis may include the following.

CUTANEOUS
- Sporotrichosis, chromomycosis, lobomycosis, mycobacterial infections, sarcoidosis, and halogenodermas.

MUCOCUTANEOUS
- Paracoccidioidomycosis, midline facial lethal granuloma, histoplasmosis, mucormycosis, rhinoscleroma, and leprosy.

POST-KALA AZAR DERMAL LEISHMANIASIS
- Leprosy, yaws, and syphilis.

VISCERAL
- Filariasis and schistosomiasis.

TREATMENT

CUTANEOUS
- First line—Pentavalent antimony—stibogluconate or meglumine antimonate (IM, IV); or pentamidine (IM, IV)

- Second line—ketoconazole (oral), or itraconazole (oral)

MUCOSAL
- First line—Pentavalent antimony—stibogluconate or meglumine antimonate (IM, IV)
- Second line—Amphotericin B (IV)

VISCERAL
- First line—Pentavalent antimony—stibogluconate or meglumine antimonate (IM, IV)
- Second line—Amphotericin B (IV), or liposomal amphotericin B, ampho B colloidal dispersion, or ampho B lipid complex (IV)
- In the United States, Pentostam (stibogluconate sodium) is the pentavalent antimonial compound available through the Centers for Disease Control in Atlanta, Ga
- Protective clothing, insect repellent, and vector control.

REFERENCES

Berman JD. Human leishmaniasis: clinical, diagnostic, and chemotherapeutic developments in the last 10 years. *Clin Infect Dis.* 1997;24:684.

Gilbert DN, Moellering Jr RC, Sande MA. *The Sanford Guide to Antimicrobial Therapy 2001*, ed 31. Antimicrobial Therapy Inc., 2001:87.

Lucchina LC, Wilson ME, Drake LA. Dermatology and the recently returned traveler: Infectious diseases with dermatologic manifestations. *Int J Dermatol.* 1997;36:167.

Martin S, Gambel J, Jackson J, et al. Leishmaniasis in the United States military. *Military Med.* 1998;163:801.

Murray HW, Pepin J, Nutman TB, et al. Tropical medicine. *BMJ.* 2000;320:490.

Pearson RD, Sousa AQ, Jeronimo SMB. Leishmania species: Visceral (kala azar), cutaneous and mucosal leishmaniasis. In: Mandell GL, Bennett JE, Dolin R, eds. *Principles and Practice of Infectious Diseases*, ed 5. Philadelphia: Churchill Livingstone, 2000:2831.

AMERICAN TRYPANOSOMIASIS

EPIDEMIOLOGY

- American trypanosomiasis, which is also known as Chagas' disease, results from infection with the protozoan parasite *Trypanosoma cruzi*.
- This parasite is found primarily in rural Mexico, Central America, and South America.
- It is estimated that 16 to 18 million people currently have chronic *T. cruzi* infection.

- The vector for transmission of the parasite is the blood-sucking Reduviidae species of the Triatoma, Rhodnius, and Panstrongylus genera. These are referred to as "kissing or cone-nose bugs."
- The reservoir for the protozoa includes: humans and domestic and wild animals.
- The transfusion of blood donated by individuals infected with *Trypanosoma cruzi* often results in transmission of the parasite to the donor recipient.

PATHOPHYSIOLOGY

- Infection occurs when the metacyclic, flagellated trypomastigotes are shed in reduviid bug feces at the time of a blood meal. Transmission is enhanced when the victim scratches the area of the bite. However, the trypomastigotes can invade directly through mucosal or conjunctival tissues.
- The trypomastigotes enter local cells and become intracellular amastigotes where they multiply, disseminated hematogenously, and invade smooth muscle and autonomic ganglia, which results in the development of chronic disease.

CLINICAL FEATURES

- The acute phase of Chagas' disease is characterized by the formation of an indurated papule at the bite site that may be accompanied by local swelling (chagoma), adenopathy, fever, myocarditis. When the bite occurs near the eye, periorbital edema commonly develops (Romana sign). The acute phase generally resolves spontaneously in approximately 4 to 6 weeks.
- In rare cases, *T. cruzi* can initially invade the CNS and cause meningoencephalitis.
- The chronic phase of the illness follows the acute illness by months to years and is characterized by a low-grade parasitemia, although patients are generally asymptomatic. In 10 to 30% of infected individuals, the chronic phase may manifest as irreversible cardiomyopathy with congestive heart failure, dysrhythmias, and thromboembolism; irreversible megaesophagus with dysphagia and aspiration; and irreversible megacolon with severe constipation.

DIAGNOSIS AND DIFFERENTIAL

- Acute disease is diagnosed by detection of trypanosomes in blood.
- Serologic testing can detect anti-*T. cruzi* antibodies using complement fixation, hemagglutination, indirect

immunofluorescence, and ELISA. However, false positive results can occur due to cross-reactivity with malaria, leishmaniasis, syphilis, and collagen vascular diseases.
- In the acute phase, the initial appearance of the indurated papule and local swelling may be mistaken for arthropod bites or angioedema.
- In the chronic phase, all causes of dilated cardiomyopathy, megacolon, and/or megaesophagus must be included in the differential.

TREATMENT

- Only the acute phase of Chagas' disease can be successfully pharmacologically treated with a 50% parasitologic cure rate.
- Benznidazole and nifurtimox are used in the acute phase with variable efficacy.
- Surgery can be employed for symptomatic treatment of the chronic phase of the disease (i.e., heart transplant).
- Protective clothing, insect repellent, and vector control.

REFERENCES

Benenson AS. *Control of Communicable Diseases Manual*, ed 16. Washington DC:American Public Health Association, 1995:482.

Gilbert DN, Moellering Jr RC, Sande MA. *The Sanford Guide to Antimicrobial Therapy 2001*, ed 31. Antimicrobial Therapy Inc., 2001:90.

Guerrant RL, Walker DH, Weller PF. *Tropical Infectious Diseases; Principles, Pathogens and Practice*. Philadelphia: Churchill Livingstone, 1999.

Kirchhoff LV. *Trypanosoma* species (American trypanosomiasis, Chagas' disease): Biology of trypanosomes. In: Mandell GL, Bennett JE, Dolin R, eds. *Principles and Practice of Infectious Diseases*, ed 5. Philadelphia:Churchill Livingstone, 2000:2845.

Kirchhoff LV. American trypanosomiasis (Chagas' disease) — a tropical disease now in the United States. *N Engl J Med.* 1993;329:639.

World Health Organization. *Weekly Epidemiol Rec.* 2000; 75:9.

AFRICAN TRYPANOSOMIASIS

EPIDEMIOLOGY

- Human African trypanosomiasis is also known as African sleeping sickness.

- African sleeping sickness results from transmission by the Glossina tsetse fly of two distinct species of protozoa found in different regions of Africa. These species of protozoa are *Trypanosoma brucei gambiense* in West and Central Africa and *Trypanosoma brucei rhodesiense* in East and Southern Africa.
- It has been established that the reservoir for *T. b. rhodesiense* is primarily domestic cattle, in contrast to a human reservoir for *T. b. gambiense*.
- It is estimated to have over 100,000 new infections reported per year.

PATHOPHYSIOLOGY

- The infected tsetse fly bites a human victim. The metacyclic trypomastigote leaves the salivary gland of the tsetse fly to enter the human at the site of the bite. The trypanosomes invade and mature in the blood and lymphatics of the human and eventually invade the central nervous system. This organism does not have an amastigote form.
- Once transmission has been successfully completed, the infection progresses rapidly with *T. b. rhodesiense* and can be fatal within weeks to months if untreated.
- In contrast, *T. b. gambiense* produces a more chronic infection that can persist for several years but is also fatal if not treated.

CLINICAL FEATURES

T. B . GAMBIENSE
- The bite site may cause a chancre to develop, which may be tender. This chancre may or may not heal spontaneously. The chancre may be followed later by fever and lymphadenopathy. The late stage or CNS stage, is characterized by fever, headache, and signs of meningoencephalitis. The CNS stage may be preceded by a long, asymptomatic stage.

T. B. RHODESIENSE
- It causes an acute illness characterized by fever and constitutional symptoms and signs of meningoencephalitis.

DIAGNOSIS AND DIFFERENTIAL

- Diagnosis can be made by detection of parasites in blood smears or tissue aspirates.
- Lumbar puncture can be performed to assess for parasitic invasion of the CNS.

- Serologic testing can be performed to detect antitrypanosomal antibodies using immunofluorescence and hemagglutination.
- The differential diagnosis includes malaria and a variety of febrile illnesses.

TREATMENT

- Early infection is treated with suramin, pentamidine, or eflornithine.
- CNS involvement should be treated with eflornithine for infection with *T. b. gambiense* and melarsoprol for *T. b. rhodesiense*.
- Melarsoprol is the most dangerous of the medications used to treat sleeping sickness because it can cause a potentially fatal encephalopathy. This occurs in less than 10% of treated cases.

REFERENCES

Barrett MP. Problems for the chemotherapy of human African trypanosomiasis. *Curr Opin Infect Dis.* 2000;13:647.

Benenson AS. *Control of Communicable Diseases Manual*, ed 16. Washington DC:American Public Health Association, 1995:482.

Gilbert DN, Moellering Jr RC, Sande MA. *The Sanford Guide to Antimicrobial Therapy 2001*, ed 31. Antimicrobial Therapy Inc., 2001:90.

Guerrant RL, Walker DH, Weller PF. *Tropical Infectious Diseases; Principles, Pathogens and Practice.* Philadelphia: Churchill Livingstone, 1999.

Kirchhoff LV. Agents of African trypanosomiasis (sleeping sickness). In: Mandell GL, Bennett JE, Dolin R, eds. *Principles and Practice of Infectious Diseases*, ed 5. Philadelphia: Churchill Livingstone, 2000:2853.

Murray HW, Pepin J, Nutman TB, et al. Tropical medicine. *Br Med J.* 2000;320:490.

Welburn SC, Ferve EM, Coleman PG, et al. Sleeping sickness. *Trends Parasitol.* 2001;17:19.

11 BLISTERING DISEASES

Jo-David Fine

INHERITED BLISTERING DISEASES

EPIDERMOLYSIS BULLOSA

EPIDEMIOLOGY

- Epidermolysis bullosa (EB) is a rare, inherited disorder encompassing at least 20 different phenotypes, which has no gender or ethnic predilections.
- The overall incidence of inherited EB in the United States, based on findings of the National EB Registry, is approximately 19 per one million live births. The corresponding prevalence of this group of diseases is approximately eight per one million.
- The most common type of EB is EB simplex, accounting for at least 60% of all cases within the American-based National EB Registry. Similarly, about two-thirds of all EB simplex patients have the localized variant referred to as Weber–Cockayne disease.

PATHOPHYSIOLOGY

- All forms of inherited EB result from genetic mutations, which may arise within any of at least 10 genes encoding for structural proteins within the epidermis or the skin basement membrane zone.
- The types of mutations (i.e., point mutations; premature termination codons; missense or nonsense mutations) and modes of transmission (autosomal dominant vs autosomal recessive; homozygous vs compound heterozygous mutations) vary among three different EB subtypes, and may help to explain the variability in phenotype observed among the many types and subtypes of EB that have been reported to date.
- The different levels of skin cleavage characteristic of the three different EB types (i.e., simplex, junctional, dystrophic) correspond with the ultrastructural locations of specific proteins targeted for genetic mutation in inherited EB. Most of these "targeted" proteins normally reside within the skin dermoepidermal junction.
- The skin dermoepidermal junction (DEJ) is a specialized type of basement membrane that separates the epidermis from the underlying dermis. It is best defined either by transmission electron microscopy or by immunohistochemical staining with antibodies that recognize specific components of the DEJ. Associated proteins include bullous pemphigoid antigens 1 and 2; plectin, laminins 1, 5, and 6; uncein; $\alpha_6\beta_4$ integrin, collagens type 4 and 7; chondroitin-6-sulfate proteoglycan; and heparan sulfate proteoglycan. Ultrastructurally, the DEJ is comprised of two regions: an electron sparse one (lamina lucida), which is in direct apposition with the overlying basal keratinocyte cell membrane, and an electron dense one (lamina densa), which separates the lamina lucida from the uppermost papillary dermis. The DEJ also has several associated ultrastructures, visible only via electron microscopy, which include the hemidesmosome, subbasal dense plate, anchoring filament, and anchoring fibril.
- Blisters within nearly every subtype of EB simplex, for example, arise within the basilar keratinocyte. In contrast, blisters in junctional EB arise within the lamina lucida, and in dystrophic EB, the blisters arise within the sublamina densa region of the uppermost papillary dermis.
- The associated ultrastructural features seen in different subtypes of EB also correspond closely with the locations of those targeted proteins that contribute to the structural integrity of these ultrastructures. Keratin filaments may appear disarrayed, clumped, reduced in number, or even absent in some subtypes of EB simplex. Junctional EB skin may show qualitative or quantitative changes (i.e., reduction or absence) in both hemidesmosomes and subbasal dense plates. Anchoring filaments, which normally reside within the lamina lucida, may be similarly reduced in number or absent in more severely affected patients with junctional EB. Anchoring fibrils, which normally attach the lamina densa to the papillary dermis, may be reduced in number and/or rudimentary in structure in milder forms of recessive dystrophic EB, and completely absent in the skin of patients with severe generalized recessive dystrophic EB.
- EB simplex results from usually autosomal dominantly transmitted mutations in either of two keratins, K5 or K14, which are those paired keratins present primarily within basilar keratinocytes. More severely affected subtypes of EB simplex are associated with mutations within the more structurally unstable portions of the K5 and K14 genes.

- The most severe subtype of junctional EB (JEB), so-called Herlitz JEB, results from severe mutations within any of the three genes encoding for the three chains of laminin-5, a macromolecule that spans the lamina lucida and plays a key role in the maintenance of epidermal attachment to the underlying dermis and also presumably contributes to the composition of hemidesmosome, the subbasal dense plate, and the anchoring filament. A somewhat milder subtype of JEB, so-called non-Herlitz JEB (also known as generalized atrophic benign EB or GABEB), arises from less structurally severe mutations within the genes for either laminin-5 or bullous pemphigoid antigen-2. A rare form of generalized JEB that is associated with congenital pyloric atresia (JEB-PA) results from mutations in the genes encoding for either of the two chains of $\alpha_6\beta_4$ integrin.
- All forms of dystrophic EB presumably arise from mutations within the gene encoding for type VII collagen, which is the main biochemical component of the anchoring fibril.
- A rare form of EB simplex associated with muscular dystrophy arises from mutations within the gene encoding for plectin, a known component of both skeletal muscle and the cytoplasmic portion of the hemidesmosome.
- Patients with dystrophic EB also are known to have increased levels of a tissue collagenase that degrades type VII collagen and, therefore, presumably contributes to collagenolysis within the uppermost portion of the dermis in these patients.

CLINICAL FEATURES

- All types and subtypes of inherited EB have mechanically fragile skin, resulting in blister formation and erosions following even the most minimal traction or trauma to the skin.
- The extent of skin involvement, as well as the anatomic sites of predilection, vary among the many subtypes of EB.
- The frequency of occurrence of specific cutaneous findings also varies among the three major EB types (simplex, junctional, and dystrophic) and subtypes. The combined absence of milia, nail dystrophy, and scarring is more suggestive of simplex than nonsimplex types of EB, although any or all of these may still occur in some EB simplex subtypes, especially in the more severe, generalized ones (i.e., Koebner; Dowling–Meara).
- Milia are present in virtually every patient with dystrophic EB, although they may also commonly arise in junctional EB.

- Nail dystrophy and atrophic scarring are typical features of dystrophic EB, but also occur in the majority of patients with junctional EB.
- Exuberant granulation tissue, most commonly in periorificial array, is nearly pathognomonic of Herlitz JEB, but may not be present within the first year of life.
- Mitten deformities (pseudosyndactyly) of the hands and feet most commonly arise in dystrophic EB, especially in patients with the severe, generalized subtype of recessive dystrophic EB known as Hallopeau–Siemens disease. This finding may occur as early as within the first year of life in a minority of these patients. By young adulthood nearly every Hallopeau–Siemens patient will have developed at least localized partial pseudosyndactyly.
- Herpetiform grouping of vesicles or bullae is a characteristic feature of the Dowling–Meara subtype of generalized EB simplex. This finding is not a constant one, but instead may be most obvious when disease activity is not at its worst.
- Confluent keratodermas of the palms and soles also eventually result by young adulthood in most patients with Dowling–Meara disease. More localized calluses are common findings on the palms and soles of most patients with each of the other subtypes of EB simplex, to include even the most localized variant (Weber–Cockayne disease), although they may not be present until young adulthood. They tend to be painful, since they overlie recurrent blisters. Other cutaneous findings that may occur in some patients with inherited EB include hypotrichosis, scarring alopecia of the scalp, and postinflammatory hypo- or hyperpigmentation.
- Virtually any epithelial-lined or surfaced tissue may be involved in more severely affected types and subtypes of EB. Commonly affected tissues include the oral cavity (which may be associated with microstomia or ankyloglossia, primarily in recessive dystrophic EB; enamel hypoplasia in JEB), esophagus (leading to stricture or stenosis, primarily in JEB and dystrophic EB), urethra (leading to stricture or stenosis, primarily in JEB and recessive dystrophic EB), the upper airway (leading to partial or complete airway obstruction in infants and young children, primarily with JEB but also rarely in Dowling–Meara EB simplex), and the external surface of the eye (primarily in recessive dystrophic EB, which may result in corneal scarring and rarely in partial or complete blindness).
- Other organs or tissues that may be involved in some types or subtypes of EB include skeletal muscle (in EB simplex associated with muscular dystrophy), stomach (in the JEB-pyloric atresia syndrome), and bone marrow (characterized by severe, secondary,

multifactorial anemia, especially in patients with Herlitz-JEB and Hallopeau–Siemens recessive dystrophic EB).

- Severe to profound growth retardation may arise in some children with EB, especially those with Herlitz-JEB and Hallopeau–Siemens recessive dystrophic EB, as a result of chronic nutrient malabsorption across extensive areas of inherently abnormal small intestinal mucosa.
- Death from failure to thrive is a risk for infants and small children with more severe forms of generalized EB, especially those with the Herlitz subtype of JEB, Hallopeau–Siemens subtype of recessive dystrophic EB, and Dowling–Meara EB simplex.
- Death from bacterial sepsis is a low but real risk during infancy in more severely affected subtypes of EB, to include both subtypes of JEB, Dowling–Meara EB simplex, and Hallopeau–Siemens recessive dystrophic EB.
- Patients with primarily Hallopeau–Siemens disease are at some risk for the eventual development of renal failure, the result of either post-streptococcal glomerulonephritis or renal amyloidosis.
- Patients with recessive dystrophic EB are at major risk for the development of at least one skin-derived squamous cell carcinoma on or after about age 12 years. The risk of these tumors varies by subtype of recessive dystrophic EB, with nearly every patient with Hallopeau–Siemens, and most patients with non-Hallopeau–Siemens disease, eventually developing at least one of these tumors during young or later adulthood. Multiple primary squamous cell carcinomas is the rule in these patients. Rare patients with JEB are also at risk for developing a squamous cell carcinoma. Squamous cell carcinomas that arise in the setting of EB are almost always well differentiated histologically. Despite this, however, they tend to recur and then spread at least regionally, despite initial aggressive wide excision.
- In the setting of Hallopeau–Siemens disease, most patients will die of metastatic squamous cell carcinoma within 5 years of the diagnosis and surgically adequate excision of his or her first cutaneous squamous cell carcinoma. About 20% of all non-Hallopeau–Siemens recessive dystrophic EB patients will similarly die of squamous cell carcinoma.
- There is a small but significant (i.e., nearly 3%) cumulative risk of malignant melanoma arising within the first decade of life in patients with Hallopeau–Siemens disease, although none has yet been reported to have recurred or metastasized.
- There may be an increased risk of basal cell carcinomas in mid- to late adulthood in some patients with generalized EB simplex.

DIAGNOSIS AND DIFFERENTIAL

- The diagnosis of inherited EB is quite straightforward in any nontoxic-appearing newborn or infant who has mechanically fragile skin and blisters. Further differentiation into major EB types (i.e., simplex, junctional, or dystrophic) or subtype, however, is exceedingly difficult (if not impossible) on clinical grounds alone, in the absence of a confirmed diagnosis in a previously affected family member. More sophisticated testing, based on skin biopsies, is mandatory in every apparently sporadic (or otherwise undefined) case of inherited EB.
- Routine histology is worthless in the setting of inherited EB, since it may be impossible to accurately distinguish between even intraepidermal and subepidermal blistering at the light microscopic level.
- The gold standard for the diagnosis of inherited EB remains transmission electron microscopy, since it permits precise determination of the ultrastructural site of skin cleavage, as well as assessment for the presence of additional ultrastructural changes that may be present within lesional skin in its keratin filaments, hemidesmosomes, subbasal dense plates, anchoring filaments, or anchoring fibrils.
- An equally useful and accurate diagnostic approach is antigenic immunofluorescence mapping. In addition, this latter approach allows assessment of the relative expression of specific skin basement membrane proteins, including laminin-5, uncein, and type VII collagen, which may further assist in subclassification and prognostication.

TREATMENT

- There still is no specific systemic or topical therapy for EB.
- It is hoped, however, that gene therapy may ultimately become a reality for at least some forms of inherited EB, even if this proves not to be practical for treatment of the entire surface area of the skin or some affected extracutaneous sites.
- Current topical therapy involves the chronic use of bland antibiotic preparations (i.e., polymyxin B-bacitracin; silver sulfadiazine) followed by the application of nonadherent sterile dressings (including petroleum jelly-impregnated gauze and synthetic hydrocolloid sheets) and sterile, tubular gauze wrappings (for protective padding of active wounds and specific anatomic sites, such as the elbows and knees, which are at high risk for repeated injury). Adhesives are never to be applied to EB skin due to the inherent mechanical fragility of the skin in this disease.

- Localized areas of secondary impetigo may be treated with brief courses of topical mupirocin, a highly effective antistaphylococcal medication.
- Oral antibiotics may be used to treat areas of impetigo that do not respond to topical measures [which also include wet-to-damp compresses with conventional astringents (such as Burow's solution or normal saline)].
- Chronic pain control may involve any of the conventional analgesics, although chronic opiate therapy is to be avoided due to the risk of worsening constipation (and eventual megacolon development) and narcotic addiction. Amitriptyline may also be effective in pain management in some severely affected children and adults.
- Chronic constipation in EB may be managed with lactulose. Surgical interventions may be required to treat secondary complications that arise within the skin (skin grafting for chronic nonhealing ulcerations; excision of cutaneous malignancies), oral cavity (reconstructive dental procedures), esophagus (dilatation; colonic transposition), tracheolaryngeal tree (tracheostomy), urethra (dilatation), kidney (renal transplant), external eye (corneal transplant), and hands (mitten release).
- Meticulous surveillance for squamous cell carcinomas should begin in patients with JEB and recessive dystrophic EB on at least a yearly basis by about age 10 years. Any suspicious lesion, especially atypically nonhealing erosions or ulcerations, should be biopsied immediately and, if necessary, rebiopsied a few months later, if the first biopsy fails to reveal tumor, and yet clinically this is still deemed to be a real clinical possibility.
- Surveillance for malignant melanoma should be performed in recessive dystrophic EB, especially in patients with Hallopeau–Siemens disease, throughout childhood and at least young adulthood, since these tumors have arisen as early as age 3 years.
- Aggressive nutritional supplementation should be given to any severely affected child with EB who appears to have significant anemia and/or growth retardation. If necessary, gastrostomy placement should be implemented, since this may help to partially override underlying chronic, severe gastrointestinal malabsorption, as well as to enhance wound healing.
- Psychological support should be provided to any patient (or family) with EB needing such assistance, given the common occurrence of oftentimes severe reactional depression in patients with more severe types and subtypes of EB.

REFERENCES

Eady RA. Epidermolysis bullosa: Scientific advances and therapeutic challenges. *J Dermatol.* 2001;28:638.

Fine J-D, Bauer EA, McGuire J, Moshell A, eds. *Epidermolysis Bullosa: Clinical, Epidemiologic, and Laboratory Advances, and the Findings of the National Epidermolysis Bullosa Registry.* Baltimore:Johns Hopkins University Press, 1999.

Fine J-D, Eady RAJ, Bauer EA, et al. Revised classification system for inherited epidermolysis bullosa: Report of the Second International Consensus Meeting on Diagnosis and Classification of Epidermolysis Bullosa. *J Am Acad Dermatol.* 2000;42:1051.

McGrath JA. Keratinocyte adhesion and the missing link: From Dowling–Meara to Hay–Wells. St. John's Hospital Dermatological Society Annual Oration 2000. *Clin Exp Dermatol.* 2001;26:296.

Mellerio JE. Molecular pathology of the cutaneous basement membrane zone. *Clin Exp Dermatol.* 1999;24:25.

Uitto J, Pulkkinen L. Molecular genetics of heritable blistering diseases. *Arch Dermatol.* 2001;137:1458.

Uitto J, Pulkkinen L. The genodermatoses: Candidate diseases for gene therapy. *Hum Gene Ther.* 2000;11:2267.

ACQUIRED BLISTERING DISEASES

BULLOUS PEMPHIGOID

EPIDEMIOLOGY

- Bullous pemphigoid (BP) is an uncommon autoimmune bullous disease that occurs primarily in middle-aged or elderly individuals. Rarely, it may also occur in childhood.
- There appears to be no significant gender or ethnic predilection.

PATHOPHYSIOLOGY

- BP develops as a result of autoimmunity to bullous pemphigoid antigen-1, bullous pemphigoid antigen-2, or both.
- BP antigen-1 (BPA-1) is a 230 kD protein which forms a portion of the intracytoplasmic portion of the hemidesmosome, a structural component of the cell membrane that resides within the inferior most part of the basilar keratinocyte. The hemidesmosome is involved in the maintenance of epidermal–dermal adhesion, and provides an attachment point to K5

and K14 keratin filaments that reside within the cytoplasm of the basilar keratinocyte. It is believed that BP antigen-1 plays a role in both adhesion and migration of keratinocytes.

- BP antigen-2 (BPA-2, also known as type XVII collagen and BP-180) is a 180 kD protein that contains a collagenous domain. This protein spans the keratinocyte cell membrane at the level of the hemidesmosome, and inserts inferiorly into the lamina lucida of the underlying skin basement membrane zone. This antigen is also believed to play an important role in keratinocyte adhesion and migration across subepidermal wounds.

- Animal (murine) models suggest that autoimmunity to BPA-2 is the most important factor in the pathogenesis of bullous pemphigoid. It is unknown, however, what triggers the recognition of BPA-2 as a foreign protein and, therefore, as the target of an autoimmune response in humans. This mechanism, at least in mice, also requires the presence of functional leukocytes (especially eosinophils), mast cells, complement, and neutrophil-derived gelatinase B and neutrophil elastase.

- Mouse models involving immunization of newborn animals with purified mouse BPA-2 (or passive transfer of purified antibodies to mouse BPA-2) demonstrate that the anti-BPA-2 autoantibodies bind to the dermoepidermal junction and fix C5, a major component of the classical complement cascade. Mast cells then rapidly align along the dermoepidermal junction, recruit neutrophils, and induce neutrophil degranulation within 1 to 2 hours of passive injection of this autoantibody. These activated neutrophils release gelatinase B, which is an inactivator of α_1-proteinase inhibitor. This prevents inactivation of neutrophil elastase, which is also released from these activated inflammatory cells. Extracellular elastase then contributes to the separation of the dermoepidermal junction, and the subsequent development of macroscopic subepidermal blisters (which are clinically, histologically, and immunologically identical to those seen in humans with BP).

- Recent mouse model studies also suggest that there may indeed be a direct correlation between the level of autoantibody titer to BPA-2 (but not BPA-1) antigen and the level of clinical disease activity. This is in contrast to much older data, based on indirect immunofluorescence studies with otherwise uncharacterized human serum from BP patients, that suggested a lack of correlation with BP autoantibody levels.

- There appears to be no well-defined HLA haplotype associated with BP, suggesting a lack of immunogenetic predisposition for BP.

CLINICAL FEATURES

- The primary lesion in BP is an intact blister that arises on either normal-appearing or focally erythematous skin. The skin itself is not fragile (i.e., the Nikolsky sign, which defines the ability to induce tearing or extension of a lesion at its periphery following application of lateral mechanical traction, is characteristically absent).

- Less frequent presentations include small vesicles (vesicular pemphigoid), urticarial plaques (urticarial pemphigoid), or generalized erythroderma.

- Lesional distribution is usually bilateral and generalized. When more localized, it may favor flexural skin surfaces or, in the case of usually middle-aged, Caucasian females, the extensor aspects of the lower extremities.

- Vesicles and/or erosions may also infrequently arise within the oral cavity, although they tend to be asymptomatic, as opposed to the oral involvement seen in cicatricial pemphigoid.

- Scarring and intense postinflammatory hyperpigmentation are only rarely seen, although milia may occasionally arise, mimicking other bullous conditions.

- Intense pruritus, usually only partially controlled with systemic antihistamines, is experienced in most patients with BP.

- BP tends to be a chronic and somewhat cyclic disease, characterized by intermittent relapses.

DIAGNOSIS AND DIFFERENTIAL

- The diagnosis of BP is made on the basis of clinical findings, coupled with those of routine histology and immunopathology.

- The typical histologic findings in BP include subepidermal blister formation and the presence of eosinophils (within the blister cavity, along the dermoepidermal junction, and around dermal vasculature). The overlying epidermal roof is characteristically unremarkable. The earliest lesions, especially urticarial ones, may present primarily with only focal subepidermal vesiculation and the presence of small numbers of mast cells (the latter linearly aligned along the dermoepidermal junction). At the ultrastructural level, blister formation occurs within the lamina lucida. This may be confirmed by direct split-skin immunofluorescence.

- Direct immunofluorescence (perilesional skin) reveals the present of IgG and/or C3 in thin, linear, uninterrupted array along the dermoepidermal junction (and along the roof of an intact blister). The only exception is in the uncommon form of localized BP, which arises along the lower extremities in women; direct immunofluorescence may be negative in these particular patients.

- Direct immunoelectron microscopy reveals that the autoantibody deposition in BP resides within the lamina lucida.
- Indirect immunofluorescence (serum) demonstrates the presence of IgG class antiskin basement membrane autoantibodies, in usually moderate titers, in at least 80% of patients. These autoantibodies bind exclusively to the roof of salt-split, normal human skin.
- Indirect immunoelectron microscopy has demonstrated that BP autoantibodies bind to the hemidesmosome (to include its cytoplasmic portion).
- Although research tools, immunoblotting (serum) or ELISA may also be useful in demonstrating the presence of autoantibodies to BP-1, BP-2, or both antigens.

TREATMENT

- Localized BP may respond to topical treatment with potent corticosteroids.
- Generalized BP usually requires initial therapy with high dosage (usually about 1 mg/kg/day as a starting dose) systemic corticorticoids (usually prednisone) given as a single dose every morning. Lower starting dosages rarely work in this disease, and place the patient at risk for the same steroid-associated complications that occur with higher dosages. In some severely affected patients, a higher starting dosage may be required to induce complete remission, and rare patients may need simultaneous treatment with another systemic drug before new blisters cease to occur.
- Subsequent systemic therapy involves one or more corticosteroid-sparing agents, to include methotrexate, azathioprine, cyclophosphamide, mycophenolate mofetil, or cyclosporin.
- Rare BP patients may benefit from dapsone, although this drug is far less effective in BP than in cicatricial pemphigoid or one of the IgA-associated autoimmune bullous diseases. Infrequently, some patients may respond instead to high-dosage, systemic tetracycline and nicotinamide. This may be a particularly inviting choice in those elderly patients who may not be able to tolerate the side effects of systemic corticosteroids.
- Limited numbers of patients with severe BP have also been successfully treated with plasmapheresis or IVIG, analogous to what has been reported in pemphigus vulgaris. When the former approach is taken, concurrent immunosuppressive therapy is mandatory

to prevent a subsequent rebound in autoantibody release by the patient's immunoreactive B-cells following reduction of autoantibody levels by repeated plasmapheresis.

REFERENCES

Challacombe SJ, Setterfield J, Shirlaw P, et al. Immunodiagnosis of pemphigus and mucous membrane pemphigoid. *Acta Ondont Scand.* 2001;59:226.

Dabelsteen E. Molecular biological aspects of acquired bullous diseases. *Crit Rev Oral Biol Med.* 1998;9:162.

Huilgol SC, Black MM. Management of the immunobullous disorders. I. Pemphigoid. *Clin Exp Dermatol.* 1995;20:189.

Korman NJ. New and emerging therapies in the treatment of blistering diseases. *Dermatol Clin.* 2000;18:127.

CICATRICIAL PEMPHIGOID

EPIDEMIOLOGY

- Cicatricial pemphigoid (CP) is a rare autoimmune disease that may occur at any age.
- CP may occur in both genders and within any ethnic group.

PATHOPHYSIOLOGY

- CP most often results from autoimmunity to bullous pemphigoid antigen-2. Less frequently, it may represent an autoimmune response to laminin-5.
- Like BP, it is believed that blister formation in CP requires autoantibodies to BP antigen-2, functional leukocytes, and complement. Whether the mechanism for blister formation in CP is identical to BP at the molecular level will await the results of ongoing animal model studies.
- It is unknown why mucosal scarring is a hallmark feature in CP but not in BP, given that both result from an autoimmune response to the same tissue antigen.
- It is unclear whether any HLA type predisposes to CP, although most investigators have failed to identify any significant HLA haplotype associations.
- Older studies, based on indirect immunofluorescence testing of patients' sera, have failed to demonstrate a definite correlation between autoantibody level and clinical disease activity in this disease.

CLINICAL FEATURES

- CP most often involves the oral cavity and/or external eye. Less frequently, skin and other mucosal surfaces (urethral, larynx, esophagus, other) may also be involved.

- Onset and course of disease may be insidious, progressive, or rarely, fulminant.
- The earliest intraoral findings are focal erythema and painful erosions (desquamative gingivitis) of those portions of the gingivae closest to the surfaces of the teeth. Larger erosions (or rarely, frank vesiculation) may be seen elsewhere within the oral cavity, most notably the buccal surfaces. Significant atrophic scarring is a much later feature within the oral cavity in most patients with CP.
- The external eye (usually bilateral) may be severely involved. The earliest finding may be only focal conjunctival injection or erythema. In some patients this may progress to frank vesiculation, symblepharon, ectropion, trichiasis, corneal drying and scarring, and even eventual blindness. The course of external eye disease, like that of the oral cavity, is quite unpredictable, to include mild or self-limited disease, spontaneous remissions, or severe rapid progression.
- Laryngeal involvement, an uncommon occurrence, may present as hoarseness or chronic cough. Aphonia is a rare complication of severe laryngeal involvement, resulting in complete destruction of the vocal cords.
- Skin involvement occurs in only about a quarter of all patients. Usually, only a few blisters arise. These are associated with a tendency to heal with atrophic scarring. Although lesional or perilesional skin is not usually overtly fragile in CP, Nikolsky's sign may be positive in rare patients.
- An uncommon variant of CP, referred to as Brunsting–Perry pemphigoid, is characterized by vesiculation, erosions, crusts, and atrophic scarring. It primarily occurs on the face and scalp, and may be unassociated with mucosal disease activity. Lesions tend to be small vesicles, mimicking those of dermatitis herpetiformis, rather than the large tense blisters which are typically seen in BP.
- CP tends to be a chronic disease, characterized by spontaneous remissions and recurrences. The course of CP is difficult to predict, making assessment of the need for continued long-term immunosuppressant therapy very difficult.

DIAGNOSIS AND DIFFERENTIAL

- The diagnosis of CP is made on the basis of consistent clinical findings, the presence of subepidermal blister formation on routine histology, and (in 80% of cases) positive direct immunofluorescence. It is important to realize, however, than negative direct immunofluorescence does not by itself exclude the diagnosis of CP. Routine histology from skin in CP is indistinguishable from that of BP, that is, there is a subepidermal blister associated with eosinophils within both the blister cavity and the upper dermis. Intraoral blisters may, histologically, be difficult at times to distinguish from bullous lichen planus, and may include a mixed cellular infiltrate.
- Direct immunofluorescence, present in only about 80% of CP cases, reveals one or more immunoreactants (to include IgG, IgA, IgM, and complement) in thin, linear, continuous array along the epithelial–connective tissue junction (regardless of whether skin, oral mucosa, or conjunctiva is sampled). The presence of three or more immunoreactants is more suggestive of CP and epidermolysis bullosa acquisita than BP. Most cases, when examined by direct split-skin immunofluorescence, reveal immunoreactants along the roof rather then the base of the blister cavity, consistent with blister formation within the lamina lucida.
- Indirect immunofluorescence (serum) is positive for antiskin basement membrane autoantibodies in less than 10% of cases. When present, these antibodies (usually IgG class; less commonly, IgA) are usually of very low titer (and are easily missed if undiluted or minimally diluted serum is not examined).
- When ocular, intraoral, and skin involvement are all present, differential diagnosis is usually confined to epidermolysis bullosa acquisita, pemphigus vulgaris, and erythema multiforme.
- When only desquamative gingivitis is present, the major differential diagnosis includes pemphigus vulgaris, lichen planus, and some type of chronic irritant or allergic dermatitis.
- Exclusive involvement of the external eye, particularly when only unilateral, is difficult to diagnose on clinical grounds alone, and may suggest a wide differential diagnosis that includes virtually any ocular inflammatory process that results in scar formation.

TREATMENT

- Localized, mild involvement of the gingiva may be treated with potent topical corticosteroids under removable plastic tray occlusion.
- More extensive involvement that is still confined to the oral cavity may respond to systemic dapsone.
- Significant disease activity within the external eye is a true emergency situation, since undertreated this may result in rapid further progression, at times leading to complete blindness. As such, first-line therapy

of external eye disease involves immediate institution of high-dosage systemic corticosteroids.

- Most patients with at least moderate nonocular CP disease activity require systemic corticosteroid therapy (prednisone, with a starting dosage of 1 mg/kg/day). Response is often incomplete, however. Oral involvement is particularly difficult to manage with this approach.

- Most CP patients treated with systemic corticosteroids will also eventually require a second steroid-sparing immunosuppressant for good control. Drugs commonly employed in CP include azathioprine, cyclophosphamide, mycophenolate mofetil, and cyclosporin.

REFERENCES

Chan LS, Ahmed AR, Anhalt GJ, et al. The first consensus statement on mucous membrane pemphigoid: Definition, diagnostic criteria, pathogenic factors, medical treatment, and prognostic factors. *Arch Dermatol.* 2002;138:370.

Egan CA, Yancey KB. The clinical and immunopathological manifestations of antiepiligrin cicatricial pemphigoid, a recently defined subepithelial autoimmune blistering disease. *Eur J Dermatol.* 2000;10:585.

Fleming TE, Korman NJ. Cicatricial pemphigoid. *J Am Acad Dermatol.* 2000;43:571.

Nguyen QD, Foster CS. Cicatricial pemphigoid: Diagnosis and treatment. *Int Ophthal Clin.* 1996;36:41.

Pleyer U, Bruckner-Tuderman L, Friedmann A, et al. The immunology of bullous oculo-muco-cutaneous disorders. *Immunol Today.* 1996;17:111

HERPES GESTATIONIS

EPIDEMIOLOGY

Herpes gestationis (HG; also known as pemphigoid gestationis) is a rare autoimmune bullous disease that occurs exclusively in women, usually in association with pregnancy.

- HG tends to have its onset during the first or second trimester of pregnancy, waxes and wanes throughout pregnancy, usually flares at the time of delivery, and then usually slowly dissipates and then resolves completely many weeks or months postpartum.

- HG usually recurs with each successive pregnancy, and may appear earlier or be more clinically severe than that which occurred during a previous pregnancy. The risk of further courses of HG appears to be influenced by whether the patient's sexual partner is the same one who was responsible for the previous pregnancy.

- Individuals having experienced HG may develop clinical relapses if later treated with oral contraceptives.

- Although somewhat controversial, there does appear to be an increased risk of prematurity or still births if the mother has HG.

PATHOPHYSIOLOGY

- Patients with HG are believed to develop their disease as a result of autoantibodies to bullous pemphigoid antigen-2, although there appears to be no definite correlation between autoantibody titers and the level of clinical disease activity present.

- Although an animal or in vitro model is as yet lacking for HG, it is believed that this disease, identical to BP, is dependent on autoantibody, leukocytes, and complement.

- Patients with HG have a definite immunosusceptibility to this disease, as evidenced by nearly all being HLA-DR3 or HLA-DR4 positive.

- Experimental evidence suggests that the HLA profile of the father may play some role in the tendency for this disease to occur, although the precise mechanism is as yet unknown.

CLINICAL FEATURES

- The primary lesion in HG is a tense, clear-filled blister that arises either on normal-appearing or erythematous skin. Urticarial plaques may also be present, as occasionally can target-like lesions (mimicking erythema multiforme).

- Most commonly, lesions of HG tend to occur on the trunk and most proximal portions of the extremities. The neck and face can infrequently be involved. The upper chest and breasts tend to be relatively spared of disease activity. There is no predilection for the striae distensiae, in contrast to PUPPP (pruritic urticarial papules and plaques of pregnancy).

- A transient vesicular eruption may be seen during the newborn period in babies of mothers affected with HG, due to transplacental transmission of the offending autoantibodies to the fetus.

- Pruritus is present in most patients with HG.

DIAGNOSIS AND DIFFERENTIAL

- The diagnosis of HG is facilitated by its rather characteristic clinical findings and its time of onset. It is confirmed by light microscopy and both direct and indirect immunofluorescence studies.

- Routine histology of an intact blister reveals subepidermal cleavage (proven by electron microscopy to be within the lamina lucida) associated with eosinophils within the blister cavity, along the dermoepidermal junction, and around dermal vessels. Earlier nonbullous lesions may reveal occasional eosinophils within the epidermis (eosinophilic spongiosis).
- Direct immunofluorescence of perilesional skin reveals linear continuous deposits of IgG and/or C3 along the dermoepidermal junction.
- Indirect immunofluorescence (serum) is usually negative, whereas a complement fixation assay (HG factor) on normal human skin is usually positive for the presence, in low titer, of antiskin basement membrane autoantibodies. There is no correlation between autoantibody titer and level of disease activity.
- Differential diagnosis includes gestational erythema multiforme. Onset during late pregnancy may suggest the possibility of PUPPP.

TREATMENT

- Most HG patients require systemic therapy with medium dosage corticosteroids (i.e., prednisone at approximately 0.7 to 1 mg/kg/day) due to the severity of pruritus and the extent of blistering. Response is usually rapid. If prednisone is ineffective or contraindicated, patients may be safely treated with dapsone (unless allergic to sulfa drugs).
- Corticosteroid dosage usually must be increased during delivery or the immediate postpartum period due to the tendency for major flares of HG to occur during those specific times. The dosage may be slowly tapered over the next several weeks to a few months postpartum, and then subsequently discontinued in most HG patients. However, rare patients with HG may have persistent blistering for months, or even years, even in the absence of further pregnancies, necessitating chronic systemic therapy.
- Oral contraceptive therapy is contraindicated in patients who have a past history of HG due to the likelihood of relapse or recurrence, if such therapy is employed.
- Oral antihistamines may be beneficial in some patients, although corticosteroids usually best control the intense pruritus associated with HG.

REFERENCES

Engineer L, Bhol K, Ahmed AR. Pemphigoid gestationis: A review. *Am J Obst Gyn* 2000;183:483.

Jenkins RE, Hern S, Black MM. Clinical features and management of 87 patients with pemphigoid gestationis. *Clin Exp Dermatol.* 1999;24:255.

Shornick JK. Dermatoses of pregnancy. *Sem Cutan Med Surg.* 1998;17:172.

Wakelin SH, Black MM. The autoimmune bullous diseases. *J Roy Coll Phys.* (London) 1997;31:364.

DERMATITIS HERPETIFORMIS

EPIDEMIOLOGY

Dermatitis herpetiformis (DH) is an uncommon autoimmune vesicular disease that most often first develops during young adulthood.

- DH is more commonly seen in Caucasians than in African-Americans, due to its close association with HLA-B8 and -DR3 haplotypes (which are present only rarely in the latter ethnic population).

PATHOPHYSIOLOGY

- Although the precise mechanism by which DH occurs is unknown, it is invariably characterized by the presence of granular IgA deposits within the uppermost papillary dermis, suggesting an underlying humoral immune mechanism.
- Given the known association of celiac sprue-like changes within the small intestines of patients with DH, the known exacerbation of skin disease activity following ingestion of gluten, as well as the presence in many of serum autoantibodies to gliadin, it is believed that skin lesions in DH may represent the end result of injury induced by IgA-class autoantibodies to gluten, which then selectively deposit themselves within the uppermost papillary dermis and somehow induce blister formation.
- Since some patients with DH also have autoantibodies against reticulum, it has been postulated that the selective deposition of IgA within the papillary dermis may reflect crossreactivity of the IgA autoantibodies to this particular structural component of the extracellular matrix.
- Nearly 90% of patients with DH also characteristically have autoantibodies against smooth muscle endomysium.
- More recent studies have shown that most patients with DH, and those with celiac disease, have circulating autoantibodies against transglutaminase, an enzyme that can degrade gluten. It has also been suggested that the antiendomysial autoantibodies in DH sera cross-react with those that are reactive against

transglutaminase. As such, it is likely that transglutaminase may represent the real primary target of autoantibody response in this disease.

- C3 may also be seen within the upper papillary dermis in some DH patients, suggesting that complement activation may play some important role in the overall pathogenesis of tissue injury within DH skin lesions, possibly via recruitment of neutrophils to the dermoepidermal junction and the subsequent release of one or more proteases by these cells.

CLINICAL FEATURES

- Patients with DH characteristically complain of a burning sensation or intense localized pruritus prior to the development of their skin lesions.
- The primary lesion in DH is a small vesicle which arises on clinically normal appearing skin. Occasionally these lesions may appear hemorrhagic. Rarely, only urticarial plaques are present, making the diagnosis difficult on clinical grounds alone. Skin lesions in DH tend to be in grouped configuration, at times even annular, hence, the term "herpetiformis" to describe this disease.
- Secondary cutaneous findings include excoriations and postinflammatory hyperpigmentation.
- Skin lesions tend to arise in a characteristically symmetrical array, favoring extensor aspects of the body. Typical sites of involvement include the elbows, knees, shoulders, and buttocks. The scalp is also commonly involved. Infrequently, other distributions may occur, including generalized disease activity.
- Although most patients lack extracutaneous symptomatology, a minority of patients will also complain of diarrhea, consistent with the known histological features of celiac sprue in the small intestines of patients with DH.
- A minority of DH patients may have or will develop hypothyroidism.
- Rare patients may also have concurrent IgA nephropathy.

DIAGNOSIS AND DIFFERENTIAL

- Histology of an intact vesicle reveals subepidermal cleft formation, accompanied by the presence of collections of neutrophils (neutrophilic microabscesses) within the papillary tufts of the upper dermis.
- Direct immunofluorescence of perilesional skin reveals granular deposits of IgA within the papillary tufts. Less commonly, more discrete IgA granular deposits may be seen in rather linear fashion along the dermoepidermal junction, and/or within blood vessels of the uppermost dermis.

- C3 may also be seen infrequently, in granular array, within the same papillary tufts.
- Indirect immunofluorescence (serum), using monkey esophagus as the tissue substrate, reveals the presence of antiendomysial autoantibodies in virtually every DH patient. In contrast, autoantibodies reactive to other epidermal or basement membrane antigens are characteristically absent in patients with DH.
- Autoantibodies against transglutaminase are present in the sera of most patients with DH.
- Specialized ELISA testing of serum may reveal, in a minority of DH patients, the presence of autoantibodies to gliadin or reticulum.
- The diagnosis of DH is usually a very easy one to make on clinical grounds alone, given the highly symmetrical nature of this intensely pruritic vesicular process. When the findings are minimal or localized, other diagnoses may be considered, to include arthropod bites, contact dermatitis, scabies, or herpetic infection. Similarly, more generalized presentations of DH may suggest any of the other subepidermal autoimmune vesiculobullous diseases. Urticarial lesions may instead suggest acute or chronic urticaria, urticarial pemphigoid, and urticarial vasculitis.

TREATMENT

- Dapsone is the treatment of choice for patients with DH. It works presumably by interfering with leukocyte chemoattraction to the skin.
- Other sufones or sulfonamides may be employed, to include sulfapyridine and diasone.
- A strict gluten-free diet may, by itself, result in complete control of this disease, but complete remission may require at least 12 to 18 months of continuous dietary therapy.
- Although not a universal precipitating factor, patients with DH should be advised that they may develop clinical flares shortly after ingestion of foods that are high in iodine content (i.e., shellfish).
- Systemic and topical corticosteroids tend to work poorly in DH.
- Other possible therapies include an elemental diet and colchicine.
- None of the sulfones or sulfonamides should be employed until it is documented that the patient has a normal G-6-PD level. These drugs are absolutely contraindicated in patients with known allergy to sulfa drugs. Since methemoglobulinemia is a common side effect of such therapy, particular care should be given to its use in patients with significant coronary artery disease, or in those patients who reside in cities located at higher altitudes. The typical "pasty"

coloration of the skin in patients being treated with dapsone or a related drug may mask the presence of early hypothyroidism.

REFERENCES

Hall RP 3rd. Dermatitis herpetiformis. *J Invest Dermatol.* 1992;99:873.

Reunala TL. Dermatitis herpetiformis. *Clin Dermatol.* 2001;19:728.

LINEAR IgA DERMATOSIS

EPIDEMIOLOGY

- The prevalence of linear IgA dermatotis (LAD) is unknown, although it appears to much less common than dermatitis herpetiformis.
- There is a bimodal distribution of LAD in early childhood to mid-childhood (i.e., age 6 months to about 10 years), and adulthood. In addition, the cutaneous findings usually differ between these two age groups.

PATHOPHYSIOLOGY

- Like DH, LAD is believed to represent an IgA-mediated autoimmune disorder. At a tissue level, these two entities differ in the pattern of IgA deposition (i.e., granular in DH and homogeneous linear in LAD).
- Unlike DH, HLA immunosusceptibility does not appear to play a role in the pathogenesis of LAD.
- In contrast to DH, there are no known associations with celiac sprue in patients with LAD.
- Although still somewhat controversial, it has been suggested that adult LAD patients may be at some risk for lymphoma.

CLINICAL FEATURES

- Both subtypes of LAD are associated with intense pruritus or burning sensation of the skin.
- Patients with childhood LAD (chronic bullous disease of childhood, CBDC) characteristically develop large, tense, clear-filled blisters, arising on normal appearing skin. Individually, each blister may mimic bullous pemphigoid.
- Adults with LAD tend instead to present with small, clear-filled vesicles, which individually may mimic DH. In contrast to DH, however, lesions in adult LAD usually are not in grouped or herpetiform configuration.

- Lesions in childhood DH characteristically arise in a symmetrical array, involving the neck (in a necklace-like configuration), upper trunk, inguinal regions, genitalia, and upper thighs. Blisters tend to be present at the periphery of the lesions, with erythema and/or postinflammatory hyperpigmentation present more centrally.
- The distribution of lesions in adulthood LAD is less well defined. Usually, only a paucity of lesions is present. In contrast to DH, there is no predilection for extensor surfaces. The mid- and lower back is a common site of involvement. Scalp is rarely involved, in comparison to DH.
- There is no association with celiac sprue or thyroid disease in either form of LAD. It has been suggested that there may be an association between adult LAD and some forms of lymphoma, although too few patients have been studied to confirm this.

DIAGNOSIS AND DIFFERENTIAL

- When LAD presents in childhood with typical morphology and distribution, there really is no significant differential diagnosis, although rare patients with childhood BP or epidermolysis bullosa acquisita may have similar cutaneous findings.
- Adult-onset LAD is very difficult to diagnose solely on the basis of cutaneous features, given the lack of characteristic morphology or distribution.
- Routine histology of a lesion in LAD is usually indistinguishable from that of DH.
- Direct immunofluorescence of perilesional skin in both forms of LAD reveals homogeneous linear deposition of IgA along the dermoepidermal junction.
- Indirect immunofluorescence (sera) from children with LAD may reveal the presence of IgA antiskin basement membrane autoantibodies, which bind to the epidermal half of salt-split, human skin substrate. In contrast, sera from adult LAD patients are characteristically negative for circulating autoantibodies.

TREATMENT

- Dapsone is the treatment of choice in both forms of LAD. Caution must be used when treating young children with dapsone, due to the likelihood of significant drug-induced hemolysis, associated with temporary anemia and, rarely, with secondary splenomegaly. Dapsone therapy is contraindicated in patients who are G-6-PD deficient or allergic to sulfa.
- There appears to be no role for a gluten-free diet in either form of LAD.

- Concurrent therapy with systemic corticosteroids may be beneficial, especially in children with LAD, although corticosteroids by themselves tend not be terribly effective.

REFERENCES

Schmidt E, Zillikens D. Autoimmune and inherited subepidermal blistering diseases: Advances in the clinic and the laboratory. *Adv Dermatol.* 2000;16:113.

Wojnarowska F, Frith P. Linear IgA disease. *Devel Ophthal.* 1997;28:64.

Zillikens D, Giudice GJ. BP180/type XVII collagen: Its role in acquired and inherited disorders of the dermal-epidermal junction. *Arch Dermatol Res.* 1999;291:187.

EPIDERMOLYSIS BULLOSA ACQUISITA

EPIDEMIOLOGY

- Epidermolysis bullosa acquisita (EBA) is a rare autoimmune bullous disease that may arise at any age. It is most often seen, however, in individuals who are middle-aged or older.
- Either gender and any ethnicity may be involved.
- There are no known predisposing factors for EBA, although limited data suggest the possibility that it may possibly occur more frequently in the setting of inflammatory bowel disease, rheumatoid arthritis, or some other internal diseases.
- There is also a definite relationship between EBA and bullous lupus erythematosus, consistent with their shared autoantibody target, suggesting that these two entities may represent different poles of a disease continuum. Occasional patients with EBA have later developed systemic lupus erythematosus; whereas, patients with bullous lupus erythematosus are known to have autoantibodies to type VII collagen and have skin lesions that are clinically, histologically, and immunologically very similar or identical to those seen in EBA.

PATHOPHYSIOLOGY

- EBA results from an autoimmune response to type VII collagen (previously referred to as the EBA antigen), which is the major component of the anchoring fibril.
- An in vitro model (leukocyte attachment model) of EBA confirms that blister formation in this disease is dependent on the presence of autoantibodies to type VII collagen, functional neutrophils, and complement.

- Early lesions in EBA arise within the lamina lucida, identical to the site where blisters develop in most other bullous diseases. In EBA patients with more long-standing disease activity, however, blisters occur within the sublamina densa region of the dermoepidermal junction, consistent with secondary destruction of anchoring fibrils in such skin, leading to preferential separation just beneath the level of the lamina densa.

CLINICAL FEATURES

- The hallmark lesion in EBA is a tense subepidermal blister, which may arise either on normal-appearing skin or in an area of erythema or urticaria.
- Additionally useful cutaneous findings, which when they are present, help to distinguish EBA from BP, are milia and atrophic scarring. These findings occur in the so-called classic form of EBA, closely mimicking those seen in inherited dystrophic EB (which shares with EBA type VII collagen as the underlying molecular target of injury, thereby explaining the common clinical phenotype).
- Nikolsky-sign positivity is a characteristic feature in patients with the classical presentation of EBA, implying the presence of marked mechanical fragility of the skin. Presumably, this is a reflection of injury to anchoring fibrils within such skin.
- Infrequently, patients with EBA may present with cutaneous features that are clinically indistinguishable from those of BP, that is, tense blisters in the absence of milia or scar formation. This may explain why prior to development of tests to identify EBA, at least 5% of patients previously diagnosed with BP, as later identified and restudied via sera banks, were later shown to have EBA.
- Rare patients with EBA may also present with clinical findings most suggestive of CP or porphyria cutanea tarda.
- The oral cavity is commonly involved in EBA. Findings may include intact blisters, erosions, and scar formation, and may be associated with severe symptomatology.
- The external eye, esophagus, urethra, anus, and other epithelial-lined or surfaced organs may also be involved, analogous to inherited dystrophic EB.
- Rare EBA patients may also develop partial web formation of the hands and feet, analogous to inherited dystrophic EB.

DIAGNOSIS AND DIFFERENTIAL

- Routine histology from lesional skin in EBA most commonly reveals subepidermal blister formation, in association with the presence of neutrophils, both along the dermoepidermal junction and within the blister cavity. These findings alone may be confused with dermatitis herpetiformis, although neutrophils tend to accumulate within more discrete microabscesses within the upper papillary dermis in DH skin. Rarely, the dermal infiltrate within lesional skin in EBA is cell-poor.

- The diagnosis of EBA is most precisely confirmed by the results of direct immunofluorescence and indirect split-skin immunofluorescence studies.
- Perilesional skin in EBA is characterized via direct immunofluorescence by the presence of linear deposits of one or more immunoreactants (to include IgG, IgA, complement, and fibrin) along the dermoepidermal junction.
- Nearly every patient with EBA will also have detectable antiskin basement membrane autoantibodies (so-called EBA autoantibodies; mainly IgG class) within their serum. This is best demonstrated via split-skin indirect immunofluorescence technique (SS-IIF), rather than by IIF on intact tissue substrates.
- As determined via SS-IIF, autoantibodies in EBA bind exclusively to the dermal portion of salt-split, normal human skin, readily distinguishing this disease from BP.
- EBA autoantibodies recognize epitopes on type VII collagen.
- Direct immunoelectron (IEM) microscopy of perilesional skin in EBA reveals the presence of electron-dense deposits of immunoreactants within the uppermost papillary dermis, associated with evidence of destruction of anchoring fibrils. Indirect IEM confirms that EBA autoantibodies bind to portions of the anchoring fibrils.
- The differential diagnosis of a patient with the classical type of EBA is dystrophic EB. The latter can be usually readily eliminated by medical history (since EBA is acquired, and only rarely occurs in infancy or early childhood) and family history (if positive for other affected family members). Patients without the classical presentations of EBA suggest a much wider differential diagnosis, to include bullous lupus erythematosus, bullous pemphigoid, cicatricial pemphigoid, dermatitis herpetiformis, erythema multiforme, and porphyria cutanea tarda.

TREATMENT

- Given the rarity of localized cutaneous disease activity in EBA, initial therapy is usually systemic prednisone (at a dosage of 1 to 1.25 mg/kg/day). More severely affected patients may require up to 2 mg/kg/day. Even then, only a subset of EBA patients respond completely to prednisone therapy by itself.
- Most EBA patients require concurrent treatment with a second systemic drug (to include azathioprine, cyclophosphamide, mycophenolate mofetil, cyclosporin, or dapsone) to induce complete remission and to provide a steroid-sparing effect.
- IVIG may be employed, as may photopheresis. Other therapies reportedly beneficial include colchicine and methotrexate.

REFERENCES

Engineer L, Ahmed AR. Emerging treatment for epidermolysis bullosa acquisita. _J Am Acad Dermatol._ 2001; 44:818.

Gammon WR, Briggaman RA. Epidermolysis bullosa acquisita and bullous systemic lupus erythematosus. Diseases of autoimmunity to type VII collagen. _Dermatol Clin._ 1993;11:535.

Zillikens D. Acquired skin disease of hemidesmosomes. _J Dermatol Sci._ 1999;20:134.

PEMPHIGUS

EPIDEMIOLOGY

- Pemphigus includes several autoimmune bullous diseases characterized by intraepidermal blister formation. The two main types of pemphigus are pemphigus foliaceus and pemphigus vulgaris. Subtypes of each exist (pemphigus vegetans as a subtype of pemphigus vulgaris; pemphigus erythematosus as a subtype of pemphigus foliaceus). An IgA-mediated variant of pemphigus and drug-induced variants of pemphigus vulgaris also exist. Although precise epidemiological data are lacking, each type and subtype of pemphigus is rare, with the exception of the endemic form of pemphigus foliaceus, which occurs in South America.
- All forms of pemphigus may occur at any age, but tend to occur most often in late adulthood. Both genders may be involved.
- Although pemphigus may occur in any ethnic background, the vulgaris form is particularly associated with Ashkenazi Jews.
- There are several reported HLA associations with pemphigus vulgaris. Specific HLA haplotypes predisposing to pemphigus vary among different ethnic groups (i.e., different haplotypes have been reported in Caucasians in the United States, in Ashkenazi Jews, and in native Japanese).
- One variant of pemphigus foliaceus, referred to as fogo sevalgem (wildfire), is endemic in rural Brazil.

Most often seen in patients who reside along the river banks in the Amazon region of Brazil, some epidemiologic data have suggested the possibility that this form of pemphigus may be triggered by chronic bites from black flies, leading to autoantibody formation as a result of antigenic mimicry.

- One variant of pemphigus vulgaris, known as pemphigus paraneoplastica, arises in the setting of internal malignancies (most commonly non-Hodgkin's lymphoma, chronic lymphocytic leukemia, and Castleman's disease).

PATHOPHYSIOLOGY

All forms of autoimmune pemphigus (i.e., excluding familial benign pemphigus of Hailey–Hailey) result from autoimmunity to one or more structural antigens within the epidermis.

- The target antigen in pemphigus vulgaris in desmoglein-3 (Dsg-3), a 130 kD protein that is present along keratinocyte cell surfaces primarily within the lower half of the epidermis.
- The target antigen in pemphigus foliaceus is Dsg-1, a 160 kD cell surface protein on keratinocytes.
- There are multiple target antigens in pemphigus paraneoplastica, to include bullous pemphigoid antigen-1, Dsg-1, Dsg-3, plectin, desmoplakin 1 and 2, periplakin, and envoplakin.
- The target antigen in the "subcorneal pustular dermatosis" subtype of IgA pemphigus is desmocollin. The target in the other subtype (intraepidermal neutrophilic) of IgA pemphigus is as yet unknown, although the desmogleins do not appear to be involved.
- Earlier human keratinocyte cell culture studies with pemphigus vulgaris autoantibody confirm that epithelial dysadhesion in pemphigus vulgaris is critically dependent on the presence of pemphigus autoantibodies but independent of complement. Complement fixation, however, accentuates this process.
- A mouse model of pemphigus, involving passive transfer of large amounts of purified pemphigus autoantibodies into newborn mice, confirms that the mechanism of blister formation in pemphigus vulgaris and pemphigus foliaceus is autoantibody dependent but inflammatory cell independent.
- Clinical disease activity in pemphigus is directly correlated with pemphigus autoantibody level.

CLINICAL FEATURES

- All forms of pemphigus vulgaris are characterized by flaccid blisters and marked mechanical fragility of the epidermis (as confirmed by the presence of a positive Nikolsky-sign in perilesional skin).
- Pemphigus foliaceus, a more superficial form of pemphigus, more often presents with crusts and erosions than frank blisters.
- IgA pemphigus may present with pustules, in addition to vesicles or blisters.
- Patients with pemphigus paraneoplastica typically present with erosive mucositis, conjunctivitis, and generalized blistering of the skin. Clinically, these patients often resemble erythema multiforme, rather than more typical forms of pemphigus. Disease activity may improve if the underlying tumor responds to surgery or chemotherapy.
- Healing in pemphigus vulgaris is typically associated with marked postinflammatory hyperpigmentation, a finding not usually seen in other autoimmune bullous diseases (with the possible exception of epidermolysis bullosa acquisita).
- The oral cavity is commonly involved in pemphigus vulgaris. Painful erosions may arise anywhere within the oral cavity, to include the tongue and hard and soft palates, and are associated with marked phagodynia. When extensive, it may mimic severe erythema multiforme. When mild and confined to the gingivae, it may mimic cicatricial pemphigoid.
- Other epithelial-lined organs may also be involved in pemphigus vulgaris, to include the external eye, esophagus, bladder, urethra, and external female genitalia.
- Pemphigus vulgaris may rarely be associated with concurrent thymoma or myasthenia gravis.
- With the exception of drug-induced pemphigus, most other forms tend to be very chronic; spontaneous remission is infrequent. Untreated, pemphigus vulgaris is associated with high mortality, due to bacterial sepsis from widespread denudation of the skin. Unfortunately, chronic immunosuppressant therapy, especially if involving systemic corticosteroids, commonly results in drug-induced complications (i.e., osteoporosis and vertebral fractures secondary to chronic prednisone therapy). Drug-induced pemphigus usually remits shortly after withdrawal of the offending drug.

DIAGNOSIS AND DIFFERENTIAL

- Pemphigus vulgaris, when localized and confined to the oral cavity, may be confused with localized erythema multiforme. Although CP also typically involves the oral cavity, lesions in the latter disorder tend to favor the gingivae and buccal mucosal surfaces. Pemphigus foliaceus, when confined to the face, may mimic poorly responsive seborrheic dermatitis.

- Photodistributed pemphigus foliaceus should suggest the possibility of pemphigus erythematosus (Senear–Usher disease), a variant of pemphigus that arises in the setting of systemic lupus erythematosus.
- Routine histology of lesional skin in both major types of pemphigus demonstrates keratinocyte dysadhesion (acantholysis). Blister formation occurs within the suprabasilar layer in pemphigus vulgaris, leaving a single layer of keratinocytes (tombstoning) along the base of the blister. In pemphigus foliaceus, blisters arise subcorneally.
- Routine histology in pemphigus paraneoplastica reveals features of pemphigus vulgaris (i.e., suprabasilar cleavage), in combination with focal keratinocyte dyskeratosis and an interface or lichenoid infiltrate.
- Direct immunofluorescence (of perilesional skin) in both pemphigus vulgaris and pemphigus foliaceus reveals crisp cell surface staining throughout the epidermis with IgG and, to a lesser extent, complement.
- Direct immunofluorescence in pemphigus paraneoplastica reveals both pemphigus intraepidermal staining and a usually smudged linear deposition of IgG along the dermoepidermal junction (the latter consistent with erythema multiforme).
- Indirect immunofluorescence of serum in pemphigus vulgaris and foliaceus reveals the presence of circulating autoantibodies that bind to the cell surfaces of the entire epidermis or epithelium of normal tissue substrates (i.e., normal human skin; monkey esophagus). In the setting of pemphigus paraneoplastica, rat bladder is a more useful tissue substrate, since pemphigus vulgaris autoantibodies tend not to bind to this particular tissue, whereas pemphigus paraneoplastica autoantibodies avidly bind it.

TREATMENT

- Localized pemphigus may respond to topical applications of high-potency corticosteroids or to intralesional corticosteroid injections.
- Patients with more generalized pemphigus are usually treated initially with high dosage prednisone (i.e., 1.25 to 1.50 mg/kg/day). Since only very rare patients respond quickly and completely to systemic corticosteroids as single drug therapy, most patients are also soon begun and later maintained on a second steroid-sparing immunosuppressant (to include azathioprine, methotrexate, cyclophosphamide, cyclosporin, or mycophenolate mofetil).
- Dapsone infrequently may prove to be helpful second- or third-line therapy, concurrent with treatment with one or more other systemic medications.

- Plasmapheresis, with or without concurrent intravenous pulse therapy with corticosteroids or cyclophosphamide, is an effective approach to treatment. It is usually performed in conjunction with some type of concurrent systemic immunosuppressant therapy, to prevent a rapid rebound in autoantibody production.
- IVIG has been similarly shown to be effective in patients with generalized pemphigus vulgaris.

REFERENCES

Amagai M. Autoimmunity against desmosomal cadherins in pemphigus. *J Dermatol Sci.* 1999;20:92.

Anhalt GJ. Paraneoplastic pemphigus. *Adv Dermatol.* 1997;12:77.

Challacombe SJ, Setterfield J, Shirlaw P, Harman K, Scully C, Black MM. Immunodiagnosis of pemphigus and mucous membrane pemphigoid. *Acta Odont Scand.* 2001; 59:226.

Nishikawa T, Hashimoto T, Shimizu H, Ebihara T, Amagai M. Pemphigus: From immunofluorescence to molecular biology. *J Dermatol Sci.* 1996;12:1.

Stanley JR. Pathophysiology and therapy of pemphigus in the 21st century. *J Dermatol.* 2001;28:645.

Toth GG, Jonkman MF. Therapy of pemphigus. *Clin Dermatol.* 2001;19:761.

ERYTHEMA MULTIFORME AND STEVENS–JOHNSON SYNDROME

EPIDEMIOLOGY

- Erythema multiforme (EM) is a relatively common disease that affects all ages, both genders, and all ethnicities.
- EM is divided into two main subtypes. The more common one, EM minor, is confined to skin and usually oral involvement. The more uncommon and more severe variant, EM major (also known as Stevens–Johnson syndrome), involves skin, external eye, oral mucosa, and often other epithelial-lined tissues.
- EM major usually evolves from EM minor, but may occur de novo.
- The most common cause of EM is herpes simplex infection of the skin. There are numerous other precipitating causes, including virtually any infectious agent or drug.

PATHOPHYSIOLOGY

- There is no well-characterized animal or in vitro model for either form of EM. Despite this, it has been hypothesized that EM results from a primarily cyto-toxic T cell-mediated autoimmune response.

• Lesional skin specimens from the majority of patients with EM minor have detectable herpes simplex antigens within keratinocytes, suggesting a causal relationship.

CLINICAL FEATURES

• The hallmark lesion in EM is a target lesion that is an erythematous, circular macule of variable size that resembles a bulls-eye. The center of this lesion may be macular, papular, or vesiculobullous. A common site for the target lesion is the palm. Multiple target lesions may occur.

• Skin involvement may be localized or generalized in EM minor, and is generalized in EM major.

• Cutaneous pain is a characteristic feature.

• The eruption in EM is pleomorphic, hence, the name "multiforme." Lesions may include macules, papules, urticarial or non-urticarial plaques, vesicles, bullae, petechiae, and purpura.

• EM major (Stevens–Johnson syndrome) is character-ized by widespread cutaneous lesions of EM, in con-junction with conjunctivitis, widespread oral disease activity (erythema, blisters, erosions, and necrotic epithelial slough), and constitutional symptoms (to include fever, chills, and generalized weakness). Large areas of skin and oral mucosa may become denuded. Other organs may be involved, including the upper gastrointestinal tract, lower genitourinary tract, and lungs (resulting in pneumonitis).

• The skin in EM is typically Nikolsky sign-negative, readily contrasting it with toxic epidermal necrolysis. An uncomplicated course of EM minor, if untreated, lasts 7 to 14 days, although it may still be associated with significant discomfort. EM minor may recur if the patient is rechallenged with the same (or cross-reacting) drug or if the inciting infection recurs. EM minor, which is associated with herpes simplex infec-tion, for example, typically recurs within a few days of the beginning of a new episode of herpes.

• The course of EM major is variable, but usually lasts for at least several weeks, and is usually associated with severe morbidity. There is a low risk of mortality associated with EM major, particularly when it occurs in children and the elderly.

DIAGNOSIS AND DIFFERENTIAL

• The diagnosis of EM is usually quite straightforward, especially when target lesions are present. In the absence of obvious target (or targetoid) lesions, the diagnosis of EM should still be suspected in any erup-tion of rather acute onset that is morphologically pleomorphic.

• Differentiation between EM major and toxic epider-mal necrolysis is more difficult, given the rather artificial diagnostic criteria that some have recom-mended. For practical purposes, especially as pertains to the risk of mortality, the Nikolsky sign is one rea-sonable variable in distinguishing between these two often overlapping diseases. When the sign is present, the patient has toxic epidermal necrolysis; when nega-tive, the patient has EM major.

• Routine histology in both forms of EM reveals focal epidermal dyskeratosis, subepidermal blister formation, and a usually mixed cellular infiltrate within the dermis.

• Direct immunofluorescence of lesional skin in EM reveals usually weak, smudged deposition of IgG and/or fibrin along the dermoepidermal junction, as well as around upper dermal vasculature. These find-ings, however, are variable and nonspecific; as such, immunofluorescence is not usually recommended as part of the diagnostic evaluation of a patient suspected of having EM, although it may be very useful in dif-ferentiating herpes gestationis from gestational EM.

TREATMENT

• Patients with EM minor are usually treated with wet compresses with an astringent agent (such as Burow's solution), followed by the application of a bland antibiotic ointment, to prevent secondary impetig-inization of open wounds.

• Patients with EM minor that is associated with recur-rent herpes simplex infection may be treated with oral antiviral agents (acyclovir; other). Prophylactic ther-apy with one of these agents may also prevent recur-rence of EM minor in this subset of patients.

• The treatment of EM major usually requires hospital-ization, to include aggressive topical care by skilled nursing staff within the equivalent of a burn unit Current clinical trials are underway to determine the potential efficacy of IVIG therapy in EM major.

• Although based on only limited case reports, it has been suggested that rare patients who experience recurrent EM major may be successfully managed by long-term immunosuppressant therapy with an agent such as azathioprine.

REFERENCES

Bachot N, Roujeau JC. Physiopathology and treatment of severe drug eruptions. *Curr Opin Allergy Clin Immunol.* 2001;1:293.

Fine JD. Management of acquired bullous skin diseases. *N Engl J Med.* 1995;333:1475.

Huff JC. Erythema multiforme and latent herpes simplex infection. *Sem Dermatol.* 1992;11:207.

Revuz J. New advances in severe adverse drug reactions. *Dermatol Clin.* 2001;19:697.

Roujeau JC. Treatment of severe drug eruptions. *J Dermatol.* 1999;26:718.

TOXIC EPIDERMAL NECROLYSIS

EPIDEMIOLOGY

- The prevalence or incidence of toxic epidermal necrolysis (TEN) in the United States is unknown. It is, however, an uncommon disease, but one that is encountered many times a year in every tertiary care hospital.
- TEN usually results from a severe hypersensitivity reaction to a systemically administered drug, although topically applied agents (i.e., sulfa-based ophthalmic preparations in a patient with known severe allergy to sulfa drugs) may also rarely result in TEN. Common offenders include sulfa drugs, phenytoin, nonsteroidal/antiinflammatory drugs, and members of the penicillin family.

PATHOPHYSIOLOGY

- There are no animal or in vitro models of TEN. The mechanism is believed to be similar or identical to those proposed for EM, however, except that the inciting factor is almost always a drug.

CLINICAL FEATURES

- TEN is characterized by the presence of widespread epidermal necrosis and sloughing of the skin. Blisters and extensive erosions are also present.
- The skin in TEN is characteristically Nikolsky sign-positive.
- Multiple extracutaneous sites are usually involved, especially the external surface of the eyes and the oral mucosa.
- Marked constitutional symptoms are invariably present.
- The risk of mortality in TEN is very high, and increases with increasing surface area involved, analogous to the risk of mortality in second-degree burns.

DIAGNOSIS AND DIFFERENTIAL

- The diagnosis of TEN is straightforward on clinical grounds alone, although determination of the inciting cause may be difficult, if not impossible, if the patient has been exposed to multiple medications.
- The only differential diagnosis in TEN is Stevens–Johnson syndrome. As discussed previously, the presence or absence of Nikolsky sign-positivity is used as the primary defining criterion, rather than the extent of surface area involved.
- Histology of lesional skin demonstrates full thickness necrosis of the epidermis, with associated subepidermal blister formation.

TREATMENT

- The treatment of TEN necessitates intensive medical and nursing care or a burn unit, with topical care identical to that given in a patient with generalized second- or third-degree burns. Supportive care involves meticulous monitoring of fluid status and transcutaneous protein loss.
- Treatment of TEN with high-dosage systemic corticosteroids remains controversial, although it is still recommended by some authorities.
- European studies have demonstrated the efficacy of IVIG therapy in TEN. Although not yet FDA-approved, it is likely that this will soon become the treatment of choice for TEN, eliminating further need for consideration of the use of systemic corticosteroids in this disease.

REFERENCES

Bachot N, Roujeau JC. Physiopathology and treatment of severe drug eruptions. *Curr Opin Allergy Clin Immunol.* 2001;1:293.

Craven NM. Management of toxic epidermal necrolysis. *Hospital Medicine.* (London) 2000;61:778.

Fine JD. Management of acquired bullous skin diseases. *N Engl J Med.* 1995;333:1475.

Paquet P, Arrese JE, Beguin Y, Pierard GE. Clinicopathological differential diagnosis of drug-induced toxic epidermal necrolysis (Lyell's syndrome) and acute graft-versus-host reaction. *Curr Topics Pathol.* 2001;94:49.

Revuz JE, Roujeau JC. Advances in toxic epidermal necrolysis. *Sem Cutan Med Surg.* 1996;15:258.

Ringheanu M, Laude TA. Toxic epidermal necrolysis in children—An update. *Clin Pediatr.* 2000;39:687.

Smoot EC III. Treatment issues in the care of patients with toxic epidermal necrolysis. *Burns.* 1999;25:439.

Wolkenstein P, Revuz J. Toxic epidermal necrolysis. *Dermatol Clin.* 2000;18:485.

BULLOUS FIXED DRUG ERUPTION

EPIDEMIOLOGY

- Fixed drug eruptions are very uncommon. Limited data exist on the incidence and prevalence of this disorder.
- Fixed drug eruptions may recur if the patient is re-exposed to the same medication.

PATHOPHYSIOLOGY

- It is assumed that fixed drug eruptions are T-cell mediated, although no models exist for this disease.

CLINICAL FEATURES

- Fixed drug eruptions have an acute onset. The primary lesion is a tender, erythematous macule, which rapidly becomes indurated and then centrally bullous.
- Most common sites of involvement are the glans penis and lips.
- Untreated, individual lesions of fixed drug eruption spontaneously resolve within usually 7 to 14 days. Marked postinflammatory hyperpigmentation, which may persist for at least many months, is a highly characteristic feature.
- Re-exposure to the inciting drug results in rapid recurrence within the same site that was previously involved. Recurrences may also include the development of additional lesions within new sites, which then also recur with subsequent disease activity.
- Common inciting drugs include tetracycline and phenolphthalein.

DIAGNOSIS AND DIFFERENTIAL

- History and evidence of recurrence within the same anatomic site, coupled with its characteristic cutaneous morphology, makes the diagnosis of recurrent fixed drug eruption rather simple.
- The initial occurrence of a fixed drug eruption, especially early in the evolution of the solitary lesion, may, however, suggest a differential diagnosis to include an arthropod bite reaction and localized erythema multiforme.
- Histology reveals findings that may mimic those seen in an early lesion of erythema multiforme. Older lesions, however, also have marked pigment incontinence within the upper dermis, helping in the confirmation of the correct diagnosis.

TREATMENT

- Treatment of isolated lesions of fixed drug eruption involves use of high-potency corticosteroid creams and, if a blister is present, wet compresses with an astringent solution.
- Treatment of a patient with widespread lesions of fixed drug eruption, especially if associated with significant pain, may include the use of systemic corticosteroids until the eruption has cleared.
- The most important facet in the management of a patient with fixed drug eruption is determination of the inciting drug and meticulous avoidance of future exposure of this medication.

REFERENCES

Lee AY. Fixed drug eruptions. Incidence, recognition, and avoidance. *Am J Clin Dermatol.* 2000;1:277.

Savin JA. Current causes of fixed drug eruption in the UK. *Br J Dermatol.* 2001;145:667.

STAPHYLOCOCCAL SCALDED SKIN SYNDROME (SSSS)

EPIDEMIOLOGY

- Staphylococal scalded skin syndrome (SSSS) is an uncommon disorder that usually arises in otherwise healthy children.
- SSSS has also rarely arisen in adults in the setting of underlying immunosuppression or renal insufficiency.
- There is no gender or ethnic predilection for this disease.

PATHOPHYSIOLOGY

- An elegant newborn mouse model of SSSS has demonstrated that this disease results from the effect of an exfoliative toxin produced by only a limited number of serotypes of *Staphylococcus aureus.*
- Administration of systemic corticosteroids to these newborn mice markedly increases the risk of death. This may correlate with the finding that SSSS may also arise in adults who are immunocompromised.
- This disorder cannot be induced in older mice. This may explain why SSSS may also arise in the setting of renal insufficiency in adult humans, since newborn mice, in contrast to older animals, have reduced glomerular filtration rates, preventing renal clearance of the exfoliative toxin.

- The level of skin cleavage in SSSS is within the subcorneal portion of the epidermis, within the same site that blisters arise in pemphigus foliaceus. This may be explained by recent studies which have demonstrated that the exfoliative toxin in SSSS is a serine protease that targets and degrades desmoglein-1, which is the target of autoimmune injury in pemphigus foliaceus.

CLINICAL FEATURES

- Children affected by SSSS usually present initially with rather localized erythema and then expands peripherally. In other children, more widespread areas of erythema may be present.
- The affected skin is very mechanically fragile, resulting in the shearing of thin sheets of epidermis following the application of even minimal lateral traction, leaving potentially large, superficially eroded areas.
- Patients may appear clinically toxic, and may be febrile.

DIAGNOSIS AND DIFFERENTIAL

- The presence of the acute onset of erythema, superficial erosions, and mechanically fragile skin in a young child strongly suggests the diagnosis of SSSS.
- Differential diagnosis primarily involves drug-induced TEN.
- Histology reveals uniform cleavage at the level of the base of the stratum corneum, in the absence of dermal inflammation.
- A rapid means of diagnosing SSSS is to determine, via frozen sections, the level of skin cleavage within an induced peel of the skin. In SSSS, cleavage is solely at the level of the stratum corneum. Cleavage within an induced peel from a patient with TEN reveals variable levels of cleavage, to include deeper, if not full-thickness, separation within the epidermis.
- Blood and wound cultures should be obtained to confirm the presence of *Staphylococcus aureus.* Although not necessary for routine clinical care of such patients, bacterial serotyping can be obtained from selected reference laboratories, if there are epidemiologic needs for such data.

TREATMENT

- Conventional therapy with a systemic antistaphylococcal drug is the treatment of choice for SSSS.

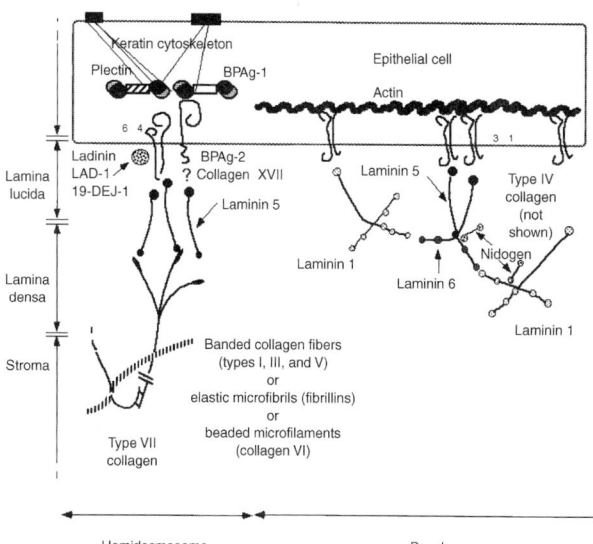

FIGURE 11.1 Model of the hypothetical relationships of molecules within the dermal-epidermal junction basement membrane. The illustration depicts monomeric laminin 5 as the bridge between the transmembrane hemidesmosomal integrin $\alpha_6\beta_4$ and the type VII collagen NC-1 domain. The tight binding of laminin 5 to $\alpha_6\beta_4$ and to type VII collagen provides the primary resistance to frictional forces. The transmembrane collagen BPAg-2 also participates in this stabilization, but its extracellular ligand is not yet known. The lamina lucida proteins 19-DEJ-1 (uncein), ladinin, and LAD-1 are drawn in the region of the exodomains of BPAg-2 and $\alpha_6\beta_4$, but this is entirely speculative. Within the epithelial cell, the transmembrane elements bind the proteins of the hemidesmosomal dense plaque, BPAg-1 and plectin, which then associate with the cytokeratins. Indirect evidence suggests that BPAg-2 binds BPAg-1, and integrin $\alpha_6\beta_4$ binds plectin. The laminin 5-6 complex is shown within the basement membrane between hemidesmosomes, bound by integrin $\alpha_3\beta_1$, where it potentially functions to maintain basement membrane assembly or stability. Integrin $\alpha_3\beta_1$ may function as the link between the basement membrane and the epithelial cortical actin network. None of the molecules is drawn to scale.

- Topical care involves the use of wet dressings with an astringent agent, followed by the application of a mild antibiotic cream (i.e., one containing polymyxin B and/or bacitracin) and a nonadhesive sterile dressing.

REFERENCES

Gemmell CG. Staphylococcal scalded skin syndrome. *J Med Microbiol.* 1995;43:318.

Ladhani S. Recent developments in staphylococcal scalded skin syndrome. *Clin Micro Infection.* 2001;7:301.

Ladhani S, Evans RW. Staphylococcal scalded skin syndrome. *Arch Dis Child.* 1998;78:85.

12 CONNECTIVE TISSUE DISEASES

Jeffrey Callen

LUPUS ERYTHEMATOSUS

CHRONIC CUTANEOUS LUPUS ERYTHEMATOSUS

EPIDEMIOLOGY

- Discoid lupus erythematosus (DLE) may occur at any age but most often occurs in persons aged 20 to 40 years. The mean age is approximately 38 years.
- Male-to-female ratio of DLE is 1:2.
- DLE is slightly more common in African Americans than in Caucasians or Asians.
- The prevalence of DLE is unknown, but may be as high as 50/100,000.
- Lupus erythematosus panniculitis is much rarer than DLE, affects women more than men, and is perhaps more common in African Americans.
- Hypertrophic LE is very rare. Men and women are equally affected, and Caucasians more frequently are affected.

PATHOPHYSIOLOGY

- Genetic predisposition.
- Possible TNF alpha polymorphisms.
- Ultraviolet light exacerbates the process.

CLINICAL FEATURES

- DLE lesions frequently are characteristic.
- The primary lesion is an erythematous papule or plaque with slight to moderate scaling.
- Older lesions thicken and scale may become adherent. Pigmentary changes may develop, with hypopigmentation in the central or inactive area and hyperpigmentation at the active border.
- Dilation of follicular openings occurs with a keratinous plug, termed follicular plugging or patulous follicles.
- Resolution of the active lesion results in atrophy and scarring.
- The scalp is a common area of involvement, and permanent alopecia may result.

- Patients with DLE often are divided into two subsets: localized and widespread. Localized DLE occurs when the head and neck only are affected, while widespread DLE occurs when other areas are affected, regardless of whether disease of the head and neck is seen. Patients with widespread involvement often have hematologic and serologic abnormalities, are more likely to develop SLE, and are more difficult to treat.

VARIANTS OF CCLE

- Mucosal surfaces may be affected by lesions that appear identical to DLE of the skin or by lesions that may simulate lichen planus.
- Palms and soles may be affected, but this occurs in fewer than 2% of patients.
- DLE lesions may become hypertrophic or verrucous. This subset is manifested by wartlike lesions, most often on the extensor arms.
- Lupus panniculitis is a subcutaneous form of chronic CLE that may be accompanied by typical DLE lesions or may occur in patients with SLE.

DIAGNOSIS AND DIFFERENTIAL

- Clinical-pathologic correlation is usually sufficient. Characteristic histopathologic alterations observed in chronic cutaneous LE include (1) vacuolar alteration of the basal cell layer and (2) an inflammatory cell infiltrate (usually lymphocytic) around vessels (perivascular), around appendiceal structures (periappendiceal), and in a subepidermal location. Epidermal changes, such as atrophy, are common, and follicular plugging is often observed. An abundance of mucin often is seen within the dermis.
- Occasionally immunofluorescence microscopy is useful, but there are false-positive and false-negative test results and careful correlation is necessary.
- DLE must be differentiated from lichen planus, psoriasis vulgaris, actinic keratosis, tinea corporis/capitis, and subacute cutaneous lupus erythematosus.
- Lupus panniculitis must be differentiated from other panniculitides.
- Hypertrophic LE must be differentiated from warts, keratoacanthomas, and squamous cell carcinomas.

TREATMENT

- Assess patient for potential systemic lupus erythematosus. Serologic testing, CBC, urinalysis.
- Reassure patient if results are negative.
- Cosmetics—cover-up makeup, wigs.
- Smoking cessation.
- Sunscreen application—broad-spectrum, high sun protective factor (SPF). Sun protective measures.
- Topical corticosteroids—select an agent that is appropriate for the site being treated.
- Intralesional injection of corticosteroids in recalcitrant lesions is locally effective.
- Antimalarial agents—hydroxychloroquine, chloroquine, or quinacrine. Appropriate ophthalmologic evaluation is needed for patients on hydroxychloroquine and chloroquine.
- Alternative agents—topical: retinoids, tacrolimus. Systemic: thalidomide, methotrexate, azathioprine, mycophenolate mofetil, auranofin, dapsone, retinoids.

SUBACUTE CUTANEOUS LUPUS ERYTHEMATOSUS

EPIDEMIOLOGY

- The male-to-female ratio of cutaneous lupus erythematosus (CLE) is approximately 1:4.
- SCLE is more common in Caucasians (85%).
- SCLE typically occurs in patients aged 15 to 70 years. The mean age is approximately 43 years.
- Of patients with CLE, 10 to 50% have SCLE.
- Approximately one half of patients with SCLE have four or more of the criteria for classification as SLE, but in these patients, the disease is less severe, although in individual patients the full range of severity and end-organ dysfunction is possible. By definition, skin lesions heal without scarring or atrophy but may leave residual dyspigmentation.

PATHOPHYSIOLOGY

- SCLE occurs in genetically predisposed individuals.
- Most often patients have human leukocyte antigen B8 (HLA-B8), DR3 (HLA-DR3), DRw52 (HLA-DRw52), and DQ1 (HLA-DQ1). In addition they often have TNF-α polymorphisms.
- A strong association exists with anti-Ro (SS-A) auto-antibodies.
- The cutaneous reaction is believed to be related to ultraviolet (UV) light modulation of autoantigens, epidermal cytokines, and adhesion molecules, with resultant keratinocyte apoptosis.

CLINICAL FEATURES

- SCLE often begins as a papular eruption. Often the process is asymptomatic, but mild pruritus may occur. Photosensitive distribution is common.
- The papules coalesce and form annular plaques or scaly plaques.
- Approximately 50% of SCLE patients have accompanying joint involvement. Arthralgias are common, often symmetrical, and usually affect small joints such as hands and wrists.
- Patients commonly complain of fatigue.
- Some patients have Sjögren's syndrome, while others note dryness of their eyes (keratoconjunctivitis sicca) and/or mouth (xerostomia).
- Patients may manifest symptoms of SLE; therefore, the history should include an assessment for symptoms of pleuritis, pericarditis, neurologic involvement, and renal impairment.

CLINICAL VARIANTS
- Psoriasiform.
- Annular (or polycyclic).
- Drug-induced SCLE: reported most commonly with hydrochlorothiazide, but also calcium channel blockers, ACE inhibitors, terbinafine and other drugs.
- Tumid lupus erythematosus (TLE) involves a deeper more nodular lesion in which little or no scaling is seen. These lesions heal without scarring, yet they are chronic and some authors prefer to classify these patients within the chronic cutaneous LE subset.
- Annular erythema of Sjögren's syndrome has been felt by some authors to be a distinct entity in Japanese and Polynesian patients. It has been this author's opinion that this is a variant of SCLE.
- A variant including erythema multiforme-like lesions in association with DLE and chilblains may exist, but it is not clear whether this is a distinct entity. Some have termed this Rowell's syndrome.
- Neonatal lupus erythematosus (NLE) most often manifests as a nonscarring form of LE. Skin lesions are worsened by UV light and usually resolve by age 4 to 6 months. Some patients with NLE have congenital heart block. Patients with complete heart block eventually may require a pacemaker, may die suddenly, or may develop heart failure. NLE also may be manifested by cytopenias, and if thrombocytopenia is present, the neonate may have petechiae. Lastly, hepatosplenomegaly also may occur. Except for

congenital heart block, all other manifestations resolve without intervention within 4 to 6 months.

DIAGNOSIS AND DIFFERENTIAL

- The diagnosis of SCLE is confirmed by clinical-pathologic correlation. Skin biopsy reveals similar features to those observed in chronic cutaneous LE, but there is less prominent follicular plugging and less frequent epidermal atrophy. Although patients frequently have antibodies to Ro (SS-A), their presence is not diagnostic and their absence is not exclusionary. Immunofluorescence microscopy is useful only in selected patients and the findings must be interpreted within the context of the clinical findings.
- Disorders to be excluded include polymorphous light eruption, dermatomyositis, psoriasis, lichen planus, tinea corporis, erythema annulare centrifugum, and sarcoidosis.

TREATMENT

- Assess patient for potential systemic lupus erythematosus: serologic testing, CBC, urinalysis.
- Reassure patient if results are negative.
- Cosmetics—cover-up makeup, wigs.
- Smoking cessation.
- Stop any drug that may be implicated as inducing or exacerbating the disease.
- Sunscreen application—broad spectrum, high SPF. Sun protective measures.
- Topical corticosteroids—select an agent that is appropriate for the site being treated.
- Intralesional injection of corticosteroids in recalcitrant lesions is locally effective.
- Antimalarial agents—hydroxychloroquine, chloroquine, or quinacrine. Appropriate ophthalmologic evaluation is needed for patients on hydroxychloroquine and chloroquine.
- Alternative agents—topical: retinoids, tacrolimus. Systemic: thalidomide, methotrexate, azathioprine, mycophenolate mofetil, auranofin, dapsone, retinoids.

CUTANEOUS DISEASE IN SYSTEMIC LUPUS ERYTHEMATOSUS

EPIDEMIOLOGY

- SLE prevalence ranges from 17 to 48 cases per 100,000.
- The highest prevalence of SLE occurs in patients aged 40 to 60 years.
- The male-to-female ratio of SLE is approximately 1:10.

PATHOPHYSIOLOGY

- Multifactorial etiology involving a genetic predisposition, hormonal influences, and environmental factors including sunlight and drugs.

CLINICAL FEATURES

- Acute cutaneous LE—malar rash or photo-induced erythema. Heals without scarring.
- Vasculitis—may be large, medium, or small vessel vasculitis.
- Mucinosis—may occur within lesions of cutaneous LE, or may occur in otherwise normal skin.
- Porphyria cutanea tarda may be more common in LE patients. When it does occur, there are therapeutic implications for both the LE and the PCT.
- Sjögren's syndrome may occur in LE.
- Livedo reticularis and pyoderma gangrenosum-like leg ulcers may occur in patients with primary antiphospholipid antibody syndrome (APS) or in patients with secondary APS.
- Bullous lesions of LE are histopathologically nonspecific. These lesions often signify active SLE.

DIAGNOSIS AND DIFFERENTIAL

- The American College of Rheumatology has created a set of criteria for the classification of SLE. These criteria are often misused as diagnostic criteria; however, when the patient has 4 or more of the 11 criteria either concurrently or at any time in their lives they are considered to have SLE. The criteria include serologic abnormalities (ANA and other positive tests), photosensitivity, malar rash, discoid LE rash, polyarthritis, renal abnormalities such as proteinuria or hematuria, cytopenias, and CNS disease such as seizures or psychosis.
- Bullous LE—epidermolysis bullosa acquisita (EBA), porphyria cutanea tarda (PCT), pseudoporphyria.
- Serologic abnormalities are frequent in patients with systemic lupus erythematosus. Virtually all patients have a positive antinuclear antibody. The pattern may be predictive of other antibodies that may be present, but patterns have become less important with the availability of multiple other more specific antibodies. Anti-nDNA antibodies a specific for lupus erythematosus and high levels seem to correlate with disease

activity, particularly renal disease. Anti-Sm antibodies also are specific for SLE and correlate with disease activity. Anti-U$_1$RNP is found more in patients that have features that overlap with scleroderma. Anti-Ro (SS-A) and anti-La (SS-B) antibodies occur, particularly in patients who also have Sjögren's syndrome.

TREATMENT

- Bullous LE—dapsone.
- APS—aspirin, anticoagulants.
- Vasculitis—corticosteroids and/or immunosuppressive agents.

REFERENCES

Black DR, Hornung CA, Schneider PD, Callen JP. Frequency and severity of systemic disease in patients with subacute cutaneous lupus erythematosus. *Arch Dermatol.* 2002;138:1175.

Callen JP, Hughes AP, Kulp-Shorten CL. Subacute cutaneous lupus erythematosus induced or exacerbated by terbinafine: A report of 5 cases. *Arch Dermatol.* 2001;137: 1196.

Callen JP, Klein J. Subacute cutaneous lupus erythematosus. Clinical, serologic, immunogenetic, and therapeutic considerations in seventy-two patients. *Arthritis Rheum.* 1988; 31:1007.

Martens PB, Moder KG, Ahmed I. Lupus panniculitis: Clinical perspectives from a case series. *J Rheumatol.* 1999; 26:68.

Sontheimer RD. The lexicon of cutaneous lupus erythematosus—a review and personal perspective on the nomenclature and classification of the cutaneous manifestations of lupus erythematosus. *Lupus.* 1997;6:84.

Sontheimer RD, Thomas JR, Gilliam JN. Subacute cutaneous lupus erythematosus: A cutaneous marker for a distinct lupus erythematosus subset. *Arch Dermatol.* 1979;115:1409.

DERMATOMYOSITIS

EPIDEMIOLOGY

- The incidence of dermatomyositis/polymyositis (DM/PM) has been estimated at 5.5 cases per million. However, it appears that the incidence is increasing.
- Dermatomyositis may cause death due to muscle weakness or cardiopulmonary involvement. Patients with an associated cancer may die from the malignancy.
- Most patients with DM survive, in which case they may develop residual weakness and disability. In children with severe disease, contractures can develop if they do not receive physical therapy.

- Caucasians are more frequently affected. However, the rise in the incidence for African Americans is greater than that for Caucasians.
- Women are affected twice as often as men.
- DM can occur at any age. The most frequent age at onset is in the fifth and sixth decades.
- Several cases of drug-induced disease have been reported. Dermatomyositis-like skin changes have been reported with hydroxyurea in patients with chronic myelogenous leukemia or essential thrombocytosis. Other agents that may trigger the disease include penicillamine, statin drugs, quinidine, and phenylbutazone.

PATHOPHYSIOLOGY

- Recent studies of the pathogenesis of the myopathy have been controversial. Some suggest that the myopathy in DM and PM are pathogenetically different, with DM being due to a vascular inflammation. Other studies of cytokines suggest that the processes are similar. The pathogenesis of the cutaneous disease is poorly understood.

CLINICAL FEATURES

- Patients often present with skin disease as one of the initial manifestations. In approximately 40% of the patients, the skin disease may be the sole manifestation at the onset. Muscle disease may occur concurrently, may precede the skin disease, or may follow the skin disease by weeks to years.
- Patients often notice an eruption on exposed surfaces. The disease is often pruritic, and sometimes, intense pruritus may disturb sleep patterns. Patients also may complain of a scaly scalp or diffuse hair loss.
- Muscle involvement is manifest by proximal muscle weakness. Patients often begin to note fatigue of their muscles or weakness when climbing stairs, walking, rising from a sitting position, combing their hair, or reaching for articles in cabinets that are above their shoulders. Muscle tenderness may occur but is not a regular feature of the disease.
- Systemic manifestations may occur; therefore, the review of systems should assess for the presence of arthralgias, arthritis, dyspnea, dysphagia, arrhythmias, and dysphonia.
- Malignancy is possible in any patient with dermatomyositis, but it is much more frequent in adults over 60 years of age.
- Children with DM may have an insidious onset that defies diagnosis until the dermatologic disease is clearly observed and diagnosed. Calcinosis is a complication

of juvenile DM but is rarely observed at the onset of disease.

- Characteristic and possibly pathognomonic cutaneous features of dermatomyositis are heliotrope rash and Gottron papules.
- The heliotrope rash consists of a violaceous to dusky erythematous rash with or without edema in a symmetrical distribution involving periorbital skin. Sometimes this sign is quite subtle and may involve only a mild discoloration along the eyelid margin.
- Gottron papules are found over bony prominences, particularly the metacarpophalangeal joints, the proximal interphalangeal joints, and/or the distal interphalangeal joints. They may also be found overlying the elbows, knees and/or feet. The lesions consist of slightly elevated, violaceous papules and plaques. There may be a slight scale and on some occasions there is a thick psoriasiform scale.
- Several other cutaneous features are characteristic of the disease despite not being pathognomonic. They include the following:
  - Malar erythema.
  - Poikiloderma in a photosensitive distribution, such as the extensor surfaces of the arm, the "V" of the neck, or the upper back (Shawl sign).
  - Violaceous erythema on the extensor surfaces.
  - Nailfold changes consist of periungual telangiectases and/or a characteristic cuticular change with hypertrophy of the cuticle and small, hemorrhagic infarcts with this hypertrophic area.
  - Scalp involvement in dermatomyositis is relatively common and is manifest by an erythematous to violaceous, psoriasiform dermatitis.
- Dermatomyositis-sine myositis, also known as amyopathic dermatomyositis (ADM), is diagnosed in patients with typical cutaneous disease in whom there is no evidence of muscle weakness and who repeatedly have normal serum muscle enzyme levels. Some patients with ADM when studied will have an abnormal ultrasound, magnetic resonance imaging, or muscle biopsy. These patients have muscle involvement but may still be classified as having ADM. Since many of the ADM patients are not evaluated beyond clinical and enzymatic studies, many feel that the ADM patient represents a systemic process requiring systemic therapies.
- There are patients whose myositis resolves following therapy, but whose skin disease remains as an active, important feature of the disease. These patients are not said to have ADM, despite the fact that at this point in time the skin is the major and often only manifestation of their disease. There is also a small subset of patients who never develop myositis, despite having prominent cutaneous changes. Rarer cutaneous manifestations include vesiculobullous, erosive lesions, as well as an exfoliative erythroderma. Biopsy from these patients reveals an interface dermatitis similar to biopsy of heliotrope rash, Gottron papules, poikiloderma, or scalp lesions. These cutaneous manifestations may be more common in patients with an associated malignancy.
- A variety of other cutaneous lesions have been described in patients with DM or PM that do not reflect the interface changes observed histopathologically with the pathognomonic or characteristic lesions. These include panniculitis and urticaria, as well as changes of hyperkeratosis of the palms known as "mechanic's hands." Other findings include cutaneous mucinosis, follicular hyperkeratosis, hyperpigmentation, ichthyosis, white plaques on the buccal mucosa, cutaneous vasculitis, and a flagellate erythema.
- Joint swelling occurs in some patients with dermatomyositis. The small joints of the hands are the most frequently involved. The arthritis associated with DM is nondeforming.

DIAGNOSIS AND DIFFERENTIAL

- The diagnosis of DM is confirmed by careful correlation between the clinical findings and laboratory tests.
- Amyopathic DM is often a difficult diagnosis because it simulates subacute cutaneous lupus erythematosus. Many of these patients are pruritic and the lesions often occur over the bony prominences. Studied carefully, many of these patients will be found to have subtle muscle abnormalities on MR imaging, electromyogram, or muscle biopsy.
- Muscle enzymes are often abnormal at some time in the course of patients with dermatomyositis, except in those with the "amyopathic" variant. The most common enzyme to order is the creatine kinase, but aldolase levels and other tests such as AST and LDH also may yield abnormal results. At times, the elevation of the enzymes precedes clinical evidence of myositis. Thus if a patient who is presumably stable develops an elevation of a previously normal enzyme, the clinician should assess the possibility of a flare of the muscle disease.
- Electromyography is a means of detecting inflammation of the muscles and has at times been useful for the selection of a site for muscle biopsy. This test is less commonly ordered now.
- Muscle biopsy, either open or by a needle, may enhance the ability of the clinician to diagnose dermatomyositis. It is also sometimes useful to differentiate steroid myopathy from active inflammatory myopathy when patients have been on corticosteroid therapy but are still weak.

- Several serologic abnormalities have been identified, but their routine use has not yet been delineated. As a group these antibodies have been termed myositis-specific antibodies (MSAs).
- A positive antinuclear antibody is common in patients with dermatomyositis. Anti-Mi-2 is highly specific for dermatomyositis, but it lacks sensitivity as only 25% of the patients with dermatomyositis demonstrate this abnormality. Anti-Jo-1 is associated with pulmonary involvement but is more frequent in patients with polymyositis than dermatomyositis.
- MRI may be useful for assessing the presence of an inflammatory myopathy in patients without weakness. It is also useful to differentiate a steroid myopathy from continued inflammation. Lastly, it may serve as a guide for selection of a site for a muscle biopsy.
- Skin biopsy reveals an interface dermatitis that is difficult to differentiate from lupus erythematosus.
- A systemic evaluation should be conducted in all patients at the time of diagnosis and should include a chest x-ray, esophageal motility, pulmonary function tests, and an electrocardiogram.
- An age-appropriate evaluation for a possible malignancy should be performed at the time of diagnosis and annually for the first 3 years. Female patients should be screened for ovarian cancer. After that time, patients should be evaluated for malignancy at intervals similar to any other person of the same age and sex.
- Dermatomyositis must be differentiated from lupus erythematosus, lichen planus, lichen myxedematosus, psoriasis, rosacea, seborrhea, pityriasis rubra pilaris, and sarcoidosis.

TREATMENT

SKIN DISEASE
- Skin disease is treated in a similar manner to cutaneous lupus erythematosus with slight modifications.
- Assess patient for potential systemic disease.
- Sunscreen application—broad spectrum, high SPF. Sun protective measures.
- Topical corticosteroids—select an agent that is appropriate for the site being treated. Usually I use 1% hydrocortisone ointment except on the scalp.
- Antimalarial agents—hydroxychloroquine, chloroquine, or quinacrine. Appropriate ophthalmologic evaluation is needed for patients on hydroxychloroquine and chloroquine. About one third of patients with DM will develop a drug reaction to these agents; therefore they should be warned of this possibility.
- Alternative agents—topical: tacrolimus. Systemic: thalidomide, methotrexate, mycophenolate mofetil, dapsone, retinoids.

MUSCLE DISEASE
- Muscle disease is treated with systemic therapies.
- Corticosteroids: prednisone 1 to 2 mg/kg per day, or an equivalent.
- Immunosuppressive agents—azathioprine (1 to 2 mg/kg per day depending on the results of thiopurine methyl transferase testing), methotrexate, cyclophosphamide, cyclosporin, mycophenolate mofetil.
- Intravenous immune globulin 1 g/kg per day for 2 days each month for at least 6 months.

ASSOCIATED DISEASE
- Malignancy—removal or appropriate chemotherapy.
- Pulmonary disease may respond to corticosteroids and/or immunosuppressive agents.
- Cardiac disease may respond to corticosteroids and/or immunosuppressive agents.
- Esophageal disease—proximal disease involves the striated muscle and may respond to therapy for the muscles, but distal disease is managed by change in dietary habits and antireflux, antacid therapy.

REFERENCES

Callen JP. Dermatomyositis. *Lancet.* 2000;355:53.

Caproni M, Cardinali C, Parodi A, et al. Amyopathic dermatomyositis: A review by the Italian group of immunodermatology. *Arch Dermatol.* 2002;138:23.

Dalakas MC, Illa I, Dambrosia JM, et al. A controlled trial of high-dose intravenous immune globulin infusions as treatment for dermatomyositis. *N Engl J Med.* 1993;329:1993.

Douglas WW, Tazezlaer HD, Hartman TE, et al. Polymyositis-dermatomyositis-associated interstitial lung disease. *Am J Respir Crit Care Med.* 2001;164:1182.

Euwer RL, Sontheimer RD. Amyopathic dermatomyositis (dermatomyositis sine myositis). Presentation of six new cases and review of the literature. *J Am Acad Dermatol.* 1991;24:959. See comments.

Hill CL, Zhang Y, Sigurgeirsson B, et al. Frequency of specific cancer types in dermatomyositis and polymyositis: A population-based study. *Lancet.* 2001;357:96.

Jorizzo JL. Dermatomyositis: Practical aspects. *Arch Dermatol.* 2002;138:114.

Kasteler JS, Callen JP. Low-dose methotrexate administered weekly is an effective corticosteroid-sparing agent for the treatment of the cutaneous manifestations of dermatomyositis. *J Am Acad Dermatol.* 1997;36:67. See comments.

Kasteler JS, Callen JP. Scalp involvement in dermatomyositis. Often overlooked or misdiagnosed. *JAMA.* 1994;272:1939.

Sontheimer RD. Cutaneous features of classic dermatomyositis and amyopathic dermatomyositis. *Curr Opin Rheumatol.* 1999;11:475.

Woo TY, Callen JP, Voorhees JJ, et al. Cutaneous lesions of dermatomyositis are improved by hydroxychloroquine. *J Am Acad Dermatol.* 1984;10:592.

Zieglschmid-Adams ME, Pandya AG, Cohen SB, Sontheimer RD. Treatment of dermatomyositis with methotrexate. *J Am Acad Dermatol.* 1995;32:754.

SCLERODERMA

LOCALIZED SCLERODERMA

EPIDEMIOLOGY

- The prevalence of localized scleroderma has been estimated to be 27 cases per million.
- Several variants exist—linear morphea, plaque-type morphea, generalized morphea, and morphea profunda.
- The frequency of subtypes varies between adults and children—linear scleroderma is most common in children whereas plaque-type morphea is most common in adults.
- Morphea is more prevalent in children; Caucasians may be slightly more frequently affected.
- There is an overlap with lichen sclerosus et atrophicus, particularly in children with plaque-type morphea.
- Morphea is often self-limiting, but residual deformity is possible or growth retardation may occur.

PATHOPHYSIOLOGY

- Unknown.
- Overproduction of collagen and glycosaminoglycans by dermal fibroblasts.
- Possible causes: autoimmune dysregulation of fibroblast activity, vascular aberrations of the endothelial cells with abnormal cytokine production.

CLINICAL FEATURES

- Plaque-type morphea—localized induration of the skin. Sometimes there is hyperpigmentation. In patients with overlapping features of lichen sclerosus, there is surface change of epidermal atrophy with hyperkeratosis.
- Generalized morphea—generalize plaques of morphea.
- Linear scleroderma (morphea)—may occur on the extremities, or on the face. On the face it is often referred to as "En coup de sabre."
- Some patients have deep-tissue involvement and a resulting facial hemiatrophy known as Parry–Romberg syndrome may appear. The relationship between morphea and the Parry–Romberg syndrome is controversial.
- Morphea profunda is characterized by involvement in the deep tissues of the panniculus.

- Several other variants are rare, but have been reported, such as bullous morphea, keloidal morphea, and pansclerotic morphea.
- There may be some relationship of morphea to the atrophoderma of Pasini and Perini.
- These patients rarely have evidence of systemic scleroderma, and they do not have Raynaud's phenomenon. There are rare cases in which the patient eventually develops systemic scleroderma.

DIAGNOSIS AND DIFFERENTIAL

- There are no tests that confirm the diagnosis of morphea.
- Skin biopsy is similar in morphea and systemic sclerosis and reveals homogenization of collagen bundles. The epidermis can be either normal or atrophic with loss of rete ridges. In the early inflammatory stage, there is often a perivascular lymphohistiocytic infiltrate in the reticular dermis and the fibrous trabeculae of subcutaneous tissues. Numerous plasma cells may also be present. The dermis is typically edematous, with collagen bundle swelling in lower reticular dermis. In the late sclerotic stage, the inflammatory infiltrate usually becomes absent. Collagen bundles become thick, dense, homogenous, and eosinophilic, with collagen changes extending to the upper dermis and possibly also involving the panniculus, fascia, and muscle. Hair follicles, sweat glands, and subcutaneous fat are progressively lost as collagenous material accumulates.
- Frequent abnormalities include an eosinophilia, positive antinuclear antibodies, positive anti-single-stranded DNA antibodies, and positive anti-histone antibodies.
- Radiographic studies may be abnormal if deeper tissues are involved.
- Must be differentiated from systemic scleroderma and sclerodermoid syndromes.

TREATMENT

- Reassure the patient and family that the process is benign and often self-limited.
- Topical agents—corticosteroids, calcipotriene.
- Phototherapy—UVA-1.
- Systemic therapy—methotrexate, vitamin D_3.

SYSTEMIC SCLEROSIS

EPIDEMIOLOGY

- Female to male ratio is 4:1.

- The peak incidence is in the fourth decade of life.
- No racial predilection exists.

PATHOPHYSIOLOGY

- Genetic predisposition.
- Unknown etiology.
- Multifactorial—genetics, environmental, vascular reactivity, immunologic aberration.
- Excess production of collagen with resultant fibrosis.

CLINICAL FEATURES

- History—tightening of the skin, joint pains, Raynaud's phenomenon, shortness of breath, cough, dysphagia.
- Physical examination—sclerodactyly, telangiectasia, calcinosis.
- May be divided into limited and generalized forms. CREST (calcinosis, Raynaud's, esclerodactyly, and telangectasia) is a variant of the limited form.

DIAGNOSIS AND DIFFERENTIAL

- There is no diagnostic test for scleroderma.
- The skin biopsy findings are similar to those observed in localized scleroderma.
- Differentiate from sclerodermoid syndromes— eosinophilic fasciitis, eosinophilia–myalgia syndrome, scleromyxedema, chronic graft-versus-host disease.
- CREST may sometimes mimic hereditary hemorrhagic telangiectasia.
- Skin biopsy is rarely necessary.
- Evaluation of the patient should include CXR, pulmonary function studies, esophageal motility, EKG, serologic tests (ANA, anti-centromere antibody, anti-topoisomerase I antibody).

TREATMENT

- Raynaud's phenomenon—smoking cessation, cold avoidance, nitroglycerin ointment, calcium channel blockers, prostacyclin, lorsartan.
- Anti-fibrotic therapy is not of proven benefit— colchicine, potaba, penicillamine, photopheresis, interferon.
- Immunosuppressive agents, particularly cyclophosphamide, appear to be beneficial for the lung involvement.
- Aggressive antihypertensive therapy for patients with kidney disease.

REFERENCES

Cunningham BB, Landells ID, Langman C. Topical calcipotriene for morphea/linear scleroderma. *J Am Acad Dermatol.* 1998;39:211.

Dutz J. Treatment options for localized scleroderma. *Skin Therapy Lett.* 2000;5:3.

Dziadzio M, Denton CP, Smith R, et al. Losartan therapy for Raynaud's phenomenon and scleroderma: Clinical and biochemical findings in a fifteen-week, randomized, parallel-group, controlled trial. *Arthritis Rheum.* 1999;42:2646.

Elst EF, Van Suijlekom-Smit LW, Oranje AP. Treatment of linear scleroderma with oral 1,25-dihydroxyvitamin D3 (calcitriol) in seven children. *Pediatr Dermatol.* 1999;16:53.

Girardi M, Schaffer JV. Morphea. In: James WD, Elston D, eds. *Medicine Dermatology.* www.emedicine.com.

Sapadin AN, Fleischmajer R. Treatment of scleroderma. *Arch Dermatol.* 2002;138:99.

Seyger MM, van den Hoogen FH, de Boo T. Low-dose methotrexate in the treatment of widespread morphea. *J Am Acad Dermatol.* 1998;39:220.

Stege H, Berneburg M, Humke S. High-dose UVA1 radiation therapy for localized scleroderma. *J Am Acad Dermatol.* 1997;36:938.

Uziel Y, Feldman BM, Krafchik BR, et al. Methotrexate and corticosteroid therapy for pediatric localized scleroderma. *J Pediatr.* 2000;136:91.

Vierra E, Cunningham BB. Morphea and localized scleroderma in children. *Semin Cutan Med Surg.* 1999;18:210.

White B, Moore WC, Wigley FM, et al. Cyclophosphamide is associated with pulmonary function and survival benefit in patients with scleroderma and alveolitis. *Ann Intern Med.* 2000;132:947.

EOSINOPHILIC FASCIITIS

EPIDEMIOLOGY

- Equal occurrence in men and women.
- The peak incidence is in the fourth decade of life; however childhood cases have been reported.
- Caucasians are predominantly affected.

PATHOPHYSIOLOGY

- Unknown etiology.
- Multifactorial—possible genetic factors, environmental factors may play a role, such as *Borrelia burgdorferi* infection. "Excessive" exercise is often associated with the onset of disease. Immunologic aberration.

CLINICAL FEATURES

- History—tightening of the skin usually in the proximal extremities with sparing of the hands and fingers. Joint pains. Raynaud's phenomenon is absent. Malaise, myalgias, and fever are common.
- Physical examination—tight, bound-down skin with a peau d'orange appearance; sclerodactyly is absent; carpal tunnel syndrome occurs in about 20% of patients.
- Laboratory findings—peripheral eosinophilia, hypergammaglobulinemia.
- Eosinophilic fasciitis has been associated with aplastic anemia.

DIAGNOSIS AND DIFFERENTIAL

- There is no diagnostic test for eosinophilic fasciitis.
- Differentiate from sclerodermoid syndromes—morphea, systemic sclerosis, eosinophilia–myalgia syndrome, scleromyxedema, chronic graft-versus-host disease.
- Skin biopsy should be a deep incisional biopsy that includes the fascia.
- Evaluation of the patient should include complete blood count, muscle-derived enzymes, and serum protein electrophoresis. ANA and rheumatoid factor are occasionally positive.

TREATMENT

- Systemic corticosteroids 0.5 to 1 mg/kg per day.
- For nonresponders, consider hydroxychloroquine, methotrexate, or cyclosporine.

EOSINOPHILIA—MYALGIA SYNDROME

EPIDEMIOLOGY

- 83% of reported patients are women.
- The median age is 48, with a range of 4 to 85 years.
- 94% of reported patients are white.

PATHOPHYSIOLOGY

- Exposure to L-tryptophan-containing compounds.

CLINICAL FEATURES

- History—diffuse rash, tightening of the skin, morphea-like lesions, alopecia. Raynaud's phenomenon is absent. Myalgias are almost universal. Shortness of breath is common. Neuropathy is frequent. Joint pain occurs in three fourths of patients.
- Physical examination—peau d'orange changes are common, groove sign is often present (indentation along the course of the veins).

DIAGNOSIS AND DIFFERENTIAL

- There is no diagnostic test for eosinophilia–myalgia syndrome.
- Differentiate from sclerodermoid syndromes—eosinophilic fasciitis, systemic scleroderma, scleromyxedema, chronic graft-versus-host disease, dermatomyositis.
- Skin biopsy should be a deep incisional biopsy that includes the fascia.
- Evaluation of the patient should include CBC, hepatic derived enzymes, CXR, electromyogram, pulmonary function studies, electrocardiogram.

TREATMENT

- Discontinue L-tryptophan.
- Corticosteroid therapy—0.5 to 1 mg/kg per day of prednisone or equivalent.
- Immunosuppressive agents have been tried in nonresponsive patients.
- Death is possible even with adequate therapy.

REFERENCES

Arya V, Arbesfeld DM, Schwartz RA, Quartarolo N. Eosinophilia-myalgia syndrome. *eMedicine J.* Feb. 6, 2002.

Varga J, Kahari VM. Eosinophilia–myalgia syndrome, eosinophilic fasciitis and related fibrosing disorders. *Curr Opin Rheumatol.* 1997;9:562.

13 SUBCUTANEOUS DISORDERS

Luis Requena
Evaristo Sánchez-Yus

PANNICULITIS

EPIDEMIOLOGY

- The panniculitides are a group of heterogeneous inflammatory diseases involving the subcutaneous fat. All of them exhibit similar clinical features that consist of erythematous nodules generally located on the lower limbs. Therefore, the clinical findings are often not enough for differential diagnosis among them, and a biopsy is usually necessary to establish the specific diagnosis.
- In order to reach a histopathologic diagnosis, the first step is to classify the panniculitis as a primarily septal or primarily lobular panniculitis, according to the structures where the inflammatory infiltrate is more abundant (Table 13–1). The inflammatory changes can involve both areas, but a representative section often permits a classification into mostly septal or mostly lobular. In septal panniculitis, the disease involves mainly the connective tissue septa that separate the fat lobules. In lobular panniculitis, the inflammatory process invades the fat lobules.
- The second step is to assess whether vasculitis is present. If it is, the size and the nature of the involved blood vessel must be determined.
- The third step will be to identify the nature of the cells present in the inflammatory infiltrate. Table 13–2 summarizes, in order of frequency, the most common panniculitides according to the age of the patient.

REFERENCES

Requena L, Sánchez Yus E. Panniculitis. Part I. Mostly septal panniculitis. *J Am Acad Dermatol*. 2001;45:163.
Requena L, Sánchez Yus E. Panniculitis. Part II. Mostly lobular panniculitis. *J Am Acad Dermatol*. 2001;45:325.

PRIMARILY SEPTAL PANNICULITIS WITH VASCULITIS

- Etiologic individual entities include leukocytoclastic vasculitis, superficial thrombophlebitis, and cutaneous polyarteritis nodosa.

PATHOPHYSIOLOGY

- Cutaneous leukocytoclastic vasculitis can present with subcutaneous erythematous nodules when the involved vessels are those of the connective septa of the subcutaneous fat. As in other forms of leukocytoclastic vasculitis, the lesions result from the deposition of immune complexes in the vessel walls with activation of the complement system.
- In superficial thrombophlebitis, the involved vessels are the large veins of the septa in the upper subcutis. It can be caused by a hypercoagulable stage, either primary or secondary. Venous insufficiency of the lower extremities is usually the only precipitating factor.
- Cutaneous polyarteritis nodosa is a vasculitis involving the arteries and arterioles of the septa of subcutaneous fat with little or no evidence of systemic disease.

CLINICAL FEATURES

- Leukocytoclastic vasculitis: In addition to the subcutaneous nodules, the patient usually shows the typical purpuric papules on the lower extremities, as the process commonly involves the postcapillary venules of the superficial dermal plexus.
- Superficial thrombophlebitis: Erythematous, tender subcutaneous nodules arranged in a lineal fashion, with a cord-like thickening of the subcutis along the involved vein, located on the lower limbs. The locations of the nodules change from one day to another because multiple segments of the vein may be involved. Hence the term migratory is applied to describe this disorder. In some cases, superficial migratory thrombophlebitis is a paraneoplastic condition.

159

TABLE 13–1   Histopathologic Classification of the Panniculitides

MOSTLY SEPTAL PANNICULITIDES

With vasculitis
Small vessels—venules: Leukocytoclastic vasculitis

Large vessels
Veins: Superficial thrombophlebitis
Arteries: Cutaneous polyarteritis nodosa

Without vasculitis

Lymphocytes and plasma cells mostly
With granulomatous infiltrate in septa: Necrobiosis lipoidica
No granulomatous infiltrate in septa: Subcutaneous morphea

Histiocytes mostly—granulomatous infiltrate

Mucin in center of palisaded granulomas: Subcutaneous granuloma annulare

With fibrin in center of palisaded granulomas: Rheumatoid nodule

With large areas of degenerated collagen, foamy histiocytes, and cholesterol clefts: Necrobiotic xanthogranuloma

Without mucin, fibrin, or degenerated collagen, but with radial granulomas in septa: Erythema nodosum

MOSTLY LOBULAR PANNICULITIDES

With vasculitis
Large vessels–Arteries: Erythema induratum of Bazin

Without vasculitis
Few or no inflammatory cells
Necrosis at the center of the lobule: Sclerosing panniculitis
With vascular calcification: Calciphylaxis, oxalosis
With needle-shaped crystals in adipocytes: Sclerema neonatorum

Lymphocytes predominant
With superficial and deep perivascular dermal infiltrate: Cold panniculitis

With lymphoid follicles, plasma cells, and nuclear dust of lymphocytes: Lupus panniculitis

With lymphocytes and plasma cells: Panniculitis in dermatomyositis

Neutrophils predominant
Extensive fat necrosis with saponification of adipocytes: Pancreatic panniculitis

With neutrophils between collagen bundles of deep reticular dermis: α_1-antitrypsin deficiency

With bacteria, fungi or protozoa identifiable by specialized stains: Infective panniculitis

With foreign bodies: Factitial panniculitis

Histiocytes predominant (granulomatous)
No crystals in adipocytes: Subcutaneous sarcoidosis, traumatic panniculitis, lipoatrophy

With crystals in adipocytes: Subcutaneous fat necrosis of newborn, poststeroid panniculitis

With cytophagic histiocytes: Cytophagic histiocytic panniculitis

• Cutaneous polyarteritis nodosa presents with bilateral tender erythematous nodules, livedo reticularis, and ulceration of the lower limbs. Usually there are mild constitutional symptoms, with low-grade fever, arthralgias, myalgias, malaise, and fatigue, but

TABLE 13–2   Most Common Panniculitides (in order of frequency, according to age of patient)

ADULTS

Erythema nodosum
Erythema induratum of Bazin
Traumatic panniculitis
Sclerosing panniculitis
Superficial thrombophlebitis
Infective panniculitis

CHILDREN

Erythema nodosum
Cold panniculitis
Subcutaneous granuloma annulare

NEWBORNS

Subcutaneous fat necrosis of the newborn

absence of significant systemic involvement. In contrast to systemic polyarteritis nodosa, laboratory evidence of immunologic abnormalities (ANA, ANCA, rheumatoid factor, cryoglobulins, or decreased complement level) is lacking. In a small portion of patients there is mild renal involvement and serologic evidence of hepatitis B infection, cryoglobulinemia, and peripheral neuropathy.

DIAGNOSIS AND DIFFERENTIAL

• Leukocytoclastic vasculitis shows necrosis of endothelial cells, fibrin deposition, neutrophils, and nuclear dust within the walls of the small blood vessels in the connective tissue septa of the subcutaneous fat.
• In superficial thrombophlebitis the affected vessel shows luminal thrombosis and an inflammatory infiltrate within its wall. In early lesions the inflammatory cell infiltrate is mostly composed of neutrophils, whereas in later stages there are lymphocytes, histiocytes, and occasional multinucleated giant cells.
• Cutaneous polyarteritis nodosa is more of an inflammatory than a thrombotic process. Characteristically, the tunica intima of the involved artery exhibits an eosinophilic ring of fibrinoid necrosis, giving a target-like appearance to the vessel.

TREATMENT

• For treatment of leukocytoclastic vasculitis, see Chapter 4. Cutaneous ulcers can be managed with relative rest and local measures.
• Evaluating the response to treatment of patients with cutaneous polyarteritis nodosa is difficult because the course of the disease fluctuates. Mild cases may be

managed with nonsteroidal anti-inflammatory drugs or low doses of prednisone (20 mg/d).

REFERENCES

Daoud MS, Hutton KP, Gibson LE. Cutaneous periarteritis nodosa: A clinicopathologic study of 79 cases. *Br J Dermatol.* 1997;136:706.

Samlaska CP, James WD. Superficial thrombophlebitis: I. Primary hypercoagulable states. *J Am Acad Dermatol.* 1990; 22:975.

PRIMARILY SEPTAL PANNICULITIS WITHOUT VASCULITIS

- Individual entities include erythema nodosum, necrobiosis lipoidica, morphea profunda, subcutaneous granuloma annulare, rheumatoid nodule, and necrobiotic xanthogranuloma.

ERYTHEMA NODOSUM

EPIDEMIOLOGY

- Erythema nodosum is the most common clinico-pathologic variant of septal panniculitis. The process can occur at any age, but most cases appear between the second and fourth decades of life, with a peak of incidence between 20 and 30 years of age. It is three to six times more frequently in women than in men.

PATHOPHYSIOLOGY

- Although there are considerable geographic variations, streptococcal infections are the most frequent etiologic factor for erythema nodosum in children; whereas drugs, sarcoidosis, and inflammatory diseases of the bowel are the most common associated disorders in adults. Table 13–3 summarizes a literature review of the described etiologic factors of erythema nodosum.
- Erythema nodosum is considered to be a hypersensitivity response to a wide variety of inciting factors. The variability of possible antigenic stimuli that can induce erythema nodosum indicates that this disorder is a cutaneous reactive process. Erythema nodosum probably results from the formation of immune complexes and their deposition in and around venules of the connective tissue septa of the subcutaneous fat. Circulating immunocomplexes and complement activation have been recorded in patients with erythema nodosum. Direct immunofluorescence studies have shown deposits of immunoglobulins in the blood vessels walls of the septa of subcutaneous fat. However, some studies have failed to demonstrate circulating immunocomplexes in patients with erythema nodosum, and a type IV delayed hypersensitivity reaction has been suggested to play an important role in the pathogenesis of this disorder.

CLINICAL FEATURES

- The typical eruption of erythema nodosum is characterized by a sudden onset of symmetrical, tender, erythematous, warm nodules and raised plaques usually located on the shins, ankles, and knees. Often the lesions are bilaterally distributed. At first, the nodules show a bright red color and are raised slightly above the level of the skin. In few days, they become flat, with a livid or purplish color. Finally, they exhibit a yellow or greenish appearance often taking on the look of a deep bruise ("erythema contusiformis"). Ulceration is not a feature of erythema nodosum, and the nodules heal without atrophy or scarring.
- Acute bouts of erythema nodosum are associated with fever of 38 to 39° C, fatigue, malaise, arthralgia, headache, abdominal pain, vomiting, cough, or diarrhea. The eruption generally lasts 3 to 6 weeks, but persistence beyond this time is not unusual and recurrences are frequent.

DIAGNOSIS AND DIFFERENTIAL

- The clinical picture is characteristic in most cases and a biopsy is not required.
- If histologic confirmation is desired, erythema nodosum shows the stereotypical picture of a mostly septal panniculitis with no vasculitis. The septa of the subcutaneous fat are always thickened and variously infiltrated by inflammatory cells that extend to the periseptal areas of the fat lobules. The composition of the inflammatory infiltrate in the septa varies with time. In early lesions, edema, hemorrhage, and neutrophils are responsible for the septal thickening; whereas fibrosis, periseptal granulation tissue, lymphocytes, and multinucleated giant cells are the main findings in late-stage lesions of erythema nodosum.
- A histopathologic hallmark of erythema nodosum is the presence of the so-called Miescher's radial granulomas, which consist of small, well-defined nodular aggregations of small histiocytes around a central stellate or banana-shaped clef.

TABLE 13–3   Etiologic Factors in Erythema Nodosum

INFECTIONS

Bacterial Infections

Atypical mycobacterial infections
Borrelia burgdorferi infections
Boutonneuse fever
Brucellosis
Campylobacter infections
Cat-scratch disease
Chancroid
Chlamydia psittaci infections
Corynebacterium diphteriae infections
Escherichia coli infections
Gonorrhea
Leptospirosis
Lymphogranuloma venereum
Meningococcemia
Moraxella catarrhalis infections
Mycoplasma pneumoniae infections
Pasteurella pseudotuberculosis infections
Propionibacterium acnes
Pseudomona aeruginosa infections
Q fever
Salmonella infections
Shigella inflections
Streptococcal infections
Syphilis
Tuberculosis
Tularemia
Yersinia infections

Viral Infections

Cytomegalovirus infections
Hepatitis B
Hepatitis C
Herpes simplex
HIV infection
Infectious mononucleosis
Measles
Milker's nodules
Orf
Parvovirus B19 infections
Varicella

Fungal Infections

Aspergillosis
Blastomycosis
Coccidioidomycosis
Dermatophytes
Histoplasmosis
Sporotrichosis

Protozoal Infections

Amebiasis
Ancylostomiasis
Ascariasis
Giardiasis
Hydatidosis
Hookworm infestation
Sparganum larva
Toxoplasmosis
Trichomoniasis

DRUGS

Acetaminophen
Actinomycin-D
All-trans retinoic acid
Aminopyrine

TABLE 13–3 (*Continued*)

DRUGS

Amiodarone
Amoxicillin
Ampicillin
Antimony
Arsphenamine
Azathioprine
Bromides
Busulfan
Carbamazepine
Carbenicillin
Cefdinir
Chlordiazepoxide
Chlorotrianisene
Chlorpropamide
Ciprofloxacin
Clomiphene
Codeine
Cotrimoxazole
D-penicillamine
Dapsone
Diclofenac
Dicloxacillin
Diethylstilbestrol
Disopyramide
Echinacea herbal therapy
Enoxacin
Erythromycin
Estrogens
Fluoxetine
Furosemide
Glucagon
Gold salts
Granulocyte colony-stimulating factor
Hepatitis B vaccine
Hydralazine
Ibuprofen
Indomethacin
Interleukin-2
Iodides
Isotretinoin
Leukotriene-modifying agents (zileuton and rafirlukast)
Levofloxacin
Meclofenamate
Medroxyprogesterone
Meprobamate
Mesalamine
Methicillin
Methimazole
Methyldopa
Mezlozillin
Minocycline
Naproxen
Nifedipine
Nitrofurantoin
Ofloxacin
Omeprazole
Oral contraceptives
Oxacillin
Paroxetine
Penicillin
Phenylbutazone
Phenytoin
Piperacillin
Progestins

TABLE 13–3 (Continued)

DRUGS

Propylthiouracil
Pyritinol
Sparfloxacin
Streptomycin
Sulfamethoxazole
Sulfixoxazole
Sulfonamides
Sulfosalazine
Thalidomide
Ticarcilin
Trimethoprim
Typhoid vaccination
Verapamil

MALIGNANT DISEASES

Adenocarcinoma of the colon
Carcinoma of the uterine cervix
Hodgkin's disease
Leukemia
Non-Hodgkin's lymphoma
Pancreatic carcinoma
Postradiotherapy for pelvic carcinoma
Renal carcinoma
Sarcoma
Stomach cancer

MISCELLANEOUS CONDITIONS

Acne fulminans
Adul Still's disease
Ankylosing spondylitis
Antiphospolipid antibody syndrome
Behçet's syndrome
Berger's disease
Chronic active hepatitis
Coeliac disease
Colon diverticulosis
Crohn's disease
Diverticulitis
Granulomatous mastitis
IgA nephropathy
Jellyfish sting
Lupus erythematosus
Pregnancy
Radiotheraphy
Recurrent polychondritis
Reiter's syndrome
Rheumatoid arthritis
Sarcoidosis
Sjögren's syndrome
Smoke inhalation
Sweet's syndrome
Systemic lupus erythematosus-like syndrome due to C4 deficiency
Takayasu's arteritis
Ulcerative colitis
Vogt–Koyanagi disease
Wegener's granulomatosis

- Initial evaluation of a patient with erythema nodosum should include complete blood count, determination of the sedimentation rate, antistreptolysin O (ASO) titer, urinalysis, throat culture, intradermal tuberculin test, and chest roentgenogram. A high ASO titer is seen in those cases of erythema nodosum associated with a sore throat streptococcal infection. Usually, a significant change in ASO titer of at least 30% in two consecutive determinations performed in 2 to 4-week intervals indicates recent streptococcal infection. When the etiology is in doubt, a sample of blood should be serologically investigated for the bacterial, viral, fungal, or protozoal infections more prevalent in that area. In those cases suspected of being tuberculous, an intradermal tuberculin test should be performed. A chest x-ray should be performed in all patients with erythema nodosum to rule out pulmonary diseases as the cause of the cutaneous reactive process. Radiologically demonstrable bilateral hilar lymphadenopathy with febrile illness and erythema nodosum with no evidence of tuberculosis characterize Löfgren's syndrome, which in most cases represents an acute variant of pulmonary sarcoidosis with a benign course.

TREATMENT

- Treatment should be directed to the underlying associated condition, if identified.
- Usually, nodules of erythema nodosum regress spontaneously in a few weeks, and bed rest is often sufficient.
- Aspirin and nonsteroidal anti-inflammatory drugs, such as indomethacin or naproxen, may be helpful to enhance analgesia and resolution. If the lesions persist longer, potassium iodide in a dosage of 400 to 900 mg daily, or a saturated solution of potassium iodide, 2 to 10 drops in water or orange juice three times per day, has been reported to be useful.

REFERENCES

García-Porrúa C, González-Gay MA, Vázquez-Caruncho M, et al. Erythema nodosum. Etiologic and predictive factors in defined population. *Arthritis Rheum.* 2000;43:584.

Sánchez Yus E, Sanz Vico MD, de Diego V. Miecher's radial granuloma. A characteristic marker of erythema nodosum. *Am J Dermatopathol.* 1989;11:434.

Schulz EJ, Whiting DA. Treatment of erythema nodosum and nodular vasculitis with potassium iodide. *Br J Dermatol.* 1976;94:75.

OTHER SEPTAL PANNICULITIS WITHOUT VASCULITIS

CLINICAL FEATURES

NECROBIOSIS LIPOIDICA

- Necrobiosis lipoidica is described in detail in Section 14. Involvement of the subcutis in necrobiosis lipoidica is always a deep extension of the dermal process, and there are no descriptions of necrobiosis lipoidica involving only the subcutaneous fat.

MORPHEA PROFUNDA

- Morphea profunda presents as indurated plaques or nodules that remain stable or enlarge progressively and often heal with subcutaneous atrophy and residual hyperpigmentation. The lesions have a predilection for appearing on the shoulders, upper arms, and trunk. Eosinophilic fasciitis, also named Shulman's syndrome, is regarded as a variant of scleroderma characterized by a sudden onset, sometimes following intense physical activity, of symmetrical induration of the skin and subcutaneous tissues of the limbs. Usually, there is a gradual improvement of the lesions, even without any treatment, and complete recovery is seen after some years.

SUBCUTANEOUS GRANULOMA ANNULARE

- Subcutaneous granuloma annulare is an uncommon clinicopathologic variant of granuloma annulare that appears more frequently in children and young adults. Subcutaneous nodules, with no inflammatory appearance at the skin surface, are preferably located on the anterior aspects of the lower legs, hands, head, and buttocks.

RHEUMATOID NODULES

- Rheumatoid nodules appear as deeply situated nodules, with firm consistency on palpation, and with no inflammatory changes on the skin surface. The most frequently involved areas are the elbows and fingers. Approximately 20% of the patients with rheumatoid arthritis have rheumatoid nodules in the vicinity of the joints. These patients present more aggressive forms of the disease. A rare variant of multiple rheumatoid nodules involving the fingers with little or no articular disease is named rheumatoid nodulosis.

NECROBIOTIC XANTHOGRANULOMA

- Necrobiotic xanthogranuloma can present with multiple large indurated plaques, sharply demarcated, with yellow-violaceous coloration and tendency to ulceration. The most common involved areas are the periorbital regions of the face. Necrobiotic xanthogranuloma appears in patients with paraproteinemia, mostly of IgG kappa type, and cases associated with multiple myeloma and other lymphoproliferative disorders have been recorded.

DIAGNOSIS AND DIFFERENTIAL

- Necrobiosis lipoidica shows an inflammatory infiltrate involving the full thickness of the dermis and extending to the subcutaneous fat. Palisading granulomas with histiocytes surrounding areas of degenerated collagen can be seen within the widened septa.
- Morphea profunda shows marked fibrous thickening of the septa of subcutaneous fat, which appear eosinophilic and sclerotic. Consequently to the thickening of the septa, collagen also replaces the fat normally present around the eccrine coils, giving the misimpression that sweat glands have ascended into the dermis. Inflammatory infiltrate is only present in active lesions and it consists of aggregations of lymphocytes, with lymphoid follicle formation, surrounded by plasma cells at the junction of the thickened septa and the fat lobules.
- Subcutaneous granuloma annulare shows areas of necrobiosis with peripheral palisading granulomas involving the septa of the subcutis. The central necrobiotic areas contain increased amounts of connective tissue mucin and nuclear dust of neutrophils between the degenerated collagen bundles. The peripheral ring is composed of epithelioid histiocytes arranged in palisaded fashion and some multinucleated giant cells.
- Rheumatoid nodules show large areas of necrobiosis surrounded by palisaded granulomas involving the dermis and subcutaneous fat. In the central necrobiotic area appears an eosinophilic granular or fibrillary material containing fibrin. At the periphery, there is a well-organized palisade of elongated histiocytes and multinucleated giant cells.
- Necrobiotic xanthogranulomas show large areas of necrobiosis alternating with granulomatous inflammation involving both the deeper dermis and the subcutaneous fat. Histiocytes, many of them with foamy cytoplasm, cholesterol crystals, and multinucleated Touton-type giant cells are also present.

TREATMENT

- Treatment of necrobiosis lipoidica is discussed in Chapter 14.
- Morphea profunda usually has a poor response. In same cases there is resolution or improvement of the lesions with locally injected triamcinolone. Penicillamine has been associated with resolution in some cases.
- Like in other variants of granuloma annulare, lesions of subcutaneous granuloma annulare have an

unpredictable course, and therefore evaluating the response of different treatments is difficult. Sometimes spontaneous regression occurs.

- Rheumatoid nodules are usually asymptomatic and surgical excision is only indicated in ulcerated or painful lesions.
- Treatment of necrobiotic xanthogranuloma is directed to the associated paraproteinemia. Melphalan with or without associated prednisolone has resulted in temporary clearing of the cutaneous lesions. Plasmapheresis may reduce the level of circulating monoclonal IgG with healing of cutaneous ulcers.

PRIMARILY LOBULAR PANNICULITIS WITH VASCULITIS

ERYTHEMA INDURATUM OF BAZIN (NODULAR VASCULITIS)

EPIDEMIOLOGY

- In some countries, tuberculosis is the main etiologic factor for erythema induratum of Bazin-nodular vasculitis. *Mycobacterium tuberculosis* DNA has been demonstrated in biopsy specimens of cases of erythema induratum of Bazin by polymerase chain reaction techniques.
- In other areas, identical lesions to those of erythema induratum of Bazin-nodular vasculitis have been described unrelated to tuberculosis. In these cases, slowing of the blood flow and thrombosis of small vessels of the lower legs are probably the predominant etiologic factors.

PATHOPHYSIOLOGY

- Pathogenesis of erythema induratum of Bazin-nodular vasculitis is probably related to the deposition of immune complexes in the blood vessels of the fat lobules. Stasis, vascular damage from previous thrombophlebitis, and cold may predispose to the inflammatory response and necrosis of adipocytes. Lymphatic insufficiency may also be important. Some authors have proposed that erythema induratum of Bazin-nodular vasculitis is a hypersensitivity reaction of T lymphocytes requiring antigen presentation by dendritic cells.

CLINICAL FEATURES

- Typical erythema induratum of Bazin appears in middle-aged women as erythematous subcutaneous nodules and plaques on the posterior aspects of the lower legs. Erythrocyanosis, heavy column-like calves, erythema surrounding follicular openings, and cutis marmorata are frequently associated changes and may be predisposing factors.
- Although nonulcerated lesions may heal without scarring, often subcutaneous nodules become adherent to the skin surface and ulcerate. Healing of these ulcers is a slow process resulting in atrophic scars.
- Erythema induratum of Bazin is more frequent in obese women with some degree of venous insufficiency of the lower extremities, and subcutaneous nodules with ulceration develop mostly during the cold months of the winter. The course is protracted and recurrent episodes over years, even decades, are common. Individual lesions tend to involute, but new crops appear at irregular intervals.

DIAGNOSIS AND DIFFERENTIAL

- Evaluation of a patient with erythema induratum of Bazin-nodular vasculitis should include complete blood count, determination of the sedimentation rate, intradermal tuberculin test, and chest roentgenogram. Most patients show raised erythrocyte sedimentation rate and a nonspecific polyclonal increase of gammaglobulin titers. In those cases related to tuberculous infections, there is a strong positive reaction to the Mantoux test.
- Erythema induratum of Bazin is a mostly lobular panniculitis. At an early stage, the fat lobules are punctuated throughout by discrete collections of inflammatory cells, mostly neutrophils. In fully developed lesions, epithelioid histiocytes, multinucleated giant cells, and lymphocytes give a granulomatous appearance to the fat lobule. When intense vascular damage is present, there are extensive areas of caseous necrosis and the lesion show all histopathologic attributes of tuberculosis. Controversy persists about the nature of the involved vessel. Ziehl-Neelsen stain and immunohistochemical investigations for *Mycobacterium tuberculosis* are invariably negative in lesions of erythema induratum of Bazin-nodular vasculitis.

TREATMENT

- In those cases in which there is a strong positive reaction to the Mantoux test or *Mycobacterium tuberculosis* DNA is demonstrated in the cutaneous biopsy specimen by polymerase chain reaction techniques, a full course of 9 months of antituberculous triple-agent therapy is recommended.

- Potassium iodide has been reported as an effective and rapid symptomatic treatment for erythema induratum of Bazin-nodular vasculitis.
- Supporting bandages, bed rest, and treatment of the venous insufficiency of the lower extremities are also helpful. Nonstereoidal anti-inflammatory drugs may be used to improve painful ulcers.

REFERENCE

Baselga E, Margall N, Barnadas MA, et al. Detection of *Mycobacterium tuberculosis* DNA in lobular granulomatous panniculitis (erythema induratum-nodular vasculitis). *Arch Dermatol.* 1997;133:457.

PRIMARILY LOBULAR PANNICULITIS WITHOUT VASCULITIS

SCLEROSING PANNICULITIS (LIPODERMATOSCLEROSIS)

PATHOPHYSIOLOGY

- In the original description, this process was thought to be an infectious disease related to unusual acid-fast bacteria, but subsequent studies failed to identify any bacteria in the cultures of the lesions. Currently, venous insufficiency of the lower extremities is considered to be the main etiologic factor of sclerosing panniculitis. Venous insufficiency leads to sludging in the lobular capillaries, which results in ischemia and necrosis of the central portion of the fat lobule. Postphlebitic syndrome resolves with extensive deep fibrosis and sclerosis, resulting in atrophy of the subcutaneous fat.

CLINICAL FEATURES

- The process is more frequent in middle-aged or elderly obese women.
- Wood-like indurated plaques with erythema, edema, telangiectasia, and hyperpigmentation involving the lower legs with a stocking distribution. The involved area of the lower extremity has an inverted bottle

deformity secondary to extensive deep fibrosis and sclerosis resulting in atrophy of the subcutaneous fat.
- The condition is usually associated with chronic venous insufficiency, arterial ischemia, and previous episodes of thrombophlebitis. Often, tortuous dilated varicose veins are seen above the indurated area of the leg.

DIAGNOSIS AND DIFFERENTIAL

- Biopsy findings show in early stages a sparse inflammatory infiltrate mostly composed of lymphocytes between the collagen bundles of the septa and areas of ischemic necrosis at the center of the fat lobule, manifested as pallor and small anucleated adipocytes. In later stages the septa appear thickened and fibrotic, resulting in dramatic atrophy of the subcutaneous fat. The periphery of the fat lobule often shows lipophagic granuloma with scattered lymphocytes and plasma cells. In old lesions, sclerosis of the septa is the main histopathologic finding, with small size fat lobules due to lypophagic fat necrosis and fatty microcysts with foci of membranocystic change. Changes of stasis dermatitis are present in the superficial dermis, with proliferation of capillaries and venules in the papillary dermis; there is also fibrosis, and abundant hemosiderin deposition.

TREATMENT

- Standard measures for venous insufficiency of the lower extremities, including compression stockings, have been useful but not curative.
- Some cases improved rapidly and consistently with the anabolic steroid stanozolol.

REFERENCE

Jorizzo JL, White WL, Zanolli MD, et al. Sclerosing panniculitis. A clinicopathologic assessment. *Arch Dermatol.* 1991;127:554.

CALCIPHYLAXIS

PATHOPHYSIOLOGY

- The main feature of this disorder is the calcification of cutaneous vessel walls resulting in necrosis and ulceration.
- Calciphylaxis is usually associated with chronic renal failure and most of these patients have abnormalities

of calcium–phosphorus metabolism, with elevated serum calcium and phosphorus levels, often in the context of the secondary hyperparathyroidism.

CLINICAL FEATURES

- Cutaneous lesions consist of violaceous, mottled to reticulated patches and plaques resembling livedo reticularis. Lesions evolve into necrotic, indurated plaques and nodules, resulting in large and deep non-healing ulcers associated with significant tenderness, ischemic digital pain, and in some cases, gangrene of the digits, necessitating amputation. The lesions exhibit bilateral symmetry and distal parts of the extremities, thighs, and buttocks are the most frequently involved sites.

DIAGNOSIS AND DIFFERENTIAL

- Serum calcium and phosphorus levels are usually elevated in patients with calciphylaxis, often in the context of the secondary hyperparathyroidism associated with renal failure. Most patients show elevated parathyroid hormone (PTH) levels, although these levels are not correlated to the onset of cutaneous lesions. Radiographs often show "pipe stem" calcification of arteries and arterioles.
- Histopathologic study of the cutaneous lesions demonstrates calcium deposition in the walls of small-to-medium diameter blood vessels of the deep dermis and subcutaneous fat, associated with lobular fat necrosis, intralobular calcification, and inflammatory infiltrate of neutrophils, lymphocytes, and foamy histiocytes.

TREATMENT

- The prognosis of calciphylaxis is poor and there is an 80% mortality rate.
- In some patients, parathyroidectomy with normalization of abnormal calcium and phosphorus serum levels stopped the progression of the disease.
- In the patients with chronic renal failure undergoing hemodialysis, a diet poor in calcium and phosphorus, binding agents, and low-calcium hemodialysis is recommended.

REFERENCE

Oh DH, Eulau D, Tokugawa DA, et al. Five cases of calciphylaxis and a review of the literature. *J Am Acad Dermatol.* 1999;40:979.

SCLEREMA NEONATORUM

PATHOPHYSIOLOGY

- Most of the cases are described in low-weight premature newborns during the course of a wide variety of severe illnesses, particularly serious infections, congenital heart disease, and other major developmental defects. This disorder is rare nowadays because of improvement of neonatal care.
- It has been postulated that the ratio of saturated to unsaturated fatty acids is relatively high in the adipose tissue of all neonates, and that this ratio is even higher in infants with sclerema neonatorum.
- The prognosis is poor, and most of the infants affected with sclerema neonatorum die within a few days.

CLINICAL FEATURES

- Cutaneous lesions appear during the first days of life, beginning on the buttocks and thighs in the form of diffuse yellow-white woody induration of the skin that rapidly extends to involve large areas of the body surface and results in immobility of the extremities.

DIAGNOSIS AND DIFFERENTIAL

- The most characteristic feature is the presence of radially arranged, needle-shaped clefts within the adipocytes, and occasionally, in the cytoplasm of some of the few multinucleated giant cells present in the sparse inflammatory infiltrate.
- In contrast with subcutaneous fat of the newborn, in lesions of sclerema neonatorum the inflammatory infiltrate is characteristically lacking.

TREATMENT

- Treatment of sclerema neonatorum is primarily that of the underlying disease.
- Systemic corticosteroids are ineffective, but repeated exchange transfusions may reduce mortality.
- Infants who survive the episode of sclerema neonatorum show a normal appearance.

COLD PANNICULITIS

PATHOPHYSIOLOGY

- Cold panniculitis is also more frequent in infants following exposure to severe cold. Examples of this variant of panniculitis have been also described in the cheeks of children sucking ice cubes, ice packs, or popsicles, and during the cold months of winter in the thighs or buttocks of women who ride horses wearing too tight trousers that obstruct the blood supply to the subcutaneous fat (equestrian panniculitis).

CLINICAL FEATURES

- The affected areas appear as indurated erythematous plaques with ill-defined margins. If the involved area is kept warm, the plaques slowly soften and resolve in some days without scarring.

DIAGNOSIS AND DIFFERENTIAL

- Biopsies of cold panniculitis show a mostly lobular panniculitis with an inflammatory infiltrate of lymphocytes and histiocytes in the fat lobule.

TREATMENT

- Cold panniculitis resolves if further exposure to cold is avoided.
- In horse riders, looser trousers should be recommended.

REFERENCE

Ter Poorten JC, Hebert AA, Ilkiw R. Cold panniculitis in a neonate. *J Am Acad Dermatol.* 1995;33:383.

LUPUS PANNICULITIS (LUPUS ERYTHEMATOSUS PROFUNDUS)

PATHOPHYSIOLOGY

- Lupus panniculitis appears in approximately 1 to 3% of patients with cutaneous lupus erythematosus. Patients with lupus panniculitis have a form of lupus erythematosus with a mild biologic behavior.

CLINICAL FEATURES

- Lupus panniculitis is more frequent in women than in men, and the lesions have a predilection for the upper arms, shoulders, face, and buttocks.

- The lesions consist of deep situated subcutaneous nodules or plaques. The surface of the nodules may show the classic features of discoid lupus erythematosus or appear as normal skin. When lesions of lupus panniculitis regress, they lead to atrophy and delling of the involved area with persistent areas of lipoatrophy. On the shoulders and upper arms the lesions are so characteristic that they allow a retrospective diagnosis of lupus panniculitis in old cases.

DIAGNOSIS AND DIFFERENTIAL

- Patients with lupus panniculitis may have extensive serologic abnormalities and ANA and anti-DNA antibodies may sometimes be present, but only a few patients with lupus erythematosus profundus have systemic lupus erythematosus.
- In over half of the cases there are epidermal and dermal changes of discoid lupus erythematosus. In the other half of the cases, the changes are confined to the subcutaneous fat, with no anomalies in the dermis or epidermis. They consist of a mostly lobular panniculitis with inflammatory infiltrate predominantly composed of lymphocytes. A characteristic feature, found in over one half of the patients, is the presence of lymphoid follicles. Collagen bundles of subcutaneous septa appear hyaline and sclerotic.

TREATMENT

- Topical treatment with potent creams of corticosteroids under occlusion has been reported as helpful in lesions of lupus panniculitis, but often a systemic course of corticosteroids or hydroxychloroquine is necessary.
- Dapsone has been also reported as an effective treatment.

REFERENCE

Sanchez NP, Peters MS, Winkelmann RK. The histopathology of lupus erythematosus panniculitis. *J Am Acad Dermatol.* 1981;5:673.

PANCREATIC PANNICULITIS

PATHOPHYSIOLOGY

- This variant of panniculitis appears in approximately 2 to 3% of all patients with pancreatic diseases, and it has been mostly described in association with acute and chronic pancreatitis. There are also reports of pancreatic panniculitis in patients with pancreatic carcinoma. In some patients with pancreatic panniculitis the skin lesions are the presenting features of the pancreatic disease.

- Pancreatic enzymes, mostly lipase, that escape to the blood from the inflamed pancreas are responsible for the subcutaneous fat necrosis in enzymatic panniculitis. The finding of pancreatic lipase in the areas of subcutaneous necrosis, and the immunohistochemical demonstration of the enzyme with antilipase monoclonal antibodies within the necrotic adipocytes, support the pathogenic role of pancreatic lipase inducing fat necrosis.

CLINICAL FEATURES

- The cutaneous lesions appear as erythematous subcutaneous nodules that spontaneously ulcerate and exude oily brown material that results from liquefaction necrosis of the adipocytes. The distal parts of the lower extremities, around the ankles and knees, are the most frequently affected sites.
- The onset of subcutaneous fat necrosis in pancreatic diseases is often accompanied by acute arthritis that results from necrosis in periarticular fat tissue. In rare instances it is associated with necrosis of the abdominal fat, pleural effusions, mesenteric thrombosis, and leukemoid reaction with eosinophilia.

DIAGNOSIS AND DIFFERENTIAL

- Increased levels of serum amylase and lipase are useful indicators of pancreatic inflammation. Some patients also have peripheral eosinophilia.
- The lesions of pancreatic panniculitis show a mostly lobular panniculitis with intense necrosis of the adipocytes. In fully developed lesions there is coagulative necrosis of the adipocytes, which leads to ghost adipocytes. Ghost adipocytes are adipocytes that have lost their nuclei and show a finely granular and basophilic material within their cytoplasm due to calcification.

TREATMENT

- Treatment of pancreatic panniculitis is primarily directed to the underlying pancreatic disease. Sometimes, complete resolution of the symptoms occurs when pancreatic anomaly is surgically corrected.

- Those cases associated with pancreatitis tend to resolve when the inflammatory episode of the pancreas regresses. In contrast, subcutaneous nodules of pancreatic panniculitis in patients with pancreatic carcinoma tend to be more chronic and persistent, with lesions, in areas beyond the lower extremities.

REFERENCE

Dahl PR, Su WPD, Cullimore KC, Dicken CH. Pancreatic panniculitis. *J Am Acad Dermatol.* 1995;33:413.

ALPHA-1-ANTITRYPSIN DEFICIENCY PANNICULITIS

PATHOPHYSIOLOGY

- Clinical manifestations of α_1-antitrypsin deficiency (α_1-protease inhibitor deficiency) only appear in homozygous patients. A heterozygotic person with PiMS or PiMZ phenotype usually shows moderate deficiency of α_1-antitrypsin, whereas homozygous patients with phenotype PiZZ have severe α_1-antitrypsin deficiency with serious clinical manifestations, including emphysema, hepatitis, cirrhosis, vasculitis, angioedema, and panniculits. In these patients, the liver produces the proenzyme of a1-antitrypsin, but this proenzyme is not released.

CLINICAL FEATURES

- Cutaneous lesions of α_1-antitrypsin deficiency panniculitis consist of subcutaneous nodules mostly located on the lower extremities; but often other areas of the skin such as arms, trunk, and face are also involved. The earliest lesions resemble cellulitis with a tendency to ulcerate and exude oily material that represents necrotic adipocytes.

DIAGNOSIS AND DIFFERENTIAL

- Quantitative measurements of serum levels of α_1-antitrypsin and enzyme phenotyping confirm the diagnosis.
- Biopsies show a mostly lobular panniculitis with severe necrosis of the fat lobules. A frequent histopathologic feature consists of the presence of neutrophils between collagen bundles of the reticular dermis. Occasionally, the intense inflammatory infiltrate of neutrophils causes collagenolysis and degeneration of elastic tissue

with destruction of the septa of the subcutis. The necrotic fat lobules then appear "floating" and surrounded by neutrophils.

TREATMENT

- In homozygous patients with severe forms of the disease, presenting with severe emphysema and liver failure, the only therapeutic possibility is supplemental infusion of exogenous α_1-proteinase inhibitor concentrate, in a dose of 60 mg/kg intravenous per week, or a liver transplantation.
- At the present moment, the production of α_1-antitrypsin by genetic engineering is being investigated.

REFERENCE

Smith KC, Su WPD, Pittelkow MR, Winkelmann RK. Clinical and pathologic correlations in 96 patients with panniculitis, including 15 patients with deficient levels of alpha-1-antitrypsin. *J Am Acad Dermatol.* 1989;21:1192.

INFECTIVE PANNICULITIS

PATHOPHYSIOLOGY

- Several bacteria or fungi may cause lobular panniculitis as the main clinical manifestation. The most frequent microorganisms causing panniculitis are *Streptococcus pyogenes, Staphylococcus aureus,* Pseudomonas sp., Klebsiella, *Nocardia sp.,* atypical mycobacteria, *Mycobacterium tuberculosis, Candida sp., Fusarium sp., Histoplasma capsulatum, Cryptococcus neoformans, Actinomyces israelii, Sporothrix schenckii, Aspergillus fumigatus,* and the fungi causing chromomycosis.

CLINICAL FEATURES

- Most infective panniculitis occur in immunosuppressed patients. In these patients, panniculitis may appear with primary or secondary skin lesions. Primary cutaneous infections arise either from direct physical inoculation or at the site of an occlusive dressing at an indwelling catheter. Secondary cutaneous infections develop from either direct extension, usually on the chest wall in patients with pulmonary infections, or from hematogenous dissemination.

DIAGNOSIS AND DIFFERENTIAL

- In immunosuppressed patients, microorganisms are numerous and they may be identified in tissue sections with the routine hematoxylin-esosin stain or with special stains (Gram's, periodic acid-Schiff, Ziehl-Neelsen, and so forth).
- In patients with preserved immune response, the microorganisms are sparse and often cannot be identified with special stains; thus the diagnosis must be established by a positive culture of the lesion or serologic studies.
- Because anti-BCG immunostaining shows cross-reactivity with many bacteria and fungi as well as its high sensitivity and minimal background staining, this immunostaining has been proposed as the best screening tool for detection of bacterial and fungal microorganisms in paraffin-embedded skin specimens.
- Primary and secondary infective panniculitis show different histopathologic features. In primary cutaneous infections, the epicenter of the inflammation is in the superficial dermis, and thrombosed vessels do not have intravascular organisms. In contrast, in secondary cutaneous infections, the inflammation involves only the deep reticular dermis and subcutaneous fat, and the blood vessels are thrombosed and dilated with masses of organisms expanding their lumens.

TREATMENT

- Treatment of infective panniculitis requires systemic administration of antibiotics, which should be selected according to susceptibility tests.

REFERENCE

Patterson JW, Brown PC, Broecker AH. Infection-induced panniculitis. *J Cutan Pathol.* 1989;16:183.

FACTITIAL PANNICULITIS

PATHOPHYSIOLOGY

- Factitial panniculitis results from the subcutaneous implantation of different materials for cosmetic or therapeutic reasons. These self-inflicted or iatrogenic panniculitides include those due to some drugs injected in the subcutaneous fat, such as povidone, meperidine, pentazocine, and vitamin K; and substances used to augment the size of breasts or genitalia or to correct facial wrinkles or other contour abnormalities, such as paraffin or silicone.

- Psychiatric patients with personality aberrations have been reported with self-inflicted panniculitis due to subcutaneous injections of the most unsuspected substances including acids, alkalis, mustard, milk, microbiologically contaminated material, urine, and feces.

CLINICAL FEATURES

- The diagnosis may be suggested by the special personality of the patient.
- Subcutaneous nodules of panniculitis and ulceration, sometimes with chronic and recurrent nature, appear on easily accessible areas of the skin. In some patients there may be fever and systemic symptoms secondary to the superinfection of the lesions.

DIAGNOSIS AND DIFFERENTIAL

- Factitial panniculitis is a primarily lobular panniculitis, with an inflammatory infiltrate predominantly composed of neutrophils in early lesions and a more granulomatous infiltrate in late-stage lesions. Sometimes polarization of the slide can identify the refractile foreign material causing the panniculitis.
- Some histopathologic findings may be helpful to identify the nature of the foreign material. For example, silicone injections used for cosmetic reasons may produce granulomatous reaction characterized by foamy histiocytes that contain multiple vacuoles in their cytoplasm and multinucleated giant cells surrounding polygonal translucent angulated foreign bodies, which represent impurities in silicone.

TREATMENT

- Patients with self-inflicted factitial panniculitis are mentally disturbed and psychiatric treatment is usually required.

TRAUMATIC PANNICULITIS

PATHOPHYSIOLOGY

- Traumatic panniculitis may result from accidental blunt trauma in several areas of the skin or in women with large breasts, in which the excessive breast weight favors the trauma of mammary subcutaneous fat.

CLINICAL FEATURES

- Lesions of traumatic panniculitis appear as indurated nodules deeply situated in the subcutaneous tissue covered by normal or erythematous skin.
- *Lipoatrophia semicircularis* is a variant of traumatic panniculitis that consists of a semicircular band-like atrophy of the subcutaneous fat involving half of the circumference of the anterolateral aspects of the thighs of women who repeatedly knock their thighs against the desk or the chair because of working habits.
- *Mobile encapsulated lipoma* is another lesion that may be also considered a residual stage of traumatic panniculitis. It consists of well-demarcated movable nodules that appear in the subcutis of lower limbs, elbows, or hips after trauma.

DIAGNOSIS AND DIFFERENTIAL

- Biopsy of traumatic fat necrosis shows cystic spaces of variable size and shape within the fat lobule, as a consequence of confluent necrosis of the fat cells, surrounded by variable degrees of fibrosis and hemorrhage.

SUBCUTANEOUS FAT NECROSIS OF THE NEWBORN

PATHOPHYSIOLOGY

- Newborns have a relatively large body surface in comparison with their weight and a greater ratio of saturated to unsaturated fatty acids than in adult fat, and these two factors favor the release caused by minor trauma of hydrolases that induce breakdown of unsaturated fatty acids.
- Infants affected by subcutaneous fat necrosis of the newborn often have hypercalcemia of unknown origin. Other etiologic factors that have been postulated include obstetrical trauma and induced hypothermia for cardiac surgery.

CLINICAL FEATURES

- Indurated plaques or subcutaneous nodules with a predilection for the buttocks, shoulders, cheeks, and thighs that appears in newborns during the first days of life.

DIAGNOSIS AND DIFFERENTIAL

- Subcutaneous fat necrosis of the newborn is a mostly lobular panniculitis, with a dense inflammatory infiltrate composed of lymphocytes, histiocytes, lipophages, multinucleated giant cells, and sometimes eosinophils interspersed among the adipocytes of the fat lobule.
- Cells with finely eosinophilic granular cytoplasm that contain narrow needle-shaped clefts radially arranged replace many adipocytes. These needle-shaped clefts represent crystals of triglycerides of the adipocytes.
- Histopathologic features identical to those of subcutaneous fat of the newborn may be seen in poststeroid panniculitis. Important for the differential diagnosis, in the lesions of sclerema neonatorum the inflammatory infiltrate is lacking.

TREATMENT

- In contrast to sclerema neonatorum, infants with subcutaneous fat necrosis of the newborn have an excellent prognosis and the subcutaneous plaques and nodules spontaneously regress in few days with no sequela.
- Etidronate, a diphosphonate, has been proposed as an effective treatment for the associated hypercalcemia.

CYTOPHAGIC HISTIOCYTIC PANNICULITIS

- Two different processes are included under this term: one is an authentic panniculitis, namely cytophagic histiocytic panniculitis, and the other is a lymphoma with clinical appearance of panniculitis, the so-called subcutaneous panniculitis-like T-cell lymphoma.

CLINICAL FEATURES

- Patients with cytophagic histiocytic panniculitis have a prolonged clinical course of the disease over the years, but most of them undergo a terminal state characterized by hemocytophagocytosis involving the bone marrow.
- Pannicultic lymphoma is a high-grade aggressive lymphoma. In these patients the lymphoproliferative process and genotypic studies have demonstrated monoclonality of the atypical lymphocytes involving the fat lobule.

PATHOPHYSIOLOGY

- These two different diseases have in common a histopathologic finding, the presence of cytophagocytosis in the subcutaneous fat that may extend to the bone marrow. In the subcutis, there is mostly a lobular panniculitis with histiocytes showing cytophagocytosis, the so-called "bean-bag" cells.
- The cases of subcutaneous panniculitis-like lymphoma show neoplastic lymphocytes, with marked atypia and large and hyperchromatic nuclei involving the fat lobule.

TREATMENT

- Most patients with cytophagic histiocytic panniculitis show a favorable response to immunosuppressive therapy with prednisone or cyclosporine.
- Patients with subcutaneous panniculitis-like T-cell lymphoma have a poor prognosis with early death despite aggressive treatment with chemotherapy and radiotherapy.

REFERENCE

Craig AJ, Cualing H, Thomas G, et al. Cytophagic histiocytic panniculitis—a syndrome associated with benign and malignant panniculitis: Case comparison and review of the literature. *J Am Acad Dermatol.* 1998;39:721.

DISORDERS ERRONEOUSLY CONSIDERED AS SPECIFIC VARIANTS OF PANNICULITIS

WEBER–CHRISTIAN DISEASE

- Weber–Christian disease is the term that has been classically used to refer to cases of mostly lobular panniculitis without vasculitis, and systemic manifestations including fever and involvement of visceral fat tissue.
- This term should be abandoned because now a more specific diagnosis may be rendered in most of the cases. Many patients originally diagnosed with Weber–Christian disease were later reclassified when other variants of lobular panniculitis, including erythema induratum of Bazin-nodular vasculitis, pancreatic

panniculitis, and α_1-antitrypsin deficiency panniculitis, became recognized.

REFERENCE

White JW, Winkelmann RK. Weber–Christian panniculitis: A review of 30 cases with this diagnosis. *J Am Acad Dermatol.* 1998;39:56.

ROTHMANN–MAKAI DISEASE

- Rothmann–Makai disease used to describe cases of relapsing nodular panniculitis similar to that of Weber–Christian disease, but with no fever or other systemic manifestations. Rothmann–Makai disease is also an obsolete term that is no longer used.

LIPOMEMBRANOUS OR MEMBRANOCYSTIC PANNICULITIS

- Lipomembranous panniculitis is a histopathologic pattern, but not a specific variant of panniculitis. The histopathologic features include the presence of cystic spaces in the fat lobule that result from necrosis of the adipocytes. The cystic spaces are lined with a homogeneous eosinophilic membrane with convoluted projections into the cystic cavity.
- Lipomembranous features can be seen in different types of panniculitis (late-stage lesions of sclerosing panniculitis, erythema nodosum, deep morphea, lupus panniculitis, and so forth).

REFERENCE

Alegre VA, Winkelmann RK, Aliaga A. Lipomembranous changes in chronic panniculitis. *J Am Acad Dermatol.* 1988; 19:39.

EOSINOPHILIC PANNICULITIS

- Eosinophilic panniculitis is a term used to refer cases of septal or lobular panniculitis in which eosinophils predominate in the inflammatory infiltrate.
- Eosinophilic panniculitis is also a histopathologic pattern rather than a distinct entity. It has been described in several types of panniculitis and other inflammatory disorders involving the skin.

REFERENCE

Winkelmann RK, Frigas E. Eosinophilic panniculitis: A clinicopathologic study. *J Cutan Pathol.* 1986;13:1.

LIPOATROPHY

PATHOPHYSIOLOGY

- Lipoatrophy refers specifically to a loss of subcutaneous fat due to a previous inflammatory process involving the subcutis. Lesions of localized lipoatrophy have been described as residual lesions of different types of panniculitis, as a result of subcutaneous injections of corticosteroids, and as a consequence of pressure and compression by tight clothes near the ankles, on the thighs, over the sacrum, on abdominal skin, and on the extremities.
- Localized lipoatrophy has received different names according its clinical appearance and location, including annular lipoatrophy, abdominal lipoatrophy, and semicircular lipoatrophy

CLINICAL FEATURES

- The clinical appearance of lypoatrophy varies from a dimple area of the skin to extensive disfiguring lesions.
- In those cases secondary to subcutaneous injections, there is a definite tendency to spontaneous recovery.

DIAGNOSIS AND DIFFERENTIAL

- In most cases the histopathologic findings are those of lipophagic granuloma surrounding a small-sized fat lobule, with perilobular fibrosis.

TREATMENT

- Cases of localized lipoatrophy secondary to lesions of panniculitis have shown some improvement with oral and topical corticosteroids, but it is questionable whether the effect is due to corticosteroids or to spontaneous improvement of the lesions with time.
- In some cases in which residual lipoatrophy produced an important cosmetic deformity, improvement was achieved with reconstructive surgery.

LIPODYSTROPHY

PATHOPHYSIOLOGY

- Lipodystrophy means an absence of subcutaneous fat with no evidence of inflammation. Lipodystrophy may be congenital or acquired, and clinical variants include total, partial, and localized forms of lipodystrophy.

CLINICAL FEATURES

- Total lipodystrophy consists of congenital or acquired complete loss of subcutaneous tissue involving diffusely all body surfaces. Acquired total lipodystrophy is usually associated with hepatomegaly, hyperglycemia, hyperlipemia, hypermetabolism, and other endocrinologic and metabolic disorders.
- Partial lipodystrophy usually begins on the face and is manifested by a symmetric loss of facial fat with or without atrophy of the subcutaneous fat of arms and upper trunk, the process named cephalothoracicobrachial lipodystrophy.

- Other forms of partial lipodystrophy include unilateral variants of facial lypodystrophy, some of them related to *Borrelia burgdoferi* infections, and localized lipodystrophy involving only the subcutaneous fat of the abdominal wall or the neck.
- Some patients with partial lipodystrophy present associated immunologic anomalies or autoimmune diseases.

DIAGNOSIS AND DIFFERENTIAL

- In fully developed lesions, biopsies of lipodystrophy show absence of subcutaneous fat with deposition of new collagen and with no evidence of inflammation.

TREATMENT

- Lipodystrophy shows a poor response to treatment. In localized forms, the lesions tend to recede over time, restoring some of the lost subcutaneous tissue.

14 DERMAL INFILTRATES

Franco Rongioletti
Paolo Romanelli

GRANULOMA ANNULARE

- Granuloma Annulare (GA) is a benign, cutaneous, inflammatory disorder of unknown etiology that is usually self-limited. Its presentation most commonly involves the hands and feet.

EPIDEMIOLOGY

- Although it can start at any age, GA is predominantly a disease of children and young adults. In a series of 208 patients, the onset was prior to age 30 in over two-thirds of the cases. Females were affected twice as often as males.

PATHOPHYSIOLOGY

- Several hypotheses as to the pathogenesis of GA lesions have been put forward based on histologic evidence of lymphocytic involvement and the presence of various cytokines and cellular products. They are as follows: (1) a vasculitis leading to necrotizing changes, (2) trauma-induced necrobiosis, (3) monocyte release of lysosomal enzymes causing necrobiotic degeneration, and (4) a type IV lymphocyte-mediated delayed hypersensitivity reaction causing degenerative changes.

CLINICAL FEATURES

- Localized GA is the most common form, typically presenting with a limited number of asymptomatic, arcuate, skin-colored or red purple dermal papules varying from 1 to 5 mm in diameter. Spontaneous resolution occurs in 50% of the patients; however, the lesions may take as long as 2 years to show involution.
- Generalized GA (disseminated) presents with hundreds or thousands of relatively small 1 to 2-mm glossy skin-colored papules. The papules may be solitary or they may coalesce. This variant has been shown to have an associated increased prevalence in HLA-Bw3 as well as HLA-A29 individuals, and it tends to be distributed primarily over the trunk. The scalp and palmar and plantar surfaces are usually not involved. Spontaneous resolution is less common.
- Perforating GA is characterized by small, superficial, skin-colored papules often with a central umbilication. This type is more commonly distributed over the hands and fingers.
- Subcutaneous or nodular GA presents as larger superficial or deep, skin-colored lesions.

DIAGNOSIS AND DIFFERENTIAL

- Diagnosis can be based on characteristic clinical manifestations; however, biopsy is recommended when the lesions have a clinically nondistinctive presentation.
- GA is often mistaken for tinea corporis. It may also be difficult to differentiate from perforating sarcoidosis because of their similar clinical appearance and the possibility of their coexistence. Furthermore, it may be confused with lichen planus, papular mucinosis, and erythema giant cell granuloma, which present with skin-colored to slightly erythematous discrete papules in an annular configuration similar to GA. However, the lack of necrobiosis on pathology is typically a distinguishing feature. Histologically, the localized form of GA is sometimes difficult to distinguish from cutaneous tuberculosis.
- Perforating GA may resemble annular lichen planus or verruca plana. The subcutaneous or nodular presentation may be confused with pseudorheumatoid nodules in children and rheumatoid nodules in adults.

TREATMENT

- Granuloma annulare is a cosmetic disease in that it is rarely symptomatic and usually has no medical consequence. The cosmetic disfigurement may be severe or mild. Although the disease is usually self-limited, a wide array of treatment methods has been employed, supposedly to hasten resolution. These include topical vitamin E and x-ray therapy, cryotherapy, laser destruction, and intralesional injection of triamcinolone. Of these, the last seems the most effective.

• Potent topical glucocorticoids suppress the disease. Glucocorticoids applied topically under occlusion or incorporated into tape may also be employed, but side effects such as atrophy of the nearby skin can occur. Psoralen plus ultraviolet (PUVA) therapy may improve the eruption and apparently even cure it. This is probably the treatment of choice for patients with widespread disease, since it is quite effective and relatively safe, at least over the short term of treatment. Acitretin alone or given during PUVA treatments may be effective.

• Systemic treatment with pentoxifylline, nicotinamide, niacinamide, isotretinoin, salicylates, chlorpropamide, potassium iodide, thyroxine, aspirin, dipyridamole, dapsone, and antimalarials has been advocated and sometimes seems to work, but spontaneous resolutions make evaluation of treatment difficult. Systemic glucocorticoids improve appearance, but risks almost always outweigh benefits.

• Treatment with low doses of chlorambucil is probably effective but only very rarely justified because of severe side effects such as induction of leukemia and bone marrow suppression.

REFERENCES

Smith MD, Downie JB, Di Costanzo D. Granuloma annulare. *Int J Dermatol.* 1997;36:326.

Wells KS, Smith MA. The natural history of granuloma annulare. *Br J Dermatol.* 1963;75:199.

NECROBIOSIS LIPOIDICA

EPIDEMIOLOGY

• Necrobiosis lipoidica diabeticorum (NLD) has a distinctive clinical appearance, unusual histopathologic features, and is strongly associated with diabetes mellitus; its cause, however, remains unknown. Multiple treatment approaches have been attempted without consistent results. In this section, we discuss the spectrum of clinical features, histopathologic findings, theories on pathogenesis, differential diagnosis, and reported therapeutic options for this challenging problem.

• NLD is closely associated with diabetes mellitus. Despite the high prevalence of diabetes mellitus in patients with NL, necrobiosis is relatively uncommon in diabetic patients; the reported prevalence is 3 per 1000. The female to male ratio is 3:1. The age of onset ranges from birth to 76 years, with an average age of 30 years in diabetic patients and 41 years in nondiabetic patients. Fifty percent of patients with NL demonstrate other diabetic end-organ damage. Spontaneous remissions occur in 13 to 19% of patients between 1 and 34 years after onset; however, residual scarring and atrophy remain.

PATHOPHYSIOLOGY

• The precise correlation between NLD and diabetes remains unresolved. The disease was first described in patients with well-established diabetes but subsequently reported in patients without evident diabetes. However, despite the lack of full concordance, NLD seems to be a valid marker for diabetes. Because NLD occurs in both insulin-dependent and non-insulin-dependent diabetes, its pathogenesis cannot be related to genetic factors, underlying autoimmune disease, or other causes of diabetes. It can be reasonably assumed that the granulomatous response is secondary to alterations in dermal collagen. This may be secondary to arteriolar changes deep into and within the areas of collagen degeneration. It has been hypothesized that increased platelet aggregation may be a trigger factor in the vascular changes.

CLINICAL FEATURES

• Typical lesions of NLD occur on the pretibial skin as irregular, ovoid plaques with a violaceous, indurated periphery and a yellow central atrophic area. Superficial telangiectases and scattered hyperkeratotic plugs are often noted. The lesions can start as small, firm, red-brown papules that slowly enlarge and develop the typical violet-brown center.

• They are usually multiple and bilateral, 16% of patients have only one plaque, and 50% have four to eight. Ulceration occurs in approximately 35% and is often precipitated by minor trauma.

DIAGNOSIS AND DIFFERENTIAL

• Although the clinical appearance of classic NLD is distinctive, early or atypical NLD can be difficult to recognize. Early NLD and GA can be virtually indistinguishable. As the lesions enlarge they become more distinctive. The typical location of GA on the dorsa of hands, fingers, and feet is helpful in distinguishing the two. Pigmented pretibial patches occur in diabetic patients as flat, atrophic, hyperpigmented lesions without the typical red or yellow coloration of NLD. Sarcoidosis can appear similar to NLD. Rheumatoid nodules can also have a clinical appearance similar to NLD, but generally the lesions appear as subcutaneous nodules on the extensor aspects of the joints in the setting of severe arthritis. Necrobiotic xanthogranuloma is characterized by yellow, indurated plaques and nodules with atrophy and ulceration that involve the periorbital areas; they are always associated with paraproteinemia.

TREATMENT

- A consistently effective treatment for NL has yet to be found. It is well accepted that the behavior of NLD does not relate to diabetic glycemic control. Reported effective treatment for NLD have included a variety of topical, oral, and surgical approaches, none universally effective. Potent topical corticosteroids applied to early lesions or the inflammatory rim surrounding well-established NLD lesions are thought to help in controlling disease progression. Intralesional injections of corticosteroids into the active border of NLD lesions are also thought to be helpful.

REFERENCE

Lowitt MH, Dover JS. Necrobiosis lipoidica. *J Am Acad Dermatol.* 1991;25:735.

ATROPHIC/DEGENERATIVE DISEASES

ANETODERMA

- Anetoderma (macular atrophy) is a rare cutaneous condition, perhaps more frequent in central Europe, characterized by a circumscribed area of slack skin associated with loss of normal elastic fibers.

PATHOPHYSIOLOGY

- The pathogenetic mechanism is unknown. Focal elastolysis may be secondary to the release of elastases from inflammatory cells.

- Complement activation may be involved as C3 is deposited on the remaining elastic fibers.
- Decreased elastin production and decreased elastase inhibitor have also been postulated. The elastin rather than the fibrillin of elastic fibers appears reduced.

CLINICAL FEATURES

- Anetoderma may be classified as either primary or secondary. Primary anetoderma occurs when there is no underlying associated disease, and in the past it has been subclassified into a Jadassohn–Pellizzari type, which is preceded by inflammation, and a Schwenninger–Buzzi type, in which the lesions appear without preceding inflammation. This is now of historical interest only, because both lesions may occur in the same patient and the prognosis and histology are identical in the two types.
- Secondary anetoderma occurs in association with another disease including lupus erythematosus, antiphospholipid syndrome, sarcoidosis, borreliosis, syphilis, leprosy, tuberculosis, HIV infection, and some skin tumors such as pilomatricomas or cutaneous lymphomas. Anetoderma induced by penicillamine has also been reported.
- In all forms of anetoderma, round to oval, atrophic localized patches of a few centimeters in diameter, primarily involving the upper trunk and upper arms, develop progressively over many years. Individual lesions may bulge outwards or be slightly depressed. They can be herniated inwards with fingertip pressure.
- The numbers of lesions may range from a few to over a hundred. Familial cases have been reported. In secondary anetoderma, atrophic patches do not always develop at the site of the known inflammatory lesions.

HISTOPATHOLOGY

- In inflammatory (early) lesions, a perivascular infiltrate with CD4 lymphocytes and occasionally plasmocytes, histiocytes, eosinophils, and neutrophils is seen. In chronic noninflammatory lesions, elastic tissue is sparse or lost in both the midreticular dermis and sometimes the papillary dermis.

DIAGNOSIS AND DIFFERENTIAL

- Anetoderma must be differentiated from cutis laxa, postinflammatory elastolysis, mid-dermal elastolysis, focal dermal hypoplasia, atrophoderma, atrophic scars (postvaricella or acne), connective tissue nevi, neurofibromas, and other focal conditions that exhibit either a clinical laxity or a histologic reduction in elastic fibers. Primary anetoderma is diagnosed only by excluding the presence of any of the disorders associated with secondary anetoderma.

TREATMENT

- No treatment is beneficial once the atrophy has developed. Surgical excision of cosmetically unacceptable lesions may be considered. Therapy of secondary anetoderma is directed at prevention of lesions of the underlying disorder.

REFERENCE

Kasper RC, Wood GS, Nihal M, LeBoit PE. Anetoderma arising in cutaneous B-cell lymphoproliferative disease. *Am J Dermatopathol.* 2001;23:124.

LICHEN SCLEROSUS ET ATROPHICUS

- Lichen sclerosus et atrophicus (LSA) is a chronic inflammatory condition resulting in white, atrophic lesions that has a predilection for the anogenital area.

EPIDEMIOLOGY

- Lichen sclerosus et atrophicus is more common in women between the fifth and sixth decades of age, but children are also affected. The exact prevalence is unknown; an incidence of 14 per 100,000 per year has been estimated. It is uncommon in black people.

PATHOPHYSIOLOGY

- The cause of LSA is unknown, but genetic susceptibility and a link with autoimmune disorders have been suggested. A relationship with morphea and lichen planus has been reported. The spirochete Borrelia and the human papillomavirus have been suggested but not substantiated as infective triggers.

CLINICAL FEATURES

- LSA most commonly involves the anogenital area (85 to 98%), with extragenital lesions in 15 to 20% of patients. The lesions are characterized by shiny, flat, white-ivory papules that coalesce to form atrophic plaques with possible teleangectasies, purpura, erosions, and blisters. Follicular hyperkeratosis and sclerosis may occur. In women, genital lesions may appear as a figure-of eight pattern around the vulva and anus.
- Intractable pruritus may lead to secondary lichenification. Soreness, dyspareunia, and dysuria are the other common symptoms, but some patients are asymptomatic. In men, the glans penis and foreskin are usually affected (balanitis xerotica obliterans). Presenting symptoms are itching, soreness, and difficulty in retracting the foreskin (phymosis).
- Progression to destructive scarring may occur in both sexes. LSA carries an increased risk of developing vulval cancer and is linked with cancer of the penis, although the incidence is low. In prepubertal girls, LSA may be confused with changes seen in sexual abuse. Boys most commonly present with LSA of the prepuce, which can be ameliorated by circumcision.
- Extragenital sites commonly affected include the upper part of the trunk, neck, inner thighs, axillae, shoulders, and wrists. Extragenital LSA may occur in pre-existing scars, areas of previous trauma, and at the sites of pressure (Koebner phenomenon). In patients with diffuse disease, it is not uncommon to see LSA overlap with morphea. Some patients with LSA have coexisting autoimmune diseases including alopecia areata, vitiligo, thyroid disorders, and diabetes.

HISTOPATHOLOGY

- Histologic features are specific and consist of follicular plugging, epidermal atrophy, hydropic degeneration of the basal layer, a pale-staining homogeneous zone in the upper dermis with dilated capillaries, and a lymphocytic infiltrate below the homogenized area. Elastic tissue is reduced in the pale-staining papillary dermis.

DIAGNOSIS AND DIFFERENTIAL

- Genital LSA should be distinguished from erosive lichen planus, cicatricial pemphigoid, and lichen simplex. Morphea and chronic radiodermatitis are the main differential diagnosis for extragenital lesions. Histopathology is usually distinctive, though changes of morphea and LSA may coexist in a same specimen. Sclerosis of the reticular dermis and subcutaneous septa favors morphea. Radiodermatitis may be distinguished by a sclerotic dermis and pleomorphic fibroblasts.

TREATMENT

- Potent topical steroids provide relief in genital LSA. There is no effective treatment for extragenital LSA. Surgery is not part of routine treatment but it is useful to relieve symptoms of scarring and to treat possible malignant lesions.
- Circumcision may be curative if the condition involves the foreskin. LSA may improve or heal spontaneously in girls after puberty.

REFERENCE

Powell JJ, Wojnarowska F. Lichen sclerosus. *Lancet.* 1999; 353:1777.

EHLERS–DANLOS SYNDROMES

EPIDEMIOLOGY

- The Ehlers–Danlos syndromes (EDS) are a genetically, biochemically, and clinically diverse group of heritable connective tissue disorders with joint laxity and skin hyperextensibility. There are no accurate estimate figures for the prevalence of Ehlers–Danlos syndrome. If all forms of the syndrome are combined, the prevalence may be as high as 1 in 5000.

PATHOPHYSIOLOGY

- The concept that EDS is a disorder of fibrillar collagen metabolism is well supported by identification of specific defects in the collagen biosynthetic pathway that produce clinically distinct forms of EDS. These are briefly reviewed here and in Table 14–1. For more complete reviews of collagen biochemistry and clinical aspects of EDS, the reader is directed to recent reviews. There are three fundamental mechanisms of disease known to produce EDS: deficiency of collagen-processing enzymes, dominant-negative effects of mutant collagen alpha chains, and haploinsufficiency. The two known examples of deficient enzyme activity leading to EDS are lysyl-hydroxylase deficiency and procollagen peptidase deficiency. In the first case, the inability to hydroxylate lysine residues precludes normal intermolecular cross-linking of collagen trimers, and in the second instance, the absence of procollagen peptidase prevents normal proteolytic cleavage of the NH2-terminus of procollagen chains. In both circumstances the morphology and strength of the collagen fibril is compromised, explaining the

TABLE 14–1   The Ehlers–Danlos Syndromes

VILLEFRANCE CLASSIFICATION (1997)	BERLIN CLASSIFICATION (1988)	CLINICAL FEATURES	INHERITANCE	BIOCHEMICAL DEFECTS
Classical type	I Gravis II Mitis	Soft, hyperextensible skin; easy bruising; thin, atrophic scars; hypermobile joints; varicose veins; prematurity of affected newborns	AD	Mutations in proα1(V) or proα2(V) chains of type V collagen (COL5A1, COL5A2) in some families
Hypermobility type	III	Soft skin; large and small joint hypermobility	AD	Not known
Vascular type	IV Arterial-ecchymotic	Thin, translucent skin with visible veins; easy bruising; absence of skin and joint extensibility; arterial, bowel, and uterine rupture	AD	Mutations in COL3A1: Abnormal type III collagen synthesis, secretion, or structure
Kyphoscoliosis type	VI	Soft skin; muscle hypotonia; scoliosis: joint laxity; hyperextensible skin	AR	Lysyl hydroxylase deficiency; mutations in PLOD gene
Arthrochalasia type	VIIA, VIIB Arthrochalasia multiplex	Congenital hip dislocation; severe joint hypermobility; soft skin with or without abnormal scarring	AD	Deletion of exons from type I collagen genes that encode the aminoterminal propeptide cleavage site of COL1A1 (type A) or COL1A2 (type B)
Dermatosporaxis type	VIIC	Severe skin fragility; sagging, redundant skin	AD	Recessive mutations in type I collagen N-peptidase
Other variants[a]				

AD = autosomal dominant; AR = autosomal recessive; XLR = X-linked recessive.
[a]Includes rare forms (types V, VIII, and X) from the 1988 Berlin Classification that have only been described in a few families.

severe and early clinical findings. Because half-normal enzyme activity is sufficient for normal collagen processing, both of these conditions are recessive.

CLINICAL FEATURES

EDS TYPE I

- EDS type I, also known as the gravis form, is characterized by joint laxity, hyperextensibility of skin, poor wound healing, and autosomal dominant inheritance. The skin is soft and velvety and can be stretched easily. The dermis is fragile and is easily bruised. Scars after trauma or surgical procedure are thinned and atrophic and may stretch considerably after healing, having a characteristic "cigarette paper" appearance. Molluscoid pseudotumors are present at the extensor surfaces of joints, in the feet, and on the shins. About half of affected individuals are delivered prematurely because of premature rupture of fetal membranes, presumably due to abnormalities in the structure of fetal tissues. A significant number of individuals with EDS type I have cardiac defects, most commonly mitral valve prolapse. A few patients have dilatation and occasionally rupture of the ascending aorta or proximal pulmonary artery. Musculoskeletal features include joint hyperextensibility in all patients and a fairly high frequency of scoliosis and pes planus (flat feet). The joint hypermobility can be associated with the onset of osteoarthritis in the third or fourth decade of life.

EDS TYPE II

- EDS type II is clinically similar to EDS type I, except that the skin is less fragile and scar formation more closely approximates normal. Ultrastructural findings show thickened collagen fibrils in skin, similar to findings in the dermis in patients with EDS type I. Since the molecular basis of this disorder is similar to EDS type I, it has been proposed that EDS types I and II be merged as a single entity.

EDS TYPE III

- EDS type III is characterized by hyperextensibility of large and small joints, soft velvety skin, and autosomal dominant inheritance. Individuals with EDS type III have normal scarring and do not have stretchy skin. Molluscoid pseudotumors are absent.

EDS TYPE IV

- EDS type IV is an autosomal dominant condition characterized by thin translucent skin with easy bruisability but normal scar formation. In fair-skinned individuals, subcutaneous vasculature is easily visible beneath the skin. Affected individuals are at high risk for life-threatening rupture of the large intestine, uterus, or medium-sized arteries.

EDS TYPE V

- EDS type V is a rare X-linked disorder characterized by mild skin hyperelasticity, mildly abnormal scarring, and joint hyperextensibility. Female carriers are asymptomatic. There is only a single large, well-documented family with EDS type V in the literature. This disorder clinically resembles EDS type II except that the latter disorder has autosomal dominant inheritance.

EDS TYPE VI

- The cardinal feature of lysil hydroxylase deficiency are neonatal onset of joint laxity, kyphoscoliosis, and hypotonia. These features are found in virtually all patients. Ocular fragility, which was observed in the original reports of lysyl hydroxylase deficiency, was found in only a minority of patients. Skin fragility, easy bruisability, and dermal hyperextensibility occur to some extent in most patients with EDS type I. Individuals with EDS type VI, like those with EDS IV, are at risk of having a potentially catastrophic arterial rupture.

EDS TYPE VII

- EDS type VII (arthrochalasia multiplex) is characterized by extreme joint laxity, multiple joint dislocations, and congenital hip dislocations that are difficult to repair surgically. Dermal features in these patients include tissue fragility and widened scars.

EDS TYPE VIII

- EDS type VIII is a rare autosomal dominant condition characterized by soft, hyperextensible skin, abnormal scarring, easy bruising, hyperextensible joints, and generalized periodontitis.

EDS TYPE X

- EDS type X is represented by a single family in which two siblings of unaffected parents had joint hyperextensibility, mitral valve proplapse, easy bruisability, and poor wound healing.

REFERENCES

Mao JR, Bristow J. The Ehlers–Danlos syndrome: On beyond collagens. *J Clin Invest.* 2001;107:1063.

Wenstrup RJ. Abnormal collagen fibril biology in the Ehlers–Danlos syndrome. *Prog Dermatol.* 2001;35:1.

PSEUDOXANTHOMA ELASTICUM

- Pseudoxanthoma elasticum (PXE) (Grönblad–Stramberg syndrome) is an inherited disorder of elastic tissue that most frequently affects the skin, retina, and arterial walls.

EPIDEMIOLOGY

- PXE has been estimated to have a prevalence of about 1 in 100,000 to 160,000 with no gender predominance.

PATHOPHYSIOLOGY

- PXE is linked to mutations of the gene encoding the transmembrane transporter protein ABCC6 on chromosome 16p13.1. The primary pathophysiologic process is the calcification of the elastic fibers resulting from altered metabolism of mesenchimal cells such as fibroblasts and smooth muscle cells. Other matrix constituents (collagen, proteoglycans) are also altered.

CLINICAL FEATURES

- The most common presentation involves yellowish papules confluent into plaques with a cobblestone appearance on the lateral aspect of the neck and on flexural areas of the skin (axillae, antecubital and popliteal fossae, inguinal region). These lesions resemble "plucked-chicken skin." Redundant folds of the skin may develop in more advanced cases. In the mouth the lesions may mimic Fordyce spots.
- The onset of symptoms usually occurs in the second decade of life. The retinal changes are referred to as angioid streaks, which are tears in Bruch's membrane beneath the retina and occur in roughly 85% of patients.
- Arterial elastic calcification occurs in peripheral, coronary, and gastrointestinal tract vessels and result in claudication, hypertension, angina, and gastrointestinal hemorrhages.
- PXE is a genetically heterogeneous disease with different forms and much controversy over inheritance patterns. The majority of cases appear to be autosomal recessive with early onset (average age 13 years), but a classification of PXE into at least five genetic groups has been proposed: two autosomal dominant types and three autosomal recessive types. Dominant

type I shows a flexurally distributed "peau d'orange" rash, severe atherosclerosis, and severe retinopathy with early blindness. Dominant type II is much less severe with a slight canary-yellow macular rash, minimal vascular involvement, and mild retinal changes. Recessive type I resembles the dominant type I, although vascular and retinal degeneration are milder. Recessive type II shows generalized cutaneous laxity without systemic complications. Recessive type III occurs in patients of Afrikaner descent and shows moderate skin and cardiovascular changes, but after the third decade a severe visual impairment may develop.
- There is a group of acquired and localized variants of PXE with skin lesions that are clinically and histologically similar to classic hereditary PXE but are not located in typical flexural sites and are not associated with retinal or cardiovascular disease. The term perforating calcific elastosis has been suggested for some of these cases. One form has been described in black, obese, multiparous, hypertensive women with periumbilical lesions; another form can be precipitated by repeated rubbing of calcium salts into damp skin.

HISTOPATHOLOGY

- Histologic sections stained with hematoxylin and eosin show fragmented, clumped, and basophilic elastic fibers in the middle and deep reticular dermis. A von Kossa stain demonstrate calcification of these elastic fibers. Calcification of the elastic laminae of visceral blood vessels accounts for the hemorrhagic complications and vascular occlusions seen in PXE.

DIAGNOSIS AND DIFFERENTIAL

- The diagnosis of PXE is based on the presence of clinically and histologically characteristic lesions in flexural areas. Other heritable forms of dermatochalasis such as cutis laxa and dermatofibrosis lenticularis disseminata (Buschke–Ollendorf) must be excluded. Several nonheritable conditions may also mimic PXE. PXE-like papillary dermal elastolysis is a clinically similar condition seen on the sides of the neck in the elderly and considered as a manifestation of intrinsic skin aging; histopathology, however, shows only loss of the elastic fibers in the papillary dermis. In solar elastosis, the degeneration of elastic fibers is histologically different without calcification and lies in the upper dermis.

TREATMENT

- There is currently no known therapy for PXE. Cosmetic plastic surgery may improve the appearance of the skin lesions. Restriction of dietary calcium remains controversial. Complications from vascular involvement must be prevented or dealt with by the appropriate specialist. Genetic counselling is important.

REFERENCES

Pukkinen L, Nakane A, Riugfeil F, Uitto J. Identification of ABCC6 pseudogenes on human chromosome 16p: Implications for mutation detection in pseudoxanthoma elasticum. *Hum Genet.* 2001;109:356.

Sherer DW, Sapadin AN, Lebwohl MG. Pseudoxanthoma elasticum: An update. *Dermatology.* 1999;199:3.

CUTIS LAXA

- Cutis laxa is a disorder of elastic tissue that may be inherited or acquired.

EPIDEMIOLOGY

- This is a rare disease and the inherited form seems to be more common than the acquired type.

PATHOPHYSIOLOGY

- In the congenital form, there is a defective elastic fiber formation involving both the elastin and the microfibrils of the elastic fibers that appears to be due to different mutations in exon 30 of the elastin gene. An alteration of fibulin-5, which is a protein essential to stabilize and organize elastic fibers in the tissues, has been recently proposed. In the acquired form, an immunologic basis has been suggested with an increased elastase activity and destruction of the elastic fibers. In X-linked cutis laxa, a defect in copper metabolism, probably due to mutations in the copper-transporting ATPase gene, has been found.

CLINICAL FEATURES

- The skin is flaccid and hangs loosely as though it were too large for the body, giving the appearance of premature aging. In addition to the sagging appearance, the skin does not spring back when pulled out.
- The facial appearance is often referred to as a bloodhound facies. Involvement of the eyelids includes blepharochalasis. These manifestations are common to all types of cutis laxa. What differentiates the various inherited or acquired types are the associated conditions.

INHERITED FORMS

- Inherited cutis laxa include a heterogeneous group of conditions both clinically and genetically. Two autosomal recessive, one autosomal dominant, and one X-linked recessive forms may be considered. In the commoner autosomal recessive form, cutis laxa is associated with emphysema. Generalized skin laxity is evident at birth, with a typical facies characterized by downward-slanting palpebral fissures, a hooked nose, sagging cheeks, and a long upper lip. In addition to a severe pulmonary emphysema, hernias, diverticula, and aortic ectasia are important complications. Death often occurs before age 2 years. In the rarer, less severe recessive type, cutis laxa is associated with a retarded psychomotor development, corneal clouding, and ligamentous laxity. The autosomal dominant form presents a clinical picture milder than the recessive variety. Lax skin may develop at any age, and sometimes is the only abnormality, with a normal life expectancy. In other cases there are systemic manifestations such as emphysema, pulmonary stenosis, diverticula, and herniae. X-linked cutis laxa, formerly known as Ehlers–Danlos syndrome type IX, is characterized by mild joint laxity, hernias, bladder diverticula, and cranial occipital exostoses.

ACQUIRED FORMS

- Acquired cutis laxa may be generalized or localized and may develop de novo or following inflammatory skin conditions such as angioedema, drug reactions (penicillin, isoniazid), erythema multiforme, Sweet's syndrome, and lupus erythematosus. It has also been described in association with sarcoidosis, syphilis, myeloma, lymphoma, Klippel–Trenaunay syndrome, complement deficiency, and nephrotic syndrome. Musculoskeletal, cardiovascular, pulmonary, and gastrointestinal manifestations have been reported. The localized variant may have an exclusive acral distribution. Postinflammatory elastolysis with cutis laxa is a rare form described in black children and probably represent an unusual reaction resulting in skin laxity secondary to an arthropod bite.

HISTOPATHOLOGY

- Sections stained with hematoxylin-eosin look normal but with elastic tissue stain, the elastic fibers are diminished or absent throughout the dermis. The remaining elastic fibers are short and fragmented. In the inflammatory stage of acquired cutis laxa an infiltrate with lymphocytes and neutrophils is seen.

DIAGNOSIS AND DIFFERENTIAL

- Differential diagnosis of cutis laxa include other conditions associated with wrinkled sagging skin such as anetoderma, a recessive form of psedoxanthoma elasticum, perifollicular elastolysis, mid-dermal elastolysis, and granulomatous slack skin (a form of cutaneous T-cell lymphoma).

TREATMENT

- There is no effective treatment for cutis laxa other than corrective surgery. Most of the medical management is directed toward the extracutaneous manifestations.

REFERENCES

Bouloc A, Godeau G, Zeller J, et al. Increased fibroblast activity in acquired cutis laxa. *Dermatology.* 1999;198:346.

Yawagisawa H, Davis EC, Starcher BC, et al. Fibulin-5 is an elastin-binding protein essential for elastic fibre development in vivo. *Nature.* 2002;415:168.

ATROPHODERMA OF PASINI–PIERINI

- Atrophoderma of Pasini–Pierini is an uncommon form of dermal atrophy, usually appearing as one or more well-demarcated, depressed areas.

PATHOPHYSIOLOGY

- The cause is unknown. It is considered an abortive, atrophic variant of morphea. A clear relationship with *Borrelia burgdorferi* has never been proven.

CLINICAL FEATURES

- Atrophoderma of Pasini–Pierini is characterized by asymptomatic, single or multiple, sharply but often irregularly demarcated, brown or gray depressed patches on the trunk, mainly the back. The patches enlarge very slowly for years before stabilizing. Both inflammatory and sclerotic changes are absent. A unilateral and segmental distribution has been described. All ages may be affected (youngsters in particular), and there is a slight female predominance.

HISTOPATHOLOGY

- The histologic changes are slight and adjacent normal skin is needed for comparison. There is a hyperpigmentation of the basal layer. In well-developed plaques, homogenization of the collagen with diminished interbundle spaces, slight fibrosis, and an inflammatory T-cell perivascular infiltrate is seen. Elastic fibers have been reported both as normal or clumped.

DIAGNOSIS AND DIFFERENTIAL

- Differentiation from morphea, possibly an academic exercise, is made on clinical and histologic grounds.

TREATMENT

- None is specific. Antibiotics (penicillin, tetracyclines) in the early stages and PUVA have helped some patients. The lesions can resolve spontaneously.

REFERENCE

Kencha D, Blaszczyk M, Jablonska S. Atrophoderma Pasini–Pierini is a primary atrophic abortive morphea. *Dermatology.* 1995;190:203.

STRIAE DISTENSAE

- Striae distensae (stretch marks) are very common in Caucasians and occur in most adult women, as they readily develop at puberty or during pregnancy.

PATHOPHYSIOLOGY

- The development of striae is related to a continuous and progressive stretching of the skin that induces changes in the components of the extracellular dermal matrix, including fibrillin, elastin, and collagen. Excessive adrecortical activity, genetic factors, inherited defects of the connective tissues (Marfan syndrome), pregnancy, and sudden weight gain are important factors.

CLINICAL FEATURES

- Striae are linear scars, several centimetres long and 1 to 10 mm wide that follow cleavage lines transverse to the direction of greatest tension. Initially, they appear as raised, pink/purple linear lesions without depression, but with time they become paler, depressed, and finely wrinkled. The commonest sites are the outer aspect of the thighs, the buttocks, and the breasts in women.
- Striae may develop on the shoulders in young male weight lifters. In Cushing's syndrome or after systemic steroid therapy, striae may be larger and more widely distributed, while after topical steroids they occur particularly on the flexures. In pregnancy the striae are more conspicuous on the abdomen.

HISTOPATHOLOGY

- The histology is that of a scar. Under a flattened epidermis, the collagen bundles are thin and arranged parallel to the skin surface. Elastic tissue has been reported both as increased and reduced. Early lesions are rarely biopsied and show some inflammatory changes around dilated capillaries.

DIAGNOSIS AND DIFFERENTIAL

- The diagnosis is simple. In linear focal elastosis the lesions are yellow and palpable; this entity, however, is considered a keloidal repair of a stria.

TREATMENT

- There is no effective treatment. Adolescents may be reassured that in time the striae will become less evident. Some beneficial effects with topical tretinoin have been reported.

REFERENCE

Watson RE, Parry EJ, Humphries D, et al. Fibrillin microfibrils are reduced in skin exhibiting striae distensae. *Br J Dermatol.* 1998;138:931.

MID-DERMAL ELASTOLYSIS

- Mid-dermal elastolysis is an acquired form of elastic fiber loss in the mid-dermis.

PATHOPHYSIOLOGY

- The etiology is unclear, although damage of elastic fibers and unmasking of antigenic epitopes may result in a T-cell mediated immune response with cytokine and elastase production, leading to destruction of elastic tissue. A controversy exists about the role of sun exposure.

CLINICAL FEATURES

- In mid-dermal elastolysis, the most common changes are asymptomatic, well-demarcated, oval to round patches of fine wrinkles on the trunk or extremities. Erythema and urticaria may precede or accompany the wrinkles. A minority of cases also show perifollicular papules due to looseness of the skin around hair follicles. The condition is more often seen in young and middle-aged women.

HISTOPATHOLOGY

- There is a selective loss of elastic fibers in the mid-dermis. A T cell-lymphocytic perivascular infiltrate with phagocytosis of elastic fibers by histiocytes and giant cells is often present.

TREATMENT

- None is specific. Topical tretinoin may improve the lesions.

REFERENCES

Boyd AS, King LE. Middermal elastolysis in two patients with lupus erythematosus. *Am J Dermatopathol.* 2001;23:136.

Rebora A, Parodi A, Rongioletti F. Mid dermal elastolysis and pseudoxanthoma elasticum-like papillary dermal elastolysis. *Br J Dermatol.* 1995;132:487.

THE CUTANEOUS MUCINOSES

- The cutaneous mucinoses are a heterogeneous group of disorders in which an abnormal amount of mucin accumulates in the skin either diffusely or focally. Mucin is a normal component of the dermal connective tissue produced in small amounts by fibroblasts. It is a jelly-like, amorphous mixture of proteoglycans (formerly called acid mucopolysaccharides) whose most important component is hyaluronic acid. Mucin plays a major role in maintaining the salt and water balance of the dermis. A light blue staining between the separated collagen bundles or empty spaces is a good clue for mucin deposition.
- Inasmuch as the causes of these condition are unknown, the cutaneous mucinoses can be divided into two groups: (1) primary (distinctive) cutaneous mucinoses, in which mucin deposition is the main histologic feature resulting in clinically distinctive lesions; and (2) disorders associated with histologic deposition of mucin (secondary mucinoses), in which mucin is only an incidental finding.
- The primary cutaneous mucinoses are further subdivided into dermal and follicular mucinoses, according to the site of mucin deposition.

PAPULAR MUCINOSIS AND SCLEROMYXEDEMA

- Papular mucinosis (lichen myxedematosus, scleromyxedema) is a chronic, idiopathic disorder characterized by lichenoid papules, nodules, and/or plaques due to mucin dermal deposition and a variable degree of fibrosis in the absence of thyroid disease. Papular mucinosis includes two clinicopathologic subsets: a generalized papular and sclerodermoid form (also called scleromyxedema) with monoclonal gammopathy and systemic, even lethal, manifestations; and a localized papular form that does not run a disabling course. Some cases of papular mucinosis share intermediate or atypical features between scleromyxedema and the localized forms.

EPIDEMIOLOGY

- The generalized and sclerodermoid form, termed scleromyxedema, is an uncommon disease. It affects middle-aged adults without sex predilection. The localized form is also rare, but its prevalence is underestimated.

PATHOPHYSIOLOGY

- The pathogenesis of papular mucinosis is unknown. The significance of the monoclonal gammopathy in scleromyxedema remains in doubt. Paraprotein levels do not correlate with either the extent or the progression of the disease.

CLINICAL FEATURES

- In scleromyxedema, a widespread symmetric eruption of 2 to 3 mm, firm, waxy, closely spaced papules is most commonly located on the hands, forearms, face, upper trunk, and thighs. Papules are commonly arranged in a linear fashion; the skin nearby is shiny and its appearance resembles scleroderma. The glabella is typically involved with deep longitudinal furrowing.
- Erythema, edema, and a brownish discoloration may be also present in the involved areas. Itching is not uncommon. The mucous membranes and the scalp are spared. As the condition progresses, erythematous and infiltrated plaques may develop with skin stiffening, sclerodactyly, and decreased motility of the mouth and joints. Scleromyxedema is almost always associated with a paraproteinemia. The monoclonal gammopathy is usually IgG-lambda. Even though a mild plasmocytosis may be found in the bone marrow, scleromyxedema progresses to multiple myeloma in less than 10% of cases.
- Scleromyxedema has a number of internal manifestations including muscular, neurologic, rheumatologic, pulmonary, renal, and cardiovascular disorders. Dysphagia, proximal muscle weakness due to myositis, disturbances of the central nervous system leading to unexplained coma, peripheral neuropathy, arthropathies, carpal tunnel syndrome, restrictive or obstructive pneumopathy, and scleroderma-like renal disease may accompany or follow the cutaneous manifestations.
- In the localized papular mucinosis the patients exhibit small, firm, waxy papules (or nodules and plaques produced by the confluence of papules) confined only to a few sites (usually upper and lower limbs and trunk) without sclerotic features, paraproteinemia, systemic involvement, or thyroid disease. This entity may be observed in HIV-infected individuals.

HISTOPATHOLOGY

- Scleromyxedema is characterized by a triad of microscopic features including a diffuse deposit of mucin in the upper and midreticular dermis, an increase in collagen deposition, and a marked proliferation of irregularly arranged fibroblasts. The follicles may be atrophic, and a slight perivascular, superficial, lymphoplasmocytic infiltrate is often present. The elastic fibers are fragmented and decreased in numbers. Mucin may fill the walls of myocardial vessels and the interstitium of the kidney, pancreas, adrenals, and nerves.
- The changes in the localized form are not as characteristic. Mucin accumulates in the upper and midreticular dermis; fibroblast proliferation is variable.

DIAGNOSIS AND DIFFERENTIAL

- Histopathology helps distinguish the localized mucinosis from several papular eruptions that have a similar appearance, such as granuloma annulare, lichen amyloidosis, lichen planus and other lichenoid eruptions. Scleromyxedema should be distinguished from systemic scleroderma and scleredema by the presence of papules and the presence of a monoclonal gammopathy.

TREATMENT

- The treatment of scleromyxedema is disappointing. Melphalan, originally used to treat the associated plasma cell dyscrasia, produced some clinical improvement. It has, however, been implicated in 30% of the reported deaths due to hematologic malignancies and septic complications. Other chemotherapeutic agents have been tried, such as cyclophosphamide and methotrexate, with no better results. Systemic steroids may be effective but the results are often temporary.
- Electron-beam and spot radiotherapy, extracorporeal photochemotherapy, PUVA, retinoids, cyclosporin, and plasmapheresis, have all produced some improvement without treating the underlying disease. Intravenous gammaglobulin and autologous stem cell transplantation seem to be promising therapies. On the other hand, spontaneous improvement with resolution, even after 15 years, has been described.
- Localized papular mucinosis does not require therapy, and a wait-and-see approach is recommended. Topical corticosteroids may be of some benefit.

RETICULAR ERYTHEMATOUS MUCINOSIS

- Reticular erythematous mucinosis (REM) (synonyms: plaque-like cutaneous mucinosis, REM syndrome, midline mucinosis) is a persistent, photoaggravated, erythematous reticular or plaque-like eruption in the midline of the back or chest.

EPIDEMIOLOGY

- REM is a worldwide, rare disorder occurring most often in middle-aged women, although men and children are not spared. Sunlight may be a causal or promoting factor.

CLINICAL FEATURES

- Reddish macules and papules merge into reticulate annular or plaque-like, slightly pruritic lesions in the midback or chest, at times spreading to the abdomen. Sun exposure worsens the eruption, but it has also been reported as beneficial. Phototesting may reproduce REM lesions. REM is not associated with systemic diseases and altered laboratory tests. Oral contraceptives, menses, and pregnancy may trigger or exacerbate REM.

HISTOPATHOLOGY

- The epidermis is normal. Interstitial deposits of small amounts of mucin are seen in the upper dermis, along with a perivascular and, at times, perifollicular lymphocytic infiltrate. Vascular dilation is present. Direct immunofluorescence is negative, but granular deposits of IgM, IgA, and C3 have been seen at the dermoepidermal junction.

DIAGNOSIS AND DIFFERENTIAL

- Lupus erythematosus shows involvement of the epidermis histologically and deposits of IgG and C3 at the dermo-epidermal junction. An unusual form of lupus erythematosus known as lupus erythematosus tumidus can be impossible to distinguish microscopically from REM, but clinically presents as scattered smooth-topped papules. Jessner's lymphocytic infiltration usually lacks mucin deposits. Seborrheic dermatitis is a scaling disorder that involves the scalp and face; mucin is absent.

TREATMENT

- Antimalarials are usually effective in clearing the lesions in 2 to 4 weeks. Sunscreens should be used. REM may clear spontaneously even after 15 years.

SCLEREDEMA

- Scleredema is a symmetrical diffuse induration of the upper part of the body due to the thickened dermis and deposition of mucin.

EPIDEMIOLOGY

- The disease is rare, affects all races, and is seen more often in females. Diabetes is considered a pathogenetic factor. Streptococcal hypersensitivity, injury to lymphatics, and paraproteinemia may also play a role.

CLINICAL FEATURES

- There are three types of scleredema. The first type affects mostly middle-aged females, but also children. It is preceded by fever, malaise, and by an infection, usually streptococcal, of the upper and lower respiratory tract. The skin of the cervicofacial region suddenly hardens, spreading to the trunk and proximal upper limbs. The face is expressionless, and opening the mouth and swallowing are difficult because of involvement of the tongue and pharynx. This type usually resolves in a few months.
- The second type shares the same clinical features, but has a subtler onset without preceding illness and persists for years. This type is more frequently associated with a monoclonal gammopathy.
- The third type occurs mainly in obese middle-aged males with insulin-dependent diabetes (scleredema diabeticorum). The onset is subtle and the disorder persistent. Erythema and induration of the back are common.
- Serositis, dysarthria, dysphagia, myositis, ocular and cardiac abnormalities, and parotiditis may occur in all forms. There may be also associated rheumatoid arthritis, Sjögren's syndrome, myeloma, and HIV infection. Scleredema causes little morbidity besides the limitation of movement. Type 1 may clear in 6 months to 2 years, whereas the other types last longer.

HISTOPATHOLOGY

- The principal alteration in scleredema is thickening of the reticular dermis, with large collagen bundles separated from each other by clear spaces filled with mucin and causing fenestration of the dermis. There is a sparse perivascular lymphocytic infiltrate. Mucin also accumulates in skeletal muscle and in the heart.

DIAGNOSIS AND DIFFERENTIAL

- The early edematous stages of systemic scleroderma may be confused with scleredema. Raynaud's phenomenon and acrosclerosis characterize scleroderma. Scleromyxedema differs in that it presents with papules rather than diffuse dermal induration.

TREATMENT

- Therapy is unnecessary for type 1 scleredema because it is often self-limiting. Regression in scleredema associated with diabetes or monoclonal gammopathy is more uncommon, and no specific treatment is available. The control of glycemia does not have any influence on the skin. Pulse therapy with cyclophosphamide and steroids by mouth, PUVA, electron-beam therapy, and cyclosporine have all been anecdotally reported of benefit.

PRETIBIAL MYXEDEMA

- Localized or pretibial myxedema is a cutaneous induration of the shins due to mucin deposition, associated with hyperthyroidism (most commonly due to Graves' disease) or occurring after thyroidectomy.

EPIDEMIOLOGY

- Graves' disease is seven times more common in women and occurs usually in the third and fourth decades of life. Localized myxedema is one of the signs of Graves' disease along with goiter, exophthalmus, thyroid acropathy, and high blood levels of thyroid stimulating hormone receptor antibody. It is found in 1 to 5% of patients with Graves' disease, but in up to one fourth of patients with exophthalmus. Rarely, localized myxedema occurs in Hashimoto's thyroiditis without thyrotoxicosis, in hypothyroidism following treatment of Graves' disease, and even in euthyroid patients.

- A serum factor could incite fibroblasts to produce mucin. Fibroblasts in the lower extremities have been found to be more sensitive to this factor than fibroblasts of other areas of the body. An insulin-like growth factor, local trauma, and lymphatic obstruction due to mucin deposition may also play a role.

CLINICAL FEATURES

- Localized myxedema develops as erythematous to skin-colored, sometimes purple-brown or yellowish, waxy, indurated, peau d'orange, nodules or plaques. Usually, they are located on the anterolateral aspect of the legs or feet.
- Localized myxedema may also present as a diffuse nonpitting edema on the shins or feet evolving into elephantiasis. More rarely, localized myxedema may affect the face, shoulders, upper limbs, lower abdomen, or scars. Large plaques are often painful and pruritic. Hypertrichosis and hyperhidrosis may be present in pretibial myxedematous skin.

HISTOPATHOLOGY

- Large quantities of mucin are deposited in the reticular dermis, causing collagen bundles to separate and the dermis to thicken. A bordering zone of normal collagen is also observed. There is a perivascular and periadnexal lymphocytic infiltrate with mast cells and large stellate fibroblasts. Elastic fibers are reduced. The epidermis is often papillated, hyperplastic, and hyperkeratotic.

DIAGNOSIS AND DIFFERENTIAL

- Lichen simplex chronicus, lymphedema, elephantiasis, and hypertrophic lichen planus lack mucin deposition and are usually not seen in the setting of thyroid disease.

TREATMENT

- Steroids administered under occlusive dressings or delivered by intralesional injection may help. Skin grafting is followed by relapses. Plasmapheresis and gradient pneumatic compression have been of benefit. Therapy of hyperthyroidism does not improve the cutaneous lesions and often localized myxedema develops

after its onset. Localized myxedema may also clear spontaneously (average of 3.5 years).

MUCOUS (MYXOID) CYSTS

DIGITAL MUCOUS CYST

- Mucous digital cyst occurs at any age, mostly in women, as a cystic nodule, seldom wider than 2 cm, on the distal interphalangeal joint of a finger. Clear viscous material comes out when punctured, but older lesions may be solid. The adjacent nail may show a longitudinal furrow.
- There are two main sources of mucin, namely the synovial cells and the dermal fibroblasts. Cysts derived from the synovial cells are located over the joints, while those derived from fibroblasts are located between the interphalangeal joints.

HISTOPATHOLOGY

- Mucous cyst is not a true cyst. It shows a large deposit of mucin, some clefts, and vascular spaces.

TREATMENT

- Excision, incision and drainage, CO_2 laser vaporization, aspiration of the content, intralesional steroids, or sclerosant agents are commonly used, but relapses are frequent.

MUCOUS CYST OF THE ORAL MUCOSA (MUCOCELE)

- Mucoceles are single, dome-shaped, translucent, blue-whitish cysts that contain a viscous fluid. They are usually located on the inner surface of the lower lip or on the floor of the mouth. Most are smaller than 1 cm in diameter and wax and wane over several months. Mucoceles result either from the rupture of a salivary gland duct or from retention of mucus due to obstruction of a duct.

HISTOPATHOLOGY

- Mucin-filled spaces are intermixed with inflamed granulation tissue; in older lesions, large cystic spaces develop. Mucoceles contain sialomucin produced by epithelial cells.

TREATMENT

- The lesion can be excised or treated with cryotherapy. It may resolve spontaneously.

PINKUS FOLLICULAR MUCINOSIS (ALOPECIA MUCINOSA)

EPIDEMIOLOGY

- This uncommon inflammatory disorder has a predilection for children and young adults. Although follicular keratinocytes have been considered as the source of the mucin, an etiologic role for cell-mediated immune mechanisms has been proposed. Very recently, it has been considered a form of localized mycosis fungoides.

CLINICAL FEATURES

- Pinkus follicular mucinosis is an idiopathic benign form, not linked with lymphoma. It presents as an acute or subacute eruption occurring in children and young adults characterized by one or several tumid plaques of grouped follicular papules limited to the face and scalp with alopecia. Nodules, annular lesions, folliculitis, and acneiform eruptions have also been described.

PATHOPHYSIOLOGY

- Mucin accumulates within the follicular epithelium and sebaceous glands causing keratinocytes to disconnect. In more advanced lesions, the follicles are converted into cystic spaces containing mucin, inflammatory cells, and altered keratinocytes. A perifollicular infiltrate of lymphocytes, histiocytes, and eosinophils is seen.

DIAGNOSIS AND DIFFERENTIAL

- The main differential diagnosis is with follicular mucinosis associated with lymphoma, mainly mycosis fungoides. Pinkus follicular mucinosis usually occurs in children and young adults as a solitary plaque on the scalp and face and is self-limited. Although no single histologic criterion has been shown to predict the development of a lymphoma, the presence of a band-like, atypical lymphocytic infiltrate in the upper dermis with significant epidermotropism is more commonly seen in mycosis fungoides. However, the recent finding of a monoclonal rearrangement of the T-cell receptor both in Pinkus follicular mucinosis and in lymphoma-associated follicular mucinosis suggests that the former may represent a form of localized cutaneous T-cell lymphoma.

TREATMENT

- There is no specific treatment and a wait-and-see approach is recommended since many cases of follicular mucinosis resolve spontaneously in 2 to 24 months. Topical, intralesional, and systemic steroids; PUVA; x-rays; dapsone; antimalarials; indomethacine; mynocycline; oral isotretinoin; interferon-α_{2b}, and UVA1 phototherapy have been reported as beneficial. The disease, however, heals spontaneously in most cases.

REFERENCES

Cerroni L, Finch-Puches R, Bach B, Kerl H. Follicular mucinosis. *Arch Dermatol.* 2002;138:182.

Feasel AM, Donato ML, Duvic M. Complete remission of scleromyxedema following autologous stem cell transplantation. *Arch Dermatol.* 2001;137:1071.

Rongioletti F, Rebora A. Cutaneous mucinoses. Microscopic criteria for diagnosis. *Am J Dermatopathol.* 2001; 23:257.

Rongioletti F, Rebora A. Updated classification of papular mucinosis, lichen myxedematosus and scleromyxedema. *J Am Acad Dermatol.* 2001;44:273.

Rongioletti F, Rebora A. The new cutaneous mucinoses. A review with an up-to-date classification of cutaneous mucinoses. *J Am Acad Dermatol.* 1991;24:265.

AMYLOIDOSIS

EPIDEMIOLOGY

- Amyloidosis is not a single disease but a term for diseases that share a common feature: the extracellular deposition of pathologic insoluble fibrillar proteins in organs and tissues. In the mid-19th century, Virchow adopted the botanical term "amyloid," meaning starch or cellulose, to describe abnormal extracellular material seen in the liver at autopsy. The epidemiology of amyloidosis is difficult to define precisely, since the disease is often undiagnosed or misdiagnosed and selection bias potentially makes data from tertiary referral centers unrepresentative. The age-adjusted incidence of amyloidosis is estimated to be 5.1 to 12.8 per million person-years, which means that there are approximately 1275 to 3200 new cases annually in the United States.

PATHOGENESIS

- The process by which precursor proteins produce fibrils appears to be multifactorial and to differ among the various types of amyloid. In amyloidosis, the demonstration that substitutions of particular amino acids at specific positions in the light-chain variable region occur at significantly higher frequencies than in nonamyloid immunoglobulins has led to the suggestion that these replacements destabilize light chains, increasing the likelihood of fibrillogenesis. Amyloid fibrils consist of various proteins such as monoclonal kappa or lambda light chains in primary amyloidosis (AL), protein A in secondary amyloidosis (AA), transthyretin (prealbumin) in familial or senile systemic amyloidosis, beta2-microglobulin (beta2M) in dialysis-associated amyloidosis, and keratin in localized cutaneous amyloidosis. All Types of amyloid stain positively with Congo red, thioflavin T, or the metachromatic stains and contain amyloid P component.

PRIMARY LOCALIZED CUTANEOUS AMYLOIDOSIS (PLCA)

- PLCA comprises macular, lichen, and the rare nodular forms. Fibrils in macular and lichen amyloidosis do not bind antibodies to protein AA or prealbumin. The concept has arisen of focal epidermal damage and filamentous degeneration of keratinocytes, followed by apoptosis and conversion of filamentous masses (colloid bodies) into amyloid material in the papillary dermis, perhaps with a contribution from the dermal-epidermal junction. In support of this theory is the fact that dermal amyloid deposits in these forms of PLCA cross-react immunohistochemically with keratin.

LOCALIZED CUTANEOUS AMYLOIDOSIS

- Nodular (tumefactive) cutaneous amyloidosis may be seen with lesions similar to those described for primary cutaneous amyloidosis or with firm, subcutaneous nodules up to several centimeters in diameter. They are brown-pink, waxy nodules often with overlying telangiectasias. They occur on the face, extremities, trunk, or genitalia and can appear atrophic anetodermic, or bullous, possibly from dermal destruction of elastic and collagen fibers.The nodular variant is the rarest of the cutaneous amyloidosis. Lichen amyloidosis commonly is seen as red-brown pruritic, reticulated hyperkeratotic papules on the shins with a subsequent spread to the dorsa of the feet and thighs. It occurs more commonly in persons of Chinese ancestry. Macular amyloidosis is seen as gray-brown pruritic patches anywhere on the trunk or extremities, but especially on the upper back. Small papules percent of cases of primary and myeloma-associated disease.

SECONDARY LOCALIZED CUTANEOUS AMYLOIDOSIS

- Deposition of insignificant microscopic amounts of amyloid in relation to a variety of cutaneous lesions is the most common type of localized cutaneous amyloidosis. Reported predisposing condition include intradermal nevi, sweat gland tumors, pilomatrixoma, dermatofibroma, seborrheic keratosis, solar elastosis, and PUVA treatment.

PRIMARY SYSTEMIC CUTANEOUS AMYLOIDOSIS

- In amyloidosis, a plasma-cell dyscrasia related to multiple myeloma, clonal plasma cells in the bone marrow produce immunoglobulins that are amyloidogenic. In affected patients, 5 to 10% of bone marrow plasma cells have clonal dominance of a light-chain isotype, and in addition produce urinary free monoclonal light chain (commonly termed Bence Jones proteins) of the dominant kappa or lambda isotype.

SECONDARY SYSTEMIC CUTANEOUS AMYLOIDOSIS

- The secondary amyloidoses are due to amyloid formed from serum amyloid A (SAA), an acute-phase protein produced in response to inflammation. There are several SAA proteins, and in humans, AA amyloid deposits consist of fragments of at least five different molecular forms. With the virtual abolition of chronic infectious diseases such as tuberculosis, osteomyelitis, and bronchiectasis in the Western Hemisphere, AA amyloidosis is rarely seen. However, it still occurs in patients with rheumatoid arthritis, inflammatory bowel disease, and untreated familial Mediterranean fever.

CLINICAL FEATURES

SYSTEMIC CUTANEOUS AMYLOIDOSIS

- Primary and myeloma-associated amyloidosis most commonly occur in elderly men. Patients may have nonspecific constitutional symptoms, macroglossia, carpal tunnel syndrome, or edema. Less common presentations include sicca syndrome, the "shoulder pad sign" (amyloid deposits in soft tissues around the shoulders), and a rheumatoid arthritis-like deposition in small joints. Gastrointestinal bleeding, peripheral neuropathies, and cardiac involvement also occur. Congestive heart failure or arrhythmias account for death in about 40% of patients with systemic amyloid. Skin or mucous membrane lesions are seen in 40% or fewer of cases. The most common lesion is purpura, seen in 15 to 17% of patients. It occurs after minor trauma (pinch purpura), particularly in areas such as eyelids, axilla, umbilicus, and anogenital regions. Facial purpura can occur after a Valsava maneuver or proctoscopy. Purpura results from amyloid deposition in vessel walls; the deposits can leave cutaneous vessels thickened and cordlike. Facial plaques may coalesce, resulting in a leonine appearance; a sclerodermatous infiltration may occur. Bullous lesions, alopecia, and cutis laxa have also been reported in association with systemic amyloidosis.

DIAGNOSIS AND DIFFERENTIAL

- The diagnosis of cutaneous amyloidosis evidently depends on the histochemical, immunohistochemical, or ultrastructural demonstration of amyloid material in a skin biopsy specimen. Biopsy of even clinically normal forearm skin has been reported positive in up to 50 tissue; jejunal biopsy is positive in about two thirds of patients, but gingival biopsy in only 19%. Gastric biopsy may produce a higher yield than rectal biopsy in AL-type amyloidosis. 96% of hepatic and 90% of renal and of splenic percutaneous needle biopsies are positive. Bone marrow aspiration may be positive in up to 45% of cases. Electrocardiography, echocardiography, angiocardiography, technetium scanning, and endomyocardial biopsy are useful in the diagnosis of amyloid heart disease. Computed tomography, ultrasound examination, and Doppler analysis of blood flow may be useful in renal amyloidosis. Sural nerve biopsy in patients with peripheral neuropathy, synovial fluid analysis in patients with arthropathy, and examination of tissue removed at carpal tunnel decompression, may be helpful. Scanning with I-labeled serum amyloid P component enables specific localization and imaging of amyloid deposits in vivo.

TREATMENT

SYSTEMIC CUTANEOUS AMYLOIDOSIS

- Most reports on the treatment of primary and myeloma-associated amyloidosis have been anecdotal, and responses to treatment are difficult to assess because of poor correlation between amyloid load and organ function. A comprehensive review of recent chemotherapy trials has recently been published. Cytotoxic chemotherapy is the mainstay of treatment, and is aimed at controlling the aberrant plasma cell population and the amount of amyloid precursor light chains. Melphalan, prednisone, colchicine, penicillamine, azathioprine, vincristine, and cyclophosphamide have been used to control systemic disease. Melphalan, combined with prednisone and possibly colchicine, appears to offer possible benefit in the treatment of amyloidosis. However, significant bone marrow toxicity limits the value of this treatment. Disease regression and prolonged survival were seen in a small number of patients treated with alkylating-agent-based chemotherapy. Supportive therapy, cardiac and renal transplantation, and dialysis have also been described. Colchicine was found to improve life expectancy in one study of 53 patients with AL-type amyloidosis. Experimental disaggregation of primary AL amyloid lambda chain fibrils was performed in vitro in recent report that used $alpha_1$-antitrypsin and may have future therapeutic implications. Future treatment approaches may include more aggressive chemotherapy, myeloablation, and autologous bone marrow transplantation. Recent investigations into the treatment of systemic amyloidosis include immunotoxins directed against the precursor of the amyloidogenic plasma cells. Colchicine is the treatment of choice in familial Mediterranean fever.

LOCALIZED CUTANEOUS AMYLOIDOSIS

- Lichen amyloidosis has been reported to respond to dermabrasion, topical DMSO, and Retinoids, although these were anecdotal reports. One etretinate failure has also been reported. Anecdotal reports of improvement in pruritus and flattening of papules with topical DMSO for lichen amyloidosis have been published, but failure has also been reported. Topical steroids and antipruritics have not provided relief to most patients. Macular amyloidosis was treated with UVB with some symptomatic relief. Well-controlled studies are limited in number, and satisfactory overall treatment is lacking at present for all forms of cutaneous amyloidosis. Nodular lesions of primary localized cutaneous amyloidosis have been treated with excision and the carbon dioxide laser, although recurrences can be expected with both. Electrodessication and curettage provided an acceptable cosmetic result in one case report. The final pathway in the development of amyloidosis is the production of amyloid fibrils in the extracellular matrix.

REFERENCES

Falk R, et al. The systemic amyloidoses. *New Engl J Med.* 1997;337:898.

Touart D, et al. Cutaneous deposition diseases. *J Am Acad Dermatol.* 1998;39:149.

MASTOCYTOSIS

EPIDEMIOLOGY

- Mastocytosis encompasses a range of disorders characterized by overproliferation and accumulation of tissue mast cells. The clinical signs vary depend on local accumulation of mast cells in different organs and the effects of their mediators. Mast-cell disease is most commonly seen in the skin, but the skeleton, bone marrow, gastrointestinal tract, and central nervous system may also be involved. The prevalence is unknown. The occurrence of cutaneous mastocytosis is estimated as one case in every 1000 to 8000 dermatology outpatient visits. Familial occurrences are unusual and the disorder occurs equally in both sexes and all races.
- Determining the prevalence of mastocytosis in the general population is problematic because patients without cutaneous lesions may not be diagnosed correctly. Even the incidence and prevalence of cutaneous mastocytosis are unknown because most cases are self-limited and probably unreported. Most patients are children; more than half have lesions by the age of 6 months. There is a second peak of incidence in the late third and early fourth decades of life.

PATHOGENESIS

- Mast cells are widely distributed and present in nearly every organ, mainly close to blood and lymphatic vessels, peripheral nerves, and epithelial surfaces. This location allows the mast cell to fulfill various regulatory, protective, and inflammatory functions. Mast cells develop from pluripotent bone-marrow progenitor cells that express CD34 antigen, and are dispersed as precursors, which undergo proliferation and maturation in specific tissues. Normal mast cell development requires an interaction between mast-cell growth factor, a cytokine, and c-kit receptors, which are expressed by mast cells at their different developmental stages. Mast-cell growth factor binds the protein product of the c-kit proto-oncogene. In addition to stimulating mast-cell proliferation, mast-cell growth factor stimulates proliferation of melanocytes and melanin synthesis. Mast cells may be activated by IgE-mediated and IgE-independent mechanisms, resulting in the release of many different preformed chemical mediators that are stored in secretory granules, and also synthesis of membrane-derived lipid metabolites and inflammatory cytokines. Episodic release of mast-cell mediators by cells that have undergone abnormal proliferation leads to a wide range of symptoms. Why mast cells proliferate and accumulate in mastocytosis is unknown. Proliferation may represent reactive hyperplasia or a neoplastic process, but this is not clear. Dysregulation or abnormalities of the c-kit receptor or excessive production of its ligand could, theoretically, produce disordered mast-cell proliferation. Increased production of the soluble form of mast-cell growth factor has been seen in cutaneous mastocytosis lesions. Raised concentrations of mast-cell growth-factor may lead to mast-cell accumulation and the hyperpigmentation typical of cutaneous mastocytosis. Since this factor also affects melanocytes, a mutation in c-kit that causes constitutive activation and expression of c-kit by mast cells in the skin and spleen was identified in two mastocytosis patients. Mast cells from both sources contained the same mutation, which indicates clonal proliferation and a possible role in the pathogenesis of mastocytosis. Mutations have not been detected in pediatric mastocytosis.

CLINICAL FEATURES

- The skin is the most commonly involved organ. Lesions, such as urticaria pigmentosa, result from local mast-cell infiltration. Any form of mastocytosis may have cutaneous lesions. Patients with systemic mastocytosis may present with intractable pruritus, dermographism, or flushing, but without any evidence of specific skin lesions. Although an absence of skin involvement seems to be associated with a more aggressive disease course, this feature is not a reliable marker of outcome. When present, cutaneous lesions evolve independently of the course of systemic disease. The true frequency of systemic mastocytosis without cutaneous involvement is unknown. The cutaneous forms tend to appear in childhood, are associated with a good prognosis, and resolve spontaneously in many cases.

• While most mytocytosis are indolent in nature, an aggressive form with eosinophilia is recognized. Mastocytosis can also be associated with lymphoreticular malignancies and a mast cell leukemia has been reported.

CUTANEOUS MASTOCYTOSIS

• Urticaria pigmentosa is the most common skin manifestation in children and adults. Urticaria, dermographism, and a variable degree of itching may also be present. The lesions are reddish-brown macules, papules, and plaques, which may be scattered over the whole body, with the highest density on the trunk. Telangiectases, petechiae, or ecchymoses may occur in the lesions. Urtication of lesions from mild trauma, such as rubbing or scratching, is known as Darier's sign and reflects mast-cell degranulation and release of inflammatory mediators. Association of urticaria pigmentosa with systemic mastocytosis has been found in 14 to 100% of cases in various studies.

• Diffuse cutaneous mastocytosis is a rare form that generally occurs in children younger than 3 years. Most of the skin in infiltrated by mast cells and becomes thickened, with exaggeration of normal skin markings; or the skin may become uniformly covered with minute papules of a yellow or cream color that give the appearance of grained leather. Nodules, tumors, or papules may also be present. Itching is often generalized and intense and dermographism is common. Round, tense, extensive bullae during the neonatal period can suggest an initial diagnosis of diffuse cutaneous mastocytosis. Although this disorder typically resolves spontaneously, serious complications, such as flushing, hypotension, gastrointestinal bleeding, severe diarrhea, or shock, may occur because of the enormous mast-cell load. These patients are also at a higher risk of systemic involvement or persistence of the disease beyond adolescence.

• Solitary mastocytomas represent localized disease; they are rare, and usually occur in infants younger than 6 months. Lesions appear as solitary or multiple macules, plaques, or nodules that measure up to 3 to 4 cm in diameter, and may show hyperpigmentation and urticate with stroking. In most cases, the lesions spontaneously resolve or are cured by excision. Both the localized and diffuse forms of cutaneous mastocytosis can develop transient vesicles or bullae.

• The rarest form of cutaneous mastocytosis is telangiectasia macularis eruptiva perstans, which consists of widespread, telangiectatic, ill-defined macules on a tan to brown background. This disorder occurs primarily in adults and is limited to the skin.

DIAGNOSIS AND DIFFERENTIAL

• In many cases a diagnosis of cutaneous mastocytosis can be made by a thorough history and skin examination, with identification of characteristic macular, telangiectatic, papular, or nodular lesions and demonstration of Darier's sign. A skin biopsy to identify dermal mast cell infiltrates is the most common confirmatory test. In most cases, a diagnosis can be made with certainty by an experienced histopathologist, with the exception of lesions of TMEP, in which the histologic changes may be subtle and the number of mast cells may appear to be within the upper limits of normal. At the time of skin biopsy, the infiltration of local anesthetic adjacent to the lesion rather than directly into it, and the use of anesthetic without epinephrine, may avoid making histologic identification of mast cells more difficult. Because of degranulation, special handling of tissue and examination of Giemsa-stained sections (1 mm thick) of Epon embedded material may be necessary to establish the diagnosis in difficult cases. In patients with symptoms affecting the skeletal system, a radiologic survey has been recommended; this may also apply to patients with extensive cutaneous involvement regardless of the presence of systemic symptoms. The goal is to identify asymptomatic bony lesions early and thereby prevent an unnecessarily extensive evaluation if bony changes are discovered incidentally later in life.

• In cases in which tissue infiltration by mast cells is not obvious, biochemical determination of mast-cell mediator release can be used to support a diagnosis of suspected mast-cell disease. Taken at one point in time, currently available tests cannot differentiate between mediator release associated with anaphylaxis or other massive degranulation events, and mediator release associated with mast-cell disease.

• The finding of chronically elevated levels of mast-cell mediators in the proper clinical setting, however, may help establish a diagnosis of mast-cell disease. The different mast-cell products that can be measured include tryptase, histamine and its metabolites, prostaglandin D_2 metabolites, and heparin. Systemic effects caused by high levels of circulating heparin are rare in patients with mastocytosis; measurement of heparin has not been useful as a diagnostic tool. The serum level of the mast-cell granule-associated enzyme tryptase can be measured by radioimmunoassay and is elevated in patients with mastocytosis. Patients with systemic mastocytosis usually have a chronic elevation of the histamine metabolite N-methylhistamine, reflecting not only high levels of histamine but perhaps an alteration in the metabolism of histamine in these patients as well. Tryptase levels, however, may be more useful than histamine levels because the latter may also be elevated in hypereosinophilic states. Metabolites of prostaglandin D_2 in the urine can be measured by mass spectroscopy and correlate well with levels of histamine metabolites. However, this test is not widely available.

TREATMENT

- Therapy can be directed at blocking mast-cell degranulation or the effects of mast-cell mediators on organs. Treatment is aimed only at relieving symptoms and does not alter the course of the disease. Patients should avoid triggering factors, such as ingestion of aspirin or alcohol, use of nonsteroidal anti-inflammatory agents, and exposure to pressure, friction, or extremes in temperature. Opioid analgesic, such as morphine, codeine, and pethidine, can produce severe, adverse reactions. Agents known to activate mediator release directly such as dextran and radiologic contrast dyes should also be avoided. The possibility of anaphylaxis after an insect sting, such as from a bee or wasp, is worrisome. General anaesthesia can be potentially hazardous. Histamine-releasing medications should be avoided.

- Histamine antagonists are the mainstay of therapy. Cutaneous symptoms, such as flushing, pruritus, and urticaria, mediated primarily by H_1 receptors, can be controlled with H_1-antihistamines. H_2 antagonists control oversecretion of gastric acid, which is an important factor in the development of gastritis and peptic ulcer disease. H_2 antihistamines are often not effective in controlling diarrhea, but anticholinergics may provide relief. Although no specific antihistamine provides a significant advantage, combined H_1-receptor blockade increases efficacy by complete inhibition of histamine effects. In addition, cautious use of aspirin to inhibit prostaglandin D_2 production by mast cells relieves recurrent flushing that is unresponsive to H_1-blockers and H_2-blockers. High doses of aspirin to achieve plasma salicylate concentrations of 1.45 to 2.17 mmol/L are necessary to control symptoms, but this should be reached gradually since aspirin can provoke mast-cell activation and severe hypotension in a small number of patients.

- Oral cromolyn sodium, although poorly absorbed, relieves cutaneous and central nervous system symptoms,

reduces diarrhea and abdominal pain, and is useful in patients who are unresponsive to other treatments. Until effective treatment for chronic disease is established, patients should carry injectable epinephrine for self-administration to abort attacks, and wear medical alert bracelets in case of massive mast-cell mediator release associated with shock, in which epinephrine and volume repletion are critical.

- Various other drugs have limited effect in the treatment of mastocytosis. Systemic corticosteroids can help in severe skin disease, malabsorption, or ascites. Topical steroids under occlusive dressings for limited periods or intralesional injection may transiently decrease numbers of mast cells to clear lesions and improve symptoms. Photochemotherapy with psoralens and ultraviolet-A irradiation results in decreased pruritus and fading of lesions. Relapse of symptoms eventually occurs after therapy is stopped, and its use is, therefore, limited. Interferon alpha may control the signs and symptoms of widespread systemic mastocytosis, but requires further investigation. When present, associated hematologic disorders should be treated appropriately.

REFERENCES

Golkar L, Bernhard JD. Mastocytosis. *Lancet*. 1997;349: 1379.

Longley J, et al. The mast cell and mast cell disease. *J Am Acad Dermatol*. 1995;32:545.

LIPOID PROTEINOSIS

EPIDEMIOLOGY

- Lipoid proteinosis, also referred to as hyalinosis cutis et mucosae or Urbach–Wiethe disease (UWD), was first described in 1929 by Urbach, a dermatologist, and Wiethe, an otolaryngologist. It is a rare autosomal recessive deposition disorder in which masses of hyaline-like material are deposited in the skin, mucous membranes, brain, and other internal organs. Most patients are of European descent, including South African descendants of German or Dutch immigrants. The deposits are primarily found in the walls of small blood vessels and lying freely in the papillary dermis. Ultrastructurally, reduplication of the basement membrane of vessels and occasionally the dermoepidermal junction is seen.

PATHOGENESIS

- Ultrastructural studies reveal that two separate substances are present in the eosinophilic hyaline seen in lesions of UWD (true hyaline of fibroplast origin, and reduplicated basement membranes produced by multiple cells). One study revealed peculiar cytoplasmic inclusions in lesional fibroblasts and cytoplasmic vacuolization, suggesting the possibility of a lysosomal storage disease. The inclusions contained granular, electron-dense structures, the nature of which remains unknown. They do not occur in normal skin.
- Biochemical studies suggest high levels of carbohydrates within the inclusions, again supporting the possibility of a lysosomal storage disease, although no recent data are available to confirm this. The hyaline deposits in the papillary dermis and around vessels may contain increased amounts of an uncharacterized noncollagenous glycoprotein secreted by fibroblasts. Studies of gene expression in cultured fibroplasts from patients with UWD have been performed with molecular hybridization with various procollagen complementary DNA probes. Abnormal expression of procollagen genes was observed with a decreased type I/III procollagen mRNA ratio. This was primarily caused by decreased type I procollagen mRNA levels. It is possible that other collagen genes are overexpressed in this disorder. Although a markedly reduced proliferative capacity of fibroplasts has been reported, it remains unclear whether the primary underlying disorder is an abnormality of collagen metabolism.

CLINICAL FEATURES

- The first clinical sign of the disease is often hoarseness, caused by infiltration of vocal cords of the laryngeal mucosa, that develops by the time of birth or during early childhood. Skin lesions usually appear shortly afterward or simultaneously. Clinical signs may be precipitated by a minor infection or vaccination.
- Papular, nodular, or diffuse yellow waxy papules are located on the face, the axillae, and the scrotum. Skin lesions resembling pitted acne scars may be located not only on the face but also in non-acne-prone regions. Other lesions of the face resemble solar elastosis because of the deposition of yellow material inducing a marked thickening of the skin with deep wrinkles.
- The classic and most easily recognizable sign, although not always present, is the beaded arrangement of waxy papules along the eyelids. Lesions on the scalp may occur and cause alopecia. The tongue is often firm, and its mobility may be limited. The tonsils and other areas in the oral cavity may be infiltrated. A yellow discoloration of the lips is characteristic. Hyperkeratosis is observed on the palm and dorsum of the hands and on the elbows, knees, and buttocks, possibly related to frequent trauma in these locations.

DIAGNOSIS AND DIFFERENTIAL

- Lipoid proteinosis has to be differentiated from other diseases related to the deposition of amorphous material in the dermis. The differential diagnosis applies at both clinical and histopathologic levels. Porphyria, mainly erythropoietic protoporphyria, is a photosensitive disorder that shows deposition of a PAS-positive material around the blood vessels mainly in sun-exposed areas. Light sensitivity is, however, not a feature of lipoid proteinosis, and the observation of lesions in nonexposed sites aids the diagnosis. Furthermore, xanthoma cells never occur in lipoid proteinosis.
- Amyloidosis may resemble lipoid proteinosis. Its development is often more progressive and accompanied by involvement of the kidneys, heart, and other tissues. Amyloid deposition may occur in the skin of lipoid proteinosis patients.

TREATMENT

- There is no known cure for UWD. Anecdotal reports of treatment successes are difficult to evaluate because of the fluctuating course of the disease. One report of clinical and histologic regression after dermabrasion is of interest. Oral DMSO has also been reported to be effective. Surgical resection of plaques on vocal cords may improve hoarseness. Supportive treatment, especially anticonvulsants, should be considered.

REFERENCE

Touart DM, Sau P. Cutaneous deposition disease (part one). *J Am Acad Dermatol.* 1998;39:149.

Xanthomas

EPIDEMIOLOGY

- Xanthomas are localized infiltrates of lipid-containing histiocytic foam cells that usually are of lipoprotein metabolism. The lipids found accumulating in the foam cell of xanthomas (as well as atheromas) are primarily free and esterified, but occasionally other sterols and triglycerides accumulate in significant amounts in certain xanthomas.

PATHOPHYSIOLOGY

- Plasma lipoproteins are a polydisperse collection of particles composed of lipids (cholesterol, triglycerides, and phospholipids) and specific proteins called apolipoproteins. Lipoproteins serve as lipid-transporting aggregates in the blood plasma. Since the major lipids transported are triglycerides and cholesterol, which are very insoluble in the watery milieu of the plasma and tissues, the apoproteins and phospholipids provide excellent emulsifying properties by which these lipid moieties are solubilized.
- The plasma lipoproteins may be divided into five major classes on the basis of their physical and chemical properties: (1) chylomicrons, (2) very-low-density lipoproteins (VLDLs or prebeta lipoproteins), (3) intermediate-density lipoproteins (IDLs or remnant lipoproteins), (4) low-density lipoproteins (LDLs or beta lipoproteins), and (5) high-density lipoproteins (HDLs or alpha lipoproteins). Elevation of certain plasma lipoproteins levels (chylomicrons, VLDLs, IDLs, and LDLs) are seen in association with xanthomas. Much of the lipid constituent of xanthomas is derived from the plasma. In many instances the occurrence of skin xanthoma is related directly to the degree of elevation in one or more of the lipoproteins just mentioned. Xanthomas, particularly eruptive and tuberous forms, have been reported to wax and wane in parallel to fluctuations in serum lipoproteins.
- Radioisotopic tracer studies also have demonstrated that lipoproteins find their way directly into cutaneous lesions. Further, correlative lipid analytic and electron microscopic studies on experimental and human xanthomas suggest that lipoproteins permeate the walls of dermal capillaries and are then phagocytized by dermal histiocytes that evolve into foam cells.
- There is a close relationship between xanthomas and atheroma formation in patients with certain forms of hyperlipoproteinemia; foam cells are seen in both types of lesions. Atheromas, like xanthomas, contain large quantities of free and esterified cholesterol and the cholesterol ester fatty acid patterns in human atheromas are like those found in xanthomas, suggesting similar modes of deposition; this explains the high incidence of premature atherosclerosis seen in patients with various kinds of xanthomatosis.

CLINICAL FEATURES

- The clinical variants of xanthomas are tendinous, planar, tuberous, eruptive, and disseminated.
- Tendinous xanthomas arise in tendons, ligaments, and fascia and are noted initially as deeply situated, smooth, firm nodules of various sizes with normal-appearing skin, freely movable over the surfaces. Tendinous xanthomas occur most frequently in the extensor tendons of the hands, knee, elbows, and achilles tendons. These patients often have abnormal lipoprotein metabolism and coronary artery disease.
- Planar xanthomas occur in several areas of the body, but they are always yellow, soft, and either macular or slightly elevated plaques. The most commonly encountered planar lesion, xanthelasma or xanthelasma palpebrarum, occurs on the eyelids. Although these xanthomas are suggestive of underlying hypercholesterolemia when seen in persons under 40 to 50 years of age, only about one half of patients will have plasma lipid elevations.
- Tuberous xanthomas appear as yellow to red nodules with a predilection for extensor surfaces of the body (e.g., elbows, knees, knuckles, and buttocks), as well as the palms. Early in their evolution these dermal xanthomas appear as small, soft papules that can be easily mistaken for eruptive xanthomas. Later they coalesce, enlarge, and become firm, with increasing fibrosis. Such xanthomas indicate a systemic alteration in lipid metabolism involving cholesterol and/ or triglycerides. Atherosclerosis is found in these patients.
- Eruptive xanthomas are characterized by small, yellow, cutaneous papules, 1 to 4 mm in diameter, with an erythematous halo around the base. They appear suddenly in crops over pressure points and extensor surfaces of the arms, legs, and buttocks. These forms of xanthomas develop exclusively in the presence of hyperlipemic or lactescent plasma because of the presence of high concentrations of triglycerides in the plasma. Hypertriglyceridemia may also be accompanied by lipemia retinals, abdominal pain, and occasionally acute pancreatitis.
- Xanthoma disseminatum lesions are rare but distinctive papulo-nodular, red-yellow lesions that slowly become dark mahogany brown with age. In contrast to tuberous and eruptive xanthomas, xanthoma disseminatum lesions have a predilection for the flexural creases, mucous membranes, central nervous system, cornea or sclera, and occasionally bone. Mucosal lesions may result in nasopharyngeal stricture, causing dysphagia and laryngeal obstruction with hoarseness and dyspnea. Xanthomatous lesions of the tuber

cinereum, infundibulum, and pituary gland occasionally cause diabetes insipidus. Serum lipids are normal in xanthoma disseminatum. This disease is therefore thought to result from local tissue metabolic derangements, probably a primary proliferation of histiocytic elements with secondary accumulations of lipid (cholesterol).

DIAGNOSIS AND DIFFERENTIAL

- Finding xanthomas mandates a careful history and physical examination, with attention directed to the familial incidence of xanthomas or premature atherosclerotic cardiovascular disease, as well as lipemia retinalis, arcus senilis, and hepatosplenomegaly in the patient.
- The first step in the diagnosis of hyperlipoproteinemia is the quantitative measurement of both cholesterol and triglyceride levels in plasma of the fasting patient. At least two fasting plasma lipid samples should be abnormal before lipoprotein studies should be undertaken.
- Ancillary laboratory tests are necessary to distinguish the various diseases that may cause secondary hyperlipoproteinemias and xanthomas. Evaluation of thyroid, liver, and renal function will help in diagnosing many of the secondary diseases. Generalized planar xanthoma may be associated with paraproteinemias (myeloma, lymphoma, cryoglobulinemia, macroglobulinemia); therefore, such patients require a more extensive evaluation.

TREATMENT

- Dietary manipulation alone often is effective in lowering blood lipid levels in most primary hypercholesterolemia; however, optimal diet alone rarely achieves more than a 20% reduction in cholesterol levels.
- When dietary restrictions and weight reduction are ineffective, a number of agents may be added to the therapeutic regimen, but it is important to stress to the patient that the prescribed diet should be maintained while on these drugs.

REFERENCE

Parker F. Xanthomas and hyperlipidemias. *J Am Acad Dermatol.* 1985;13:1.

15 CUTANEOUS ULCERS

Ysabel M. Bello
Anna F. Falabella

VENOUS INSUFFICIENCY

EPIDEMIOLOGY

- Venous insufficiency is the most common cause of leg ulcers, accounting for approximately 80 to 90%. Approximately 20% of the patients with venous leg ulcers have associated mixed arterial and venous insufficiency.
- Limited epidemiologic studies are available from the United States. However, the prevalence of venous ulcers in Europe is between 0.15 and 1% of the population. The prevalence of venous ulcers increases progressively with age, and there is no significant difference between men and women at any age.
- Venous insufficiency is associated with a history of leg injuries, phlebitis, and prior deep venous thrombosis. Deep venous thrombosis may be silent, or may occur during or after pregnancy or surgery.

PATHOPHYSIOLOGY

- The venous system of the lower extremities is comprised of deep, superficial, and communicating veins. One-way valves in the venous system and the calf muscle pump assist the return of venous blood to the heart against gravity and prevent retrograde blood flow. A diseased venous system (faulty or dysfunctional valves or venous obstruction), or failure of the calf muscle pump, causes sustained venous hypertension.
- Venous ulcers are thought to result from venous hypertension. Several hypotheses, including white blood cell margination, growth factor trapping, and oxygen/nutrient barrier by pericapillary fibrin cuffs, have been proposed to explain how venous hypertension leads to ulceration. In fact, all three may be involved in the formation of venous ulcers.
- Concomitant systemic alteration in fibrinolysis could contribute to the hypotheses mentioned and has been identified in patients with venous ulcers and venous disease.

CLINICAL FEATURES

- Patients with venous insufficiency complain of aching and swelling of the legs, more severe at the end of the day, exacerbated by dependency and relieved by leg elevation.
- Lower leg edema, hyperpigmentation (secondary to deposition of hemosiderin), hypopigmentation, eczematous changes (venous dermatitis), and presence of varicose veins and lipodermatosclerosis (induration and fibrosis of the dermis and subcutaneous tissue) are signs of venous insufficiency. Peripheral pulses are usually palpable, unless edema is severe.
- Superficial ulcer with irregular, shaggy borders usually located on the gaiter area (2.5 cm above the malleoli to the point at which the calf muscles become prominent posteriorly).

DIAGNOSIS AND DIFFERENTIAL

- Clinical signs as described are helpful in the diagnosis of venous ulcers. Duplex ultrasound scanning is a noninvasive vascular study used to confirm the site and extent of venous disease. Other noninvasive assessment procedures include Doppler ultrasound, air plethysmography, and photo-plethysmography.
- Arterial disease needs to be ruled out because the management of a venous ulcer will change if there is concomitant arterial disease. Pain with leg elevation, presence of diminished or absent pulses, necrotic eschar on the ulcer bed, and distal location of the ulcer suggest arterial disease. Determination of the ankle brachial pressure index (ABI), which is the ratio of systolic pressure between the ankle and the arm using a hand-held Doppler device, will help determine arterial blood flow to the limb. It should be measured before initiation of compression therapy.
- Other causes such as neuropathic ulcers or pyoderma gangrenosum should be excluded.

TREATMENT

- Compression therapy is the gold standard treatment for venous ulcers. However, it should not be applied if there is evidence of moderate or severe arterial disease (ABI less than 0.8). Compression therapy may be delivered using graduated compression stockings; elastic, non-elastic, or multilayer compression bandages; and orthotic compression devices and compression pumps.
- Leg elevation above the level of the heart for a few hours per day and at night is a helpful adjuvant therapy. However, it is difficult to implement in ambulatory patients.
- Wound dressings are frequently used in conjunction with compression therapy to relieve pain, debride necrotic tissue, promote granulation tissue formation and stimulate wound healing. For heavily exuding ulcers, hydrofiber, alginate, or foam dressings are recommended; for moderately exuding ulcers, hydrocolloid or foam dressings can be used; for mildly exuding ulcer, hydrocolloid or hydrogel dressings; for dry ulcer, hydrogel dressing; for contaminated or infected ulcers, cadexomer iodine or nanocrystalline silver dressings; for malodorous ulcers, activated charcoal dressing or metronidazole gel are effective.
- Good wound care and compression therapy will heal up to 50% of venous ulcers. For slow-to-heal or large venous ulcers, other therapies such as skin grafting (pinch grafting, or split-thickness skin grafting) or bioengineered skin substitutes are available. Graftskin, a human skin equivalent composed of neonatal keratinocytes and fibroblasts cultivated in bovine type I collagen (Apligraf), has been approved by the Food and Drug Administration for venous ulcer treatment. New skin substitutes, as well as other therapeutic modalities and growth factors, may have a role in the future management of venous ulcers.
- A systemic pharmacologic agent, pentoxifylline (a methyl-xanthine derivative), has been reported to accelerate healing of venous leg ulcers compared to placebo at a dose of 800 mg three times per day. Side effects include gastrointestinal upset and dizziness.
- Systemic antibiotics are recommended only in the presence of cellulitis or infection, guided by bacterial culture and sensitivity.
- Once the ulcer is healed, patients should be instructed to use well-fitted compression stockings every day and replace them every 4 to 6 months. Early intervention after recurrence is also recommended.
- If venous insufficiency affects the superficial veins only, stripping of the affected veins may prevent ulcer recurrence. If incompetence is limited to the perforating veins, a new less invasive procedure, subfascial endoscopic perforating surgery, might be beneficial in preventing recurrence.

REFERENCES

Bello YM, Phillips TJ. Management of venous ulcers. *J Cutan Med Surg.* 1998;3(suppl 1):6.

Falanga V. Care of venous leg ulcers. *Ostomy/Wound Manage.* 1999;45(suppl 1A):33S.

Kirsner RS. Venous Ulcer. *Conn's Current Therapy.* New York:Saunders, 1999.

Phillips TJ. Current approaches to venous ulcers and compression. *Dermatol Surg.* 2001;27:611.

Valencia IC, Falabella AF, Kirsner R, Eaglstein WH. Chronic venous insufficiency and venous leg ulceration. *J Am Acad Dermatol.* 2001;44:401.

ARTERIAL ULCERS

EPIDEMIOLOGY

- Abnormal arterial blood flow in the extremities or peripheral vascular disease affect 30% of the adult population and two thirds of all the cases are asymptomatic. It rarely affects the upper extremities.
- Peripheral vascular disease is infrequent until middle age, and then its prevalence increases dramatically. The prevalence is slightly higher in men than women, but this difference balances after middle age.
- Cigarette smoking, hypertension, hypercholesterolemia, and diabetes are risk factors for developing arterial disease.
- Peripheral vascular disease has been associated with coronary artery disease and cerebrovascular disease.

PATHOPHYSIOLOGY

- Peripheral vascular disease is mainly caused by atherosclerosis (degenerative disease of large vessels consisting of the accumulation of cholesterol plaques, cells, matrix fibers, and tissue debris), which progressively narrows the vessel lumen, creating interference or obstruction of blood flow.

CLINICAL FEATURES

- Decreased peripheral pulses, leg pallor on elevation of the extremity, leg rubor on dependency of the extremity, slow toenail growth, loss of leg and foot hair, and unilateral cool extremity may suggest asymptomatic peripheral vascular disease.

- Symptomatic patients may have a history of intermittent claudication (pain or aching in the calves, thighs, or buttocks) that occurs while walking and is relieved by rest. Rest pain is present in more severe stages of the disease, worsened when the leg is elevated and relieved by dependency.
- Painful ulcers with well-demarcated borders or "punched-out" appearance, located over the toes, interdigital spaces, dorsum of the foot, and at sites subjected to trauma or rubbing from footwear are clinical signs of peripheral vascular disease. The ulcer base is pale, and it can be covered with necrotic eschar. Tendon exposure is usually observed in arterial ulcers.

DIAGNOSIS AND DIFFERENTIAL

- Arterial disease can be detected by a simple, noninvasive calculation of the ankle brachial index (ABI). The ankle systolic pressure should be equal to or greater than the brachial artery systolic pressure. Measurements of ABI between 0.5 and 0.8 are consistent with moderate peripheral arterial disease and claudication, while values less than 0.5 are consistent with severe disease.
- Segmental leg pressure may allow diagnosing peripheral vascular disease and localizing the level of obstruction.
- Analysis of arterial waveform by Doppler or pulse volume recording may be useful when patients have calcified, noncompressible vessels.
- An arteriogram is often necessary particularly when vascular surgery is being contemplated.
- Magnetic resonance angiography is an alternative to conventional angiography if more diagnostic information is needed before a planned revascularization procedure.

TREATMENT

- Surgical reestablishment of an adequate vascular supply is recommended whenever possible. The patient should be referred for a vascular surgical evaluation.
- General recommendations include smoking cessation with the offer of nicotine replacement combined with behavioral modification therapy. Adequate control of associated hypertension, hypercholesterolemia, and diabetes should be implemented.
- Conservative management includes local wound care and limb protection. Wounds should be kept moist by

the use of hydrogel dressings to prevent additional cell death; management of pain and infection should be initiated as needed.

- Cilostasol (Pletal), a type III phosphodiesterase inhibitor approved for use in intermittent claudication, has been shown to bring about significant improvement in pain and walking distance at a dose of 100 mg twice daily. It is metabolized by the cytochrome P-450 system, and caution is therefore required regarding possible drug interactions. Adverse events include headache, diarrhea, and dizziness.
- Gene therapy may be an option in the future, especially for patients who are not candidates for surgical reconstruction.

REFERENCES

Bello YM, Phillips TJ. Chronic leg ulcers: Types and treatment. *Hosp Pract.* 2000;35:101.

Federman DG, Trent JT, Froelich CW, et al. Epidemiology of peripheral vascular disease: A predictor of systemic vascular disease. *Ostomy/Wound Manage.* 1998;44:58.

Weiner SD, Reis ED, Kerstein MD. Peripheral arterial disease. Medical management in primary care practice. *Geriatrics.* 2001;56:20.

NEUROPATHIC ULCERS

EPIDEMIOLOGY

- Neuropathic ulcers are most common in diabetic patient, but could be the sign of other diseases such as Hansen's disease, syringomyelia, spinal dysraphism, tabes dorsalis, spinal cord injuries, or hereditary sensory/autonomic neuropathies.
- Peripheral neuropathy is the cause of diabetic foot ulcers in 60 to 70% of cases, whereas peripheral vascular disease is the cause of diabetic foot ulcer in 15 to 20% of cases. Both conditions are present in 15 to 20% of patients with diabetic foot ulcers.

PATHOPHYSIOLOGY

- Neuropathy (motor and sensory) occurs as a complication of prolonged glucose elevation. Sensory neuropathy leads to loss of protective function. Neuropathic ulcers are the result of unrecognized repetitive trauma because of lack of protective sensation in the foot. An ulcer frequently starts from a minor wound related to improper fitted shoes, traumatic trimming of the toenails, foreign body from walking barefoot, or burns from immersion of the foot in a hot bath.

CLINICAL FEATURES

- History of numbness, paresthesias, or burning lancinating pain.
- Deep ulcer surrounded by a thick white rim of callus, located on weight-bearing areas or areas subject to trauma, such as on the sole of the foot particularly over the metatarsal heads, toes, or heels.

DIAGNOSIS AND DIFFERENTIAL

- Assessment of the presence or absence of protective sensation by the use of a monofilament, which is pressed against the foot with enough pressure to bend, is recommended by the American Diabetic Association. Sensation should be measured at 10 different sites on the foot at least once a year. Risk of ulcer formation exists when there is a failure to feel the monofilament at 4 or more different sites.
- Vascular evaluation includes palpation of pulses. Absence of pulses may indicate ischemia and requires vascular surgical consultation. ABI has been demonstrated to be unreliable as a measure of ischemia in diabetic patients.
- Diabetic foot ulcers should be assessed for infection. Infection is suggested by local redness, swelling, purulent drainage, sinus tract formation or crepitation, hyperglycemia, fever, chills, and leukocytosis. However, these symptoms and signs may be absent in two thirds of patients with infection. Infections in diabetic patients frequently present as recalcitrant hyperglycemia and malaise. Diabetic patients often have underlying osteomyelitis that is clinically unsuspected. If the ulcer probes to bone, osteomyelitis should be considered. The standard to diagnose osteomyelitis is bone biopsy. Culture-based antibiotic therapy should be initiated.

TREATMENT

- Preventive measures are the most important interventions in diabetic patient management. These include patient and family education, regular foot inspection, routine podiatric care, regular trimming of callus, well-fitting shoes, running shoes with molded inserts, avoidance of walking barefoot, treatment of fungal infection, smoking cessation, and blood glucose control.

- Pressure relief can be achieved by off-loading the pressure from the ulcer site, by the use of total contact cast, bed rest, walker, wheelchair, or crutches; plus surgical shoes, half-shoes, customized sandals, or felted foams.
- Aggressive sharp debridement of callous and devitalized tissue to a healthy bleeding base is recommended, as well as the use of hydrogel dressings as primary dressings.
- Other advanced therapies approved by the FDA for the treatment of diabetic foot ulcers include Graftskin (a bilaminate human skin equivalent), Dermagraft (a dermal matrix with viable living allogeneic fibroblast), and Becaplermin (a topical gel formulation of recombinant human platelet-derived growth factor).
- Maximizing arterial flow by restoration of arterial supply should be performed when necessary and possible.
- Diabetic patients with leg ulcers are at high risk of developing severe complications and may require amputation. Therefore, implementation of early, aggressive treatment is necessary. Hospitalization and intravenous antibiotics are required when there is evidence of progressing cellulitis, lack of response to oral antibiotic therapy, systemic signs of infection, abscess formation, or osteomyelitis.

REFERENCES

American Diabetes Association. Consensus development conference on diabetic foot wound care. *Diabetes Care.* 1999; 22:1354.

Browne AC, Sibbald RG. The diabetic neuropathic ulcer: An overview. *Ostomy/Wound Manage.* 1999;45(S1A):6S.

PRESSURE ULCERS

EPIDEMIOLOGY

- The prevalence of pressure ulcers in hospitalized patients ranges from 3 to 11%. The prevalence of intraoperative acquired pressure ulcers is 8.5%, after at least 3 hours of surgery. In long-term care settings, a high prevalence (15 to 25%) is observed because of a larger at-risk population.
- More than 70% of pressure ulcers occur in patients older than 70 years of age. However, younger patients with cerebral palsy, multiple sclerosis, or spinal cord injury are also at risk.
- Risk factors that predispose a person to develop pressure ulcers include prolonged immobilization (bed or

chair bound), sensory deficit that impedes perception of pain from prolonged pressure, poor nutrition, and circulatory disturbances.

PATHOPHYSIOLOGY

- Pressure, shearing forces, friction, and moisture are the major factors involved in the development of pressure ulcers.
- A constant pressure of 70 mm Hg results in tissue damage. Pressure over bony prominences can cause severe deep tissue trauma, with little superficial damage.
- Shearing forces result from sliding and displacement of two opposing surfaces. The lack of tensile strength in the subcutaneous tissue makes it vulnerable to mechanical forces.
- Friction, the force that resists relative motion between two surfaces in contact, is frequently observed when patients are pulled across bedsheets.
- Moisture as a result of perspiration, as well as fecal or urinary incontinence, increases the possibility of ulcer formation.

CLINICAL FEATURES

- Pressure ulcers can present in several stages:
  Stage I: Nonblanchable erythema with intact skin.
  Stage II: Partial-thickness skin loss.
  Stage III: Full-thickness skin loss with damage that does not extend through the fascia.
  Stage IV: Full-thickness skin loss with damage to muscle, bone or supporting structures.

DIAGNOSIS AND DIFFERENTIAL

- Osteomyelitis can be present in nonhealing pressure ulcers. If osteomyelitis is suspected, a bone scan should be obtained. If it is abnormal, bone biopsy and culture are needed.
- Squamous cell carcinomas have been reported to occur in approximately 0.5% of pressure ulcers.

TREATMENT

- Daily inspection of the patient's skin and assessment of sites at risk for developing pressure ulcers is required.
- Reduction of pressure, shearing, and friction forces. Bedridden patients should be repositioned at least every 2 hours, and the head of the bed should be kept

at the lowest possible level of elevation. Chair-bound patients should be moved every hour, and patients should be taught to shift their weight every 15 minutes. Pressure-reducing mattresses or chair cushions are helpful, and pillows or foam wedges should be used to protect bony prominences. Lifting devices, such as a trapeze, should be used to move patients.
- Local wound care includes debridement of necrotic tissue, wound cleansing using saline solution, application of dressings that maintain a moist wound environment, and keeping the surrounding skin dry. Hydrofiber or calcium alginate dressings can be used if there is exudate, while hydrogel dressing is an option if the wound is dry.
- High bacterial colonization, chronic subclinical infection, underlying osteomyelitis, and inadequate pressure relief should be addressed if ulcers do not improve.
- Nutritional status of patients with pressure ulcers should be evaluated and improved if necessary.
- Oxandrolone, an anabolic (protein-building) steroid, has been approved by the FDA at doses up to 20 mg/d to promote weight gain in patients with severe weight loss due to extensive surgery, chronic infections, or severe trauma.
- Vacuum-assisted closure (VAC) is a relatively new technique that has been shown to be effective in the treatment of pressure ulcers.
- Surgical management includes primary closure, skin flaps, myocutaneous flaps, skin grafts, tissue expansion, and skin substitutes.

REFERENCE

Kanj LF, Wilkin SVB, Phillips TJ. Pressure ulcers. *J Am Acad Dermatol.* 1998;38:517.

PYODERMA GANGRENOSUM

EPIDEMIOLOGY

- The incidence of pyoderma gangrenosum (PG) is not known. PG may occur at any age, but it mainly affects adults; there is no sex predilection.
- PG may be idiopathic but it is associated with systemic disease in more than 50% of all cases. The most common associated systemic disease is inflammatory bowel disease. PG has also been associated with rheumatoid arthritis, Felty's syndrome, osteoarthritis, sacroileitis, myeloid leukemia, multiple myeloma,

Waldenstrom's macroglobulinemia, polycythemia rubra vera, myelofibrosis, lymphoma, HIV disease, chronic active hepatitis, hidradenitis suppurativa, and hypo or hyperthyroidism.

PATHOPHYSIOLOGY

- The pathophysiology of PG is unclear. A phenomenon called pathergy, in which the patient develops a new lesion at sites of trauma, is common in PG.

CLINICAL FEATURES

- Ulcer with a purplish-blue, undermined rolled border, with a cribriform or honeycomb-like base appearance. Ulcers may be single or multiple, involving any area of the body, with predilection for the legs.
- Several clinical variants of PG have been described: ulcerative, pustular, bullous, and vegetative. The pustular form appears to be most commonly seen in patients with inflammatory bowel diseases, while the bullous form has an association with myelodysplastic disease.

DIAGNOSIS AND DIFFERENTIAL

- Diagnosis depends on clinical appearance because the histopathologic changes are not specific and there are no known serologic or hematologic markers for this condition. Detailed history, meticulous physical examination, and skin biopsy for cultures (bacterial, fungal, and/or viral) are essential to rule out other causes of cutaneous ulceration.

- Once other diagnoses have been ruled out, the diagnosis of PG can be made based on history and clinical presentation.

TREATMENT

- Aggressive surgical debridement is not recommended; in fact, it can be detrimental.
- Management of the associated disease and specific local and/or systemic therapy are recommended.
- Local therapy includes wound cleansing, use of moisture-retentive dressings, topical or intralesional corticosteroids, cromolyn sodium, and tacrolimus ointment.
- Systemic therapy includes corticosteroids, which can be given orally or in a pulse intravenous form, and other immunosuppressive agents such as dapsone, colchicine, clofazimine, hydroxychloroquine, methotrexate, azathioprine, cyclophosphamide, and cyclosporine. Infliximab, a monoclonal antibody that binds specifically and with high affinity to free and membrane-bound tumor necrosis factor alpha, has been reported to be effective in patients with inflammatory bowel disease and concomitant pyoderma gangrenosum or psoriasis.

REFERENCES

Bennett Ml, Jackson JM, Jorizzo JL, et al. Pyoderma gangrenosum. A comparison of typical and atypical forms with an emphasis on time to remission. Case review of 86 patients from 2 institutions. *Medicine.* 2000;79:37.

Falabella A, Falanga V. Uncommon causes of ulcers. *Clin Plast Surg.* 1998;25:467.

Powell FC, Su WP, Perry HO. Pyoderma gangrenosum: Classification and management. *J Am Acad Dermatol.* 1996;34:395, quiz, 410.

16 PIGMENTARY DISORDERS

Melissa C. Lazarus
Francisco Kerdel

- Pigmentation of skin results from the incorporation of the melanin-containing melanosomes, produced by the melanocytes, into the keratinocytes in the epidermis and their ensuing degradation. In darker-pigmented individuals, the melanosomes are larger, more heavily melanized, and the melanosomes undergo degradation at a slower rate than in lighter-skinned individuals. Melanin is produced by the hydroxylation of tyrosine to 3,4-dihydroxyphenylalanine (DOPA) by the enzyme tyrosinase. Tyrosinase subsequently oxidizes DOPA to dopaquinone, leading to the formation of melanin (eumelanin and pheomelanin). Eumelanins produce the dark brown and black pigments while pheomelanins produce the red and yellow pigments. The combinations of these pigments produce skin color. People with light-complexioned skin mostly produce pheomelanin, while those with dark-colored skin mostly produce eumelanin.
- Once the melanin is made within the melanosomes, it then migrates into the melanocyte's dendrite tips. Each melanocyte is in contact with several neighboring keratinocytes, forming an "epidermal melanin unit." The melanin found in these melanocytes is then incorporated into other keratinocytes of the epidermal melanin unit or into the dermis by a process that is still poorly understood.
- Pigmentation can be affected by many different processes, resulting in either hyperpigmentation or hypopigmentation. In many cases, these changes in pigment are due to alterations in melanin production at any stage in the pathway.

REFERENCE

Baumann L. *Cosmetic Dermatology: Principles and Practice.* New York:McGraw-Hill, 2002.

HYPERPIGMENTATION

ACANTHOSIS NIGRICANS

- Acanthosis nigricans is a nonspecific reaction pattern that may accompany diabetes; obesity; excess corticosteroids; pineal tumors; endocrine disorders; drugs such as nicotinic acid and estrogens; and underlying cancer.
- There are three types of acanthosis nigricans (types I, II, and III).
- Acanthosis means hyperplasia of the stratum spinosum of the epidermis.

EPIDEMIOLOGY

- More common in women than men, although can be seen in both sexes and in all races.
- More common in obese patients.

PATHOPHYSIOLOGY

- During the process there is papillary hypertrophy, hyperkeratosis, and an increased number of melanocytes in the epidermis.
- Type I (associated with malignancy) may result from secretion of tumor products with insulin-like activity or transforming growth factor alpha, which stimulates keratinocytes to proliferate.
- Epidermal changes may be due to hypersecretion of a pituitary peptide or nonspecific growth promoting effects of hyperinsulinemia.

CLINICAL FEATURES

- Acanthosis nigricans is characterized by symmetrically distributed hyperpigmentation and papillary hypertrophy, which may give the lesion a velvety appearance.
- The regions of the body most commonly affected are the face, neck, axillae, groin, external genitals, inner aspect of the thighs, umbilicus, anus, and flexor surface of the ankles and knees.
- Patches are generally gray, brownish, or black in color.

TYPE I: ACANTHOSIS NIGRICANS ASSOCIATED WITH MALIGNANCY

- Type I is usually associated with adenocarcinoma, with the stomach as the most common site of malignancy, followed by lung and breast. Cancer in several other areas of the body has also been reported.
- In approximately one third of patients, the skin lesions accompany the clinical manifestations of cancer. Acanthosis nigricans has also been reported to precede (18%) or follow (22%) the onset of cancer. In several cases, skin lesions have disappeared with successful removal of the tumor.

TYPE II: FAMILIAL ACANTHOSIS NIGRICANS

- Type II is present at birth and accentuated at puberty. It is extremely rare and is inherited in an autosomal dominant manner.

TYPE III: ACANTHOSIS NIGRICANS ASSOCIATED WITH OBESITY, INSULIN-RESISTANT STATES, AND ENDOCRINOPATHY

- Type III is the most common type of acanthosis nigricans.
- Usually presents on the skin of the sides of the neck, axillae, and groin.
- Occurs in obesity, with or without endocrine disorders. When associated with obesity, the process is often referred to as *pseudoacanthosis nigricans*.
- Acanthosis nigricans is also seen in endocrine disorders such as acromegaly and gigantism, Stein–Leventhal syndrome, diabetes mellitus, hypothyroidism, Addison's disease, Cushing's syndrome, hyperandrogenic states, and hypogonadal syndromes.
- Many other insulin-resistant states present with acanthosis nigricans, and can be divided into two subtypes, A and B.
- Type A is also known as the HAIR–AN syndrome.
- It is due to a defect in the insulin receptor, or postreceptor pathways. It is more common in young children with hyperandrogenic manifestations.
- It is named for its associated symptoms: HA (hyperandrogen), IR (insulin resistance), and AN (acanthosis nigricans).

- Type B is due to a defect in which autoantibodies to the insulin receptor are present. It is seen in middle-aged patients with autoimmune diseases.
- Both types are more common in African-American women.

DIAGNOSIS AND DIFFERENTIAL

- All forms of acanthosis nigricans are similar histologically. The epidermis undulates sharply to form numerous repeating peaks and valleys. Variable hyperplasia may be seen, along with hyperkeratosis and slight basal cell layer hyperpigmentation without melanocytic hyperplasia.
- Type I should be highly suspected if widespread lesions develop in a nonobese male over the age of 40.
- Differential diagnosis includes ichtyosis hystrix, Gougerot–Carteaud syndrome, Dowling–Degos' disease, acropigmentation of Kitamura, and Haber's syndrome.

TREATMENT

- Lesions are usually asymptomatic and do not require treatment; however, patients should be examined for possible underlying causes.
- Lesions associated with obesity usually improve with weight loss.
- Reducing thicker lesions in areas of maceration may decrease odor and promote comfort for patients.
- Lesions may be softened by the use of Lac-Hydrin (12% lactic acid cream) applied as needed.
- Retinoids may be effective in the treatment of acanthosis nigricans. Retinoic acid (Retin-A cream or gel) applied each day, or less often if irritation occurs, can be effective. Oral isotretinoin (Accutane) has also been reported to be useful; however skin lesions recur when the drug is discontinued.
- Type I may regress with removal of malignancy.
- Type II is generally accentuated at puberty, and at times regresses when the patient is older.

REFERENCES

Braverman IM. Skin manifestations of internal malignancy. *Clin Geriatr Med.* 2002;18:1.

Darmstadt GL, Yokel BK, Horn TD. Treatment of acanthosis nigricans with tretinoin. *Arch Dermatol.* 1991;127:1139.

Elmer KB, George RM. HAIR–AN syndrome: A multisystem challenge. *Am Fam Physician.* 2001;63:2385.

Paron NG, Lambert PW. Cutaneous manifestations of diabetes mellitus. *Prim Care.* 2000;27:371.

Schwartz RA. Acanthosis nigricans. *J Am Acad Dermatol.* 1994;31:1.

MELASMA

- Melasma is also known as chloasma or "mask of pregnancy."
- It is a very common condition that is usually seen in women of childbearing age.

EPIDEMIOLOGY

- 90% of patients are women.
- More common in people of Hispanic, Indo-Chinese, and Asian origin, although all races can be affected.
- Most apparent in skin types IV to VI.

PATHOPHYSIOLOGY

- The cause of melasma is unknown, although multiple factors are implicated in the disease.
- Factors implicated include exposure to ultraviolet and visible light, use of oral contraceptives, pregnancy, estrogen-progesterone therapy, thyroid dysfunction, medications (such as the antiepilepsy drugs hydantoin and Dilantin), genetic predisposition, and cosmetics.

CLINICAL FEATURES

- Presents as irregularly shaped, but often distinctly defined, blotches of light to dark-brown pigmentation usually seen on the upper lip, nose, cheeks, chin, forehead, and sometimes neck.
- Three patterns are recognized clinically.
- The centrofacial pattern, which is the most common, involves the cheeks, forehead, upper lip, nose, and chin.
- The malar pattern affects the nose and cheeks.
- The mandibular pattern.
- Most commonly seen in sun-exposed areas.

DIAGNOSIS AND DIFFERENTIAL

- Can be divided into three types based on Wood's light examination.
- Epidermal type (brown), with increased melanin in basal and suprabasal epidermis, causes accentuation with Wood's light examination.
- Dermal type (blue-gray), with melanin-laden macrophages in a perivascular distribution in the superficial and deep dermis, does not accentuate with Wood's light examination.
- Mixed type (brown-gray), has elements of both epidermal and dermal types, and appears a deep brown color. It only accentuates with Wood's light exam in the areas with epidermal component.

TREATMENT

- The therapeutic objective of treatment is to retard the proliferation of the melanocytes, inhibit the formation of melanosomes, and promote the degradation of melanosomes.
- Treatment must include a good high-SPF sunscreen with UVA protection, which should be worn throughout the day, and sun avoidance. UVA screens for car and home windows, and protective clothing, such as hats, are a great addition to a topical treatment regimen.
- Topical treatments may include hydroquinone 2 to 4%, low-potency steroids, azelaic acid, kojic acid, arbutin, hydroxy acids, and retinoids.
- Melasma is a chronic disorder that can be frustrating to patients and physicians because it is often very difficult to treat.

REFERENCES

Griffiths CE, Finkel LJ, Ditre CM, et al. Topical tretinoin (retinoic acid) improves melasma. A vehicle-controlled, clinical trial. *Br J Dermatol.* 1993;129:415.

Lawrence N, Cox SE, Brody HJ. Treatment of melasma with Jessner's solution versus glycolic acid: A comparison of clinical efficacy and evaluation of the predictive ability of Wood's light examination. *J Am Acad Dermatol.* 1997;36:589.

Pandya AG, Guevara IL. Disorders of hyperpigmentation. *Dermatol Clin.* 2000;18:91.

Sanchez NP, Pathak MA, Sato S, et al. Melasma: A clinical, light microscopic, ultrastructural, and immunofluorescence study. *J Am Acad Dermatol.* 1981;4:698.

INCONTINENTIA PIGMENTI

- Also known as Bloch–Sulzberger syndrome.

EPIDEMIOLOGY

- X-linked dominant disease; therefore usually lethal in males.

- Over 700 cases have been reported, with 97% being female.
- Rare reports of male patients with the disease may be explained by the XXY genotype (Klinefelter syndrome), a postzygotic mutation, a half-chromatid mutation, or an unstable permutation.

PATHOPHYSIOLOGY

- X-linked dominant disease with gene locus Xq28.

CLINICAL FEATURES

- There are four stages of the disease.
  - Stage I: Vesicular (age, birth to 2 weeks). Presents with vesicles and bullae in a linear arrangement on the trunk, extremities, and scalp with erythematous macules and papules.
  - Stage II: Verrucous (age, 2 to 6 weeks). Presents with streaks of hyperkeratotic papules and pustules on extremities.
  - Stage III: Hyperpigmentatuin (age, 3 to 6 months). Presents with swirls and whorls of hyperpigmentation following Blaschko's lines.
  - Stage IV: Hypopigmentation (age, 20s to 30s). Presents with hypopigmentation replacing hyperpigmentation seen in stage III with or without follicular atrophy.
- Other cutaneous findings include scarring alopecia (30%) and dystrophic nails (5 to 10%).
- Extracutaneous findings are seen in 70 to 80% of patients. Most commonly involved are the teeth (66%), eyes (25 to 35%), and central nervous system (30%).
  - Most common dental finding: partial anodontia (43%) and pegged teeth (30%).
  - Most common eyes changes: strabismus and cataracts.
  - Most common CNS findings: seizures (13%), mental retardation (12%), and spastic paralysis (11%).

DIAGNOSIS AND DIFFERENTIAL

- Differential diagnosis includes epidermolysis bullosa, epidermolytic hyperkeratosis, impetigo, herpes simplex virus infection, hypomelanosis of Ito, and congenital syphilis.
- Skin biopsy of vesicular stage will show intradermal vesicles with abundant eosinophils and spongiosis.
- Verrucous stage may show hyperkeratosis, acanthosis, papillomatosis, and necrotic keratinocytes.

Hyperpigmentation stage may show melanin in melanophages in the upper dermis.
- Peripheral eosinophilia can be seen in infancy.

TREATMENT

- There is no treatment for incontinentia pigmenti.
- Patients should be followed by a dermatologist, dentist, ophthalmologist, and neurologist if symptomatic.
- Mothers of children born with incontinentia pigmenti should be examined carefully to allow for genetic counseling.
- Patients have a normal life span.
- Women with the disease are believed to have a more difficult time conceiving and an increased rate of spontaneous abortions.

REFERENCES

Dutheil P, Vabres P, Cayla MC, Enjolras O. Incontinentia pigmenti: Late sequelae and genotypic diagnosis. A three-generation study of four patients. *Pediatr Dermatol.* 1995; 12:107.

El-Benhawi MO, George WM. Incontinentia pigmenti: A review. *Cutis.* 1988;41:259.

Sahn EE, Davidson LS. Incontinentia pigmenti: Three cases with unusual features. *J Am Acad Dermatol.* 1994;31:852.

Sidbury R, Paller AS. Dermatologic clues to inherited disease. *Pediatr Clin North Am.* 2000;47:825.

ERYTHEMA (PIGMENTATIO) AB IGNE

- Erythema ab igne (EAI), or redness from fire, is a reticulated erythema and hyperpigmentation in an area of the body subjected to radiant heat.
- It was initially described on the shins of women huddled around peat fires.
- It is now more often associated with overuse of heating pads and has also been described as an occupational disease in blast furnace workers and on the feet of those exposed too long to vehicle heaters.

EPIDEMIOLOGY

- Most common on the legs of women; however, can be seen in any patient with heat exposure.

PATHOPHYSIOLOGY

- Erythema ab igne is caused by repeated, chronic exposure to moderate heat from an external heat source such as a wood stove, fireplace, electric blanket, electric heater, hot water bottle, or hot compress without the production of a burn.

- The exposure results in cutaneous hyperthermia in the range of 43 to 47°C, which results in histologic changes similar to those seen in sun-damaged skin.
- Although the pathogenic mechanisms are poorly understood, one study showed that moderate heat may act synergistically with ultraviolet radiation to denature DNA in squamous cells in vitro.

CLINICAL FEATURES

- Erythema ab igne begins as a mottling caused by local hemostasis.
- Usually presents with a distinctive cutaneous eruption in a reticular pattern. It initially appears as bands of erythema, but with repeated exposure, brown hyperpigmentation develops.
- All of the various stages are usually seen in a patch, with color varying from pale pink to dark purplish-brown.

DIAGNOSIS AND DIFFERENTIAL

- Careful history can help to make the diagnosis.
- The eruption must be differentiated from livedo reticularis, which is more purple in color.
- Acanthosis nigricans, livedoid vasculitis, and poikiloderma atrophicans vasculare (cutaneous T-cell lymphoma) must also be considered.

TREATMENT

- Patients must be counseled that cessation of heat exposure is essential. After removal of heat, the patches tend to disappear gradually; however, sometimes the pigment is permanent.
- The use of bland emollients may be helpful.
- Hyperpigmentation may be reduced by treatment with Kligman's formula (hydroquinone 5%, retinoic acid 0.1%, and dexamethasone 0.1%).
- Early changes, such as erythema and little or no hyperpigmentation, may resolve within several months. The pigmentation, which is caused by melanin, may fade in time or may be permanent.
- Thermal keratosis, squamous cell carcinoma in situ, and squamous cell carcinoma have been reported within these lesions; therefore patients must be educated to monitor for changes.

REFERENCES

Dvoretzky I, Silverman NR. Reticular erythema of the lower back. Erythema ab igne. *Arch Dermatol.* 1991;127:405.
Finlayson GR, Sams WM Jr, Smith JG Jr. Erythema ab igne: A histopathological study. *J Invest Dermatol.* 1966;46:104.
Meffert JJ. Environmental skin diseases and the impact of common dermatoses on medical readiness. *Dermatol Clin.* 1999;17:1.
Meffert JJ, Davis BM. Furniture induced erythema ab igne. *J Am Acad Dermatol.* 1996;34:516.
Page EH, Shear NH. Temperature-dependent skin disorders. *J Am Acad Dermatol.* 1988;18:1003.
Shahrad P, Marks R. The wages of warmth: Changes in erythema ab igne. *Br J Dermatol.* 1977;97:179.

POSTINFLAMMATORY HYPERPIGMENTATION

- Also known as postinflammatory pigment alteration (PIPA). Can occur due to a variety of skin disorders.

EPIDEMIOLOGY

- Although it appears most frequently among patients with darker skin types, it can afflict people of any skin type on any area of the skin.

PATHOPHYSIOLOGY

- Postinflammatory hyperpigmentation is a consequence of increased melanin synthesis in response to a cutaneous insult or injury.

CLINICAL FEATURES

- PIPA can result from minor conditions such as acne, eczema, and allergic reactions; as well as more serious cutaneous events such as burns, surgeries, trauma, and treatments such as chemical peels and laser resurfacing.
- The color of the lesions ranges from light brown to black, with a lighter brown appearance if the pigment is within the epidermis and dark gray to blue if the pigment is located in the dermis.
- Epidermal lesions tend to be well circumscribed, with accentuated borders observed with Wood's lamp examination; while dermal lesions are poorly

circumscribed and do not accentuate with a Wood's lamp examination. Lesions tend to darken in color with UV exposure.

- On histopathology, numerous melanophages are found in the superficial dermis. An infiltrate of lymphohistiocytes may be seen around dermal papillae and superficial blood vessels.

DIAGNOSIS AND DIFFERENTIAL

- The diagnosis is made clinically in a patient with a history of preceding inflammation in the affected area.

TREATMENT

- Because the condition is due to inflammation and injury, only nonirritating topical products such as hydroquinone, kojic acid, and retinoids are potentially useful to treat this condition. Unfortunately, these agents have minimal efficacy.
- Patients should be counseled that the best treatment approach is sun avoidance, sunscreen use, and patience.
- PIPA phenomenon tends to recur in susceptible individuals.
- In general, these lesions resolve in time.

REFERENCES

Kim NY, Pandya AG. Pigmentary diseases. *Med Clin North Am.* 1998;82:1185.
Pandya AG, Guevara IL. Disorders of hyperpigmentation. *Dermatol Clin.* 2000;18:91.

DRUG-INDUCED HYPERPIGMENTATION

- Drug-induced alterations in pigment can cause significant concern in patients (Table 16–1).

TABLE 16–1   Medications Implicated in Hyperpigmentation

ACTH	
Amiodarone	Doxorubicin
Antimalarials	Hydantoins
Bleomycin	Minocycline
Busulfan	Oral contraceptives
Chlorpromazine	Phenacetin
Clofazimine	Procarbazine
Cyclophosphamide	Zidovudine

EPIDEMIOLOGY

- Incidence varies with each drug type.
- Relatively common with certain drugs.

PATHOPHYSIOLOGY

- A variety of mechanisms, depending on the medication, have been implicated: an increase in melanin (ACTH, phenytoin, estrogen/progesterone, antimalarials, bleomycin); an increase in hemosiderin (minocycline, antimalarials); and an increase in exogenous pigment due to metabolites (minocycline, amiodarone).

CLINICAL FEATURES

- Each drug reaction presents with a different clinical picture. Some examples are given here.
- Antimalarials can cause pseudo-ochronosis, a patchy slate-gray pigmentary alteration confined to cartilaginous structures.
- Amiodarone can cause hyperpigmentation of the face and sun-exposed areas.
- Bleomycin is known to cause a distinctive linear "flagellate" pattern of hyperpigmentation, which is usually seen on the trunk.
- Minocycline can cause pigmentary deposition in the skin, nails, bones, and teeth.
- Other chemotherapeutic agents, such as cyclophosphamide, busulfan, daunorubicin, and doxorubicin are known to cause hyperpigmentation.

DIAGNOSIS AND DIFFERENTIAL

- Differential diagnosis includes melasma.

TREATMENT

- Discontinuation of medication.
- Symptoms usually resolve with removal of medication; however, this is not always possible due to other illnesses.

REFERENCES

Fitzpatrick JE. New histopathologic findings in drug eruptions. *Dermatol Clin.* 1992;10:19.
Sicari MC, Lebwohl M, Baral J, et al. Photoinduced dermal pigmentation in patients taking tricyclic antidepressants:

Histology, electron microscopy, and energy dispersive spectroscopy. *J Am Acad Dermatol.* 1999;40:290.

Susser WS, Whitaker-Worth DL, Grant-Kels JM. Mucocutaneous reactions to chemotherapy. *J Am Acad Dermatol.* 1999;40:367.

Hypopigmentation

ALBINISM

- Albinism is a heritable disorder that affects the skin, hair follicles, and eyes.

EPIDEMIOLOGY

- Tyrosinase-negative albinism (OCA-1) is seen in approximately one in 28,000 blacks and one in 39,000 Caucasians.
- Tyrosinase-positive albinism (OCA-2) is the most common form of albinism. It is seen in one in 15,000 blacks and one in 37,000 caucasians.
- TRP-1-related albinism (OCA-3) has been described only in black patients. Incidence is not known.
- In all forms, incidence is equal in males and females.

PATHOPHYSIOLOGY

- Albinism is associated with either an abnormality of melanosome maturation, numbers, or distribution with the melanocytes and keratinocytes; or an abnormality in the enzymes of the melanosomes.
- OCA-1 is inherited in an autosomal-recessive pattern. Mutations in both copies of the tyrosinase gene are seen, and produce the classic clinical picture with total lack of melanin.
- OCA-1 can be subclassified, but all types have in common a defective tyrosinase activity. Tyrosinase activity is the rate-limiting enzyme in the synthesis of melanin.
- OCA-2 has been traced back to mutations in the P gene on chromosome 15q, the human homologue of the murine pink-eyed dilution (p) gene.
- Genetic research suggests that the neurologic symptoms in these patients may result from the loss of genes adjacent to the P gene, which encodes receptors for the vital neurotransmitter gamma-aminobutyric acid.
- OCA-3 is an autosomal recessive disorder caused by mutations in the tyrosine related protein 1 (TRP-1) on chromosome 9.
- In these patients, pigmentation changes are due to the formation of brown rather than black melanin.

CLINICAL FEATURES

- Oculocutaneous albinism is differentiated into 10 variants based on genetic defect. The most common include types I, II, and III.
- Skin color may vary from pink to light brown in all types.
- Photophobia, decreased visual acuity, and nystagmus are often associated with all types, but to varying degrees.

TYPE I

- Type I (OCA-1), historically called tyrosinase-negative oculocutaneous albinism, is most common in caucasians.
- Patients have white hair, milky white skin, and pale, translucent irides, which may appear pink or red.
- Ocular abnormalities are associated and include decreased visual acuity, nystagmus, and strabismus.
- On electron microscopy, melanosomes devoid of melanin can be seen in structurally normal melanocytes.

TYPE II

- Type II (OCA-2), historically known as tyrosinase-positive oculocutaneous albinism (OCA), is most common in black populations.
- Typically, hair follicles in these patients have the ability to produce pigment. The ocular involvement seems to be proportional to the iris and cutaneous hypopigmentation.
- On electron microscopy melanin is present, but melanocytes are developmentally arrested at an early stage.

TYPE III

- Type III (OCA-3) presents with light brown hair, light brown skin, and blue/brown irides.

DIAGNOSIS AND DIFFERENTIAL

- Diagnosis of albinism can usually be made clinically.
- Chromosome analysis may be used to classify albinism.
- Historically, the hair bulb incubator test for tyrosinase activity has been used.

TREATMENT

- Patients should be counseled on sun avoidance behavior: long sleeves, broad-spectrum sunscreen, hat with brim, UVB-blocking sunglasses.

- Patients should be followed by a dermatologist with skin cancer screenings every 6 months, and by an ophthalmologist.
- OCA-2 has been associated with Prader–Willi syndrome, and with Angelman syndrome due to a link to chromosome 15q, involving deletions of the paternal or maternal allele, respectively; therefore, patients should be evaluated for other defects.
- Vision remains the same or worsens with age.
- Skin and hair do not improve with age.

REFERENCES

Dohil MA, Baugh WP, Eichenfield LF. Vascular and pigmented birthmarks. *Pediatr Clin North Am.* 2000;47:783.

Russell-Eggitt, I. Albinism. *Ophthalm Clin North Am.* 2001;14.

VITILIGO

- Vitiligo is a depigmenting disorder characterized by amelanotic macules resulting from a loss of melanocytes.

EPIDEMIOLOGY

- Vitiligo affects approximately 2% of the worldwide population regardless of race, ethnic background, or gender.
- There is a positive family history in at least 30% of cases.
- Approximately 50% of cases begin before age 20.

PATHOPHYSIOLOGY

- It has been suggested that there is some genetic mechanism involved in the etiology of vitiligo, and that it is polygenic in nature.
- Although the mechanism has yet to be determined, it may be due to autoimmunity, neurohumoral factors, and autocytotoxicity.

CLINICAL FEATURES

- There are four main types of vitiligo.
- Type A is the more common type, and is also known as generalized vitiligo.
- It has a fairly symmetric pattern of white macules with well-defined borders. Borders may have a red halo (inflammatory) or a rim of hyperpigmentation.

- The loss of pigmentation in type A may not be apparent in fair-skinned individuals, but it may be disfiguring in dark-skinned patients.
- Initially the disease is limited, but it then progresses slowly over years.
- Commonly involved sites in type A include the backs of the hands, the face, and body folds, including the axillae and the genitalia. White areas are also common around body orifices.
- Koebner's phenomenon is often seen.
- Type B is also known as segmental vitiligo.
- It is characterized by one or several macules in one band on one side of the body, and is rarely associated with distant vitiligo macules.
- It is rarely associated with further evolution of the disease.
- Focal vitiligo is included in type B, and is characterized by one or several macules in a single site; however, this may be an early evolutionary stage of another type.
- Universal vitiligo applies to cases where the entire body is depigmented.
- Acrofacial vitiligo is a pattern of depigmentation that affects distal fingers and facial orifices.
- Most patients with vitiligo have no other associated findings; however, it has been reported to be associated with alopecia areata, hypothyroidism, Addison's disease, Graves' disease, pernicious anemia, insulin-dependent diabetes mellitus, uveitis, chronic mucocutaneous candidiasis, the polyglandular autoimmune syndromes, and melanoma.
- Thyroid disorders are the most commonly associated disorder, reported in as many as 30% of vitiligo patients.
- Halo nevi are common.
- On histology, there is a complete absence of melanocytes. There is usually no inflammatory component.

DIAGNOSIS AND DIFFERENTIAL

- Examination with the Wood's light accentuates the hypopigmented areas and is useful for examining patients with light complexions. The axillae, anus, and genitalia should be carefully examined as these areas are frequently involved but often clinically not visible without Wood's light examination.
- Although the diagnosis of vitiligo generally is made clinically, a biopsy occasionally may be helpful to differentiate it from other hypo pigmentary disorders.
- Differential diagnosis includes lupus erythematosus, pityriasis alba, piebaldism, pityriasis versicolor, chemical leukoderma, leprosy, nevus depigmentosus, nevus anemicus, tuberous sclerosis, and postinflammatory leukoderma.

TREATMENT

- The most common methods of treating the disorder include cosmetics, topical and intralesional corticosteroid therapy, and psoralen ultraviolet light (PUVA) therapy.
- Some new and emerging treatments include phototherapy, topical tacrolimus, surgical grafting techniques, and melanocyte transplants.
- Depigmentation may be an option in some patients.
- There is the possibility that the use of cytokines and growth factors that may mimic the actions of phototherapeutic agents at the cellular level and use of immunomodulators may prove to be helpful.
- Vitiligo can cause patients to feel anxious or depressed about their skin condition. Patients should be referred to the Vitiligo Foundation, or to a mental health professional if needed.
- Patients should be evaluated for other associated diseases.
- Spontaneous repigmentation occurs only in 15 to 25% of cases.
- Many patients feel embarrassed. Physicians should be especially alert to the effects of disfigurement.
- Vitiligo in childhood in usually segmental in distribution, and is associated with more frequent autoimmune and endocrine abnormalities, high incidence of premature graying in the families, and a poor response to PUVA therapy.

REFERENCES

Drake LA, Dinehart SM, Farmer ER, et al. Guidelines of care for vitiligo. American Academy of Dermatology. *J Am Acad Dermatol.* 1996;35:620.

Halder RM, Young CM. New and emerging treatments for vitiligo. *Dermatol Clin.* 2000;18:79.

Kovacs SO. Vitiligo. *J Am Acad Dermatol.* 1998;38:647.

Löntz W, Olsson MJ, Moellmann G, Lerner AB. Pigment cell transplantation for treatment of vitiligo: A progress report. *J Am Acad Dermatol.* 1994;30:591.

HYPOMELANOSIS OF ITO

- Hypomelanosis of Ito used to be known as incontinentia pigmenti achromians because the lesions suggest the "negative image" of incontinentia pigmenti; however, they are now proven not to be related.

EPIDEMIOLOGY

- Female to male ratio is about 2.5 to 1.
- Hypomelanosis of Ito is an extremely rare condition that is not inherited.

PATHOPHYSIOLOGY

- Chromosomal mosaicism is believed to be the reason that the phenotype of hypomelanosis of Ito is so varied. Certain genes, namely, those on 9q33-qter, 15q11-q13, and Xp11, have been implicated in hypomelanosis of Ito; however, no consensus exists about the identity of the exact gene.
- No inflammatory changes or vesiculation are seen before the development of hypopigmentation.

CLINICAL FEATURES

- Skin lesions are usually seen during the first year of life (70%) and may be noticeable at birth (54%).
- Usually presents with small (0.5 to 1-cm) hypopigmented or white macules coalescing to form reticulated patches along Blaschko's lines.
- The macules cover more than 2 dermatomes and are often on both sides of the body; however, they are not symmetrically distributed.
- The palms, soles, and mucous membranes are spared.
- Three fourths of affected individuals also have associated anomalies of the central nervous system, hair, teeth, eyes, nails, internal organs, or musculoskeletal system. Mental retardation and seizures are the most common findings.

DIAGNOSIS AND DIFFERENTIAL

- A Wood's lamp exam enhances the pattern of the lesion, especially in Caucasian patients.
- Differential diagnosis includes the fourth stage of incontinentia pigmenti, tuberous sclerosis, linear and whorled nevoid hypermelanosis, nevus depigmentosus, and segmental vitiligo.

TREATMENT

- There is no treatment for the cutaneous findings; however, camouflage may be used to cosmetically treat patient.
- Hypopigmentation may fade with time.
- Patients should be examined by specialists if needed for other findings.
- Death is rare. Morbidity depends on severity of the associated abnormalities.

REFERENCES

Donnai D, Read AP, McKeown C, Andrews T. Hypomelanosis of Ito: A manifestation of mosaicism or chimerism. *J Med Genet.* 1988;25:809.

Glover MT, Brett EM, Atherton DJ. Hypomelanosis of Ito: Spectrum of the disease. *J Pediatr.* 1989;115:75.

Hamada T, Saito T, Sugai T, Morita Y. Incontinentia pigmenti achromians (Ito). *Arch Dermatol.* 1967;96:673.

Nehal KS, PeBenito R, Orlow SJ. Analysis of 54 cases of hypopigmentation and hyperpigmentation along the lines of Blaschko. *Arch Dermatol.* 1996;132:1167.

Pascual-Castroviejo I, Roche C, Martinez-Bermejo A, et al. Hypomelanosis of ITO. A study of 76 infantile cases. *Brain Dev.* 1998;20:36.

PIEBALDISM

- Piebaldism is a congenital disorder also known as partial albinism.

EPIDEMIOLOGY

- Incidence equal in males and females.
- Equal incidence in all races.
- Occurs in fewer than one in 20,000 births.

PATHOPHYSIOLOGY

- Piebaldism is an autosomal dominant syndrome caused by a mutation in the c-kit protooncogene on chromosome 4q12, which encodes the cellular transmembrane tyrosinase kinase for mast/stem cell growth factor.
- Pigmentation abnormalities are a result of a permanent localized absence of melanocytes and melanosomes or reduced numbers of abnormally large melanocytes.
- The pattern of depigmentation is thought to be due to defective melanocyte proliferation or migration from the neural crest during development.

CLINICAL FEATURES

- Characteristic clinical features include a white forelock (80 to 90%) and a patchy, sharply demarcated, absence of skin pigment that occur most frequently on the forehead, anterior scalp, ventral trunk, elbows, and knees.
- Areas of hyperpigmentation within depigmented areas and on normal skin are another characteristic feature of piebaldism.

DIAGNOSIS AND DIFFERENTIAL

- Differential diagnosis includes vitiligo, nevus depigmentosus, and Waardenburg syndrome.
- Piebaldism can be distinguished from vitiligo by the presence of lesions from birth, the hyperpigmented macules, and the static course.
- Waardenburg's syndrome shares similar features, including a white forelock; however, these patients usually also demonstrate facial dysmorphism and sensorineural hearing loss.

TREATMENT

- Some patients may respond to treatment with autologous cultured melanocyte grafts.
- Patients must be counseled to use sunscreen daily.
- Various methods of camouflage can be used to cosmetically treat patients. White forelocks can be camouflaged using hair dye. Hyperpigmented areas can be lightened using hydroquinone or monobenzyl ether of hydroquinone. Dermablend can be used to camouflage depigmented areas.
- The patients have a normal life span.
- Pigmentary alterations are usually permanent and stable over the lifetime.

REFERENCES

Sidbury R, Paller AS. Dermatologic clues to inherited diseases. *Pediatr Clin North Am.* 2000;47:825.

Tomita Y. The molecular genetics of albinism and piebaldism. *Arch Dermatol.* 1994;130:355.

Ward KA, Moss C, Sanders DS. Human piebaldism: Relationship between phenotype and site of kit gene mutation. *Br J Dermatol.* 1995;132:929.

NEVUS DEPIGMENTOSUS

- Nevus depigmentosus is a stable, congenital, group of off-white macules that follow a Blaschko's line pattern.

EPIDEMIOLOGY

- Nevus depigmentosus is found in all races and is seen equally in both men and women.
- Incidence is not known.

PATHOPHYSIOLOGY

- The lesions are not inherited, but are believed to be due to genetic mosaicism causing a developmental defect of the fetal melanocyte.
- On histologic examination, the melanocytes appear normal in number and shape.
- On electron microscopy, melanocytes show aggregated melanosomes of variable morphology and a decrease in the overall number of melanosomes.

CLINICAL FEATURES

- Presents as congenital, patchy hypopigmented macules or patches with feathery borders, often with a distinct ventral midline demarcation.
- Lesions are unilateral and typically follow one of two patterns: isolated or segmental. Those that are segmental can be either contiguous or noncontiguous.
- Lesions are found more commonly on the trunk, neck, face, and proximal extremities.
- Rarely, extracutaneous abnormalities, such as hemihypertrophy, seizures, and mental retardation, can be seen.

DIAGNOSIS AND DIFFERENTIAL

- Differential diagnosis includes segmental vitiligo and hypomelanosis of Ito.
- On Wood's lamp exam, vitiligo has a chalk-white appearance while nevus depigmentosus has an off-white appearance.

TREATMENT

- Treatment is limited to cosmetic camouflage if the patient finds it necessary.
- Periodic monitoring of the patient's neurologic development throughout childhood is recommended.
- The patch is generally stable in its relative size and distribution throughout life.

REFERENCES

Di Lernia V. Segmental nevus depigmentosus: Analysis of 20 patients. *Pediatr Dermatol.* 1999;16:349.

Dohil, MA, Baugh WP, Eichenfield LF. Pediatric dermatology: Vascular and pigmented birthmarks. *Pediatr Clin North Am.* 2000;47:783.

Lee HS, Chun YS, Hann SK. Nevus depigmentosus: Clinical features and histopathologic characteristics in 67 patients. *J Am Acad Dermatol.* 1999;40:21.

Nehal KS, PeBenito R, Orlow SJ. Analysis of 54 cases of hypopigmentation and hyperpigmentation along the lines of Blaschko. *Arch Dermatol.* 1996;132:1167.

NEVUS ANEMICUS

- Nevus anemicus is a congenital lesion that was first described by Vorner in 1906.

EPIDEMIOLOGY

- Most often seen in females.
- Prevalence is not known.

PATHOPHYSIOLOGY

- It has been suggested that the defect is due to increased sensitivity of the blood vessels to catecholamines.

CLINICAL FEATURES

- Nevus anemicus is characterized by macules of varying sizes and shapes that are paler than the surrounding skin and cannot be made red by trauma, cold, or heat.
- The patches are usually round and well defined with irregular edges. Often smaller white macules are seen beyond the border of the largest lesion.
- Most frequently observed on the chest or back, although can be found anywhere on the body.
- It resembles vitiligo but affected skin contains a normal amount of melanin.

DIAGNOSIS AND DIFFERENTIAL

- Affected skin does not respond with a flare after rubbing, but surrounding skin does respond.
- The lesion is most often confused with tinea versicolor or vitiligo. Leprosy and tuberous sclerosis can also be considered in the differential.
- Affected skin does not enhance with Wood's light and does not produce scale.
- Nevus anemicus can be distinguished by diascopy. With diascopy, the lesion becomes indistinguishable from the blanched surrounding skin.

TREATMENT

- Cosmetic camouflage if desired by patient.
- Although usually benign, nevus anemicus may be linked with certain genodermatoses, including

neurofibromatosis and phakomatosis pigmentovascularis; therefore patients should be evaluated.

- Nevus anemicus generally grows with the child and then remains unchanged over the patient's lifetime.

REFERENCES

Ahkami RN, Schwartz RA. Nevus anemicus. *Dermatology.* 1999;198:327.

Greaves MW, Birkett D, Johnson C. Nevus anemicus: A unique catecholamine-dependent nevus. *Arch Dermatol.* 1970; 102:172.

Mountcastle EA, Diestelmeier MR, Lupton GP. Nevus anemicus. *J Am Acad Dermatol.* 1986;14:628.

Requena L, Sangueza OP. Cutaneous vascular anomalies. Part I. Hamartomas, malformations, and dilation of preexisting vessels. *J Am Acad Dermatol.* 1997;37:523.

IDIOPATHIC GUTTATE HYPOMELANOSIS

- Idiopathic guttate hypomelanosis, also known as leukopathia symmetrica progressiva, is a condition seen almost universally in fair-skinned elderly people.
- It presents with white spots on the arms and legs, and is related to lack of pigmentary protection from sun and sun exposure rather than to age.

EPIDEMIOLOGY

- Guttate hypomelanosis is a very common condition most commonly seen on fair-skinned middle-aged to elderly individuals with a history of a high degree of sun exposure.
- It is more commonly seen in women beginning around age 30. However, with increasing age and sun exposure, it is found almost equally in elderly men and women.

PATHOPHYSIOLOGY

- As skin pigmentation is due to an integration of melanocyte and keratinocyte function, an acquired defect of the epidermal melanin unit results in the observed hypopigmentation. Significantly fewer dopa oxidase-positive melanocytes are seen in the lesions.
- In some studies, the affected areas show a 50% reduction in melanocytes.

CLINICAL FEATURES

- Patients present with small (2 to 5-mm) irregularly shaped and sharply defined depigmented macules, which occur chiefly on the shins and forearms.
- Lesions can also be located on the exposed areas of the hands and forearms although they are never seen on the trunk and face.
- Typical histologic findings are epidermal atrophy, patchy absence of melanocytes and melanin, flat rete ridges, and basket weave hyperkeratosis.
- In general, patients have signs of early aging and sun exposure in the same areas, including lentigines, seborrheic keratosis, and xerosis.

DIAGNOSIS AND DIFFERENTIAL

- Differential includes pityriasis alba and vitiligo, as well as postinflammatory hypopigmentation, lichenoid eruption, and pinta.

TREATMENT

- Treatment with topical retinoids, such as tretinoin, has been reported to be useful. The use of topical and intralesional corticosteroids has also been suggested.
- Dermabrasion and cryosurgery have been used to treat guttate hypomelanosis with some success.
- Patients should be advised to avoid sun exposure and suntanning in order to prevent further progression and accentuation of the disease. They should be advised to use a broad-spectrum sunscreen daily.
- Areas can be cosmetically camouflaged if patient desires.
- Although asymptomatic, this condition will progress with increasing sun exposure and, to a lesser degree, with age.

REFERENCES

Falabella R, Escobar C, Giraldo N. On the pathogenesis of idiopathic guttate hypomelanosis. *J Am Acad Dermatol.* 1987; 16:35.

Ortonne JP, Perrot H. Idiopathic guttate hypomelanosis. Ultrastructural study. *Arch Dermatol.* 1980;116:664.

Pagnoni A, Kligman AM, Sadiq I, Stoudemayer T. Hypopigmented macules of photodamaged skin and their treatment with topical tretinoin. *Acta Derm Venereol.* 1999;79:305.

Savall R, Ferrandiz C, Ferrer I, Peyri J. Idiopathic guttate hypomelanosis. *Br J Dermatol.* 1980;103:635.

Wallace ML, Grichnik JM, Prieto VG, Shea CR. Numbers and differentiation status of melanocytes in idiopathic guttate hypomelanosis. *J Cutan Pathol.* 1998;25:375.

POSTINFLAMMATORY HYPOPIGMENTATION

- Hypopigmentation, as well as hyperpigmentation, can occur after injury or insult to the skin.

EPIDEMIOLOGY

- Although more common in darkly pigmented skin, postinflammatory hypopigmentation can be seen in all skin types on any area of skin.
- Minor conditions such as acne, eczema, and allergic reactions; as well as more serious cutaneous events such as burns, surgeries, and trauma; or treatments such as chemical peels and laser resurfacing can lead to hypopigmentation.

PATHOPHYSIOLOGY

- Hypopigmentation may result as a response of the skin to inflammation or injury.

CLINICAL FEATURES

- Hypopigmented macule at the sight of previous injury or inflammation.

DIAGNOSIS AND DIFFERENTIAL

- Diagnosis can be made based on history.
- Differential diagnosis includes atopic dermatitis and vitiligo. The diagnosis of atypical nevus must also be considered.

TREATMENT

- No treatment is necessary.
- Cosmetic camouflage can be used, although these lesions usually resolve with time.
- Pigmentary alteration may persist for weeks to months; however, patients can be reassured that these lesions are usually temporary.
- Patients must be advised that the phenomenon tends to recur in susceptible individuals.

PITYRIASIS ALBA

- Also known as pityriasis streptogenes, furfuraceous impetigo, pityriasis simplex, pityriasis sicca faciei, and erythema streptogenes.

EPIDEMIOLOGY

- The disease is most common in children ages 3 to 16 years. Up to one third of school-aged children may have this disorder.
- The disease seems to be more common in patients with a history of atopy.

PATHOPHYSIOLOGY

- The cause is unknown, although it appears to be associated with atopy.
- Hypopigmentation is believed to be caused by mild dermal inflammation and the UV screening effect of the scaly skin.

CLINICAL FEATURES

- Presents with multiple hypopigmented round or oval scaling patches of the face, upper arms, neck, or shoulders.
- Lesions are usually more noticeable in dark-skinned individuals, and often appear after suntanning in lighter-skinned individuals.
- Lesions usually range in size from 0.5 to 2 cm in diameter but may be larger, especially on the trunk.

DIAGNOSIS AND DIFFERENTIAL

- Differential diagnosis includes vitiligo, tinea versicolor, discoid eczema, hypopigmented mycosis fungoides, leprosy, and psoriasis.

TREATMENT

- Pityriasis alba usually resolves spontaneously and does not require treatment.
- Emollients and bland lubricant use should be encouraged.
- Low-strength corticosteroid creams, either alone or in combination with Lac-Hydrin (lactic acid 12%), have been reported to be successful in treatment.

- Healing usually occurs spontaneously within several months to a few years.
- The degree of hypopigmentation is not affected by treatment.

REFERENCES

Beltrani VS. The clinical spectrum of atopic dermatitis. Allergy Clin Immunol. 1999;104:S87.

Dhar S, Kanwar AJ, Dawn G. Pigmenting pityriasis alba. *Pediatr Dermatol.* 1995;12:197.

Galan EB, Janniger CK. Pityriasis alba. *Cutis.* 1998;61:11.

Pinto FJ, Bolognia JL. Disorders of hypopigmentation in children. *Pediatr Clin North Am.* 1991;38:991.

Vargas-Ocampo F. Pityriasis alba: A histologic study. *Int J Dermatol.* 1993;32:870.

17 CUTANEOUS MANIFESTATIONS OF SYSTEMIC DISEASE

Angeles Flórez
Manuel Cruces
Gloria P. Jiménez

SARCOIDOSIS

- Sarcoidosis is a systemic disease characterized by non-caseating granuloma formation.
- It involves mainly the skin, lymphatic system, lungs, eyes, liver, spleen, glandular tissues, central nervous system (CNS), and bones.
- It has also been known as Bernier's lupus pernio, Besnier–Boeck's disease, Boeck's sarcoid, and Schamberg's benign lymphogranulomatosis.

EPIDEMIOLOGY

- Presents between ages 20 and 40.
- Blacks are three times more likely to develop sarcoidosis than whites, and the course of the disease is more severe.
- Black females are affected twice as often as men, while white females are affected in the same proportion to white men.
- It is more prevalent in Scandinavian countries, but can occur worldwide.
- In the United States, the southeastern states and some areas of New York show the highest prevalence.

ETIOLOGY

- The etiology is still unclear.
- Sarcoidosis is generally considered an immune-mediated disease with a Th-1 profile response taking place in genetically susceptible hosts. The disease is likely to represent a granulomatous reaction to an undefined antigen.

CLINICAL FEATURES

- Skin involvement is present in up to 35% of patients and usually manifests early in the clinical course of the disease.
- Cutaneous lesions have been classified into specific or nonspecific based on histopathologic criteria.
- Cutaneous lesions are considered specific when they contain sarcoid granulomas and nonspecific when they represent a reactive process. There is a broad morphologic variety.
- Specific lesions can be maculopapular, plaque-type, subcutaneous nodules, infiltrated scars, and lupus pernio.
- Maculopapular lesions are the most frequent type of specific skin involvement. They are asymptomatic, flesh-colored to violaceous, and slightly infiltrated. They are commonly located on the face, with characteristic periorificial distribution. The nape of the neck, trunk, and extremities may also be affected. They are generally acute and considered a sign of good prognosis.
- Skin plaques are infiltrated, round or oval, purplish-red lesions occurring on the face, back, buttocks, and limbs. They can be present on the scalp and can cause scarring alopecia.
- Subcutaneous nodules are mobile, nontender lesions, which arise deep in the dermis and subcutaneous tissue without epidermal involvement.
- Quiescent scars and areas subject to chronic trauma are frequently infiltrated by sarcoid granulomas, becoming indurated and purple-colored.
- Lupus pernio is characterized by swollen, bluish-red, and indurated plaques located on the nose, ears, malar aspect of the face, and fingers. This form tends to be scarring and chronic.
- Other specific although unusual forms include erythrodermic, ichthyosiform, lichenoid, ulcerated, verrucose, atrophic, and psoriasiform sarcoidosis.

NONSPECIFIC LESIONS

- The most frequent nonspecific skin lesion is erythema nodosum. It generally presents acutely and is associated with a benign prognosis, affects younger patients, and is described as being tender, erythematous to purple-colored cutaneous nodules located on the anterior tibial area.
- Other unusual nonspecific lesions include erythema multiforme, prurigo, calcifications, and nail involvement.

THE SKIN IN ASSESSMENT FOR SYSTEMIC DISEASE

- Maculopapular lesions have been associated with acute systemic involvement such as pulmonary involvement, uveitis, parotitis, and lymph node enlargement.
- Skin plaques have been associated with chronic disease, mainly with lung, spleen, and lymph node involvement.
- Lupus pernio is frequently associated with upper respiratory tract involvement, bone cysts, pulmonary fibrosis, and chronic uveitis.
- The association of erythema nodosum and bilateral hiliar adenopathy with or without fever, iritis, uveitis, and polyarthritis is known as Lofgren's syndrome. It affects young patients and it is generally self-limited.

DIAGNOSIS AND DIFFERENTIAL

- The prognosis of sarcoidosis depends on systemic involvement, which must be ruled out in all patients with sarcoid granulomas of the skin.
- Work-up should include a complete history and physical examination, pulmonary screening (chest radiography and pulmonary function tests such as spirometry and diffusing capacity measurements), tuberculin skin test, ophthalmologic examination (slit lamp and fundoscopy), electrocardiogram, and blood analysis including a complete blood cell count, liver and renal function tests, and calcium levels.
- Angiotensin-converting enzyme levels are considered of limited value since they are neither very specific nor very sensitive, and are not a useful guide to determine the extent of systemic involvement.
- More complex investigations such as computed tomography scanning, CNS magnetic resonance imaging, and bronchoalveolar lavage should only be performed when there is firm suspicion of organ involvement.
- The differential diagnosis is vast since sarcoid can mimic almost any dermatologic entity.

HISTOPATHOLOGY

- Sarcoid granulomas are well-defined groups of epithelioid cells without necrosis.

- Lymphocytes are sparse and located at the periphery of the islands. Giant cells can be observed and may contain Schaumamn or conchoids bodies (altered lisosomes) and stellate asteroid bodies (entrapped collagen).
- The presence of polarizable foreign bodies in cutaneous lesions cannot exclude sarcoidosis.
- Stains and cultures must be performed to rule out infections with bacteria, mycobacterium, and/or fungi.

TREATMENT

- Oral steroids are the first-line treatment for sarcoidosis but are only recommended when serious systemic involvement or chronic disfiguring cutaneous lesions are present.
- Other therapies considered helpful in treating cutaneous lesions are topical or intralesional steroids, antimalarial drugs, methotrexate, cyclosporine, allopurinol, and low doses of thalidomide.
- Surgery can be useful in disfiguring refractory cases and ulcerative lesions.

REFERENCES

Cancrini C, Angelini F, Colavita M, et al. Erythema nodosum: A presenting sign of early onset sarcoidosis. *Clin Exp Rheumatol.* 1998;16:337.

Conron M, Du Bois RM. Immunological mechanisms in sarcoidosis. *Clin Exp Allergy.* 2001;31:543.

Elgart ML. Cutaneous sarcoidosis: Definitions and types of lesions. *Clin Dermatol.* 1986;4:35.

English JC III, Patel PJ, Greer KE. Sarcoidosis. *J Am Acad Dermatol.* 2001;44:725.

Johns CJ, Michelle TM. The clinical management of sarcoidosis: A 50-year experience at the Johns Hopkins Hospital. *Medicine.* 1999;78:65.

Katta R, Nelson B, Chen D, et al. Sarcoidosis of the scalp: A case series and review of the literature. *J Am Acad Dermatol.* 2000;42:690.

Losada-Campa A, de la Torre-Fraga C, Gómez de Liaño A, et al. Histopathology of nail sarcoidosis. *Acta Derm Venerol.* 1995;75:404.

Mañá J, Marcoval J, Graells J, et al. Cutaneous involvement in sarcoidosis. Relationship to systemic disease. *Arch Dermatol.* 1997;133:882.

Marcoval J, Mañá J, Moreno A, et al. Foreign bodies in granulomatous cutaneous lesions of patients with systemic sarcoidosis. *Arch Dermatol.* 2001;137:427.

Newman LS, Rose CS, Maier LA. Sarcoidosis. *N Engl J Med.* 1997;336:1224.

Young III RJ, Gilson RT, Yanase D, et al. Cutaneous sarcoidosis. *Int J Dermatol.* 2001;40:249.

NEUROCUTANEOUS SYNDROMES

- Neurocutaneous syndromes are a heterogeneous group of entities characterized by dyplasia or neoplasia of embryonic ectoderm derived tissues, mainly the nervous system, eyes, and skin.

NEUROFIBROMATOSIS

- Neurofibromatosis (NF) is a group of disorders transmitted in an autosomal dominant fashion with many cases arising from spontaneous mutations.

EPIDEMIOLOGY

- The two major forms of the disease are NF I and NF II.
- NF I, or von Recklinghausen's disease, is the most common type, representing around 85% of all cases.
- The incidence of NF I is one in 3500 live births, and 50% of cases are due to spontaneous mutations.
- The incidence of NF II in the Caucasian population is estimated at one in 35,000 to 40,000 live births.

ETIOLOGY

- Neurofibromatosis is an autosomal dominantly inherited disease, except for type IV.
- The gene of NF I is on region 17q11.2, and codes for neurofibrimin, which regulates signals transduced by Ras proteins.
- NF II is on the long arm of chromosome 22q11-q13 and encodes for merlin (schwannomin), a protein that links the actin cytoskeleton to cell surface glycoproteins and functions as a negative growth regulator; from these about 20% are considered sporadic, but they are actually mosaic for their mutation.

CLINICAL FEATURES

- NF I is characterized by the presence of hyperpigmented macules, intertriginous freckling, multiple neurofibromas, and iris hamartomas (Lisch nodules).
- NF II is defined by the following findings: hyperpigmented macules, dermal neurofibromas, and CNS tumors.
- NF III is a mixed form between NF I and NF II.
- NF IV combines widespread neurofibromas and café-au-lait macules.

- NF V is a segmental type consisting of neurofibromas and/or café-au-lait macules in a dermatomal distribution.
- NF VI is characterized by numerous café-au-lait macules without neurofibromas.
- NF VII is defined by the appearance of neurofibromas after the third decade of life.
- NF VIII represents all forms that do not fit in the previous categories. It is not yet known whether is inherited or not.
- Café-au-lait macules are well-defined, hyperpigmented macules mainly located on the trunk and extremities. They are generally the first skin sign. To be considered a criterion for diagnosis, there should be six or more lesions and they should be larger than 1.5 cm in diameter in postpubertal individuals and over 5 mm in greatest diameter in prepuberty.
- Cutaneous manifestations are critical to the diagnosis, since café-au-lait macules can be present at birth or early childhood.
- Axillary freckling (Crowe's sign) may occur also in the neck and inguinal area. Intertriginous freckling is commonly present by school age.
- NF I neurofibromas can be dermal, subcutaneous, and plexiform. NF II neurofibromas are only dermal. Dermal neurofibromas can be sesil or pedunculated, soft, flesh-colored, pink or brown lesions, which can be flattened by palpation. They can be painful.
- Subcutaneous neurofibromas are firm lesions covered by normal skin, which follow peripheral nerves and may also be painful.
- Plexiform neurofibromas are soft, diffuse, elongated, tumor-like lesions with an irregular consistency, mainly located on the neck and extremities along the course of a nerve (trigeminal, or upper cervical). These lesions are mostly present at birth, generally covered by a hyperpigmented, hairy, and thickened skin, causing cosmetic disfigurement.
- Neurofibromas are often congenital, appear around puberty, and increase in number and size during early adulthood. Xanthogranulomas and bronzing or hyperpigmentation of the skin may be present.
- Patients can develop acromegaly, cretinism, hyperparathyroidism myxedema, pheochromocytoma, precocious puberty, paralysis due to spinal neuromas, lordosis, kyphosis, pseudoarthritis, mental retardation, spina bifida malformation, and traumatic fractures.
- Neurofibromatosis type I patients are four times more prone to develop malignancies. Neurofibrosarcomas, malignant schawannomas, Wilms's tumor, rhabdomyosarcomas, gastrointestinal malignancies, and chronic myelogenous leukemia have been reported.

DIAGNOSIS AND DIFFERENTIAL

- Every patient with NF I must undergo a periodic complete physical examination with emphasis on ophthalmologic, neurologic, orthopedic, and endocrinologic evaluations.
- Lisch nodules, which are melanocytic hamartomas of the iris, are the most common manifestation of NF I and usually appear during childhood. When multiple, these lesions are pathognomonic for NF I.
- Possible complications include optic nerve glioma, brain and spinal tumors (schwannomas and astrocytomas), malignant peripheral nerve sheath tumors, scoliosis, thinning of long bone cortex with or without pseudoartrosis, sphenoid and vertebral dysplasia, and a pheochromocytoma.
- Patients with NF II should undergo periodic audiologic, neurologic, and ophthalmologic evaluations to detect vestibular schwannomas, spinal tumors, and pre-senile cataracts.
- Initial brain and spine MRIs have been recommended, and further studies should be performed according to the clinical findings.
- First-degree relatives must be examined and genetic counseling must be performed.
- Differential diagnosis includes McCune–Albright syndrome characterized by polyostotic fibrous dysplasia, irregular pigmentation of the skin, and sexual precocity. Watson syndrome, characterized by the presence of café-au-lait macules, intellectual impairment, and pulmonary stenosis, should also be considered. Proteus syndrome, which appears with cerebriform masses of palms and soles, subcutaneous masses, mesodermal malformations, hypertrophy and scoliosis, is also in the differential.

HISTOPATHOLOGY

- Café-au-lait macules and intertriginous freckles exhibit an increased number and melanin content of skin melanocytes.
- Neurofibromas consist of arborizing Schwann cells within a collagenous matrix and eosinophilic, thin wavy spindle cells with spindle-shaped nuclei.
- Mast cells and mucin are increased.
- Giant melanosomes may be seen.

TREATMENT

- Genetic counseling to identify the children at risk.
- Learning disabilities should be approached early.

- NF I patients should undergo age-specific cancer screening.
- Neurofibromas can be excised for aesthetic reasons, patient discomfort, organ involvement, or malignant transformation.
- Laser therapy with the Q-switched ruby, Q-switched Nd YAG and Q-switched alexandrite lasers have shown variable response.

REFERENCES

Evans DG, Sainio M, Baser ME. Neurofibromatosis type 2. *J Med Genet.* 2001;37:897.

Krishnan RS, Angel TA, Orengo IF, et al. Bilateral segmental neurofibromatosis: A case report and review. *Int J Dermatol.* 2001;40:401.

Neurofibromatosis conference statement. National Institutes of Health consensus development conference. *Arch Neurol.* 1988;45:575.

Pinson S, Créange A, Barbarot S, et al. Neurofibromatosis 1: Recommendations pour la prise en charge. *Ann Derm Venereol.* 2001;128:567.

Ross KL, Muckway M. Neurofibromatosis. *Dermatol Clin.* 1995;13:105.

Sehgal VN, Sharma RC. Common genodermatoses. *Int J Dermatol.* 1996;35:685.

Wolkenstein P, Frèche B, Zeller J, et al. Usefulness of screening investigations in neurofibromatosis type I. *Arch Dermatol.* 1996;132:1333.

TUBEROUS SCLEROSIS (EPILOIA, BOURNEVILLES'S DISEASE)

- Tuberous sclerosis is an autosomal dominant disorder with a high rate of spontaneous mutations.
- It is also called epiloia (epi = epilepsy, loi = low intelligence, a = adenoma sebaceum), and tuberous sclerosis complex (TBSC).
- Patients with tuberous sclerosis can presents with seizures, mental retardation, facial angiofibromas, periungual fibromas, shagreen patches, and "ash leaf" macules.
- It is characterized by a spectrum of hamartomatous malformations with particular involvement of the brain, skin, eyes, kidneys, lung, and heart, but can affect almost any organ.

EPIDEMIOLOGY

- Tuberous sclerosis presents in one in 5800 to 15,000 live births. It is a common inherited autosomal dominant disease with highly variable penetrance.

- 50% of the cases may occur as a result as spontaneous mutations.

ETIOLOGY

- Autosomal dominant with two gene mutations, namely TSC1 and TSC2.
- TSC1 and TSC2 are tumor suppressor genes.
- TSC1 is present in chromosome 9q34 and encodes hamartin a protein with no significant homology to tuberin or any other vertebrate protein.
- TSC2 presents in 6p13.3 and encodes tuberin, a putative GTPase-activating protein for rap1 and rab5.
- Hamartin and tuberin associate physically in vivo, suggesting that they function in the same complex. This interaction explains the indistinguishable phenotypes caused by mutations in either gene.

CLINICAL FEATURES

- Ash-leaf spots, adenoma sebaceum, shagreen patches, subungueal and periungueal fibromas, forehead fibrous plaques, café-au-lait spots, and molluscum fibrosum pendulum are the recognized cutaneous signs.
- Ash-leaf spots are hypomelanotic macules measuring 1 to 3 cm and usually located asymmetrically on the trunk and buttocks. They are the most frequent skin sign (found in around 90% of cases), and are best seen with Wood's lamp examination. Hypopigmented macules can be smaller and multiple adopting a confetti-like pattern.
- Adenoma sebaceum are red-pink, small papules with glistening surfaces and symmetrically distributed over the cheeks, nose, and chin. They generally develop in early childhood.
- Shagreen patches are well-defined, yellowish, elevated, cobble-stoned plaques usually located on the lumbosacral region. They usually develop during puberty.
- Subungual and periungual fibromas (Koenen's tumors) are flesh-colored lesions usually at the edge of the nail plate, more commonly seen on the toes, and present in puberty or in early adulthood.
- Forehead fibrous plaques are flesh-colored or yellowish elevated plaques, which are located on the scalp, forehead, or eyelids.
- Café-au-lait spots are hyperpigmented macules, generally solitary and more frequent on the trunk and extremities.
- Molluscum fibrosum pendulum refers to soft pedunculated fibromas mainly observed on the neck, axillae, and groin.
- Fibromas in the gums, palate, and pits in deciduous and/or permanent teeth have also been described.

HISTOPATHOLOGY

- Hypopigmented macules show a normal number of melanocytes with a reduced number and melanization of melanosomes.
- Adenoma sebaceum, forehead fibrous plaques, and Koenen's tumors are angiofibromas. Shagreen patches are connective tissue hamartomas.

DIAGNOSIS AND DIFFERENTIAL

- Cutaneous manifestations are critical to the diagnosis since ash-leaf spots frequently are the earliest manifestation, can be present at birth, and are an indication for skull x-ray evaluation. CT scan ultrasonagraphy or MRI is necessary to evaluated intracranial nodules. Funduscopic examination, hand and foot x-ray evaluation, and renal ultrasound are also indicated.
- Every patient must undergo complete physical examinations in order to assess the following involvement: CNS (brain tubers, subependimal nodules, giant cell astrocytomas, seizures, and mental retardation); ocular (retinal hamartomas); genitourinary (renal angiomyolipomas and renal cysts); cardiovascular (cardiac rhabdomyomas); skeletal (cysts and sclerotic lesions); and pulmonary (lymphangiomyomatosis).
- First-degree relatives must be examined and genetic counseling must be performed.
- Molecular analysis for TSC1 and TCS2 mutation are not regularly available.

TREATMENT

- Conventional excision, electrodessication, and laser surgery can be performed on the cutaneous lesions, but recurrence may occur requiring repeating treatments.

REFERENCES

Bernauer TA, Mirowski GW, Caldemeyer KS. Tuberous sclerosis. Part II. Musculoskeletal and visceral findings. *J Am Acad Dermatol.* 2001;45:450.

Caldemeyer KS, Mirowski GW. Tuberous sclerosis. Part I. Clinical and central.

Clinical and central nervous system findings. *J Am Acad Dermatol.* 2001;45:448.

Józwiak S, Schwartz RA, Janniger CK, et al. Skin lesions in children with tuberous sclerosis complex: Their prevalence, natural course, and diagnostic significance. *Int J Dermatol.* 1998;37:911.

Webb DW, Clarke A, Fryer A, et al. The cutaneous features of tuberous sclerosis: A population study. *Br J Dermatol.* 1996;135:1.

STURGE–WEBER SYNDROME (ENCEPHALOTRIGEMINAL ANGIOMATOSIS)

- Sturge–Weber syndrome (SWS) is a rare congenital sporadic disease. The full-blown condition consists of vascular malformations involving the trigeminal (V) areas of the face, brain, leptomeninges, and the eye.

EPIDEMIOLOGY

- The location and extent of the port-wine stain determine the risk for the development of SWS.
- 10% of patients with V1 port-wine stain will develop SWS, and 40% of these have bilateral involvement. Those with V1, V2, and V3 or bilateral port-wine stains are at highest risk (25%) of developing the syndrome.

CLINICAL FEATURES

- Port-wine stain or nevus flammeus involving the ophthalmic branch of the trigeminal nerve and less frequently the maxillary and mandibular areas defines the condition.
- Cutaneous involvement can be bilateral and disseminated.
- Neuro-ocular involvement generally develops during childhood and adolescence (seizures, mental retardation, hemiparesis, glaucoma, and choroidal hemangiomas).
- Ipsilateral choroidal angiomatosis may lead to retinal dysfunction, anterior displacement of the retina with amblyopia, retinal detachment, ectopic bone formation, and retinal degeneration.
- Ocular manifestation affects 50% of patients.
- Homolateral leptomeningeal angiomatosis, when present, may clinically manifest as epilepsy, mental retardation, hemiplegia, hemisensory defects, and homonymous hemianopsia.

HISTOPATHOLOGY

- Nevus flammeus consists of vascular ectasia without endothelial proliferation.

DIAGNOSIS AND DIFFERENTIAL

- Port-wine stain is usually present at birth. Patients must undergo neurologic and ophthalmologic evaluations soon after birth.

- Radiologic calcifications of the brain parenchyma (tram lines) are present in early childhood (after 1 year of age). CT or MRI can confirm these calcifications. Electroencephalogram usually shows brain involvement.

TREATMENT

- Laser surgery with flashlamp pumped pulsed-dye laser is the first line therapy for port-wine stain, resulting in significant fading, which may help prevent soft tissue hypertrophy.
- Cosmetic fading, cryotherapy, and conventional surgery can also be performed.

REFERENCES

Boukobza M, Enjolras O, Cambra M, et al. Sturge–Weber syndrome. The current neuroradiologic data. *J Radiol.* 2000; 81:765.
Mirowski GW, An-Ti Liu A, Stone ML, et al. Sturge–Weber syndrome. *J Am Acad Dermatol.* 1999;41:772.

ATAXIA-TELANGIECTASIA (LOUIS–BAR SYNDROME)

- Ataxia-telangiectasia is an autosomal recessive disorder defined by progressive cerebellar ataxia and oculocutaneous telangiectasias and sinovascular infection.

ETIOLOGY

- Ataxia-telangiectasia is transmitted as an autosomal recessive trait. Heterozygotes can also manifest the disease.
- The mutated ATM gene is a member of the phosphatidylinositol-3-kinase-like family of enzymes that are involved in cell-cycle control, meiotic recombination, telomere length monitoring, and DNA-damage response.
- Affected cells are hypersensitive to ionizing radiation and are defective at the G1/S checkpoint after damage.
- The ATM gene is located on chromosome 11q22.3.
- Translocations are particularly common in chromosomes 7 and 14.

EPIDEMIOLOGY

- Affected patients are believed to be 10% more likely to develop malignancies usually before the age of 15.

- Homozygous patients also have a 100 times higher risk of breast cancer.

CLINICAL FEATURES

- The ataxia is usually first noted when the child begins to walk.
- The cutaneous telangiectasias are mainly located on sun-exposed areas. Other cutaneous manifestations include pigmentary anomalies (vitiligo, premature gray hair of the scalp, mottled hyper- and hypopigmentation (café-au-lait spots), cutaneous granulomas, poikilodermatous and sclerotic lesions, xeroderma, seborrheic and atopic dermatitis, hirsutism, acanthosis nigricans, and cutaneous infections. By the time cutaneous manifestations appear, the disorder has generally been diagnosed.
- Neurologic involvement initially consisting of ataxia, arreflexia, hypotonia, and choreathetosis movements are commonly present by the second year of life, and bulbar telangiectases by ages 4 to 6 years.
- Patients may have a marked IgA deficiency, with decreased lymphocytes and small abscesses in the thymus.
- The most common types of malignancies are B-cell lymphomas and leukemias. Homozygotes have in addition a markedly increased risk for breast cancer (100 times higher) compared to heterzygotes.
- Hyperinsulinism with insulin resistance, hypogonadism with delayed sexual development, and growth retardation are possible.
- Recurrent sinopulmonary infections with eventual bronchiectasis, respiratory failure, and death are common.
- Death usually occurs by late childhood or early adolescence.

HISTOPATHOLOGY

- Telangiectasias are dilated subpapillary venous plexuses.

DIAGNOSIS AND DIFFERENTIAL

- Patients must be monitored since they have increased risk of malignancies and sinopulmonary infections.
- Prenatal diagnosis is best achieved measuring amniotic alpha-fetoprotein levels. Serum alpha-fetoprotein levels can be measured during childhood.
- Differential diagnoses include xeroderma pigmentosa and Bloom's syndrome.

TREATMENT

- Genetic counseling must be provided.
- Early detection of malignancy is mandatory.
- Telangiectasias can be treated with laser surgery.
- Early treatment of infection.

REFERENCES

Arbiser JL. Genetic immunodeficiencies: Cutaneous manifestations and recent progress. *J Am Acad Dermatol.* 1995; 33:82.

Cohen LE, Tanner DJ, Schaefer HG, et al. Common and uncommon cutaneous findings in patients with ataxia-telangiectasia. *J Am Acad Dermatol.* 1984;10:431.

Khumalo NP, Joss DV, Huson SM, et al. Pigmentary anomalies in ataxia-telangiectasia: A clue to diagnosis and an example of twin spotting. *Br J Dermatol.* 2001;144:369.

Paller AS, Massey RB, Curtis MA, et al. Cutaneous granulomatous lesions in patients with ataxia-telangiectasia. *J Pediatr.* 1991;119:917.

Smith LL, Conerly SL. Ataxia-telangiectasia or Louis–Bar syndrome. *J Am Acad Dermatol.* 1985;12:681.

ENDOCRINOPATHIES

DIABETES MELLITUS

- Cutaneous disorders affecting diabetic patients are frequent. Their exact pathogenesis is unknown, although they have been attributed to macroangiopathy, microangiopathy, and neuropathy; immunologic disturbances also play a role.
- Many disorders have been associated with diabetes. Necrobiosis lipoidica diabeticorum (NLD), diabetic bullae, diabetic dermopahty, limited joint mobility, waxy skin syndrome, sclerema diabeticorum, perforating disorders, and cutaneous infection will be discussed in this section.

NECROBIOSIS LIPOIDICA DIABETICORUM

- Necrobiosis lipoidica diabeticorum (NLD) is a well-known cutaneous marker of diabetes mellitus. Both insulin-dependent and non-insulin-dependent diabetes mellitus (IDDM and NIDDM) can manifest NLD lesions.

EPIDEMIOLOGY

- At onset of the disorder, most patients (60%) will already have established DM.
- Incidence is 3 to 7 per 1000 diabetic patients.
- Although it has been associated with severe DM, its evolution is considered independent of glycemic control.
- Preceding trauma is a possible precipitating factor.
- It is three times more frequent in females than males, and is more frequent in young patients.

CLINICAL FEATURES

- Characterized by well-defined erythematous plaques that evolve into annular lesions with a depressed, yellowish, atrophic, telangiectatic center with a raised, reddish, scaly periphery.
- The plaques may ulcerate and are generally (85% of cases) located on the lower extremities, mainly on the pretibial areas.
- Squamous cell carcinoma may occur in chronic ulcers.

HISTOPATHOLOGY

- Evolved plaques show collagen degeneration mainly in the lower dermis. Palisaded granulomatous infiltrate appears around the area of degenerated collagen. Fatty deposits are present in the upper dermis, imparting the yellowish discoloration of the lesion.

DIAGNOSIS AND DIFFERENTIAL

- Granuloma annulare can be ruled out due to the absence of mucin at the center of the granulomas.

TREATMENT

- Lesions can resolve spontaneously and a conservative approach is recommended.
- Symptomatic, active, or ulcerative lesions can be treated with topical or intralesional steroids.
- Topical bovine collagen and cyclosporine have been reported for the treatment of chronic ulcers.
- Skin grafting after excision showed some benefit while others have had recurrent ulcers within skin grafts.
- Aspirin, dypiridamole, pentoxifyline, perilesional heparin injections, intravenous prostaglandin E_1, and hyperbaric oxygen have also been anedotically reported to be useful.

DIABETIC BULLAE

- Spontaneous, noninflammatory painless blistering, most common in acral locations, which can heal spontaneously in a few weeks.

ETIOLOGY

- Neuropathy, trauma, and ultraviolet light have been reported as inciting factors to the blistering.

EPIDEMIOLOGY

- It is more frequent in adult men and has been associated with severe, chronic DM with peripheral neuropathy.

CLINICAL FEATURES

- Bullae are usually sterile, arise spontaneously, are often bilateral with a noninflamed base, and resolve without atrophy.
- Rarely, diabetic bullae are hemorrhagic blisters healing with scarring and atrophy.

HISTOPATHOLOGY

- The bullae show intraepidermal cleavage without acantholysis.
- In the case of hemorrhagic and scarring blisters the cleavage is subepidermal.
- Electron microscopic examination shows separation at the lamina lucida level.

DIAGNOSIS AND DIFFERENTIAL

- This is an uncommon but recognized marker of diabetes.

TREATMENT

- Protective measures and avoidance of infection.

DIABETIC DERMOPATHY ("SHIN SPOTS")

EPIDEMIOLOGY

- Diabetic dermopathy is the most common cutaneous lesion of DM, although it is not a specific marker for DM.

- It is more frequent in adult men and its incidence correlates with the severity of the disease.

CLINICAL FEATURES

- Presents as multiple, bilateral, reddish scaly papules, which progress into hyperpigmented, atrophic scars.
- Shin spots, as the name implies, are often located on the pretibial areas.

HISTOPATHOLOGY

- Minor collagen changes and thickening of dermal blood vessel walls are seen.

TREATMENT

- There is no specific treatment.
- Protection from trauma is recommended.

LIMITED JOINT MOBILITY AND WAXY SKIN SYNDROME

EPIDEMIOLOGY

- It occurs in 30 to 50% of diabetic patients with chronic disease.
- This disease is more common, although not exclusive, in young insulin-dependent diabetics.

CLINICAL FEATURES

- Patients present with reduction of mobility and thickening of the skin affecting the interphalangeal and metacarpophalangeal joints.
- The disorder is otherwise asymptomatic and symmetric, and it generally begins in the fifth digit.
- Involvement of the lower extremities contributes to chronic ulcerations, which is infection prone and poses a risk for limb amputation.
- It is associated with microvascular complications such as nephropathy, neuropathy, and retinopathy.

HISTOPATHOLOGY

- Thickening of dermal collagen and reduction of elastic fibers, eccrine glands, and hair follicles.

TREATMENT

- Physical therapy, surgery, and corticosteroid injection can be of benefit in some cases with severe symptoms.

SCLEREMA DIABETICORUM

EPIDEMIOLOGY

- This condition has been associated with poorly controlled NIDDM and microvascular complications in obese, middle-aged men.

CLINICAL FEATURES

- This is a chronic, symmetric, and asymptomatic disorder that primary involves the neck, shoulders, and upper trunk.
- The lesion is characterized by an overall induration with shiny skin plaques on the upper back, neck, and shoulders.

HISTOPATHOLOGY

- Thickened dermis with swollen collagen bundles separated by an accumulation of mucin.

TREATMENT

- There is no specific treatment.

PERFORATING DERMATOSES

EPIDEMIOLOGY

- The disorder has been associated with chronic renal failure and/or diabetes mellitus (IDDM and NIDDM).

CLINICAL FEATURES

- These lesions manifest as multiple, hyperkeratotic, umbilicated, itchy papules that may be linear and are mainly located on the extensor surfaces.

HISTOPATHOLOGY

- Hyperplasic epidermis with an area of transepidermal elimination of granular material mainly composed of collagen and elastic fibers.

TREATMENT

- Topical or intralesional steroids. Ultraviolet therapy and topical tretinoin for pruritus have been used with some success.

CUTANEOUS INFECTIONS

- Diabetics are more susceptible to bacterial and fungal cutaneous infections, especially in patients with poor glycemic control.
- The most frequent infections include Candida, erythrasma (an intertrigo due to *Corynebacterium minutissimum*), and bacterial infections caused by *Staphylococcus aureus* and beta-hemolytic streptococci.
- Patients who become ketoacidotic may be infected by otherwise nonpathogenic microorganisms such as Phycomycetes, and suffer from disseminated and deep fungal infections.

OTHER CUTANEOUS DISORDERS ASSOCIATED WITH DIABETES MELLITUS

- Other cutaneous disorders include neurotrophic ulcers, yellow skin, lichen planus, eruptive xanthomas, acanthosis nigricans, lipodystrophy, clear-cell syringomas, rubeosis of the face malignant external otitis resulting from pseudomonas, Dupuytren's contracture, generalized granuloma annulare, and vitiligo.

REFERENCES

Aljahlan M, Lee KC, Toth E, et al. Limited joint mobility in diabetes. *Postgrad Med.* 1999;105:99.

Huntley AC. The cutaneous manifestations of diabetes mellitus. *J Am Acad Dermatol.* 1982;7:427.

Jelinek JE. Cutaneous manifestations of diabetes mellitus. *Int J Dermatol.* 1994;33:605.

Perez MI, Konz SR. Cutaneous manifestations of diabetes mellitus. *J Am Acad Dermatol.* 1994;30:519.

HYPOTHYROIDISM

- Hypothyroidism is defined by a deficiency of thyroid hormones.

- This deficiency alters the skin by decelerating metabolic processes and decreasing skin blood flow.

EPIDEMIOLOGY

- Middle-aged females are the more frequently affected.
- ANOTHER (Alopecia, Nail dystrophy, Ophthalmic complications, Thyroid dysfunction, Hypohydrosis ephelides, enteropathy, and Respiratory tract infections) syndrome is an autosomal recessive disease that includes hypothyroidism.

CLINICAL FEATURES

- In hypothyroidism, the skin is typically hypohidrotic, waxy, cool to the touch, pruriginous, and rough.
- The skin can be pale, but an ivory-yellowish tint or carotenemia due to a bad hepatic metabolization of carotene can also be seen.
- Palmoplantar keratoderma, xeroderma, ichthyosiform skin, and keratosis pilaris are also frequent in hypothyroidism.
- Capillary fragility and dermal elastolysis may cause friction induced bullae and purpura.
- Tuberous and eruptive xanthomas can be seen in the context of hypercholesterolemia.
- Generalized myxedema is the most typical clinical sign of hypothyroidism. It presents as edematous, swollen skin most prominent in periorbital areas, lips, and acral locations.
- Generalized myxedema is caused by dermal edema and deposition of proteoglycans, mainly hyaluronic acid and chondroitin sulfate.
- The hair may be opaque and brittle. Growth rate is retarded with an increase in telogen hairs.
- Diffuse alopecia can be seen, but the classic pattern is the loss of the lateral third of the eyebrows and pubic and axillary hair.
- Nails grow slowly and are thin and brittle. In addition they can be striated and onycholysis (separation of nail plate from its bed) and koilonychia (spoon-shaped nails) may develop.

DIAGNOSIS AND DIFFERENTIAL

- T3, T4, and thyroid-stimulating hormone (TSH) tests are recommended for screening.

TREATMENT

- Thyroid replacement.

HYPERTHYROIDISM

- Hyperthyroidism is defined by the presence of excessive amounts of thyroid hormones responsible for a hypermetabolic state and increased cutaneous blood perfusion.

ETIOLOGY

- Graves' disease and Hashimoto's thyroiditis, among others.

EPIDEMIOLOGY

- Graves' disease has a peak onset between 20 and 30 years of age. The female to male ratio is 8 to 1.
- Hashimoto's thyroiditis has a peak age between 40 and 65, and females are more often affected than males.

CLINICAL FEATURES

- The skin is warm, moist, and soft.
- Erythema, mainly on the face, elbows, and palms, and episodic flushing, are characteristic.
- Localized or diffuse hyperpigmentation can be seen due to an increased release of adrenocorticotropic hormone in compensation for accelerated cortisol degradation.
- Pruritus is common.
- Pretibial myxedema is a typical clinical sign of Graves' disease. It consists of well-defined, raised, waxy, flesh-colored to violaceous plaques, generally bilateral and pretibial, although other locations are possible.
- Elephantiasis may develop. Mucin deposits in the dermis are responsible for this disorder.
- The hair is fine and soft. Diffuse alopecia can be present due to reduction of the anagen (growth) phase.
- The nails are shiny, brittle, and grow rapidly. They can develop a "scoop shovel" configuration with or without onycholysis, known as Plummer nails.
- Thyroid acropathy, which is rare condition associated with Graves' disease, is characterized by a triad of (1) clubbing of the fingers/toes, (2) periosteal proliferation of the phalanges and long bones, and (3) thickening and fibrosis of the subcutaneous tissue overlying bony structures.
- Pretibial myxedema and thyroid acropathy can persist despite functional treatment of the thyroid problem.

DIAGNOSIS AND DIFFERENTIAL

- Elevated serum levels of thyroid hormones.
- Thyroid stimulating hormone receptor antibody levels are elevated in 80% of patients.
- It can be confused clinically with acromegaly, pachydermoperiostosis, pulmonary osteoarthropathy, or osteoperiostitis, but radiologic findings are pathognomonic.
- Vitiligo is associated with hyperthyroidism in 7% of patients with Graves' disease but can be also seen in Hashimoto's thyroiditis.

TREATMENT

- Treatment of the underlying disease.

REFERENCES

Diven DG, Gwinup G, Newton RC, et al. The thyroid. *Dermatol Clin.* 1989;7:547.

Niepomniszcze H, Huaier Amad R. Skin disorders and thyroid diseases. *J Endocrinol Invest.* 2001;24:628.

PARANEOPLASTIC SYNDROMES

- This is a heterogeneous group of dermatoses associated with malignancies.
- A skin disorder is considered paraneoplastic when it is related to the existence of an internal malignancy and when the dermatosis and the malignant condition follow a parallel course. This means that cutaneous lesions improve when the malignancy is effectively treated and reappears when there is a relapse.
- The exact pathophysiology of these disorders remains unknown. Production of a specific hormone, growth factor, or unknown substance by the neoplasm, or an altered host response to cancer cell lines, have been the main mechanisms suggested.
- Some of these dermatoses can, however, occur in association with benign systemic diseases.

ERYTHEMA GYRATUM REPENS

CLINICAL FEATURES

- Eruption consisting of urticarial, erythematous bands with fine scales disposed in a polycyclic "wood grain" pattern. This disorder is migratory and rapidly changing.

- Lung, breast, uterus, gastric, and esophageal cancer have been described; less frequently: bladder, prostate, and cervical cancer as well as multiple myeloma have been reported.

NECROLYTIC MIGRATORY ERYTHEMA (GLUCAGONOMA SYNDROME)

CLINICAL FEATURES

- Eruption of cyclic, erythematous, scaling plaques with areas of blisters and crusted erosions.
- Lesions are generally located on the face, lower abdomen, groin, buttocks, thighs, and distal extremities.
- Cheilitis, angular stomatitis, painful atrophic glossitis, and deep venous thromboses can be associated.

DIAGNOSIS AND DIFFERENTIAL

- Laboratory findings include hypoaminoacidemia, elevated glucagon level, abnormal glucose tolerance, and anemia.
- This condition is associated with glucagon secreting alpha-cell pancreatic carcinoma.

ACANTHOSIS NIGRICANS

CLINICAL FEATURES

- Acanthosis nigricans has been classified into four main groups: malignant, inherited, endocrine, and idiopathic.
- Malignant acanthosis nigricans generally presents in patients after the age of 40 with a sudden onset, rapid progression, and severe involvement.
- Brownish-black and thickened plaques with a velvety texture, affecting the intertriginous body areas, characterize the disorder. It is generally symmetric and pruriginous.
- Mucosal involvement can be rarely found. Palmoplantar hyperkeratosis and florid cutaneous papillomatosis have been reported to coexist with malignant acanthosis nigricans.
- Adenocarcinoma of the stomach is the most frequently reported associated malignancy. Lung, breast, uterus, ovary, prostate, and lymphoreticular malignancies and sarcomas have also been recognized.

SIGN OF LESER–TRELAT

CLINICAL FEATURES

- Sudden onset or sudden increases in size of pruriginous seborrheic keratosis, adenocarcinoma of the gastrointestinal tract (mainly gastric), lymphoma, and breast and lung cancer have been associated. Its existence is controversial.

TRIPE PALMS

CLINICAL FEATURES

- Thickened, velvety and cobblestone palmar surfaces that have the aspect and texture of bovine foregut.
- Frequently associated with acanthosis nigricans.
- It is associated with lung and gastric cancer.

ACROKERATOSIS PARANEOPLASICA (BAZEX'S SYNDROME)

CLINICAL FEATURES

- Eruption of erythematous, violaceous, scaly plaques that occur symmetrically on acral sites.
- Nail dystrophy and paronychia are generally present.
- It is associated with squamous cell carcinoma of the upper digestive and respiratory tracts (supradiaphagmatic). Prostate carcinoma, multiple myeloma, and carcinoid tumors have also been reported.

ACQUIRED ICHTHYOSIS

CLINICAL FEATURES

- Acquired ichthyosis is clinically and histologically similar to ichthyosis vulgaris.
- It has been reported in association with lymphoproliferative neoplasms, mainly Hodgkin's disease, and less frequently with other lymphomas including leukemia and multiple myeloma.
- Lung, breast, colon, and cervical cancer, as well as Kaposi's sarcoma, have also been described.

HYPERTRICOSIS LANUGINOSA ACQUISITA

CLINICAL FEATURES

- Hypertrichosis lanuginosa acquisita is the sudden and profuse growth of lanugo-type hairs in an adult.

- These are nonmedullar, nonpigmented, silky hairs, which can grow progressively.
- Initially located on the face, they generally disseminate, sparing the palms, soles, and genital area.
- Glossitis and acanthosis nigricans can be associated.
- Lung and colorectal cancer are the most frequently associated malignancies. Uterine, breast, ovary, pancreas, gallbladder, bladder, and liver cancer and lymphomas have also been reported.

SUPERFICIAL MIGRATORY THROMBOPHLEBITIS (TROUSSEAU'S SIGN)

CLINICAL FEATURES

- Recurrent and migratory type of superficial thrombophlebitis, mainly found on the upper extremities and trunk.
- Most frequently associated with pancreatic carcinoma; also related to lung, stomach, breast, and colon cancer.

PARANEOPLASTIC PEMPHIGUS

CLINICAL FEATURES

- Polymorphous erythema multiforme-like lesions with painful mucosal blistering and erosions.
- Non-Hodgkin's lymphoma and chronic lymphocytic leukemia are the most frequently associated malignancies.
- Thymoma, sarcoma, lung and pancreatic cancers, and Castelman's tumor have also been reported.

HISTOPATHOLOGY

- Histologically this disorder is characterized by vacuolar interface dermatitis with acantholysis and necrosis of keratinocytes. Indirect and direct immunofluorescences are positive, with IgG and/or complement deposition both in epidermal intercellular spaces and along the dermoepidermal junction. Autoantibodies act against cytostructural proteins such as desmoplakin I, periplakin, envoplakin, bullous pemphigoid antigen, and other unidentified antigens.

MULTICENTRIC RETICULOHISTIOCYTOSIS

CLINICAL FEATURES

- Eruption of flesh-colored and reddish papules, sometimes with a cobblestone appearance, associated with severe, mutilating polyarthritis.
- Cutaneous involvement is generally seen on the hands, face, ears, forearms, elbows, and scalp.
- Hematologic malignancies; breast, gastric, lung, liver, and ovarian cancer; and sarcomas have been reported.

HISTOPATHOLOGY

- Skin lesions consist of histiocytic multinucleated giant cells with eosisnophilic ground-glass cytoplasm.
- Mucosal involvement is less frequent.

OTHER PARANEOPLASTIC CUTANEOUS DISORDERS

- Other dermatoses that can be paraneoplastic in nature, including erythema annulare centrifugum, dermatomyositis, amyloidosis, erythroderma, Sweet's syndrome, pyoderma gangrenosum, vasculitis, cryoglobulinemia, subacute fat necrosis, chronic erythema nodosum, and porphyria cutanea tarda.

REFERENCES

Brenner S, Tamir E, Maharshak N, et al. Cutaneous manifestations of internal malignancies. *Clin Dermatol.* 2001; 19:290.

De la Torre C, Rodríguez T, Cruces MJ. Acroqueratosis paraneoplásica de Bazex. Aportación de un nuevo caso español y revisión de la literatura. *Med Cut I L A.* 1990;18:334.

Kimyai-Asadi A, Jih MH. Paraneoplastic pemphigus. *Int J Dermatol.* 2001;40:367.

McLean DI. Cutaneous paraneoplastic syndromes. *Arch Dermatol.* 1986;122:765.

Politi Y, Ophir J, Brenner S. Cutaneous paraneoplastic syndromes. *Acta Dermatol Venereol.* 1993;73:161.

Poole S, Fenske NA. Cutaneous markers of internal malignancy. II. Paraneoplastic dermatoses and environmental carcinogens. *J Am Acad Dermatol.* 1993;28:147.

Russo G, Millikan LE. Genetic and acquired cutaneous disorders associated with internal malignancy. *Int J Dermatol.* 1995;34:749.

Worret WI. Skin signs of internal malignancies. *Int J Dermatol.* 1993;32:1.

INHERITED DISORDERS ASSOCIATED WITH MALIGNANCIES

- There are a number of genodermatoses that combine nonmalignant skin findings as well as predisposition for internal malignancy.
- The recognition of these disorders entails screening of the patient's family and genetic counseling of the patient.

NEVOID BASAL CELL CARCINOMA SYNDROME (GORLIN SYNDROME)

ETIOLOGY

- Autosomal dominant disorder that maps to chromosome 9q22.3.

CLINICAL FEATURES

- Multiple basal-cell carcinomas, odontogenic cysts, and palmar and plantar pits characterize the disease.
- Other features include skeletal abnormalities such as bifid ribs, kyphoscoliosis, and short fourth metacarpals; calcification of brain structures, mainly the falx cerebri; and a characteristic facies with frontal bossing, hypertelorism, and a prominent mandible.
- An association with medulloblastoma, melanoma, brain tumors, and ovarian fibromas has been documented; the latter can be responsible for infertility.

MULTIPLE HAMARTOMA SYNDROME (COWDEN SYNDROME)

ETIOLOGY

- Genodermatosis with an autosomal dominant pattern of inheritance.

CLINICAL FEATURES

- This syndrome is defined by a variety of hamartomatous lesions involving mainly the skin, mucosal surfaces, thyroid gland, and breast.

- Multiple facial trichilemmomas are characteristic. Other cutaneous findings include oral mucosal papillomatosis, hyperkeratotic palms and soles, lipomas, and fibromas.
- It has been associated with Down syndrome. Patients have increased risk of developing colonic polyps. Breast, thyroid, and genitourinary malignancies have been recognized.

GARDNER'S SYNDROME

ETIOLOGY

- Autosomal dominant disorder.

CLINICAL FEATURES

- Disorder characterized by multiple gastric, duodenal, and colonic polyps with high risk of malignant transformation.
- Fibromas, lipomas, epidermoid cysts, and desmoid tumors are the main dermatologic findings.
- Osteomas and a congenital hypertrophy of retinal pigment epithelium can be present.
- This condition has been associated with osteosarcoma, hepatoblastoma, periampullary adenocarcinoma of the gallbladder, and carcinomas of thyroid, bile duct, and adrenal gland.

PEUTZ–JEGHER'S SYNDROME

ETIOLOGY

- Disorder inherited as an autosomal dominant trait, the germ line mutations of the STK11/LKB1 tumor suppressor gene (19p13.30).

CLINICAL FEATURES

- This rare genetic disorder consists of gastrointestinal hamartomatous polyps, more frequent in the small intestine, and mucocutaneous hyperpigmented macules with a periorificial and acral distribution.
- These macules are very characteristic on the lips and oral mucosa. There is increased risk of breast, lung, pancreas, and gonadal malignancy. Although not as frequent as in Gardner's syndrome, carcinomas may arise in hamartomatous polyps.

MUIR–TORRE SYNDROME

ETIOLOGY

- Disease inherited in an autosomal dominant fashion.

CLINICAL FEATURES

- Disorder characterized by the association of sebaceous gland neoplasms and internal malignancies.
- Cutaneous findings include sebaceous adenomas, epitheliomas, and carcinomas, as well as keratoacanthomas.
- Gastrointestinal malignancies, mainly adenocarcinomas of the colon. Genitourinary tumors have also been reported.

FANCONI'S ANEMIA

ETIOLOGY

- Autosomal recessive syndrome associated with chromosomal instability.

CLINICAL FEATURES

- Characterized by progressive bone marrow failure resulting in pancytopenia, radius aplasia, altered thumbs, central nervous system and genital malformations, and short stature.
- Dermatologic features consist of pigmentary changes, with a reticulate hyperpigmentation often seen on the trunk and the flexures.
- Other patterns observed are guttate hyperpigmentation, freckling, and café-au-lait spots.
- Leukemia is the neoplasm most frequently associated with Fanconi's anemia.
- Other reported tumors include mucosal squamous cell carcinomas and hepatic and breast carcinomas.

BLOOM'S SYNDROME

ETIOLOGY

- Autosomal recessive genodermatosis classified as a chromosomal instability syndrome.

CLINICAL FEATURES

- Malar erythema and telangiectasias showing a lupus-like butterfly distribution are the most characteristic cutaneous finding. Other skin manifestations reported include pigmentary changes, skin atrophy, and sacral dimpling.
- Patients show short stature, typical facies (narrow face with a prominent nose), and skeletal anomalies.
- Infertility and severe immunodeficiency resulting in recurrent infections are characteristic.
- Lymphoreticular neoplasms, mainly acute leukemias and non-Hodgkin's lymphomas, squamous cell carcinomas of the head and neck, and adenocarcinomas of the colon are the malignancies most frequently associated.

DYSKERATOSIS CONGENITA

ETIOLOGY

- X-linked disease involving males (autosomal recessive and dominant forms have been reported) and associated with chromosomal instability.
- Dyskeratosis congenita (DKC) is caused predominantly by missense mutations in the DKC1 gene linked to Xq28 corresponding to dyskeratin protein; this is an important protein implicated in aplastic anemia.

CLINICAL FEATURES

- Dermatologic manifestations include the typical diagnostic triad of poikilodermatous lesions including atrophy, reticular hyperpigmentation and telangiectasia, leukoplakia of the oral mucosa, and nail dystrophy. Reticulated hyperpigmentation is most prominent on the face, neck, thighs, and back of the hands.
- Other cutaneous findings include hyperhidrosis and loss of dermatoglyphics.
- Atrophy, telangiectasias, and keratoderma of the palms and soles are also seen.
- Somatic abnormalities, such as pulmonary disease and esophageal stricture, have also been reported.
- Bone marrow failure and immune abnormalities can lead to recurrent infections and malignancy.
- Reported malignancies include upper digestive tract and squamous cell carcinomas of the skin, pancreatic adenocarcinoma, and Hodgkin's lymphomas.

HOWEL–EVANS–CLARK SYNDROME

ETIOLOGY

- Autosomal dominant syndrome.

CLINICAL FEATURES

- It associates oral leukoplakia and palmoplantar hyperkeratosis, or tylosis.
- It has been associated with esophageal carcinoma.

ADULT PROGERIA (WERNER'S SYNDROME)

ETIOLOGY

- Autosomal recessive genodermatosis associated with chromosomal instability.
- Defined by premature aging.
- The disease is associated with mutation of the WRN gene in chromosome 8p12.
- WRN is a helicase and an exonuclease and also has an associated ATPase activity.

CLINICAL FEATURES

- Skin findings are typical and include generalized xerosis and atrophy, skin carcinomas, hyperpigmentation and telangiectasias of the face and extremities, alopecia, premature gray hair, and loss of subcutaneous fat.
- Short stature, high-pitched voice, diabetes mellitus, premature arteriosclerosis, osteoporosis, and hypogonadism.
- Fibrosarcomas, leiomyosarcomas, and thyroid and liver carcinomas have been reported.

WISKOTT–ALDRICH SYNDROME

ETIOLOGY

- The Wiskott–Aldrich syndrome (WAS) is an X-linked recessive disorder, arising from mutation of the WAS-protein (WASP) gene in chromosome subband Xpl1.23.

CLINICAL FEATURES

- Defined by the association of immunodeficiency, thrombocytopenia, and atopic dermatitis. Purpura is also a frequent cutaneous sign.
- Patients suffer from recurrent infections, hemorrhage, and allergic symptoms.
- Lymphoreticular malignancies, mainly Hodgkin's disease and acute leukemia, have been reported.

BRUTON'S AGAMMAGLOBULINEMIA

ETIOLOGY

- X-linked disease defined by the inability to make functional antibodies.
- The gene is a member of the src family of protooncogenes and encodes for a novel cytoplasmic protein tyrosine kinase (PTK).

CLINICAL FEATURES

- Becomes apparent after the first 3 to 6 months of life.
- Patients suffer from recurrent infections, allergic rhinitis, asthma, and an atopic-dermatitis-like eczematous condition. Resistance to viral infections is intact.
- Growth failure, chronic diarrhea, and absence of palpable lymph nodes are characteristic.
- Associated malignancies: hematologic disorders, mainly lymphomas and leukemias.

DIAGNOSIS AND DIFFERENTIAL

- Clinical manifestations; the absent of IgA, IgM, and IgD from serum; and small amounts of IgG.

TREATMENT

- Gammaglobulin.

MULTIPLE ENDOCRINE NEOPLASIA SYNDROME, TYPE 2B (MEN 2)

ETIOLOGY

- Inherited as an autosomal dominant trait, although up to 50% of cases can be sporadic.
- MEN 2 is caused by germ line mutation in the RET proto-oncogene, and is responsible for the development of endocrine neoplasia.

CLINICAL FEATURES

- This syndrome is characterized by the association of multiple mucosal neuromas, mainly located on the lips, tongue, and buccal and ocular mucosal surfaces.
- Medullary thyroid carcinoma and a pheocromocytoma have been recognized.
- Patients have a Marfanoid body habitus.

BIRT–HOGG–DUBE SYNDROME

ETIOLOGY

- Inherited in an autosomal dominant fashion.

CLINICAL FEATURES

- The association of multiple fibrofolliculomas with trichodiscomas and acrochordon-like lesions defines it.
- It has been recognized in association with kidney neoplasias.

REFERENCES

Bale SJ, Digiovanna JJ. Cancer-associated genodermatoses and familial cancer syndromes with cutaneous manifestations. *Clin Dermatol.* 2001;19:284.

De la Torre C, Cruces MJ. Cowden's disease and Down syndrome. An exceptional association. *J Am Acad Dermatol.* 1991;25:909.

De la Torre C, Ocampo C, Doval IG, et al. Acrochordons are not a component of the Birt–Hogg–Dubé syndrome. Does this syndrome exist? Case reports and review of the literature. *Am J Dermatopathol.*1999;21:369.

De la Torre C, Ocampo C, Rodríguez T, et al. Síndrome de Werner. Afectación de tres hermanos. *Actas Dermo-Sif.* 1991;82:663.

Hildenbrand C, Burgdorf WHC, Lautenschlager S. Cowden syndrome: Diagnostic signs. *Dermatology.* 2001;202:362.

Kutlhuhan Y, et al. Dyskeratosis congenita with isolated neutropenia and granulocyte colony-stimulating factor treatment. *In. J Dermatol.* 2002;41:170.

Poole S, Fenske NA. Cutaneous markers of internal malignancy. I. Malignant involvement of the skin and the genodermatoses. *J Am Acad Dermatol.* 1993;28:1.

Sapkota GP, Boudeau J, et al. Identification and characterization of four novel phosporylation sites (Ser31, Ser 325, Th336, and Thr 366) on LKB/STK11, the protein kinase mutated in Peutz-Jeghers cancer syndrome. *Biochem J.* 2002; 362:481.

Toro JR, Glenn G, Duray P. Birt–Hogg–Dubé syndrome. A novel marker of kidney neoplasia. *Arch Dermatol.* 1999; 135:1195.

PRURITUS

- Generalized pruritus can be a symptom of diagnostic importance associated with numerous systemic diseases.

ETIOLOGY

- The most representative systemic diseases are chronic renal failure; cholestatic liver disease (primary biliary cirrhosis, cholestatic drugs such as estrogens and allopurinol, and chronic hepatitis); endocrine disturbances (hyperthyroidism, hypothyroidism, hyperparathyroidism, and carcinoid); hematologic disorders (including polycythemia vera and iron-deficiency anemia) and Hodgkin's disease; other visceral malignancies; infectious diseases (AIDS and parasitic diseases); neurologic disorders (multiple sclerosis and cerebral abscess, infarction, or tumor); and psychiatric disturbances.

DIAGNOSIS AND DIFFERENTIAL

- Every patient with systemic pruritus must undergo a detailed medical history including drug intake and physical examination.
- Work-up should include a complete blood cell count; thyroid, liver, and renal function tests; urinalysis; feces analysis for ova and parasites; and a chest x-ray.
- More complex and directed investigations should be done when a concrete disease is suspected.

TREATMENT

- In terms of therapy the most important aspect of treating systemic pruritus is to address the underlying disease, if possible.
- Concomitant therapies are based on the physiology of itch and they include emollients, topical anesthetics, selective blockers of type C (itch) fibers (such as capsaicin), ultraviolet radiation, systemic antihistamines, tricyclic antidepressants, opiate antagonists, ion exchange resins, and emotional support.

REFERENCES

Denman ST. A review of pruritus. *J Am Acad Dermatol.* 1986;14:375.

Yosipovitch G, David M. The diagnostic and therapeutic approach to idiopathic generalized pruritus. *Int J Dermatol.* 1999;38:881.

18 EPIDERMAL NEOPLASMS AND ADNEXAL TUMORS

Karynne O. Duncan

• Neoplasms of the epidermis can be categorized into those arising from the epidermis and those arising from the adnexal structures, namely the hair follicle, sebaceous glands, apocrine glands, and eccrine glands. In both categories, both benign and malignant neoplasms exist. Premalignant or precancerous lesions arising from the epidermis also occur and will be discussed. The benign, premalignant, and malignant epidermal neoplasms can be found in Table 18–1, while many of the adnexal neoplasms are summarized in Table 18–2.

BENIGN EPIDERMAL NEOPLASMS

SEBORRHEIC KERATOSIS

EPIDEMIOLOGY

• Seborrheic keratoses (SKs) are extremely common cutaneous lesions.
• They are most commonly found in older individuals, usually appearing around or after middle age.
• Lesions may be single but most often are multiple.
• They occur primarily on the trunk and face, but can also be found on the extremities and genitalia. They do not occur on the palms or soles.

PATHOPHYSIOLOGY

• The etiology and pathogenesis of SKs are unknown.

CLINICAL FEATURES

• A typical SK appears as a discrete, tan, brown, or gray, stuck-on papule with a soft verrucous surface. Other SKs may have a smoother surface with keratotic plugs evident within the papule. Still others may present as pedunculated smaller papules that clinically resemble fibroepithelial polyps. The size of these lesions is quite variable, ranging from several mm to several cm in diameter.

• Irritated or traumatized SKs can present with overlying crusting and an underlying inflammatory base.
• Several clinical variants and presentations exist. Dermatosis papulosa nigra is found predominantly on the face of African American individuals, being observed in up to a third of such adults. Lesions are mainly located on the malar cheeks, but they can also be found on the neck and upper trunk. Individual lesions appear as small, smooth, brown papules, but they may be more pedunculated when seen on the neck or upper trunk.
• Stucco keratoses are SKs that are found predominantly in a symmetric distribution on the distal portions of the lower extremities, although they can also be seen on the distal upper extremities. These lesions appear as stuck-on, gray or white, rough, small papules.
• The Leser–Trélat sign is a controversial phenomenon characterized by the eruption of numerous SKs in association with an underlying malignancy. This condition

TABLE 18–1 Epidermal Neoplasms

Benign epidermal neoplasms
   Seborrheic keratosis
   Epidermal nevus
   Clear cell acanthoma
   Keratoacanthoma

Benign epidermal cysts
   Epidermal inclusion cyst
   Trichilemmal cyst
   Steatocystoma
   Eruptive vellus hair cyst

Premalignant epidermal neoplasms
   Actinic keratosis
   Other premalignant keratoses
     Arsenical keratosis
     Hydrocarbon keratosis
     Thermal keratosis
     Chronic radiation keratosis
     Chronic scar keratosis
     PUVA keratosis
   Bowen's disease
   Bowenoid papulosis
   Erythroplasia of Queyrat
   Erythroplakia
   Leukoplakia

Malignant epidermal neoplasms
   Basal cell carcinoma
   Squamous cell carcinoma

TABLE 18–2   Adnexal Neoplasms

Follicular derived
  Benign
    Trichofolliculoma
    Dilated pore
    Pilar sheath acanthoma
    Fibrofolliculoma
    Trichodiscoma
    Trichoepithelioma
    Pilomatricoma
    Proliferating trichilemmal cyst
    Trichilemmoma

  Malignant
    Pilomatrix carcinoma
    Malignant proliferating trichilemmal tumor
    Trichilemmal carcinoma

Sebaceous gland derived
  Benign
    Nevus sebaceous
    Sebaceous hyperplasia
    Fordyce's condition
    Sebaceous adenoma
    Sebaceoma

  Malignant
    Sebaceous carcinoma

Eccrine gland derived
  Benign
    Eccrine hidrocystoma
    Syringoma
    Eccrine poroma
    Eccrine spiradenoma
    Nodular hidradenoma
    Chondroid syringoma

  Malignant
    Porocarcinoma
    Malignant eccrine spiradenoma
    Malignant nodular hidradenoma
    Malignant chondroid syringoma
    Microcystic adnexal carcinoma

Apocrine gland derived
  Benign
    Apocrine hidrocystoma
    Hidradenoma papilliferum
    Syringocystadenoma papilliferum
    Cylindroma

  Malignant
    Malignant cylindroma

is distinct from the sudden eruption of SKs on inflamed skin. The most common underlying malignancy, in roughly two thirds of cases, is an abdominal adenocarcinoma.

HISTOPATHOLOGY

- All SKs share several histopathologic features. They all show acanthosis, hyperkeratosis, and papillomatosis. Within the neoplasm two types of cells are seen, namely, the predominant basaloid cells and squamous cells. These cells comprise the acanthotic epidermis, forming interwoven tracts. Amid these tracts are cystic inclusions of horny material called horn cysts and pseudohorn cysts.
- Irritated SKs have, in addition to the above findings, characteristic whorls of eosinophilic, compressed squamous cells, also known as squamous eddies.

DIAGNOSIS AND DIFFERENTIAL

- Typical SKs are most often diagnosed by their clinical appearance. At times, however, it can be difficult to distinguish a dark brown or black SK from a melanoma and biopsy of the lesion is then necessary.
- Other entities to consider in the differential, especially when an SK is irritated or traumatized, include verruca vulgaris, squamous cell carcinoma (SCC), actinic keratosis (AK), and basal cell carcinoma (BCC).

TREATMENT

- SKs are benign neoplasms and as such, do not require treatment. Patients may request removal of these lesions for cosmetic purposes or because they become irritated. Methods of removal of SK include liquid nitrogen cryotherapy, tangential excision, light electrodessication, and curettage.
- Other malignancies, such as SCC, BCC, and melanoma have also been reported to rarely occur simultaneously within an SK lesion. Therefore, SKs with atypical features should be viewed suspiciously and biopsied for diagnosis.

EPIDERMAL NEVUS

EPIDEMIOLOGY

- Technically, epidermal nevi can be of keratinocytic, follicular, apocrine, or eccrine origin, but for the purpose of this discussion, keratinocytic-derived epidermal nevi are addressed.
- Keratinocytic nevi are also known as verrucous nevi or linear epidermal nevi.
- The incidence of all types of epidermal nevi has been estimated at roughly 1 in 1000 live births.
- These lesions most often present at birth or develop during childhood and adolescence.
- Most cases arise sporadically, but familial cases have been described for certain subtypes.
- There is no gender or racial predilection.

PATHOPHYSIOLOGY

- Epidermal nevi are essentially hamartomas that arise from the overproduction of keratinocytes. They arise from the undifferentiated basal cells in the epidermis.

CLINICAL FEATURES

- Five clinical variants of epidermal nevi exist: localized, nevus unius lateris, inflammatory linear verrucous epidermal nevus (ILVEN), systematized, and epidermal nevus syndrome. In the localized variant, typically only one lesion is present. These lesions can be seen on any body site, more commonly affecting the trunk, extremities, or head. They classically present as a well-demarcated linear array of yellowish-brown, verrucous papules or plaques. They can vary in size from small subtle lesions to more extensive growths affecting large sections of the limb or trunk.
- Nevus unius lateris refers to a linear epidermal nevus that is localized to only one side of the body. The linear distribution typically follows along the lines of Blaschko.
- ILVEN is a unilateral linear epidermal nevus distinguished clinically by its erythema and pruritus and histopathologically by the presence of inflammation and parakeratosis.
- In the systematized variant, multiple and extensive linear epidermal nevi are found along Blaschko's lines in a widespread, unilateral or bilateral, often symmetric distribution. The term *ichthyosis hystrix* is sometimes used to describe cases of extensive bilateral involvement.
- Individuals with the epidermal nevus syndrome present with a variety of systemic manifestations in addition to the cutaneous findings. They usually present with systematized and, less often, localized epidermal nevi. Systemic manifestations may include abnormalities of the skeletal, ocular, and central nervous systems.
- On occasion, basal cell carcinoma has been reported to develop within an epidermal nevus, usually one that is located on the head. Rarely has squamous cell carcinoma been reported to arise in an epidermal nevus.
- In individuals with typically more extensive epidermal nevi, who also demonstrate epidermolytic hyperkeratosis in the lesion histopathologically, there is a chance that germline keratin 1 or keratin 10 mutations exist. If such a scenario exists, offspring of that individual have the potential to develop the full-blown syndrome of epidermolytic hyperkeratosis, otherwise known as bullous congenital ichthyosiform erythroderma.

HISTOPATHOLOGY

- Characteristic findings in almost all epidermal nevi include hyperkeratosis, acanthosis, and papillomatosis, with elongation of the rete ridges.
- In some cases of localized epidermal nevi, and in many cases of systematized epidermal nevi, the histopathologic findings of epidermolytic hyperkeratosis are evident.
- ILVEN also demonstrates alternating hyperkeratosis and parakeratosis, psoriasiform hyperplasia, and mild chronic inflammation in the superficial dermis.

DIAGNOSIS AND DIFFERENTIAL

- The diagnosis can often be made based on the striking clinical appearance of these lesions. A biopsy of the lesion can help confirm the diagnosis and determine whether or not epidermolytic hyperkeratosis is present. If the latter is present on the biopsy specimen, especially in cases of widespread epidermal nevi, the likelihood of a germline mutation in keratins 1 or 10 should be considered and genetic counseling offered to that individual.
- Clinically, early and smaller epidermal nevi can sometimes be difficult to distinguish from a nevus sebaceous or larger verruca vulgaris.
- Histopathologically, especially when no clinical history is available, epidermal nevus can be difficult to distinguish from benign papilloma, hypertrophic seborrheic keratosis, old verruca vulgaris, and acanthosis nigricans. ILVEN may also be mistaken for psoriasis.

TREATMENT

- Many treatment modalities have been proposed for epidermal nevi. The main reason for treatment is primarily for cosmetic improvement, as malignant transformation is rare.
- Small epidermal nevi are best removed with full-thickness surgical excision.
- Larger and more extensive epidermal nevi are more difficult to treat. Proposed treatment modalities have included topical calcipotriene ointment, topical tretinoin and 5-fluorouracil in combination, topical steroids, dermabrasion, cryotherapy, carbon dioxide laser therapy, and oral retinoids.
- ILVEN, because of the symptoms of intense pruritus, often requires treatment. Full-thickness surgical excision provides the most definitive treatment. Other treatment modalities are similar to those described previously.

CLEAR CELL ACANTHOMA

EPIDEMIOLOGY

- Clear cell acanthoma is an uncommon epidermal neoplasm.
- It is usually a solitary lesion found on the lower legs of middle-aged or elderly individuals, although multiple lesions have occasionally been described.
- This is a benign epidermal neoplasm, although rare case reports of malignant conversion and the concomitant development of a squamous cell carcinoma have been described.

PATHOPHYSIOLOGY

- The exact pathogenesis of the clear cell acanthoma is not known. Relationships between clear cell acanthoma and varicose veins, insect bites, and trauma have been reported.
- Clear cell acanthoma is thought to derive from the epidermis.
- Excess glycogen is present in the cytoplasm of the clear cells that constitute the bulk of the neoplasm. It is this abundance of glycogen that imparts the clear cell appearance of the keratinocytes. The enzyme phosphorylase, which degrades glycogen and is normally present in the epidermis, is absent in these clear cell keratinocytes. The normal appearing basal cells demonstrate normal amounts of glycogen and phosphorylase.

CLINICAL FEATURES

- Clear cell acanthoma typically presents as a slow-growing, discrete, red, round or oval nodule or plaque. It appears stuck on the surface of the skin.
- The size of this lesion is typically 1 or 2 cm in diameter.
- It may exude a moist substance and a thin overlying crust can be seen. The surface easily bleeds with slight trauma.
- Classically, a collarette of scale is seen lining the perimeter of the lesion.
- Polypoid, giant, cystic, and atypical lesions have also been described.

HISTOPATHOLOGY

- The lesion appears sharply demarcated from the surrounding normal epidermis. There is marked epidermal psoriasiform hyperplasia and acanthosis.
- The keratinocytes within the acanthotic epidermis are distinctly pale owing to the large amount of glycogen present in them. The basal layer cells retain their normal appearance, and the acrosyringia and acrotrichia also retain their normal staining properties.
- Dilated blood vessels are seen in the papillary dermis.
- Many neutrophils and neutrophilic dust are identified within the epidermis and parakeratotic horny layer.

DIAGNOSIS AND DIFFERENTIAL

- Clinically, clear cell acanthoma must be differentiated from pyogenic granuloma or eccrine poroma. An amelanotic melanoma or SCC may also be in the clinical differential.

TREATMENT

- Because of the clinical differential, an excisional biopsy is often performed and this also constitutes treatment of the lesion.
- Tangential excision itself would be adequate treatment.
- Other treatment modalities include cryotherapy and shave excision with curettage.

KERATOACANTHOMA

EPIDEMIOLOGY

- Keratoacanthomas (KAs) are also referred to as molluscum sebaceum.
- Controversy exists as to whether or not keratoacanthomas are benign lesions or well-differentiated malignant variants of SCC.
- Two types of KA exist, the solitary and multiple variants.
- Solitary KA typically arises in elderly individuals as a single lesion, although several lesions may be present concurrently. Sites of predilection include sun-exposed areas, but any hair-bearing cutaneous surface can develop KA. They do not occur on the palms, soles, or mucous membranes, except for a subungual variant.
- Solitary KA is more common in immunocompromised individuals.
- Solitary KA has also been described as a cutaneous manifestation of Muir–Torre syndrome, along with other sebaceous neoplasms.
- Three uncommon variants of solitary KA include the giant keratoacanthoma, keratoacanthoma centrifugum marginatum, and the subungual keratoacanthoma.

- There are two clinical variants of multiple KAs, namely the multiple self-healing epitheliomas of Ferguson–Smith, and the eruptive keratoacanthomas of Grzybowski.
- In the Ferguson–Smith variant, lesions appear in childhood or adolescence on any skin surface. The face and extremities are the most common sites, and palm and sole lesions have also been described. Lesions number in the dozen to rarely the hundred range. This condition appears to be inherited in an autosomal dominant fashion. It is more common in males.
- In the Grzybowski variant, lesions do not appear until adulthood. Lesions number in the hundreds and may be seen on the mucous membranes and larynx. There is no gender predilection in this variant.

PATHOPHYSIOLOGY

- The cause of KA is not known. Chronic UVB exposure is thought to play a role in the development of the typical solitary KA. Immunosuppression also predisposes to the development of KA.
- KAs are believed to derive from the follicular infundibulum.
- In cases of multiple KAs, predisposition and genetic factors play an additional role in their development.
- As stated earlier, controversy exists as to the malignant potential of these lesions, and many people regard KAs as variants of SCC.

CLINICAL FEATURES

- Solitary KA presents as a firm, smooth, dome-shaped papule with a crateriform, eroded, volcanic-like center. Its onset is usually sudden with a rapid increase in size of the lesion over several weeks. The diameter of these lesions usually reaches 1 to 2 cm. Lesions larger than 3 cm are referred to as giant KAs. Characteristically, involution of the KA then occurs spontaneously over a roughly 6-month period. The lesion heals with a slightly depressed scar.
- Giant KA grows rapidly and can reach diameters of 5 or more cm. Destruction of underlying tissues can occur, but the majority of these lesions spontaneously involute over several months. The nose and eyelids are predominant sites for this lesion.
- KA centrifugum marginatum is a subtype of solitary KA that may reach diameters of up to 20 cm. The dorsa of the hands and legs are sites of predilection and spontaneous involution does not regularly occur. This lesion continues to expand with a characteristic rolled border and atrophic center.

- Subungual KA presents under the distal portion of the nail as an umbilicated, painful, red, swollen lesion. The thumb and index finger are common sites of presentation. Underlying erosion of the terminal phalanx is often seen on x-ray of the finger. Spontaneous involution is not typically seen.
- In the multiple self-healing epitheliomas of Ferguson–Smith, lesions present as multiple, recurrent KAs. These lesions are usually much slower to resolve and are often associated with greater tissue damage and scarring.
- In the eruptive KA variant of Grzybowski, hundreds of smaller, several mm in diameter, follicular lesions appear. They are often pruritic or painful and may become generalized.

HISTOPATHOLOGY

- A mature KA demonstrates a central keratin plug that fills a large, irregularly shaped, volcanic-like crater. On both sides of the crater, the epidermis dips down to envelope the lesion, like a cupped fist.
- The base of a mature KA is regular and even in appearance and does not extend below the eccrine sweat glands. A significant inflammatory infiltrate is typically found at the base.
- The squamous epithelium is usually well-differentiated, although atypical cells are more prevalent in younger KA lesions. Individual cells demonstrate a pale, glassy, eosinophilic cytoplasm as a result of keratinization, which is quite prominent. Many horn pearls are also seen.
- Intraepithelial neutrophilic microabscesses are commonly seen.
- Typical mitoses along the periphery of the lesion are also seen.

DIAGNOSIS AND DIFFERENTIAL

- Differentiating between KA and SCC both clinically and histopathologically can be difficult.
- The diagnosis of KA relies on a typical clinical and histopathologic presentation. Clinically, a history of rapid onset and growth of an exophytic, crateriform lesion is suggestive of a KA.
- Histopathologically, the characteristic architecture of the lesion, the keratin plug and peripheral collarette, the prominent keratinization and neutrophilic microabscesses, and the absence of atypical mitoses, favor the diagnosis of KA.
- Because the diagnosis of KA and its differentiation from SCC depend on both the architecture and cellular

characteristics of the lesion, it is essential to perform an adequate biopsy so that the specimen presented to the dermatopathologist is adequate for making the diagnosis. Removal of the entire lesion via excisional biopsy, full-thickness shave biopsy, or an elliptical incision through the entire lesion should be adequate.

- Despite these criteria, SCCs are sometimes mistaken for KAs clinically and histopathologically. When in doubt, it is best to be cautious and assume the lesion is a SCC and treat it as such.

TREATMENT

- Because of the caution needed in making the diagnosis of KA and in not missing a SCC, many experts recommend excising all KAs as if they were potentially SCC.
- Large KAs and those located in areas that are not easily removed with surgical excision, have been treated with intralesional methotrexate, intralesional bleomycin, and with topical 5-fluorouracil.
- Multiple KAs are notoriously difficult to treat. Anecdotal treatment with oral methotrexate, cyclophosphamide, and acitretin have been described, as well as with intravenous 5-fluorouracil.

BENIGN EPIDERMAL CYSTS

EPIDERMAL INCLUSION CYST

EPIDEMIOLOGY

- Other terms used for epidermal inclusion cyst (EIC) include epidermoid cyst and infundibular cyst.
- These are relatively common lesions found most often in young or middle-aged adults.
- They most often develop spontaneously on hair-bearing skin, such as on the face, scalp, neck, and upper trunk.
- EICs can also occur on the palms and soles, usually following some sort of penetrating trauma.
- Individuals usually present with one or a few EICs.
- The presence of multiple EICs should arouse suspicion for other associated disorders, such as Gardner's syndrome or pachyonychia congenita.

PATHOPHYSIOLOGY

- Spontaneously arising EICs are believed to develop from some type of damage to the hair follicle.

- Most spontaneously occurring EICs arise from the follicular infundibulum of the hair follicle. The infundibulum is the uppermost portion of the hair follicle that extends down into the opening of the sebaceous duct.
- EICs that develop on the palms and soles, secondary to trauma, are thought to arise from the implantation of epidermis into the subcutis or dermis.

CLINICAL FEATURES

- EICs classically present as indolent, smooth, round, firm, and mobile dermal or subcutaneous nodules.
- They are typically several mm to several cm in diameter.
- A clue to their diagnosis is the presence of a surface punctum.
- When an EIC ruptures, a brisk foreign body reaction ensues, owing to the release of the cyst contents into the dermis. Clinically, this reaction presents as an erythematous, tender, enlarged, fluctuant dermal or subcutaneous nodule at the site of a previously bland EIC.

HISTOPATHOLOGY

- The wall of an EIC is composed of a true epidermal lining, as also found in the follicular infundibulum of a hair follicle.
- The cyst contents consist of a horny keratin material that is arranged in laminated layers.
- In a ruptured EIC, a keratin granuloma is seen, manifesting as a foreign body granulomatous reaction, with the presence of numerous multinucleated giant cells. The cyst wall may sometimes disintegrate in such situations and only focal collections of keratin fragments remain in the dermis amid the foreign body granulomatous reaction. At other times, pseudocarcinomatous hyperplasia may develop.
- Rarely, a basal cell carcinoma, squamous cell carcinoma in situ, or true squamous cell carcinoma can develop within an EIC.

DIAGNOSIS AND DIFFERENTIAL

- EICs are most often diagnosed based on their clinical appearance, location, and the presence of an overlying punctum.
- Dermal and subcutaneous nodules without the punctum are more difficult to diagnose as an EIC, with certainty. Other entities to consider in the differential include trichilemmal cyst (especially for lesions on

the scalp), dermoid cyst, and sometimes other dermal and subcutaneous tumors.

- When the diagnosis is in doubt, the lesion should be excised and sent for histopathologic confirmation. Alternatively, a small punch biopsy specimen, obtained from the center of the lesion, can also be submitted for histopathologic diagnosis.

TREATMENT

- Typical EICs that do not bother the patient do not necessarily need to be removed. Reasons for removal of EICs include cosmetic appearance or location, frequent episodes of rupture or inflammation, discomfort to the patient, and unclear clinical diagnosis.
- To adequately remove an EIC with lower likelihood for recurrence, the entire cyst wall needs to be extracted. A small incision can be made over the cyst, usually through the punctum. Once the cyst sac is identified, it can be held with a hemostat or skin hook, while dissecting around it and removing it carefully, without expression of its contents.
- Ruptured, inflamed, or infected cysts should not be immediately excised. It is best to let the inflammatory reaction subside and the size of the cyst lessen before excision is attempted. Such lesions can be treated with intralesional corticosteroid injections, warm compresses, and, at times, oral antibiotics, to help hasten the quiescence of the inflammatory reaction. Once the cyst has been quiescent for a reasonable amount of time, excision can then be undertaken.

TRICHILEMMAL CYST

EPIDEMIOLOGY

- Trichilemmal cysts are also called pilar cysts. They have been mistakenly called sebaceous cysts in the past.
- They are less common than epidermal inclusion cysts.
- Almost 90% of trichilemmal cysts are located on the scalp.
- They are solitary in only 30% of cases, and it has been estimated that roughly 10% of individuals with trichilemmal cysts will have more than ten such lesions.
- An autosomal dominant inheritance pattern has also been noted in up to 75% of individuals.

PATHOPHYSIOLOGY

- Trichilemmal cysts are derived from the outer root sheath of the hair follicle at the level of the follicular isthmus. This portion of the hair follicle undergoes trichilemmal keratinization, a particular type of keratinization without the presence of a granular layer.
- The reason for the development of these cysts is not known.

CLINICAL FEATURES

- Trichilemmal cysts present as smooth, flesh-colored to yellowish, dome-shaped, mobile dermal nodules.
- No punctum is present, as typically found in EIC.
- Trichilemmal cysts rarely become inflamed or infected.
- Unlike EICs, trichilemmal cysts more readily pop out as one intact unit on surgical excision. The contents of the cyst have a characteristic cheesy, lamellated appearance.

HISTOPATHOLOGY

- The wall of a trichilemmal cyst consists of a lining of epithelial cells that have obvious intercellular bridges. No granular cell layer is present. The peripheral cell layer shows characteristic palisading and the cells closest to the cyst cavity appear swollen and more vertically oriented.
- The cyst cavity is composed of a homogeneous eosinophilic material.
- Foci of calcification are seen in roughly 25% of trichilemmal cysts.
- Inflamed trichilemmal cysts demonstrate inflammatory cells in the cyst lumen, but a granulomatous reaction is not seen, as in EIC.

DIAGNOSIS AND DIFFERENTIAL

- Clinically, it is difficult to distinguish a trichilemmal cyst from an EIC that does not have a punctum. Other dermal or subcutaneous tumors, such as lipoma, can also be considered in the clinical differential diagnosis.

TREATMENT

- Trichilemmal cysts are most often surgically excised because of patient concern or dislike of the lesion. They do not necessarily need to be excised.

STEATOCYSTOMA

EPIDEMIOLOGY

- Two types of steatocystoma lesions exist, namely, steatocystoma simplex and steatocystoma multiplex.

Steatocystoma simplex is a solitary, noninherited benign neoplasm. Steatocystoma multiplex is inherited in an autosomal dominant pattern and presents with multiple lesions. There is no gender predilection.

- Steatocystoma simplex is often located on the face, chest, and limbs. Presentation is typically in adults, with no gender predilection.
- Steatocystoma multiplex are typically distributed on the chest, axillae, arms, groin, and external genitalia. Presentation is usually in adolescence.
- Steatocystoma multiplex is also a potential clinical finding in pachyonychia congenita type 2.

PATHOPHYSIOLOGY

- It is believed that cyst walls of steatocystoma are derived from the sebaceous duct.
- Mutations in keratin 17 have been associated with pachyonychia congenita type 2, steatocystoma multiplex occurring on its own, and steatocystoma multiplex occurring in association with pachyonychia congenita type 2.

CLINICAL FEATURES

- Steatocystoma simplex presents as a single, well-circumscribed, asymptomatic dermal nodule.
- Steatocystoma multiplex presents as multiple, small, dome-shaped, smooth papules and nodules. They vary in size from a few mm to several cm in diameter. They are relatively firm and appear adherent to the overlying skin. The more superficial lesions may be yellowish in color.
- When present on the presternal chest area, they can become more noticeable when the chest wall is protruded such that the overlying skin is taut.
- When steatocystoma lesions are punctured, they exude a typical oily or creamy fluid, and at times small hairs.

HISTOPATHOLOGY

- The cyst walls are intricately folded. The lining of the cyst wall mimics that of the sebaceous duct where it enters the hair follicle. It is most easily recognized by the innermost, thick, hyaline-appearing cuticle. Flattened sebaceous glands are also characteristically seen within or close to the cyst wall.

DIAGNOSIS AND DIFFERENTIAL

- Steatocystoma multiplex has a striking, characteristic presentation, although multiple vellus hair cysts or EICs could also be considered in the differential.

- Histopathology is diagnostic.
- Extrusion of the oil or creamy substance on puncture is also helpful in the diagnosis.

TREATMENT

- Individuals usually seek treatment of these lesions because of their unsightly appearance.
- Multiple treatment modalities have been used for the treatment of steatocystoma multiplex, but some have proven to be inadequate and others have resulted in significant scarring. Reported treatment modalities have included radical excisions, mini-incisions with curettage removal of the cyst wall, carbon dioxide laser therapy, cryotherapy, needle aspiration, mini-incision with electrocauterization of the cyst wall, and oral retinoids.

ERUPTIVE VELLUS HAIR CYSTS

EPIDEMIOLOGY

- These lesions are usually found in children and young adults, although they can occur at any age.
- Autosomal dominant inheritance patterns have been described.
- The most common site to find these lesions is on the chest.
- Facial, congenital, and generalized variants have also been described.
- Occurrence of eruptive vellus hair cysts along with steatocystoma multiplex has been reported and some investigators consider the two entities to be variants of the same condition.
- These lesions have been found in patients with pachyonychia congenita type 2.

PATHOPHYSIOLOGY

- Eruptive vellus hair cysts are thought to arise from developmentally abnormal vellus hairs that tend to become occluded at the infundibulum, resulting in retention of hairs and thinning of the hair bulb.
- Eruptive vellus hair cysts are closely related to steatocystoma multiplex, and the two have been referred to as multiple pilosebaceous cysts.

CLINICAL FEATURES

- These lesions typically present as multiple, asymptomatic, discrete, soft, flesh-colored to reddish-brown follicular papules.

- The diameter of the lesions is small, in the 1 to 5 mm range.
- An umbilicated or crusted surface is sometimes seen.
- Squeezing of these lesions may result in extrusion of a whitish necrotic material.

HISTOPATHOLOGY

- Characteristically in the mid dermis, there is a thin-walled cyst that is lined by an infundibular-appearing epithelium. The lumen of the cyst contains laminated keratin and numerous vellus hairs.

DIAGNOSIS AND DIFFERENTIAL

- Eruptive vellus hair cysts may be mistaken for small steatocystoma multiplex lesions, comedones or small EICs, and trichostasis spinulosa.
- Closer clinical inspection of the lesions and squeezing of the lesions with expression of the hairs and necrotic material can aid in the diagnosis.
- Histopathology is diagnostic.

TREATMENT

- Treatment of these lesions is primarily for cosmetic purposes.
- Various treatment modalities have been proposed, including excision, mini-incisions with extraction or cauterization of the cyst wall, carbon dioxide, and erbium:YAG laser therapy.

PREMALIGNANT EPIDERMAL NEOPLASMS

- The definition of a premalignant or precancerous neoplasm is one that has a strong likelihood of turning into a true malignancy. The concept of a premalignant neoplasm is controversial, with some individuals accepting it and others debating its existence. For the purposes of this section, the lesions discussed are those that clinically have the potential to become invasive carcinomas and that histopathologically have atypia confined to the epidermis. Only the premalignant keratinocytic lesions are discussed. These lesions all have the potential to become invasive SCC. These premalignant lesions and

SCC are considered by many investigators to be the same disease along a spectrum from dysplasia to carcinoma in situ to invasive SCC.

ACTINIC KERATOSIS

EPIDEMIOLOGY

- Actinic keratoses (AKs) have also been called solar keratoses or senile keratoses.
- AKs are common lesions. Behind acne and dermatitis, AKs are the third most common reason for seeing a dermatologist.
- The prevalence of AKs has ranged from 25% in the United States to 40% or more in Australia.
- Risk factors for AKs include individual susceptibility factors, such as older age; male gender; phenotype of fair skin, fair hair, light-colored eyes, easy freckling, and inability to tan; immunosuppression; outdoor occupation; and certain genetic syndromes like xeroderma pigmentosum and albinism.
- The other major risk factor is cumulative ultraviolet radiation (UVR) exposure, including tanning beds, and psoralen plus ultraviolet A (PUVA) therapy. Intense UVR exposure in childhood and living closer to the equator are additional risk factors.

PATHOPHYSIOLOGY

- The most important contributing factor to the development of AKs is chronic UVR exposure. UVR, and namely ultraviolet B radiation (UVB), is responsible for the development of AKs and eventually SCC in two ways: first, it causes mutations in cellular DNA, that when unrepaired, lead to unrestrained growth and tumor formation, and second, it acts as an immunosuppressant to prevent tumor rejection.
- UVR acts as both an initiator and promoter in the development of AK and SCC. It induces signature mutations in the tumor suppressor gene, p53, within keratinocytes. Such mutated cells may or may not undergo apoptosis, or programmed cell death. Clonal expansion of these mutated cells present clinically as an AK. A second UVR induced mutation in p53 in these keratinocytes may then allow them to progress into SCC. If this second "hit" does not take place, the AK cells may persist in their current state or regress.
- Other premalignant keratinocytic lesions, similar in clinical and histopathologic appearance to AK, have been described in association with other etiologies. All of these lesions also have the potential to develop

into invasive SCC. Arsenical keratoses are premalignant lesions found in association with chronic arsenicism. Thermal keratoses are produced in the skin in response to chronic exposure to infrared radiation. Hydrocarbon or tar keratoses develop in persons who are exposed occupationally to polycyclic aromatic hydrocarbons. Chronic radiation dermatitis arises on the skin many years after exposure to ionizing radiation, such as x-ray therapy or radioactive nuclear fallout. Chronic scar keratoses can be seen arising in long-standing scars, especially burn scars.

CLINICAL FEATURES

- The majority (80%) of AKs are distributed on chronically sun-exposed sites of the body, such as the head, neck, forearms, and dorsal hands.
- The typical AK lesion presents as a 2 to 6 mm erythematous, flat, rough or scaly papule. It is usually easier to feel than to see. The size of AKs can vary, sometimes reaching up to several cm in diameter. They are most often found among a background of chronic solar damage, such as solar elastosis, dyspigmentation, yellow discoloration, wrinkles, telangiectases, and sagging skin.
- Several other clinical subtypes of AK exist. The hypertrophic AK, or HAK, presents as a thicker, scaly, skin-colored, gray or erythematous, rough papule or plaque. It sometimes presents as a cutaneous horn. It can be found on any chronically sun-exposed site, but it has a propensity for the dorsal hands.
- Actinic cheilitis represents confluent AKs on the lips, most often the lower lip. Patients with this condition present with red, scaly, chapped appearing lips, sometimes with erosions or fissures. They often complain of persistent dryness and cracking of the lips. Persistent ulcerations or induration should raise the suspicion for SCC.
- More unusual variants of AKs include the pigmented AK, spreading pigmented AK, proliferative AK, and conjunctival AK.

HISTOPATHOLOGY

- The typical flat, erythematous AK has characteristic architectural and cytologic histopathologic features. All of the primary abnormalities are confined to the epidermis, although solar elastosis and an inflammatory infiltrate can be found in the dermis. There are foci of atypical, pleomorphic keratinocytes in the basal layer, protruding as buds into the papillary dermis. The basal layer appears more basophilic, owing to the crowding of the atypical keratinocytes. Overlying these foci of atypical keratinocytes, there is irregular acanthosis, hyperkeratosis, and parakeratosis. There is notable sparing of the adnexal epithelium, with orthokeratosis overlying these regions, thus giving rise to the classic pattern of alternating orthokeratosis and parakeratosis. Cytologically, there is an increased nuclear to cytoplasmic ratio in the atypical keratinocytes.
- Histopathologic variants of AK also exist. They all share the classic features of the AK, as previously described, but with some additional findings. The HAK displays solid hyperkeratosis and parakeratosis, while cutaneous horns show massive tiers of hyperkeratosis and parakeratosis.
- An atrophic AK has very mild hyperkeratosis and a thinned epidermis that is devoid of rete ridges.
- Bowenoid AK demonstrates full epidermal dysplasia, but unlike true Bowen's disease or SCC in situ the adnexal epithelium is spared.
- In the pigmented AK, excessive amounts of melanin are seen, especially in the basal layer.
- Lichenoid AK displays a dense, band-like lymphohistiocytic infiltrate at the dermal–epidermal junction, as well as basal layer liquefactive degeneration.
- In the acantholytic variant, there are clefts of lacunae directly above the atypical keratinocytes, similar to changes seen in Darier's disease.

DIAGNOSIS AND DIFFERENTIAL

- The diagnosis of AK is made by clinical examination in most instances. The greatest dilemma is trying to distinguish an AK from a SCC. Findings of induration, larger size, ulceration, bleeding, rapid growth, and recurrence or persistence after treatment should raise the suspicion for SCC.
- The clinical differential diagnosis of AK includes other common lesions, such as benign lichenoid keratosis, seborrheic and irritated seborrheic keratoses, verruca vulgaris, SCC in situ, SCC, keratoacanthoma, BCC, porokeratosis, discoid lupus erythematosus, psoriasis, and other variants of cheilitis.
- Of the clinical variants of AK, pigmented AK is difficult to distinguish from solar lentigo and HAK from SCC.
- Histopathologically, AKs can sometimes be confused with benign lichenoid keratoses, but closer inspection should reveal that in benign lichenoid keratosis there is no cellular atypia of the keratinocytes, as in AK. An atrophic AK can sometimes be difficult to distinguish from cutaneous lupus erythematosus, but in the latter, other histopathologic features of the disease should be present. Lastly, a pigmented AK can sometimes be mistaken for a lentigo maligna, but the latter usually

has more flattening of the epidermis, an increased number of melanocytes, atypical melanocytes, and normal keratinocytes.

TREATMENT

- An AK can persist, regress, or progress into an invasive SCC. Which path a given AK will take is impossible to predict. The estimated risk of an AK progressing into SCC is not exactly known, but a range of less than 1 to 10%, up to 20% has been reported in the literature. Other studies have reported that approximately 60% of SCCs arise from a preexisting AK. In another study, up to 25% of AKs were found to regress over a 1-year period, especially in those who avoided the sun or wore sunscreen.
- AKs are also sensitive markers for predicting the future development of nonmelanoma and melanoma skin cancer in a given individual.
- Because of the risk of progression to SCC and the uncertainty of the destiny of a given AK, most dermatologists advocate the treatment of all AKs, when possible.
- A number of different treatment options are available for the management of AK. Which treatment is chosen depends on individual patient characteristics, clinician proficiency in that technique, as well as the size, number, and location of AK.
- The most common treatment method for AKs in the United States is cryosurgery with liquid nitrogen. It can be administered with a spray device or via cotton tip application. This technique is easy to learn and is best suited for patients with a limited number of discrete AKs. Hypopigmentation is the most common adverse outcome from cryosurgery. Cure rates of up to 98.8% have been reported with this technique.
- Curettage, with or without electrosurgery, is another commonly employed therapy for treating AKs. It is an ideal treatment for patients with relatively few AKs, for treatment of lesions after biopsy, and for HAKs. Scarring and dyspigmentation are common potential side effects.
- Topical 5-fluorouracil therapy is an at-home treatment regimen that is best suited for the treatment of multiple, nonhypertrophic AKs, in a very compliant patient. The patient should expect to apply the medication topically for 3 to 4 weeks. During this time, the treated skin will become uncomfortable, eroded, crusted, and superficially ulcerated. If such outcomes are achieved with good patient compliance, then cure rates of up to 93% have been reported. Much lower cure rates are seen when compliance is poor and these expected outcomes are not reached.
- Less common treatments for AK include dermabrasion, chemical peels, laser therapy, and photodynamic therapy.
- Uncommon treatments for AK include excision, interferon, topical immune response modifiers, oral and topical retinoids, alpha hydroxy acids, and topical diclofenac sodium.

BOWEN'S DISEASE

EPIDEMIOLOGY

- Bowen's disease (BD) is a form of SCC in situ that affects both the skin and mucous membranes and has the potential to progress into invasive SCC.
- BD may occur in any age in adults, but it is very uncommon in individuals less than 30 years of age. The typical patient is older than 60 years of age.
- BD is said to occur equally in males and females, but most studies report a slight preponderance in females.
- It can be located on any body site, including both sun-exposed and non-sun-exposed regions of the body. BD does have a predilection for sun-exposed surfaces, such as the head and neck and for the lower legs in females, in particular.
- The exact incidence of BD in the United States is not known, but in one population study from Hawaii, the incidence was estimated at 142 per 100,000 persons.
- Lesions of BD are usually solitary but may be multiple in up to 10 to 20% of individuals.

PATHOPHYSIOLOGY

- A number of different factors have been implicated in the etiology of BD, including a history of sun exposure, arsenic exposure, ionizing radiation, immunosuppression, and certain types of human papillomaviruses (HPV).
- HPV 16 has been detected in many cases of anogenital BD and in some cases of finger or periungual BD.

CLINICAL FEATURES

- BD typically presents as a discrete, slowly enlarging, pink to erythematous, thin plaque with well-demarcated, irregular borders and overlying scale or crust.
- Verrucous and hyperkeratotic surface changes may also be seen, and a pigmented variant of BD has been reported in less than 2% of cases.

- Individual lesions may measure up to several cm in diameter.
- Multiple lesions are not uncommon.
- Clinical variants of BD exist. Intertriginous BD can present as an oozing, erythematous, dermatitic plaque or as a pigmented patch or plaque.
- Periungual BD can present as an erythematous, scaly, thin plaque around the cuticular margin, a crusted erosion, nail discoloration or onycholysis, a verrucous plaque or as destruction of the nail plate.
- Mucosal BD can present as a verrucous or polypoid papule or plaque, erythroplakia, or as a velvety red plaque.

HISTOPATHOLOGY

- The epidermis displays full thickness atypia, including the intraepidermal portions of the adnexal structures. Involvement spans from the stratum corneum down through the basal cell layer, although the basement membrane remains intact.
- Parakeratosis and hyperkeratosis are present, as is acanthosis with complete disorganization of the epidermal architecture. At times, the hyperkeratosis and parakeratosis are so pronounced that clinically a cutaneous horn is present.
- Throughout the epidermis numerous atypical, pleomorphic, hyperchromatic keratinocytes are present, producing the characteristic "wind blown" appearance. These cells are sometimes vacuolated and display prominent pale-staining cytoplasm, reminiscent of the cells in Paget's disease.
- The upper dermis is usually infiltrated by numerous chronic inflammatory cells, including lymphocytes, plasma cells, and histiocytes.
- Several histopathologic variants of BD exist, including psoriasiform BD, atrophic BD, acantholytic BD, and epidermolytic BD.

DIAGNOSIS AND DIFFERENTIAL

- Because BD is often mistaken clinically for other entities, a biopsy is usually indicated to confirm the diagnosis histopathologically.
- Clinically, BD is often mistaken for superficial BCC, dermatitis, psoriasis or lichen planus, AK, benign lichenoid keratosis, irritated seborrheic keratosis, or amelanotic melanoma. More hyperkeratotic or verrucous lesions of BD may be difficult to distinguish from viral warts, seborrheic keratoses, or SCC. Pigmented BD can be mistaken for melanoma.

- Histopathologically, BD must be differentiated from Paget's disease, pagetoid melanoma in situ, bowenoid papulosis, and podophyllin induced changes in a wart.

TREATMENT

- The risk of BD progressing to SCC has been estimated at around 5%. Once invasive SCC occurs in BD, it has also been estimated that roughly 33% may metastasize, unless adequate therapy is initiated.
- BD, like AK, is a cutaneous marker for the high risk of future development of nonmelanoma skin cancer in that individual. BD of the vulvar region in females has also been associated with an increased risk of uterine, cervical, and vaginal cancer.
- A number of different treatment modalities are available for the treatment of BD, including excision, Mohs micrographic surgery, electrodessication and curettage, cryosurgery, topical 5-fluorouracil, topical immune response modifiers, laser therapy, ionizing radiation, and photodynamic therapy. No one treatment is right for all forms of BD. Therapy has to be guided by the size and location of the lesion, as well as by individual patient characteristics, such as age and healing capability.
- Surgical excision is generally regarded as the treatment of choice for most lesions of BD, providing that the lesion's size and location permit such a procedure. Not only can the entire lesion be removed, but the specimen can then be sent for histopathologic examination, to rule out the possibility of invasive SCC having occurred. Cure rates of 95% have been reported.
- Curettage for superficial or extensive lesions of BD is ideal because of the avoidance of wound closure issues and the relative simplicity and speed of the procedure. With curettage alone, cure rates of 60 to 95% have been reported. When electrocautery is added to curettage, these cure rates increase from 80 to 90%. Lower cure rates, in general, are expected with this procedure, given the possibility of missing BD involving the appendages.
- Topical 5-fluorouracil has been used to treat BD in a limited number of studies. Cure rates of 66 to 92% have been reported, with the highest cure rates being achieved when treatment included a margin of normal skin around the lesion and continual treatment for 6 to 16 weeks. Recurrences are more common with this technique. It may play a role in the treatment of multiple, small, thin lesions of BD, when surgery is not an option.
- The topical immune response modifier drug, imiquimod, has recently gained attention in the treatment of BD. Cure rates of 93% have been purported in the

treatment of clinically noninfiltrated patches of BD for 4 months, but further studies need to be performed for longer-term outcomes.

- Laser therapy for BD has been performed using the carbon dioxide laser, the argon laser, and the neodymium:YAG laser. They appear to be most useful in treatment of BD in difficult to treat sites, such as the finger or genitalia. These modalities are of little use if deep follicular involvement with BD is present.
- Radiotherapy using various techniques and regimens has reported cure rates of 89 to 100% with average follow-up between 6 months and 6 years. It is advantageous for the management of large or multiple lesions, especially in elderly patients who may not tolerate surgery or in patients who tend to form hypertrophic scars or keloids. The main disadvantage of ionizing radiation for treating BD is wound healing. In fact, healing after radiotherapy of BD lesions on the lower legs is so poor that it is not recommended at these sites.
- Photodynamic therapy is a new, investigational treatment for BD. Limited studies show initial promise.

BOWENOID PAPULOSIS

EPIDEMIOLOGY

- This disease is most commonly seen in sexually active young males and females.
- Sites of predilection include the penis in males and the external genitalia in females.
- This disease has also been described in extragenital locations, especially the neck and chin.

PATHOPHYSIOLOGY

- Bowenoid papulosis is caused by infection with HPV, and numerous types of HPV have been linked with bowenoid papulosis, including types 16, 18, 31 to 35, 39, 42, 48, and 51 to 54. HPV 16 is the most common, and types 16, 18, and 33 are considered the most oncogenic.

CLINICAL FEATURES

- Bowenoid papulosis presents clinically with multiple reddish-brown to violaceous-colored papules. Many lesions are verrucous and, at times, the smaller papules coalesce into plaques.

HISTOPATHOLOGY

- The epidermis is usually hyperplastic with atypia, disordered maturation, scattered mitotic figures, and dyskeratotic keratinocytes.

DIAGNOSIS AND DIFFERENTIAL

- A biopsy of the lesions is usually necessary to make the diagnosis.
- The clinical differential includes condyloma acuminata, and in fact, most lesions of bowenoid papulosis are diagnosed clinically as condyloma acuminata.
- Seborrheic keratoses and melanoma may sometimes be clinically confused with bowenoid papulosis.
- Anogenital SCC in situ, unlike bowenoid papulosis, typically presents as a slowly enlarging pink plaque.
- Unlike true SCC in situ, bowenoid papulosis lacks the full-thickness atypia throughout the epidermis. In bowenoid papulosis the atypical keratinocytes are randomly scattered throughout the epidermis and the acrotrichia are typically spared, while in SCC in situ the acrotrichia are usually involved.

TREATMENT

- The natural history of bowenoid papulosis is variable, ranging from spontaneous regression to persistence of lesions to transformation into SCC in situ and invasive SCC.
- Patients with bowenoid papulosis and their sexual partners should be followed and examined periodically because of the risk of developing SCC, cervical and vulvar neoplasia.
- Patients with persistent disease should probably undergo testing for an altered immune status.
- Treatment of bowenoid papulosis is recommended. The disease typically responds well to local therapy, although recurrences are common.
- Therapeutic options include local destructive measures, such as electrodessication and curettage, carbon dioxide laser therapy, neodymium:YAG laser, cryosurgery, and excision. Topical tretinoin, topical 5-fluorouracil, topical imiquimod, and low-dose interferon-α have also been beneficial.

ERYTHROPLASIA OF QUEYRAT

EPIDEMIOLOGY

- Erythroplasia of Queyrat (EQ) is a SCC in situ (Bowen's disease) that affects the mucosal surfaces of the penis in uncircumcised males.
- EQ occurs in uncircumcised males between the ages of 20 and 80 years, although the majority of cases occur between the third and sixth decades.

PATHOPHYSIOLOGY

- Although the exact etiology and pathogenesis of EQ is not known, several risk factors predispose to the development of this condition. These risk factors include not being circumcised, poor hygiene, smegma, heat, friction, trauma, and genital herpes simplex virus infection.
- HPV subtypes 16 and 8 have also been identified in a number of EQ lesions.

CLINICAL FEATURES

- Clinically, EQ presents as a glistening, red, velvety plaque on the glans penis, the prepuce, or the urethra.
- It typically begins as a solitary plaque in just over half of the cases, and multiple plaques in the remainder.
- Associated symptoms include localized pain, pruritus, difficulty retracting the foreskin over the glans, bleeding, and crusting.

HISTOPATHOLOGY

- The histopathology of EQ is similar to BD, as previously described. In addition, epidermal hypoplasia and a dermal infiltrate consisting of many plasma cells are also seen.

DIAGNOSIS AND DIFFERENTIAL

- The clinical differential includes other benign inflammatory conditions, such as psoriasis, lichen planus, lichen sclerosus, candidiasis, plasma cell balanitis (Zoon's balanitis), lymphogranuloma venereum, granuloma inguinale, syphilis, and fixed drug eruption.

- If the diagnosis of EQ is considered, then a biopsy specimen should be obtained.

TREATMENT

- Lesions of EQ typically persist and slowly enlarge. By the time a biopsy is initially obtained, most lesions have been present for several years.
- Progression of EQ to invasive SCC is said to be more common than with other in situ SCCs, occurring in up to a third of cases. Once invasive SCC has occurred, perhaps 20% will display evidence of regional lymph node involvement or more distant metastases.
- Prevention of EQ in uncircumcised males entails adherence to good personal hygiene and possibly early circumcision.
- Treatment options for EQ include excision, Mohs micrographic surgery, carbon dioxide laser therapy, and topical 5-fluorouracil.

ERYTHROPLAKIA

EPIDEMIOLOGY

- Erythroplakia, also known as erythroplasia, is a clinical term used to describe either an erythematous macule or patch on a mucosal surface that cannot be clinically or histopathologically categorized into any other known disease that has been caused by inflammatory, traumatic, or vascular etiologies.
- It is considered to be a premalignant lesion because of the typical findings of either SCC in situ or focally invasive SCC on histopathology.
- Erythroplakia can occur on any mucosal surface, but in over half of the cases, it involves the oral mucosa.
- Erythroplakia is considered to be the most dangerous of all the oral precancerous lesions, carrying the greatest risk of harboring an invasive SCC.
- Erythroplakia is a relatively uncommon lesion in the oral cavity. It is also said to be the least common diagnosis among the premalignant oral lesions.
- Typically, it is found in older males who have a history of tobacco and/or alcohol use.

PATHOPHYSIOLOGY

- The exact etiology of erythroplakia is not known, but the synergistic effect of alcohol and tobacco is thought to play a major role.

CLINICAL FEATURES

- Erythroplakia of the oral mucosa is most often located on the vermilion surface of the lower lip or intraorally. Intraorally, the most common sites of involvement are the lateral and ventral tongue, the floor of the mouth, and the soft palate.
- It presents as a subtle, asymptomatic, red macule or patch. It is well-demarcated from the surrounding mucosa. Its surface is usually smooth and homogeneous in color. Sometimes, the surface appears pebbled or stippled. It often feels velvety.
- It is usually less than 1.5 cm in diameter, but lesions up to 4 cm have been described.
- Erythroplakia can commonly be seen in conjunction with leukoplakia and these lesions are called erythroleukoplakia. In instances of erythroleukoplakia, it is almost always the red patches or erythroplakia that contain or progress into invasive carcinoma.

HISTOPATHOLOGY

- Histopathology of erythroplakia usually reveals findings of SCC in situ and, occasionally, focal areas of dermal invasion may also be seen.

DIAGNOSIS AND DIFFERENTIAL

- Erythroplakia is a diagnosis of exclusion. It is the clinician's responsibility to exclude all other potential causes of erythematous oral lesions before the term erythroplakia can be assigned to a particular lesion.
- Other entities to consider in the differential include acute and chronic mechanical trauma, thermal or chemical injury, candidiasis, lichen planus, chronic contact or allergic dermatitis, submucosal hemorrhage, and various forms of glossitis.
- In general terms, any erythroplakia lesion should be biopsied if the etiology is not obvious or if it does not resolve over several weeks.
- Partial or sampling biopsies of lesions of erythroplakia may unfortunately result in missing the diagnosis of these focal areas of dermal invasion. Sometimes the use of toluidine blue can aid in the diagnosis of erythroplakia by helping to identify the best site in the lesion to take the biopsy from. This metachromatic dye selectively stains areas of dysplastic epithelium. Inflammatory lesions treated with toluidine blue may also stain positively, and thus potential irritants should be discontinued at least 2 weeks prior to the staining.

TREATMENT

- The exact progression rate of untreated SCC in situ of the oral cavity to SCC is unknown.
- In high-risk individuals with lesions of erythroplakia, such as heavy smokers or drinkers, up to 80% of such lesions may harbor foci of invasive SCC.
- The definitive treatment of erythroplakia is controversial. For early dysplastic or in situ SCC, simple excision or Mohs micrographic surgery is ideal because the entire lesion can be removed and viewed histopathologically, thus confirming the diagnosis and excluding more invasive disease.
- Other treatment modalities have been used, such as laser ablation, cryotherapy, and electrocoagulation.
- Regardless of the treatment method used, all patients should be followed at regular intervals to evaluate for the possibility of a second primary lesion in the oral cavity or aerodigestive tract.
- Carcinogenic stimuli, such as tobacco and alcohol consumption, should be discontinued.

LEUKOPLAKIA

EPIDEMIOLOGY

- Leukoplakia is a fixed, mostly whitish, mucosal lesion that cannot be clinically or histopathologically categorized as any other disease.
- Leukoplakia is most often seen in the oral cavity and sometimes on the anogenital mucosal surfaces.
- Some lesions of leukoplakia are benign, while others will transform into cancer.
- As a general group, oral leukoplakias carry a 5 to 25% chance of harboring some form of dysplasia or malignancy.
- Premalignant or malignant leukoplakia lesions are most often located on the floor of the mouth, the lateral and ventral tongue, and the soft palate. Leukoplakia in these anatomic locations has an approximate 40% risk of being premalignant or malignant.
- Leukoplakia with premalignant and malignant potential has also been described in the genetic condition, dyskeratosis congenita.
- Leukoplakia can affect any age range. In terms of leukoplakia associated with carcinogenesis, the typical host is an elderly male, aged 50 to 70 years.

PATHOPHYSIOLOGY

- A variety of factors can contribute to the development of leukoplakia, including chronic trauma, infection, alcohol consumption, and tobacco use.

CLINICAL FEATURES

- Leukoplakia presents as an asymptomatic, white, asymmetric plaque that cannot be easily rubbed off.
- The surface may be soft and smooth or rough and granular.
- Some lesions may have concomitant areas of redness, and as noted earlier, this lesion is then called erythroleukoplakia. This combination lesion carries a higher risk of containing premalignancy or malignancy in it, namely in the erythematous portion.

HISTOPATHOLOGY

- Unlike with erythroplakia, lesions of leukoplakia are less likely to show malignant or premalignant histopathologic changes.
- The more common, reactive leukoplakias exhibit hyperkeratosis, acanthosis or epidermal atrophy, and chronic inflammation. Focal areas of candidiasis may also be seen.
- Some of the leukoplakias do reveal changes consistent with dysplasia, SCC in situ, and SCC.

DIAGNOSIS AND DIFFERENTIAL

- In general, all persistent lesions of leukoplakia should be biopsied to determine the true histopathologic diagnosis.
- Leukoplakia on the floor of the mouth, lateral and ventral tongue, and soft palate carries a much greater risk of being malignant or premalignant and, therefore, should be carefully evaluated and biopsied. Many experts would go so far as to recommend that all such lesions in these locations be removed completely, regardless of the histopathologic diagnosis.
- Other conditions that may present with mucosal white plaques include oral white sponge nevus, lichen planus, candidiasis, syphilis, lichen sclerosus, smoker's keratosis, Darier's disease, and cheek biting.

TREATMENT

- The prognosis for reactive leukoplakia is good, in general.
- For all leukoplakia lesions, in general, the risk of progression into SCC is around 4%, but it is higher in the high-risk anatomic sites, as stated earlier.
- Individuals with leukoplakia should be followed closely, at regular intervals, and re-evaluated should the leukoplakia persist or recur following adequate intervention.

- Treatment of leukoplakia is dependent on where it is located. Lesions on low-risk sites, such as the buccal mucosa, hard palate, and gingival mucosa, can be followed closely if histopathologic features are benign or reactive. Lesions on high-risk sites, such as the floor of the mouth, lateral and ventral tongue, and soft palate, should probably be removed completely, regardless of the histopathology.
- Removal options include surgical excision and Mohs micrographic surgery.
- Other treatment options for premalignant leukoplakia include topical 5-fluorouracil, laser ablation, and cryosurgery.
- Carcinogenic exposures should also be avoided, such as alcohol and tobacco.

MALIGNANT EPIDERMAL NEOPLASMS

- Nonmelanoma skin cancer is the most common cancer in the United States. Half of all new cancers are skin cancers. In the year 2001, it was estimated that over one million new cases of skin cancer would be diagnosed. Of the nonmelanoma skin cancers, approximately 80% are basal cell carcinomas and 20% are squamous cell carcinomas. BCC and SCC have a greater than 95% chance of cure if detected and treated early.

BASAL CELL CARCINOMA

EPIDEMIOLOGY

- BCC is the most common skin cancer in Caucasians.
- Approximately 80% of all skin cancers are BCC and roughly 80% of all nonmelanoma skin cancers are BCC.
- It has been estimated that 28% of Caucasians will develop a BCC in their lifetime, and the incidence appears to be increasing.
- BCC is more common in older individuals, with a mean age of 62 years reported in one large university study. It is more common in males.
- The major risk factor for the development of BCC is UVR exposure. Intense exposure in childhood with a history of numerous sunburns is a particular risk factor.

- A phenotype of fair skin, light-colored hair and eyes, and inability to tan increases the likelihood of developing a BCC.
- Three genetic syndromes are associated with the development of multiple BCC, namely the autosomal dominant nevoid basal cell carcinoma syndrome (NBCC), the Bazex–Dupre–Christol syndrome, and the Rombo syndrome.

PATHOPHYSIOLOGY

- There is no precursor lesion to a BCC.
- BCC is thought to derive from multipotent progenitor cells in the bulge region of the hair follicle.
- NBCC patients have been shown to have mutations in the patched1 (ptch1) gene on chromosome locus 9q22. Ptch1 is the receptor for the morphogen hedgehog (hh), which is involved in the growth and development of the skin. Sonic hedgehog (Shh) is the hh family member that is expressed in the skin.
- Approximately 20 to 54% of sporadic BCCs have also been found to have mutations in the ptch1 gene. Mutations in the genes of other members of the sonic hedgehog signaling pathway have also been found at lower frequencies.
- UVR has been shown to induce signature mutations in the ptch1 gene, and thus the interplay between ultraviolet radiation exposure and mutations in the ptch1 gene have been established.
- P53 mutations are frequent in BCC, but they are not thought to be necessary or sufficient to cause such tumors alone.
- In addition to mutations in the sonic hedgehog signaling pathway, the surrounding stroma and cellular environment, as well as the status of the immune system, play a role in the malignant growth of BCC.
- Other causative agents for BCC include ionizing radiation and chronic arsenic ingestion. BCCs are also seen in chronic scars and vaccination scars in particular.

CLINICAL FEATURES

- BCC is almost always limited to hair-bearing surfaces, with the most common site being on the face, especially the nose. It is also found on the ear and behind the ear, the eyelids, inner canthus, and on the trunk. Less commonly, it is found on the extremities, although its presence on the lower legs of women with a history of significant sun exposure in that area is not uncommon. Rarely is it found on the lip, palms, and soles. The latter two sites are sometimes affected in patients with the NBCC syndrome.

- A number of different clinical variants of BCC exist, including noduloulcerative, superficial, pigmented, morphea-like, and fibroepithelioma.
- The noduloulcerative type of BCC usually begins as a slow-growing, pink, translucent, pearly papule with overlying telangiectases. Often, as the lesion enlarges, a central ulceration will form. As the lesion then grows, this ulcer will enlarge, while the border becomes pearly and rolled. This clinical picture is referred to as the rodent ulcer. Noduloulcerative BCCs are most common on the face.
- The superficial BCC presents most often on the trunk and extremities as a pink to erythematous, flat, slightly scaly papule or plaque. A barely perceptible pearly border can sometimes be appreciated with side-lighting. Sometimes superficial ulcerations and crusts can be seen on the surface, and central smooth atrophic scarring may also be present. These tumors are also slow growing and may reach large sizes of several cm in diameter if not treated.
- Pigmented BCCs can be of the noduloulcerative or superficial variants. In addition to these clinical features, pigmented BCCs also demonstrate central black, brown, or gray pigmentation in the form of specks, dots, or globules.
- Morphea-like, or desmoplastic, BCC presents as a solitary, flat or depressed, indurated papule or plaque. It may be flesh-colored, yellow, or slightly pink in color. The surface is usually smooth and sometimes shiny. The border of this variant is typically ill-defined. This lesion grows slowly and enlarges quite a bit before any sign of ulceration occurs.
- The fibroepithelioma type of BCC, also known as Pinkus tumor, presents as a raised, often pedunculated, firm, pink to flesh-colored papule or nodule. The surface is typically smooth. Ulceration is rare. Clinically, they resemble large fibroepithelial polyps. Most commonly, this variant is seen on the back.
- NBCC syndrome is characterized by the development of numerous BCCs beginning in childhood and adolescence. Literally hundreds of BCCs can develop on the face, scalp, trunk, and extremities. The noduloulcerative and superficial variants are most commonly seen and lesions tend to initially be small. Lesions can become quite large, however, and local invasion, destruction and mutilation are also seen. Approximately half of adult patients, beginning in the second decade of life, demonstrate small palmar and plantar pits, which represent formes frustes of BCC. Abnormalities in the central nervous system and skeletal system occur in NBCC syndrome, such as frontoparietal bossing, medulloblastomas, meningiomas, odontogenic keratocysts of the jaw, bifid ribs, and calcification of the falx cerebri.

- Bazex–Dupre–Christol syndrome is thought to be X-linked and is characterized by follicular atrophoderma, milia, and BCCs. Rombo syndrome is autosomally inherited and characterized by vermiculate facial pitting, milia, and BCCs.

HISTOPATHOLOGY

- Several histopathologic variants of BCCs also exist, including the solid, adenoid, keratotic, superficial, pigmented, morphea-like, micronodular, and fibroepithelioma variants.
- In general, the cells comprising this tumor resemble the basal cells of the epidermis, although they have a larger nucleus to cytoplasm ratio and typically do not demonstrate intercellular bridging. The tumor buds off of the epidermis in many instances and the peripheral layer of the buds shows a classic palisading of the cells. The stroma adjacent to the tumor cells often appears mucinous and usually demonstrates numerous fibroblasts and areas of retraction around the tumor island.
- Circumscribed solid BCCs show collections of various sized and shaped tumor masses in the dermis. There almost always is a connection of some of these tumor masses to the overlying epidermis.
- Adenoid BCCs present histopathologically with tubular, gland-like arrangements of tumor cells, resembling a lace-like pattern.
- Keratotic BCCs demonstrate differentiation toward hair structures and histopathologically show areas of parakeratotic cells and horn cysts, with the latter representing attempts at hair shaft formation.
- Superficial BCCs show areas of buds and irregular proliferations of tumor cells attached to the epidermis as downgrowths.
- Pigmented BCCs demonstrate a large number of melanin-laden melanocytes interspersed between the tumor cells, as well as numerous melanophages in the surrounding stroma.
- Morphea-like, fibrosing, or desmoplastic BCCs show numerous small groups of tightly packed, often elongated tumor cells within a dense fibrous stroma.
- The fibroepithelioma BCC, or Pinkus tumor, presents with long, thin strands of tumor cells that are often attached to the epidermis and demonstrate extensive branching and anastomosing strands of typical tumor cells. The stroma is typically fibrous.

DIAGNOSIS AND DIFFERENTIAL

- The diagnosis of BCC is usually suspected clinically and confirmed histopathologically. For most clinically suspicious BCCs, a shave biopsy taken from the edge or rolled border will suffice for making an adequate diagnosis. For morphea-like BCCs, a punch biopsy taken from the indurated central area is often necessary to establish the diagnosis.
- Other entities are often in the clinical differential diagnosis of BCC, especially with certain clinical subtypes. Noduloulcerative BCC can sometimes be difficult to clinically distinguish from an ulcerative SCC, amelanotic melanoma, fibrous papule, trichoepithelioma, or intradermal nevus. Superficial BCC can be confused with AK, benign lichenoid keratosis, eczema, psoriasis, SCC in situ, and even amelanotic melanoma. Pigmented BCC is often clinically confused with melanoma. Included in the differential diagnosis of morphea-like BCC is scar or an isolated plaque of morphea. The fibroepithelioma BCC can be confused with a large fibroepithelial polyp, pedunculated intradermal nevus, or neurofibroma.

TREATMENT

- BCC is usually a more slow-growing tumor. It rarely metastasizes, but it can be locally invasive if not properly treated.
- The primary goal of treating these lesions is complete eradication of the BCC. Both surgical and nonsurgical treatment options exist, and the choice of which to employ depends on the location and size of the BCC, its histopathologic subtype, the patient's age and preferences, and the physician's skill.
- Surgical treatment options include cryosurgery, electrodessication and curettage, surgical excision, and Mohs micrographic surgery. Nonsurgical treatment options include topical 5-fluorouracil, topical imiquimod, photodynamic therapy, and ionizing radiation therapy.
- BCC with a higher risk of recurrence, aggressive behavior, or difficulty in eradicating include those located on the midface or ear, those larger than 2 cm in diameter, those with morpheaform or other aggressive histopathologic subtypes, recurrent BCC, clinically ill-defined lesions, and those that have been present for longer durations. Such lesions are best removed with the Mohs micrographic surgical technique, where microscopic control of the margins is performed at the time of excision. Mohs micrographic surgery has a mean 5-year recurrence rate of approximately 1%.
- Small (<2 cm on the trunk or <1 cm on the head), primary, well-demarcated, nodular or superficial BCCs located on the head (excluding the eyelids, nose, lip, and ear), neck, trunk, or extremities can be

easily treated with electrodessication and curettage. Cure rates of 90 to 98% have been reported with this technique, when used appropriately.

- Surgical excision of BCC is most effective for primary, clinically well-defined, small (<2 cm) BCCs that are located in anatomic regions that can accommodate a fair amount of tissue removal. Mohs micrographic surgery is best employed for lesions that require a more tissue sparing technique. The margins for surgical excision should be approximately 4 mm around the tumor edges. The 5-year recurrence rate for properly selected, surgically excised, primary BCC is approximately 90%.
- Cryosurgery is less often used to treat BCC. It requires a special technique and is best reserved for patients that cannot tolerate excision, electrodessication and curettage, Mohs surgery, and who are not candidates for topical therapy. Physician familiarity with this technique is necessary for optimal treatment outcome.
- Topical 5-fluorouracil, topical imiquimod, and photodynamic therapy have been used with variable success for the treatment of small, well-defined, primary, superficial BCCs, primarily on the trunk and extremities. Such treatment modalities are not yet standard and are often attempted for patients with multiple lesions.
- Ionizing radiation is sometimes used to treat BCCs in older patients, especially when the lesions are located in anatomic sites that are hard to treat with surgery. It is also a treatment option in older patients who cannot tolerate a surgical procedure.

SQUAMOUS CELL CARCINOMA

EPIDEMIOLOGY

- SCC is the second most common skin cancer in Caucasians.
- In 2001, it was estimated that over 1.3 million cases of nonmelanoma skin cancer would occur in the United States, and of these cases, roughly 20% would be SCC.
- A significant rise in the incidence of SCC has been noted in the last few decades, with one estimate of an age-adjusted incidence growing by 50 to 200% over the last 10 to 30 years.
- SCC is more common in populations closer to the equator. The incidence doubles with each 8-to-10-degree decrease in latitude.
- SCC is more common in men than in women. The lifetime risk of SCC in 1994 was 9 to 14% in men and 4 to 9% in women.
- The greatest risk factor for developing SCC is exposure to UVR, with UVB radiation from sunlight being mainly responsible and UVA exposure also adding to the risk. Exposure to PUVA therapy, ionizing radiation, and tanning beds also contribute to the risk. It appears that chronic, long-term exposure to these agents, occupational exposure, and significant exposure during childhood predispose to the development of SCC.
- Other risk factors include a phenotype of fair skin that burns easily and rarely tans, hazel or blue eyes, and blonde or red hair.
- SCC is more common in elderly individuals, with an average age of 70 years in one study, although it can be seen in younger individuals with a significant sun exposure history.
- Certain genodermatoses, such as xeroderma pigmentosum and albinism, have a higher incidence of SCC.
- Immunosuppressed individuals, such as organ transplant recipients, have a much higher likelihood of developing SCC. SCC is greater than 50 times more likely to develop in transplant recipients than in age-matched controls. SCC usually develops 4 to 7 years post-transplantation and the frequency of SCC continues to rise with time in these individuals. Interestingly, the incidence of SCC is much greater in transplant recipients than the incidence of BCC, a reversal of the normal ratio of nonmelanoma skin cancers in nontransplant individuals.
- Other predisposing conditions for the development of SCC include certain chronic and long-standing scars, ulcers or sinus tracts, hidradenitis suppurativa, and osteomyelitis. Certain chronic inflammatory conditions may also give rise to SCC, such as lichen sclerosus, discoid lupus erythematosus, dystrophic epidermolysis bullosa, and lupus vulgaris.

PATHOPHYSIOLOGY

- The actinic keratosis (AK) is the precursor lesion to SCC. A continuum exists between the development of AK, squamous cell carcinoma in situ, and SCC. In some cases, analogous to cervical carcinoma developing from cervical dysplasia, lesions of AK will progress to SCC in situ and ultimately to SCC. In other instances, lesions of AK will persist as such or even regress. It is impossible to predict which AK will persist, regress, or progress into SCC at this point in the understanding of these lesions.
- Some SCCs develop de novo and do not form from progression of AK.
- UVR, namely UVB, acts as both an initiator and promoter in the development of SCC. UVR causes signature mutations in DNA, more specifically in the p53 tumor suppressor gene. Normally functioning p53 is

responsible for the apoptosis, or programmed cell death, of ultraviolet-mutated keratinocytes in the epidermis. Most cells with one p53 mutation have enough p53 function to allow for the apoptosis of those cells, but in some cases, a small clonal proliferation of these p53 mutated keratinocytes will develop and progress, giving rise to an AK. A second UVR-induced mutation of the p53 gene in these clonally expanded atypical cells results in total loss of p53 function, further proliferation of the atypical cells, and eventual progression into SCC.

- The status of the immune system, especially locally in the skin, plays an important role in the development of SCC.
- Human papillomavirus infection has been associated with the development of SCC, particularly SCC of the palms, soles, nail unit, genitalia, lower extremities, beard area, and possibly in immunosuppressed individuals.
- Certain chemical carcinogens and other agents have been noted to cause precursor lesions to SCC, such as arsenic, tar, polycyclic aromatic hydrocarbons, ionizing radiation, and thermal heat.

CLINICAL FEATURES

- The majority of SCCs occur on the head and neck of elderly individuals. Other sites for SCC development include the dorsal hands and arms, the trunk, and the legs of women. SCC of the genitalia, subungual regions, lips, and palms and soles have also been described.
- Typical lesions present as indurated, skin-colored to pink, usually hyperkeratotic papules and plaques. Overlying ulceration, crusting, and a central keratotic plug may be present. SCC can present as a verrucous papule or plaque or as a pink papule with an overlying cutaneous horn. SCC can also appear as a smooth, pink papule or nodule without any overlying epidermal changes. The typical size of SCC ranges from 0.5 to 1.5 cm in diameter, although larger lesions definitely occur. SCC of the genitalia and subungual regions are often verrucous in appearance.
- Individuals with SCC may describe a painful sensation related to the lesion. They also commonly describe the growth as a nonhealing lesion that often bleeds with minor trauma.

HISTOPATHOLOGY

- Different variants of SCC exist, including acantholytic, adenosquamous, spindle-cell, verrucous, and mucin-producing variants. SCC can be described as well, moderately, or poorly differentiated.

- SCC represents a true, invasive carcinoma of the epidermis. The malignant proliferation of keratinocytes extends through the basement membrane of the epidermis and into the dermis. Individual neoplastic keratinocytes demonstrate varying degree of atypia and squamous differentiation. The more poorly-differentiated the SCC, the greater is the degree of cellular atypia and the less keratinization is present.

DIAGNOSIS AND DIFFERENTIAL

- Clinically, SCC can sometimes be difficult to distinguish from BCCs that have crusted or keratotic centers, hypertrophic AK, SCC in situ, warts, inflamed or irritated SK, and KA.
- Histopathologically, SCC can be difficult to distinguish from KA and pseudoepitheliomatous hyperplasia.
- SCC can be difficult to diagnose histopathologically if the biopsy specimen is inadequate, namely if the specimen does not go deep enough into the dermis to ascertain if invasion is present and to distinguish between SCC, KA, and SCC in situ. The preferred method of biopsy of suspected SCC lesions is a shave, punch, excisional, or incisional biopsy that extends well into the dermis. The specimen should also be submitted to an experienced and qualified pathologist or dermatopathologist for optimal diagnosis.
- Regional lymph node examination should be performed on patients diagnosed with cutaneous SCC, as a risk for metastasis exists.

TREATMENT

- SCC has the potential for local destruction, recurrence, and metastasis. Unlike BCC, which almost never metastasizes, primary SCC has a 5-year recurrence rate and metastatic rate of 8 and 5%, respectively. Metastatic disease portends a poor prognosis, with 10-year survival rates of less than 20% with regional lymph node involvement and less than 10% with distant metastases. Risk factors for recurrence and metastasis include large lesions (usually greater than 2 cm), location on the lip or ear, deep invasion and poor histopathological differentiation, origination in a scar or chronically damaged skin, immunosuppression, recurrent SCC, and perineural invasion.
- Because of the greater risk for recurrence and metastasis with SCC, these lesions need to be diagnosed and treated adequately and expeditiously. Treatment of SCC needs to take into account various patient and lesion-specific factors. Because recurrent SCC carries a relatively poor prognosis, every attempt should be made to completely remove the lesion at the initial treatment.

- Electrodessication and curettage, cryotherapy, and excision, when used appropriately, can effectively treat the majority of local SCCs with low risk for metastasis, namely smaller ($\leq$1 cm in diameter), well-differentiated, clinically discrete lesions in low-risk locations. In practice, electrodessication and curettage is mostly used for superficial, slow-growing, minimally invasive SCCs on the trunk or extremities. Cure rates of 90 to 96% have been reported in such instances. Cryotherapy is rarely used, but may play a role in small, low-risk SCCs in elderly individuals who would not tolerate other therapies. Excision with standard margins of 4 mm (for low-risk lesions, smaller than 2 cm in diameter) is adequate for most of these lesions when located on the trunk or extremities or on the cheek or neck, when tissue sparing is not of concern. Cure rates of around 95% have been reported with such treatment of low-risk tumors.
- Mohs micrographic surgery, a technique in which margin control is established at the time of the surgery, is an excellent treatment option for higher risk lesions and for those in anatomic locations where tissue sparing techniques are necessary. In this procedure, the entire depth and perimeter of the lesion is viewed histopathologically while the patient is still in the office, thus providing a roughly 95 to 97% adequacy in completely clearing the tumor from the skin. This treatment modality has potentially the highest rates of cure for patients with high-risk primary or recurrent SCC, ranging from 94 to 100% for primary tumors and 90 to 93% for recurrent tumors. The cure rate for excision of recurrent tumors, on the other hand, is only around 77%.
- Ionizing radiation therapy is another alternative treatment, reserved primarily for elderly patients who cannot tolerate surgery or for those lesions in tough locations where surgery might distort the surrounding tissues, such as the eyelid, ear, nose, or lips. It is generally not used in young or middle-aged individuals because of the small potential for later development of radiation-induced cutaneous malignancy. Cure rates of 85 to 95% have been reported for radiation treatment of SCC lesions less than 2 cm in diameter, with lower rates of cure being noted for more advanced lesions. Radiation therapy is also used for concomitant treatment of aggressive or recurrent SCC.
- Recurrent and metastatic SCC requires a multidisciplinary approach to treatment.

REFERENCES

Alam M, Ratner D. Cutaneous squamous cell carcinoma. *N Engl J Med.* 2001;344:975.

An KP, Ratner, D. Surgical management of cutaneous malignancies. *Clin Dermatol.* 2001;19:305.

Brash DE, Bale AE. Molecular basis of skin cancer. *Progress Dermatol.* 1997;31:1.

Callen JP, Bickers DR, Moy RL. Actinic keratoses. *J Am Acad Dermatol.* 1997;36:650.

Callen JP, Salasche SJ, Moy RL, et al. Actinic keratoses: Scientific evaluation and public health implications. *J Am Acad Dermatol.* 2000;42:S1.

Duncan KO, Leffell DJ. Epithelial precancerous lesions. In: Freedberg I, Katz S, Wolff K, et al, eds. *Dermatology in General Internal Medicine,* ed 6. New York:McGraw-Hill, 2002 (in press).

Grossman D, Leffell DJ. The molecular basis of nonmelanoma skin cancer. *Arch Dermatol.* 1997;133:1263.

Kirkham N. Tumors and cysts of the epidermis. In: Elder D, Elenitsas R, Jaworsky C, et al, eds. *Lever's Histopathology of the Skin,* ed 8. Philadelphia: Lippincott-Raven, 1997;685.

McKee PH. Tumors of the surface epithelium. In: *Pathology of the Skin,* ed 2. London:Mosby-Wolfe, 1996;14-1.

Oro AE. Progress in understanding the pathogenesis of basal cell carcinoma. *Progress in Dermatol.* 2001;35:1.

Schwartz RA. Premalignant keratinocytic neoplasms. *J Am Acad Dermatol.* 1996;35:223.

ADNEXAL NEOPLASMS

- Neoplasms that differentiate toward the adnexal structures in the epidermis fall into one of four groups (Table 18–2): those differentiating toward hair follicles, those toward sebaceous glands, those toward eccrine glands, and those differentiating toward apocrine glands. Both benign and malignant variants of these neoplasms exist, and tumors with differentiation towards more than one structure may also exist. The origin of these neoplasms is not fully understood. Several theories exist as to their pathogenesis. One theory is that these adnexal neoplasms develop from embryonic primary epithelial germ cells. Another theory is that they arise from undifferentiated, pluripotential cells that have the potential to develop into tumors with hair, sebaceous, apocrine, or eccrine structures. The other theory is that these neoplasms arise from preexisting structures. Only a few of these are discussed in detail.

FOLLICULAR DERIVED

TRICHOEPITHELIOMA

- Trichoepithelioma is an adnexal tumor with differentiation toward hair structures, namely the hair matrix and hair shaft, that can present as an isolated lesion or as multiple lesions. A giant solitary trichoepithelioma and a desmoplastic trichoepithelioma variant have also been described.

- Multiple trichoepitheliomas is inherited in an autosomal dominant fashion. During childhood and around the time of puberty, lesions begin to appear and increase in number. The lesions present as symmetric, multiple, round, small, firm, flesh-colored papules. Overlying telangiectases and late-stage ulceration is sometimes observed. Typically, they are located around the nose, nasolabial folds, cheeks, eyebrows, eyelids, and upper cutaneous lip. Multiple trichoepitheliomas have also been reported to occur simultaneously with multiple cylindromas, another autosomal dominant inherited condition known as the Brooke–Spiegler syndrome.
- Solitary trichoepitheliomas are more commonly observed and occur spontaneously. The solitary trichoepithelioma presents as a firm, flesh-colored, somewhat larger papule or nodule, usually on the face. It occurs in childhood or early adulthood.
- The giant solitary trichoepithelioma is a distinct benign variant that presents as a slow growing nodule on the face, scalp, neck, trunk, or proximal extremities. Location in the perianal region is also a favored site of occurrence. It clinically resembles the regular solitary variant but grows to sizes up to 3 or more cm in diameter. Typically, older adults are affected.
- Histopathologically and clinically, trichoepitheliomas are sometimes difficult to distinguish from keratotic appearing BCCs. In fact, many believe that BCCs and trichoepitheliomas both derive from common pluripotential cells, and that they differ only in their degree of maturation or differentiation. Characteristic histopathologic findings of trichoepitheliomas include the presence of numerous, varying sized horn cysts, and tumor islands consisting of either a lacelike network or solid aggregation of basaloid appearing cells. The stroma surrounding these tumor islands is fibrotic and closely adherent to the islands, not allowing for the typical retraction artifact seen around the tumor islands in BCC.
- The desmoplastic trichoepithelioma usually presents as a solitary growth on the face of young adults. It is more common in females. It appears as a small, indurated, umbilicated papule. Histopathologically, it differs from the classic trichoepithelioma in that it demonstrates narrow strands of tumor cells, horn cysts, and a fibrotic or desmoplastic stroma. It can sometimes be mistaken histopathologically for a microcystic adnexal carcinoma if a deep enough biopsy is not obtained. The latter, malignant neoplasm shares the findings of narrow tumor strands, horn cysts, and desmoplastic stroma, but it differs by the presence of ductal structures and a more deeply infiltrating tumor growth.

PILOMATRICOMA AND PILOMATRIX CARCINOMA

- Another name for pilomatricoma is calcifying epithelioma of Malherbe. It is an adnexal neoplasm with differentiation toward hair matrix cells.
- It most often presents as an isolated growth on the face or upper extremities of children and adolescents. A second peak for presentation in the sixth and seventh decades has also been described. An autosomal dominant inherited disorder presenting with multiple lesions has been described, and multiple pilomatricomas in association with Gardner's syndrome and myotonic dystrophy have also been noted.
- Mutations in the gene (CTNNB1) encoding beta-catenin have been described in many pilomatricomas.
- Typically, it presents as a firm, dermal or subcutaneous nodule, with overlying normal skin. Sometimes, however, the overlying skin has a bluish or red hue, and at other times, the tumor is more superficial and sharply demarcated, presenting as a red nodule.
- On histopathology of the lesion, a multilobulated tumor, situated in the dermis or subcutaneous tissue, is seen. The tumor lobules consist of two populations of cells, the more immature basaloid cells and the more mature shadow or ghost cells. In some tumors, there are areas of abrupt and complete keratinization. Calcification is also commonly seen.
- Rarely, pilomatricomas can demonstrate evidence of malignant degeneration, either de novo or on examination upon recurrence of the lesion. Occurrence of pilomatrix carcinoma is very rare, and it has been more commonly found in males. Treatment entails wide excision of the lesion. Recurrences are common, but metastases are rare, with evidence in the draining lymph nodes and lung.

TRICHILEMMOMA AND TRICHILEMMAL CARCINOMA

- Trichilemmoma is a fairly common benign neoplasm that derives from the follicular outer root sheath that can occur as a solitary growth or as multiple lesions. Multiple trichilemmomas are commonly seen in Cowden's disease.
- Solitary trichilemmoma typically presents as a small, less than 1 mm, nonspecific, skin-colored papule on the face of adults. It can sometimes appear as a warty papule or at the base of a cutaneous horn.
- The diagnosis of multiple trichilemmomas is often diagnostic of Cowden's disease, an autosomal dominant inherited condition that is also known as the multiple hamartoma syndrome. Mutations in the tumor suppressor, PTEN gene have been identified in this condition. It is characterized by the presence of numerous facial papules, which may be trichilemmomas, dermal fibromas, or acrochordons. The trichilemmomas, which are found in all patients with

Cowden's disease, present as small, skin-colored or pink-brown verrucous papules, primarily around the mouth, nose, and ears. Other associated skin findings include skin-colored or brown scaly acral keratoses, punctate keratoses of the palms and soles, and confluent papules with cobblestoning of the oral mucosa. Systemic manifestations may include thyroid adenomas or carcinoma, ovarian cysts, uterine fibroids, colonic polyps, and breast cancer. Breast cancer is very common in this condition, and since the trichilemmomas often appear before the onset of breast cancer, a timely diagnosis of Cowden's syndrome can be life-saving for affected women.

- Histopathology of trichilemmomas reveals a tumor with several lobules extending down from the surface epithelium into the dermis. Individual cells in these lobules often appear clear, owing to their differentiation toward outer root sheath cells. The periphery of these lobules often displays characteristic palisading columnar cells and a thickened basement membrane. Trichilemmal keratinization is not present, but epidermoid keratinization is often seen, frequently leading to the development of a cutaneous horn. Histopathologic differentiation from wart or eccrine poroma may at times be difficult.

- In individuals with Cowden's disease it is often necessary to obtain multiple biopsies from facial lesions in order to find the diagnostic histopathologic picture of trichilemmoma. The oral lesions in Cowden's disease are fibrous hamartomas.

- Trichilemmal carcinoma is a rare malignant tumor that is predominantly found on sun-exposed areas of the skin in elderly individuals. Such tumors have been described as red or skin-colored papules, nodules, or plaques with frequent ulceration and crusting. It typically has an indolent course with rare recurrence or metastases. Histopathologically, this tumor consists of cytologically atypical clear cells and frank invasion. Trichilemmal keratinization is frequently seen.

SEBACEOUS GLAND DERIVED

NEVUS SEBACEOUS

- Nevus sebaceous is also known as nevus sebaceous of Jadassohn. It most often appears as a solitary congenital lesion located on the scalp or face. At birth it frequently appears as a discrete, yellow to flesh-colored, hairless plaque, that is often configured in a linear array. During puberty the lesion often becomes larger and more verrucous and nodular.

- Up to 0.3% of neonates will present with a nevus sebaceous. It occurs equally in males and females.

- Much less commonly, nevus sebaceous can present as multiple, generalized plaques arranged in the lines of Blaschko. The generalized form of nevus sebaceous has been called the nevus sebaceous syndrome and has been associated with concomitant seizures and mental retardation, neurologic defects, or skeletal abnormalities.

- Nevus sebaceous can also occur concomitantly with a linear epidermal nevus.

- Nevus sebaceous is a complex lesion that is made up of abnormalities of the hair follicles, sebaceous glands, and sweat glands.

- Histopathology typically reveals an epidermis that is hyperkeratotic with marked papillomatosis. Aborted and poorly matured hair follicle structures are present. In nevus sebaceous lesions from infants, well-developed and numerous sebaceous glands are present in the neoplasm, patterning the prominence of sebaceous glands in general in such infants. In nevus sebaceous lesions from children, one typically sees a paucity of underdeveloped sebaceous glands, although incompletely developed hair structures are still present. In mature nevus sebaceous lesions in adults, numerous sebaceous glands are present high up in the dermis and not necessarily associated with a hair follicle. In many lesions, ectopic apocrine glands are located in the lower dermis.

- During adulthood, various types of adnexal neoplasms may arise within the nevus sebaceous. The most common lesions to arise are syringocystadenoma papilliferum and BCC. Less commonly found tumors include syringoma, nodular hidradenoma, trichilemmoma, proliferating trichilemmal tumor, chondroid syringoma, sebaceous epithelioma, and SCC.

- Because of the risk of developing BCC within a nevus sebaceous after puberty, many experts recommend that the nevus sebaceous be completely excised at or before puberty.

FORDYCE'S CONDITION

- Fordyce's condition represents the presence of ectopic sebaceous glands. These ectopic sebaceous glands are found on the vermilion border of the lips or on other areas of the oral mucosa. They are more prevalent in older individuals.

SEBACEOUS HYPERPLASIA

- Lesions of sebaceous hyperplasia are common benign growths that are seen on the face of middle-aged and older adults. They are most often found on the forehead, nose, and cheeks. Lesions are frequently multiple.

- Sebaceous hyperplasia presents as single or multiple, small, 2 to 3 mm, yellow, umbilicated papules. On close inspection of these lesions, individual lobules growing out from the central umbilicated region can be identified. Overlying telangiectasia is sometimes also appreciated.

- Clinically, sebaceous hyperplasia is most often mistaken for BCC.
- Histopathology reveals a single, enlarged sebaceous gland consisting of a single, wide, centrally located sebaceous duct with outgrowing numerous sebaceous lobules. The opening of the sebaceous duct corresponds to the central umbilicated area.

SEBACEOUS ADENOMA

- Sebaceous adenoma is a rare, benign tumor seen primarily on the face or scalp of older individuals.
- It is commonly found in individuals who have the Muir–Torre syndrome, and the diagnosis of a sebaceous adenoma should prompt the clinician to investigate whether or not the patient indeed has Muir–Torre syndrome.
- Sebaceous adenomas present clinically as tan, yellow, or pink-red papules or nodules. Clinically, they are often mistaken for BCC.
- Histopathology reveals a well-circumscribed lesion that is composed of immature, irregularly sized and shaped sebaceous lobules. Two cell types are present in these lobules, namely more peripheral, undifferentiated, basaloid cells, and mature sebaceous cells. Cells with intermediate maturation between these two predominant cell types are also seen, termed transitional cells.
- Along a spectrum of sebaceous maturation, sebaceous adenoma sits between the mature lesion of sebaceous hyperplasia and the less mature sebaceoma (sebaceous epithelioma).

ECCRINE GLAND DERIVED

ECCRINE HIDROCYSTOMA

- Eccrine hidrocystoma may present as an isolated growth or with multiple lesions, usually in adults.
- These lesions are typically found on the face and present as small, 1 to 3 mm, clear to blue colored, cystic papules. Eccrine hidrocystomas are most commonly found in a periorbital location, but they also have been reported to occur elsewhere, such as on the leg.
- A characteristic finding with eccrine hidrocystomas is that they may increase in size during the warm summer months and decrease in size during the colder, winter months.
- These benign neoplasms are thought to represent malformations of the eccrine ducts.
- Clinically, these lesions are difficult to distinguish from apocrine hidrocystomas.

- Histopathology reveals a solitary dermal cyst that is lined by two layers of small cuboidal cells. Unlike in apocrine hidrocystomas, there are no myoepithelial cells and typically no decapitation secretion is evident.

SYRINGOMA

- Syringomas are common benign growths that present typically as multiple lesions on the face of women. The preferred site on the face is the lower eyelid, but they may also be found on the cheeks, axillae, abdomen, and external genitalia. Typical onset is around puberty.
- An eruptive form of syringomas has also been described. In this condition, hundreds of syringomas erupt primarily on the trunk and upper extremities of young individuals.
- Syringomas present as flesh to yellow colored, small, 1- to 3-mm, soft papules.
- Syringomas are believed to represent benign growths of intraepidermal eccrine ducts.
- Histopathology reveals a normal epidermis with a dermal collection of several small duct-like structures. The walls of these ducts are lined by two rows of epithelial cells. Characteristic of these small ducts are their comma-like tails, which are reminiscent of tadpoles. The central cavity of the ducts contains an amorphous appearing substance.
- Syringoma may need to be differentiated from microcystic adnexal carcinoma and desmoplastic trichoepithelioma histopathologically. Typically, syringomas are smaller in size, lack horn cyst formation, and rarely demonstrate single filing of the epithelial cells. Also, the ductal components do not penetrate or invade deep into the dermis and subcutaneous tissue.
- Treatment of limited numbers of syringomas has been successful with carbon dioxide laser resurfacing, excision, and dermabrasion. Eruptive syringomas are difficult to treat and several techniques have been attempted with varying success, including carbon dioxide laser resurfacing, excisions, electrodessication and curettage, and dermabrasion.

ECCRINE POROMA AND POROCARCINOMA

- Eccrine poroma is a relatively common benign skin growth that most often appears on the soles or sides of the feet in middle-aged adults. Less commonly, it may appear on the hands or fingers and, rarely, is it found on other skin surfaces, such as the neck, chest, and face.
- It typically presents as a solitary, pedunculated, skin-colored to erythematous, firm papule. It is usually less than 2 to 3 cm in diameter and is most often asymptomatic. Minor trauma, however, can predispose the lesion to bleeding.
- Several clinical variants of eccrine poroma exist, including a linear and multiple variant. In eccrine

poromatosis, hundreds of eccrine poromas appear, primarily on the palms and soles, and less often in a more generalized distribution.

- Eccrine poroma derives from cells of the outer layer of the acrosyringium and the upper dermal eccrine duct.
- Histopathologic examination of an eccrine poroma reveals replacement of the lower portion of the epidermis with tumor cells that grow down into the dermis in broad anastomosing bands. There typically is a sharp cutoff between normal epidermis and tumor. Individual tumor cells are small, uniform, and cuboidal in appearance. Intercellular bridging is noticeable between these cells and they contain prominent glycogen. In most tumors, small ductal lumina are present.
- Clinically, eccrine poroma should be differentiated from amelanotic melanoma or BCC, although the latter is rare on the palms and soles.
- Malignant eccrine poroma, also known as porocarcinoma, typically develops within a long-standing eccrine poroma, although a de novo malignant variant may also occur. It most often is found on the legs and feet of elderly individuals as a verrucous nodule, plaque, or ulcerated growth. Multiple cutaneous metastases are a unique feature of this tumor. Recurrence is fairly common and more distant metastases have also been reported.
- Benign eccrine poromas are usually removed with surgical excision. Wide excision of eccrine porocarcinoma or Mohs micrographic surgery with close follow-up is recommended.

ECCRINE SPIRADENOMA AND MALIGNANT ECCRINE SPIRADENOMA

- Eccrine spiradenoma is usually a solitary benign dermal nodule that occurs in young adults. Its size may range from 1 to 5 cm in diameter and it is typically painful. The overlying surface may also have a characteristic bluish hue. There is no characteristic location for its occurrence.
- Other clinical variants of this entity include multiple eccrine spiradenomas, the appearance of large tumors in a linear configuration, and the presence of multiple smaller lesions in a zosteriform array.
- Eccrine spiradenoma derives from the dermal eccrine duct and the secretory segment of the eccrine sweat gland.
- Histopathology reveals either one large circumscribed tumor lobule or multiple smaller lobules in the dermis. There is no connection with the overlying epidermis. The individual tumor cells appear deeply basophilic, owing to their nuclear crowding. Two distinct types of cells, arranged in interconnecting bands, are present in the lobules, namely more undifferentiated peripheral cells with small dark nuclei and

central cells with larger pale nuclei. Ductal differentiation is often present.

- Clinically, this tumor may be difficult to diagnose, as other dermal cysts and tumors are in the differential. Biopsy of the lesion is diagnostic and the presence of pain and a bluish hue can aid in the clinical suspicion.
- Malignant eccrine spiradenoma is an extremely rare tumor that most often occurs from malignant degeneration of a long-standing eccrine spiradenoma. Clinically, this transformation should be suspected when a long-standing eccrine spiradenoma begins to enlarge. Generalized and lymph node metastases have been described with this malignant variant.
- It is recommended that all eccrine spiradenomas be completely excised, once the diagnosis has been made, as recurrences and malignant degeneration can occur. Malignant spiradenomas require wide excision and close follow-up.

MICROCYSTIC ADNEXAL CARCINOMA

- Another name for microcystic adnexal carcinoma is sclerosing sweat duct carcinoma.
- This is a malignant, often aggressive tumor, which characteristically appears in middle-aged or older individuals on the upper lip, nasolabial or periorbital regions, and on the scalp. Both genders appear to be affected equally.
- It may present nonspecifically as an ill-defined, indolent, skin-colored to yellow or red, firm dermal nodule or plaque. Hyperkeratosis may also be present. Symptoms, such as pain, burning, or paresthesia, may be present if perineural invasion is present.
- The exact derivation of this malignant neoplasm is not known. Some reports state that only eccrine differentiation is present, while other investigators believe both follicular and sweat gland differentiation are present.
- Histopathology reveals a poorly delineated dermal tumor that infiltrates deep into the dermis, subcutaneous tissue, and sometimes skeletal muscle or even bone. The dermis consists of a desmoplastic stroma with interspersed keratocysts, narrow epithelial strands, and small ductules.
- As stated earlier in this chapter, microcystic adnexal carcinoma can sometimes be histopathologically mistaken for a desmoplastic trichoepithelioma, especially if a superficial biopsy specimen is obtained. Microcystic adnexal carcinoma, unlike desmoplastic trichoepithelioma, invades deep into the subcutis and skeletal muscle.
- Microcystic adnexal carcinoma is an aggressive tumor that is often associated with extensive tissue destruction. Local recurrences are common, although metastatic spread is rare. Treatment is best managed with Mohs micrographic surgical excision.

APOCRINE GLAND DERIVED

APOCRINE HIDROCYSTOMA

- Apocrine hidrocystoma is a benign tumor that usually presents as a solitary, translucent, cystic papule on the face. It is typically several mm in diameter and has a bluish hue. Although the face is the most common location for its occurrence, reports of such lesions on the ears, scalp, and trunk have also been documented.
- Multiple apocrine hidrocystomas have also been reported, although much less commonly. They are part of the constellation of cutaneous findings in Schopf–Schulz–Passarge syndrome.
- Seasonal or temperature variations do not affect the morphology of apocrine hidrocystomas, as with eccrine hidrocystomas.
- Histopathology demonstrates a dermal cyst, which is lined by two rows of cells. The innermost layer of cells consists of columnar secretory cells, which exhibit decapitation secretion. The outermost layer of cells consists of elongated myoepithelial cells.

SYRINGOCYSTADENOMA PAPILLIFERUM

- Syringocystadenoma papilliferum is a benign neoplasm that most often presents as a solitary linear plaque or array of papules on the scalp or face of newborns. It may also develop later in childhood. Around the time of puberty, the lesion often grows in size and becomes more papillomatous or verrucous.
- Syringocystadenoma papilliferum may also arise within a nevus sebaceous.
- The exact derivation of syringocystadenoma papilliferum is unknown, but it is believed to derive from pluripotential cells that have the potential to develop into various structures. Both apocrine and eccrine differentiation has been noted within this lesion.
- Histopathology demonstrates one or multiple cystic invaginations extending down off of the epidermis. The distal portion of the invagination has numerous papillary projections that bulge into the cyst lumen. These papillary projections are lined by a double layer of glandular epithelium, while the upper portion of the cystic invagination appears to be lined by normal surface epithelium. A classic feature of syringocystadenoma papilliferum is the presence of numerous plasma cells within the stroma of the tumor. Multiple apocrine glands can also be seen in the dermis, beneath the cystic invagination.

CYLINDROMA AND MALIGNANT CYLINDROMA

- Cylindromas are relatively common, benign neoplasms that arise on the scalp, head, or neck of primarily adults. They can occur as solitary or multiple lesions. Solitary lesions are more common and do not appear to be inherited. They present as solitary, slow-growing, pink to red, smooth dermal nodules, typically 1 cm in diameter.
- Multiple cylindromas are inherited in an autosomal dominant fashion. The inherited condition of coexistent multiple trichoepitheliomas and cylindromas is known as the Brooke–Spiegler syndrome. Multiple cylindromas have also been reported to coexist with multiple eccrine spiradenomas. Multiple cylindromas present as numerous, dome-shaped, pink dermal nodules, primarily on the scalp. Lesions may rarely be seen on other locations, such as the face, trunk, or extremities. Their size varies from 1 to several cm in diameter. Multiple nodules that occur on the scalp can be so extensive, as to cover it like a turban, and thus such lesions are often called turban tumors.
- Cylindromas are believed to differentiate toward either apocrine or eccrine structures, with the former being thought to be more common.
- Histopathology of both solitary and multiple cylindromas reveals a dermis consisting of multiple lobules that are arranged in a jigsaw-like pattern. Each tumor island is surrounded by a hyaline sheath of variable thickness. The islands consist of two types of cells, namely an outer layer of cells with small hyperchromatic nuclei and an inner layer of cells with larger, lighter staining nuclei. Tubular lumina are also frequently present.
- Solitary cylindromas may be easily excised, but multiple cylindromas pose a more difficult treatment dilemma. Reports of initial debulking of the tumors, followed by carbon dioxide laser resurfacing, have noted some good results.
- Malignant cylindroma is a rare neoplasm that results from the malignant transformation of a preexisting cylindroma. Although it has been reported to occur in a solitary cylindroma, it is more often seen in cases of multiple cylindromas. Clinical clues to malignant transformation have included rapid growth, bleeding, or ulceration of a preexisting cylindroma. Complications of malignant cylindroma are metastases to lymph nodes, bone or viscera, and invasion into the skull with resultant hemorrhage and meningitis. Treatment with wide local excision is recommended.

REFERENCE

Elder D, Elenitsas R, Ragsdale BD. Tumors of the epidermal appendages. In: Elder D, Elenitsas R, Jaworsky C, et al, eds. *Lever's Histopathology of the Skin*, ed 8. Philadelphia: Lippincott-Raven, 1997;747.

19 MELANOCYTIC TUMORS

Rafael Botella-Estrada

- Cutaneous pigmented lesions derived from the melanocytes are a frequent cause of dermatologic consultations due to either concern for malignancy or for aesthetic reasons. Within the group of benign melanocytic lesions, the most commonly seen in daily practice are the ephelides (freckles), lentigines (sunspots), and acquired melanocytic nevi (moles).
- Certain melanocytic nevi, such as congenital melanocytic nevus, atypical melanocytic nevus, halo nevus, or nevus spilus, display some clinicopathologic characteristics that allow them to be differentiated from common acquired melanocytic nevi.
- Melanoma has drawn considerable attention in the last decades due to its sharp increase in incidence. Currently, there is no effective treatment for this tumor when it has disseminated. Therefore, while research continues, prevention, early detection, and surgery should govern the treatment of melanoma.

BENIGN MELANOCYTIC LESIONS

CAFÉ–AU–LAIT MACULES (CALM)

PATHOPHYSIOLOGY

- In a strict sense, CALMs are not melanocytic neoplasias since histologically, melanin is increased in the epidermis but the number of melanocytes is normal or only slightly augmented.

CLINICAL FEATURES

- CALMs are well-demarcated macules, light brown in color, with a diameter ranging from 2 to 20 mm. Most of them appear in infancy or early childhood.
- Multiple CALMs can be seen in several syndromes including neurofibromatosis and McCune–Albright syndrome (polyostotic fibrous dysplasia, endocrine dysfunction, and melanotic macules). Neurofibromatosis type 1 is the most characteristic of these syndromes. The presence of more than six CALMs is one of the criteria to establish the diagnosis of this disease.

DIAGNOSIS AND DIFFERENTIAL

- Differential diagnosis should be established with Becker's nevus, congenital melanocytic nevus, nevus spilus, pigmented mosaicism such as "linear and whorled nevoid hypermelanosis," ephelides, and lentigines.
- The presence of melanin macroglobules in melanocytes and/or keratinocytes is a characteristic feature of CALMs associated with neurofibromatosis, but their absence does not exclude this diagnosis. Conversely, they are not specific since they have also been described in CALMs of people without neurofibromatosis and in several other pigmentary conditions (nevus spilus, melanocytic nevi, melanotic macules of Albright syndrome, and multiple lentiginosis syndrome).

TREATMENT

- These lesions do not require treatment. However, should removal be desirable, the best results have been achieved with Q-switched lasers.

EPHELIDES

PATHOPHYSIOLOGY

- Ephelides, commonly known as freckles, are the result of an overproduction of melanin by the melanocytes to protect the skin against the deleterious effects of ultraviolet light. They are more common in individuals that tan poorly and burn easily after sun exposure (Fitzpatrick type I and II).
- Histologically, the number of melanocytes is normal, but the amount of melanin is increased at the basal layer.

CLINICAL FEATURES

- Small, usually less than 5-mm, light-brown macules that appear on sun-exposed skin, especially on nose and cheeks, after sun exposure.

LENTIGO

PATHOPHYSIOLOGY

- Two types of lentigines can be distinguished: lentigo simplex and lentigo solaris (actinic lentigo or lentigo senilis). They appear in different clinical settings: lentigo simplex usually arises in childhood, and lentigo solaris appears on sun-damaged skin of adults and elderly individuals. Lentigo solaris is a sign of photoaging and is related to ultraviolet light exposure.

CLINICAL FEATURES

- Lentigo solaris presents as a single or multiple well-circumscribed, brown macules, usually located on the face and dorsum of the hands. Rarely, they may be present at the first decade of life.
- Lentigo simplex are small, flat, brown to black macules, evenly distributed, measuring only a few mm in diameter. Multiple lesions of lentigo simplex can appear in several syndromes, such as the multiple lentigines syndrome (LEOPARD), LAMB/NAME syndrome, and Peutz–Jeghers syndrome (Table 19–1).

DIAGNOSIS AND DIFFERENTIAL

- Lentigo solaris consists of proliferations of hyperpigmented keratinocytes, with a normal or slightly increased number of melanocytes. Its frequent clinical and histologic association with the reticulated type of seborrheic keratosis has been conducive to considering lentigo solaris as a keratinocytic more than a melanocytic lesion.
- In some cases, lentigo solaris may have clinicopathologic features similar to melanoma in situ (lentigo maligna). The confinement of the melanocytes at the dermoepidermal junction, its monomorphous appearance, and their equidistant disposition are all criteria that support the diagnosis of lentigo solaris.
- Clinically, lentigo simplex can be indistinguishable from junctional nevi. The histology of lentigo simplex shows an increase in the number of the melanocytes at the basal layer, an increase in the melanin concentration in the melanocytes and the basal keratinocytes, and a slight but characteristic elongation of the rete ridges. Junctional nevus is manifested by small nests of nevus cells at the dermoepidermal junction.

TREATMENT

- Although liquid nitrogen has been widely used in the treatment of lentigo, treatment with the frequency-doubled Q-switched Nd:YAG laser is more effective and, at the same time, causes fewer unwanted side effects.

MELANOCYTIC NEVUS

EPIDEMIOLOGY

- Melanocytic nevus is a benign lesion constituted by a proliferation of nevus cells. Nevus cells are melanocytes that have lost their dendritic shape and characteristically are grouped in nests.
- Melanocytic nevi can be congenital (present since birth) or acquired. Acquired nevi have been classified according to the microcopic location of nevus cells into junctional (nests at the dermoepidermal junction), compound (nests at the dermoepidermal junction and dermis), and intradermal (majority of nests in dermis).
- It has been estimated that the average number of nevus in a white adult individual is approximately 20.

PATHOPHYSIOLOGY

- Melanocytic nevi are not static biological entities but they represent a continuum evolving from junctional nevi, in young people, to the compound and intradermal nevi, in adult life. Over the course of time, nevus cells migrate from the dermoepidermal junction to the dermis, and in this process, they also change clinically.

CLINICAL FEATURES

- Junctional nevi are flat or slightly elevated, well-demarcated, brown or black lesions of small size.

TABLE 19–1 Syndromes Associated with Multiple Lentigo Simplex

LEOPARD	(multiple lentigines syndrome): lentiginosis, electrocardiographic conduction abnormalities, ocular hypertelorism, pulmonar stenosis, abnormal genitalia, retardation of growth, and sensorineural deafness
LAMB/NAME	LAMB: lentigines, atrial and mucocutaneous myxomas, and blue nevi
	NAME: nevi, atrial myxoma, myxoid neurofibromata, and ephelides
Peutz–Jeghers:	lentigines (buccal mucosa, lips, fingers, and toes) and gastrointestinal polyps (bleeding, obstruction, intussusception, and malignant degeneration)

They usually begin to appear in childhood or adolescence.
- When nests of nevus cells penetrates into the dermis, as in compound nevus, they become elevated with respect to junctional nevi, sometimes adopting a papilomatous shape, and the color ranges from skin colored to different shades of brown to black.
- Intradermal nevi are the most frequent nevi in adults. They are usually skin-colored, round or oval exophitic lesions with a smooth or papilomatous surface.

TREATMENT

- Most acquired melanocytic nevi do not require treatment other than for purely cosmetic purposes or if they are located on areas of irritation.
- Nevi can be surgically removed with a shaved or an elliptical excision, but the cosmetic result should be carefully evaluated.

CONGENITAL MELANOCYTIC NEVUS

EPIDEMIOLOGY

- This term is reserved for those nevi present since birth. Congenital melanocytic nevi can be divided into three categories according to their greatest diameter: small (less than 1.5 cm), intermediate (1.5 to 20 cm), and giant (greater than 20 cm). This classification is useful because the likelihood of a congenital nevus to degenerate into a melanoma is proportionate to its size. The risk has been estimated between 6 and 8% for giant lesions, whereas in small and intermediate congenital nevi, it has not been well quantified but seems to be extremely low.
- Approximately, 60% of the melanomas arising in giant congenital melanocytic nevi develop during the first decade of life, with the highest rate of malignancy during the first 5 years of life.

CLINICAL FEATURES

- Congenital nevi appear as pigmented macules and evolve into darker lesions in the course of weeks. The presence of hairs are characteristic of these lesions, as well as the progressive thickening and development of a verrucous surface.
- Clinical observation will fail to detect most malignant transformations in giant nevi because the majority of

melanomas developing in giant congenital melanocytic nevi have a nonepidermal origin.

TREATMENT

- For giant nevi, prophylactic surgical excision should be recommended as soon as possible. Referral to a plastic surgery department with experience in the management of these patients is advised.
- Small and intermediate-sized congenital nevi should be monitored through childhood and their excision considered before 12 years of age. Due to the low risk of melanoma development in those nevi, follow up may be an alternative, especially when surgery may cause disfigurement or functional impairment as a consequence of the location.

ATYPICAL MELANOCYTIC NEVUS

EPIDEMIOLOGY

- This term is currently preferred to the previously used dysplastic nevi. Atypical nevi are benign melanocytic nevi that show some clinical and histologic features that may be difficult to differentiate from melanoma. Confusion has plagued this entity due to its similarity with melanoma and concern about the potential for development of melanoma.
- There is a second reason for confusion, that of the familiar dysplastic nevus syndrome. This is a rare autosomal dominant disease described by Clark in 1978. Affected individuals have numerous atypical nevi and family members with multiple dysplastic nevi or even melanoma. The risk for development of melanoma for family members with multiple dysplastic nevi but without previous history of melanoma is 184-fold compared with the general population, whereas for those patients with a previous melanoma, the risk increases to 500-fold.
- Patients with the sporadic subtype of dysplastic nevus syndrome (patients with atypical nevi outside the familial melanoma setting) also have an increased risk of melanoma, but the risk is much lower than in those persons with the familial subtype. The risk depends on the number of atypical nevi present, ranging from a two-fold risk of developing melanoma for those persons with one atypical nevus to 12-fold if 10 or more atypical nevi are present.
- In this context, it seems adequate to consider dysplastic nevi not only as a precursor, but also as a "marker" of patients at risk for melanoma. Prophylactic removal of all dysplastic nevi is not realistic and would not eliminate the risk of subsequent melanoma.

CLINICAL FEATURES

- Atypical nevi tend to be macular lesions greater than 5 mm, with irregular borders and variegated colors of brown, black, and sometimes areas of depigmentation. They tend to be located on the trunk.

DIAGNOSIS AND DIFFERENTIAL

- Clinical differential diagnosis with melanoma can be very difficult. Some atypical nevi share features with melanoma, and can be almost indistinguishable. An important clue for diagnosis of melanoma is the "ugly duckling" sign, which refers to a pigmented lesion that is different from all the others.
- Dermoscopy, when used by experienced clinicians, has been shown to increase the sensibility and specificity in the differential diagnosis with melanoma. It may be also extremely useful for follow-up of those patients with multiple atypical nevi.
- Excision of the atypical nevus for histopathologic evaluation is mandatory when a high degree of doubt exists. Histologic criteria that define atypical nevi include the presence of nests of melanocytes at the epidermal rete ridges that frequently coalesce (bridging of nests), thickened collagen bundles around and beneath the epidermal rete ridges (fibroplasia lamellar), and random cytologic atypia. In contrast, the atypical melanocytes in melanoma can be seen at higher layers of the epidermis and not only at the dermoepidermal junction, and the degree of cytologic pleomorphism is more manifested than in atypical nevi.

TREATMENT

- Atypical nevi should be excised for histopathologic evaluation. Excision can be performed by different techniques (shave, excision, punch), but it should allow the dermatopathologist to evaluate the deep and lateral aspects of the lesion.

HALO NEVUS

CLINICAL FEATURES

- Halo nevus is a benign melanocytic nevus in which a depigmented halo has developed. This depigmented halo may envelop the nevus until this latter has completely disappeared. In some cases, several nevi become surrounded by the halo simultaneous or progressively. Halo nevus is more frequent in children or young adults.

DIAGNOSIS AND DIFFERENTIAL

- Histologically, a dense lymphocytic infiltrate is admixed with nevus cells.

SPITZ NEVUS

EPIDEMIOLOGY

- Spitz nevus was described in 1948 by Sophia Spitz under the name of benign juvenile melanoma. It is also designated as nevus of spindle and epithelioid cells.
- Spitz nevus is currently considered a benign proliferation of nevus cells. It usually arises in childhood, and has attracted much attention in the dermatologic literature due to its great histologic similarity with malignant melanoma.

CLINICAL FEATURES

- Dome-shaped lesions, 3 to 10 mm in diameter, with a coloration that usually ranges from red to orange. The face is the typical location, although they can also arise on the trunk or extremities.

DIAGNOSIS AND DIFFERENTIAL

- Clinical differential diagnosis includes pyogenic granuloma, hemangiomas, cutaneous leishmaniasis, and juvenile xanthogranuloma.
- Histologically, Spitz nevus is a compound or intradermal nevus with alarming cytologic features. In about half of the cases, the cells of a Spitz nevus are pleomorphic, spindle shaped, or epithelioid, with an abundant eosinophilic-staining cytoplasm and mitoses. The silhouette of the lesion is symmetrical and well circumscribed, with a characteristic epithelial hyperplasia and hyperkeratosis. Helpful clues for the differential diagnosis with melanoma are the maturation of nevus cells (decrease in size) toward the base of the lesion in Spitz nevus, the absence of mitoses at the base, and the presence of eosinophilic round bodies (Kamino bodies) in the basal layer of the epidermis (present in more than half of Spitz nevi and rare in malignant melanoma and ordinary melanocytic nevi).

TREATMENT

- Surgical excision.

NEVUS SPILUS

CLINICAL FEATURES

- Nevus spilus, also known as speckled and lentiginous nevus, presents as a light-brown macular area containing darker lentigo-like lesions scattered on its surface. The appearance is that of multiple pigmented nevi on an area of lentiginous changes.

DIAGNOSIS AND DIFFERENTIAL

- Histologically, some areas show features similar to lentigo simplex, whereas other areas show features of junctional or compound melanocytic nevi. Malignant melanoma within a nevus spilus has been reported in fewer than a dozen of cases. Consequently, although prophylactic excision is not justified, patients should be advised to report any change they notice on a lesion of this type.

REFERENCES

Carpo BG, Grevelink JM, Grevelink SV. Laser treatment of pigmented lesions in children. *Semin Cutan Med Surg.* 1999;18:233.

Clark WH Jr, Reimer RR, Greene M, Ainsworth AM, Mastrangelo MJ. Origin of familial malignant melanoma from heritable melanocytic lesions. "The B–K mole syndrome." *Arch Dermatol.* 1978;114:732.

Greene MH, Clark WH Jr, Tucker MA, Kraemer KH, Elder DE, Fraser MC. High risk of malignant melanoma in melanoma-prone families with dysplastic nevi. *Ann Intern Med.* 1985;102:458

Grob JJ, Bonerandi JJ. The 'ugly duckling' sign: Identification of the common characteristics of nevi in an individual as a basis for melanoma screening. *Arch Dermatol.* 1998;134:103.

Landau M, Krafchik BR. The diagnostic value of café–au–lait macules. *J Am Acad Dermatol.* 1999;40:877.

Todd MM, Rallis TM, Gerwels JW, Hata TR. A comparison of 3 lasers and liquid nitrogen in the treatment of solar lentigines: A randomized, controlled, comparative trial. *Arch Dermatol.* 2000;136:841.

Tucker MA, Halpern A, Holly EA, et al. Clinically recognized dysplastic nevi. A central risk factor for cutaneous melanoma. *JAMA.* 1997;277:1439.

DERMAL MELANOCYTOSIS

- Under this term, there are several benign pigmented lesions characterized by a proliferation of melanocytes, which in their normal migration from the neural crest to their final location in the basal layer, never reach their destination and become arrested in the dermis. The characteristic blue or blue-grey color of the dermal melanocytoses is the consequence of the transmission of the black melanin color through the dermis. Histologically, melanocytes in these lesions have a spindle shape, are heavily loaded with melanin, and are intermingled between collagen bundles.

BLUE NEVUS

CLINICAL FEATURES

- Two types have classically been distinguished: common and cellular blue nevus. Common blue nevus presents as a well-defined blue or black papule, with a diameter ranging between 3 and 10 mm. It is usually located on the extensor surfaces of hand or feet. Cellular blue nevus tends to be larger and locate on the sacroiliac region.

DIAGNOSIS AND DIFFERENTIAL

- The common blue nevus shows a proliferation of dendritic melanocytes in the reticular dermis arranged in small aggregates that tend to be disposed around appendages, vessels, or nerves. In cellular blue nevus, there is a mixture of spindle and dendritic cells, with larger cells exhibiting neural differentiation.

MONGOLIAN SPOT

EPIDEMIOLOGY

- This lesion is more frequent in dark-skinned individuals, and is highly prevalent in Asians, with more than 90% of infants affected. Conversely, it is present in only 1% of white infants.

CLINICAL FEATURES

- A macular deep-blue pigmentation that appears at birth on the sacral region of some infants. In some cases, it may occupy a large area of the back, or even extend through the flanks to the abdomen.

TREATMENT

- No treatment is necessary. In most cases, Mongolian spots gradually fade away in a matter of months to few years.

NEVUS OF OTA AND NEVUS OF ITO

CLINICAL FEATURES

- Nevus of Ota, also known as nevus fuscoceruleus oph-thalmomaxillaris, is a macular lesion located on one side of the face, following the distribution of the first and/or second branches of the trigeminal nerve. The color ranges from grey to brown. The sclera is also pigmented in 65 % of cases.
- Nevus of Ito, nevus acromioclavicularis, is similar to nevus of Ota but involves the shoulder, neck, and/or arm.
- Nevus of Ota and Ito are persistent throughout life.

TREATMENT

- Q-switched lasers (ruby, neodimium-YAG, or alexandrite) have offered some hope of clearance or fading.

REFERENCE

Moreno-Arias GA, Camps-Fresneda A. Treatment of nevus of Ota with the Q-switched alexandrite laser. *Laser Surg Med.* 2001;28:451.

MALIGNANT MELANOMA

- Cutaneous malignant melanoma (MM) is a potentially lethal tumor. Melanoma originates from malignant melanocytes. Thus, it may potentially develop in any surface tissue hosting these cells. Besides the skin, melanoma has been described in the mucosal epithelia, conjunctiva, retina, and leptomeninges, although the relative frequency in all these locations is very low.

EPIDEMIOLOGY

- The incidence of cutaneous MM has risen dramatically. It is estimated that 1 of every 75 Americans born in the year 2000 will develop melanoma during their lifetime. One of the factors that has contributed to the rise in incidence is its early detection.
- Based on clinical and histologic features, there are four types of malignant melanoma: superficial spreading melanoma, acral lentiginous melanoma, nodular melanoma, and lentigo maligna melanoma. Superficial spreading melanoma accounts for 70% of all melanomas. Acral lentiginous melanoma accounts for about 5 to 8% of all melanomas in Caucasians. In other more pigmented races, such as African Americans and Asians, the global incidence of melanoma is much lower, and 35 to 90% of their melanomas belong to this type. Nodular melanomas account for 15 to 20% and lentigo maligna melanoma for 5% of all melanomas.

PATHOPHYSIOLOGY

- The etiopathogenesis of melanoma is incompletely understood. Several factors have been identified. Increased total sun exposure, as well as an intermittent pattern of exposure, have been implicated. Sunlight ultraviolet radiation causes DNA lesions, whose incorrect repair leads to DNA mutations. UVB radiation is mainly responsible for DNA lesions, but UVA is more abundant in sunlight, causes oxidative DNA damage that is potentially mutagenic, and has an immunosuppressive role. In contrast with the more common skin cancers, which are associated with total cumulative exposure to ultraviolet radiation, melanomas appear to be associated with a pattern of intermittent exposure. This fact explains the body location and the population group affected by each neoplasia. Whereas basal cell and squamous cell carcinomas arise in those areas of the body more exposed to sunlight, such as the face and the back of the hands and forearms, melanomas occur in areas exposed intermittently to the sun, such as the back in men and lower legs in women. For the same reason, people with the largest incidence in basal and squamous cell carcinomas are those exposed almost daily to sunlight, such as sailors and farmers. Melanoma, however, is more common in people exposed to sun only on weekends and vacations. The explanation for this difference seems to rely on the fact that the risk of melanoma is associated with sun exposures that induce sunburn. It has been found that the risk of melanoma in a person with five or more severe sunburns during adolescence is higher than twofold.
- Mutations in a tumor suppressor gene, CDKN2A, located on the short arm of chromosome 9, have been found in 20% of melanoma-prone families (those with three or more affected members from different parts of the world).
- The best way of preventing melanoma is to avoid sun exposure, especially midday sun (between 11 AM and 4 PM). Promoting sunscreen use that protects against UVB and UVA is an integral part of prevention programs against skin cancers. Nevertheless, the use of

sunscreens may lead to a paradoxical deleterious effect due to changes in the behavioral pattern of regular sunscreen users. It has been documented that there is a tendency to stay out much longer in the sun with sunscreen use, which compensates for or even exceeds the benefits of these agents.

- Several personal risk factors contribute to the development of melanoma. Patients with dysplastic nevus syndrome in the context of a family history of atypical nevi or melanoma have a higher risk for developing melanoma. The total number of nevi is another well-recognized risk factor, since individuals with 50 to 100 nevi have a risk of developing melanoma 3.2 times that of those patients with none to four nevi. As discussed previously, melanoma develops in 6 to 8% of giant congenital melanocytic nevi. Other well-established factors include individuals with Fitzpatrick type I skin (never tan and always burn when exposed to sun), tendency to freckling, prior history of familial or personal melanoma, and living in proximity to the Equator.
- Although melanoma tends to originate de novo, a small proportion develops from a melanocytic precursor lesion. The percentage of melanomas that develop from preexisting melanocytic nevi cannot be established according to clinical features, because what may have looked like a nevus clinically, may actually have been the earliest manifestation of a melanoma. Therefore, only histopathology may shed some light into the subject of how many melanomas develop into melanocytic nevi. Remnants of a benign melanocytic nevus have been found in 10 to 30% of melanomas.

CLINICAL FEATURES

- Visual examination is the most common method for the identification of melanoma. Of paramount importance is the ABCD rule that defines four characteristics of melanoma: A for asymmetry, B for borders irregularity, C for color heterogeneity, and D for diameter larger than 6 mm.
- Suspicion that a nevus is evolving into melanoma should be raised when some change is noticed in a preexisting nevus. Changes in size, color, surface (a nodule that develops on a flat lesion), desquamation, ulceration, or bleeding should alert about the potential malignant degeneration of a nevus.
- Superficial spreading melanoma usually presents in individuals in the fourth or fifth decades of life. May be located in any area, but it is more common on legs in women and trunk in men.
- Acral lentiginous melanoma is located on palms, soles, and the periungual and nail bed region.

- Nodular melanoma presents as a pigmented, rounded, nodule exhibiting a rapid growth because it enters directly into the vertical growth phase.
- Lentigo maligna melanoma arises from a clinical variant of melanoma in situ known as lentigo maligna or melanotic freckle of Hutchinson. Lentigo maligna is a macular lesion that grows very slowly. It develops on sun-damaged skin in the elderly, most commonly on the face, neck, or extensor forearms, and it takes many years for invasion to develop.

DIAGNOSIS AND DIFFERENTIAL

- Suspicious lesions should be carefully evaluated. Since atypical nevi frequently fulfill some of the clinical criteria (ABCD rule) used for diagnosis of melanoma, the differential diagnosis from a clinical point of view between these two entities can be difficult.
- Dermoscopy, dermatoscopy, or epiluminiscence microscopy, is a relatively new noninvasive diagnostic technique for the in vivo evaluation of pigmented skin lesions. It consists of placing mineral oil on the skin and visualizing the lesion with a hand-held dermatoscope, a stereomicroscope, or a digital imaging system. The magnification of the different systems ranges from 6 to 40X. The oil placed on the lesion eliminates surface reflection making the cornified layer transparent, which allows a better visualization of the pigmented structures of the epidermis, dermoepidermal junction, and dermis, as well as the dermal vessels. The method is based on the recognition of different structures and patterns that allow a more objective evaluation of a given lesion than the mere clinical observation with the naked eye. With appropriate training, dermoscopy has been shown to improve by 10 to 27% the sensitivity in diagnosing melanoma based on clinical features.
- If based on clinical and dermoscopy features a lesion is suspected of melanoma, a biopsy should be performed. The entire lesion should be removed to allow the pathologist a complete examination including the architectural pattern. Biopsies that do not remove the entire lesion may be only justified in cosmetic areas such as the face, and in very large pigmented lesions in which an excision with direct side to side closure would not be possible.
- The histopathologic criteria used to diagnose a melanoma may be basically divided into two categories: architectural and cytological. Architecturally, melanomas tend to be larger than 5 to 6 mm in diameter, asymmetric, with poor lateral circumscription, and the size and shape of the nests are not uniform. Melanocytes may be seen above the basal layer of the

TABLE 19–2 Proposed Stage Groupings for Cutaneous Melanoma. American Joint Committee on Cancer Staging System 2001

STAGE	CRITERIA
0	Melanoma in situ
IA	Localized melanoma, 1.0 mm, without ulceration and clark level II/III
IB	Localized melanoma, 1.0 mm, with ulceration or Clark level IV/V, or 1.01 to 2.0 mm without ulceration
IIA	Localized melanoma, 1.0 to 2.0 mm with ulceration, or 2.0 to 4.0 mm without ulceration
IIB	Localized melanoma 2.01 to 4.0 mm with ulceration, or >4 mm without ulceration
IIC	Localized melanoma >4.0 mm with ulceration
IIIA[a]	Micrometastasis in 1 to 3 nodes with primary melanoma not ulcerated
IIIB	Micrometastasis in 1 to 3 nodes with primary melanoma ulcerated, or macrometastasis in 1 to 3 nodes with primary melanoma not ulcerated, or in transit met(s)/satellite(s) without metastatic nodes with any primary melanoma
IIIC	Macrometastasis in 1 to 3 nodes with primary melanoma ulcerated or >4 mets nodes, or in transit met(s)/satellite(s) with metastatic nodes
IV	Three groups: M1a: distant skin, subcutaneous or nodal mets; M1b: lung mets; M1c: all other visceral mets or any distant mets plus elevated serum LDH

[a]A clinical and a pathologic staging are proposed. There are no stage III subgroups for clinical staging.
Adapted from Balch et al.

TABLE 19–3 Survival Rates for Melanoma According to the Pathologic Stage

PATHOLOGIC STAGE	5-YEAR SURVIVAL (%)
IA	95
IB	90
IIA	78
IIB	65
IIC	45
IIIA	66
IIIB	52
IIIC	26
IV	9 to 18

Adapted from Balch et al.

epidermis (pagetoid spreading). Cytologically, melanocytic nuclei are large and atypical. Mitoses and necrosis of melanocytes are additional cytologic features of malignant melanoma. Except for nodular melanoma, in the other three variants, a radial or horizontal growth phase precedes, sometimes for months or years, the development of the vertical growth phase. In the horizontal phase, malignant melanocytes are confined to the epidermis, and sometimes infiltrate the papillary dermis as small nests or individual cells. In the vertical growth phase, the cells invade directly the dermis forming large aggregates, and acquire capacity to metastasize.

- Histopathologic examination of melanocytic tumors may be extremely difficult. In very early lesions of melanoma in situ, an increased number of melanocytes, with nuclei that range from mildly typical to overtly atypical, are disposed at the basal layer as solitary units. Later, some of the melanocytes ascend in the epidermis. Eventually, nests of melanocytes become situated above the dermoepidermal junction. Although not present in all melanomas, one of the most characteristic histologic features of melanoma is the presence of atypical melanocytes in pagetoid distribution in the epidermis and adnexal epithelial structures.

- Once the diagnosis of melanoma has been reached, the histopathologic report must include several parameters with prognostic value: Breslow's thickness, ulceration, Clark's level, lymphocitic reaction, number of mitoses per high-power field, signs of regression, vascular or lymphatic embolization, and muscular or perineural invasion. The inclusion in pathology reports of ambiguous terms, such as dysplastic nevus with mild, moderate, or severe dysplasia, may interfere with the understanding of the benign or malignant potential of a given lesion. Thus, a fluid communication between the pathologist and dermatologist is essential.

- Currently, the most important prognostic factor for localized melanoma is Breslow's thickness, that is, the thickness of a melanoma measured with a micrometer from the granulous layer to the deepest portion of the tumor. Ulceration has been determined as the second most important pronostic factor. Clark's levels of invasion are established according to the position of melanoma cells. In level I, melanoma cells are confined to the epidermis and its appendages; in level II, the cells have broken the dermoepidermal junction, and may be found in the papillary dermis; in level III, melanoma cells fill the papillary dermis; in level IV, the reticular dermis is involved; and in level V, melanoma cells invade the subcutaneous layer. Clark's levels are more subjective and are dependent on the location of melanoma rather than the measured tumor thickness. For that reason, it has partially lost its prognostic relevance. Table 19–2 shows the final version of the American Joint Committee on Cancer Staging System for staging of cutaneous melanoma and Table 19–3 summarizes the prognosis for melanoma patients according to the new classification.

- Diagnostic work-up of a patient with melanoma: a suggested scheme for the initial diagnostic work-up and ongoing follow-up is detailed in Table 19–4. Two considerations should govern management of melanoma patients. First, routine initial and interval

TABLE 19–4   Suggested Scheme for the Initial Diagnostic Work-up and Ongoing Follow-up of Melanoma Patients

BRESLOW DEPTH (mm)	FOLLOW-UP	
	PHYSICAL EXAMINATION	CHEST X-RAY AND LABORATORY[a]
Stage I	6 mo × 2 yr; 12 mo thereafter	Initial
State IIa	4 mo × 3 yr; 12 mo thereafter	Yearly
Stage IIb	4 mo × 3 yr; 6 mo 2 yr; 12 mo thereafter	Yearly
Regional (Stage III) or distant (Stage IV) disease	3 to 4 mo × 5 yr; 12 thereafter	Every other visit × 5 yr; yearly thereafter[a]; Initial CT scans head/chest/abdomen/pelvis or PET[b] if available

[a] Laboratory: liver function tests and LDH.
[b] PET: positron emission tomography.

TABLE 19–5   Recommendations for Surgical Management of Melanoma

TUMOR THICKNESS (mm)	CLINICAL EXCISION MARGINS
In situ	0.5
<2	1
2	2

history with physical examination should direct the laboratory tests or imaging studies solicited. Second, the majority of metastases and recurrences are discovered by the patient or a family member. Thus, patient education on skin and lymph node examination is critical. Based on these recommendations, a chest x-ray, liver function tests, and serum lactate dehydrogenase (LDH) should be performed in the initial work-up of asymptomatic patients. In the absence of clinical evidence of metastatic disease, in patients with melanomas less than 1 mm, yearly chest x ray, liver function tests, and LDH, should be considered. Although this may be reasonable, in a study involving more than 800 asymptomatic patients with localized melanomas that were initially examined with chest x-rays, unsuspected metastasis was demonstrated in only 1 patient. The false-positive rate was approximately 15% and it led to costly investigations to rule out the presence of metastases, with the subsequent patient's anxiety.

- With regard to the follow-up interval, it should be considered that the thickness of primary melanoma is the main factor related to the probability of metastases, and that the majority of metastases appear in the first few years after diagnosis. Other factors that should be taken into account to establish the follow-up regimen are (1) patients with multiple melanomas, (2) family history of melanoma, and (3) presence of clinically atypical nevi. According to all these facts, follow-up two to four times per year for 2 to 3 years after diagnosis, and one to two times thereafter is recommended.

TREATMENT

- The risk of recurrence decreases as time goes by and is proportional to each stage. Decrease in survival is especially important in stages II, III, and IV, in the first 5 years after the excision. There are series with ultralate recurrent melanomas (more than 15 years elapsed from treatment), therefore, a patient should not be given certainty that the tumor is cured. Teaching patients to explore themselves, and offering optimism and support over the long term, is the most reasonable strategy.

- The treatment of choice of cutaneous melanoma is surgery. Current recommendations include the excision of a margin of normal-appearing skin around the tumor to ensure its complete removal. The recommendations for excisional margins have changed over time. Some decades ago, wide margins were excised but several prospective studies did not found any statistically significant difference in favor of the wide margins. The current American Academy of Dermatology guidelines for treatment of melanoma are summarized in Table 19–5. Excision should be performed down to the fascia but there is no need to include it. In cosmetically sensitive areas such as the face, margins can be reduced to preserve the function of certain structures such as the eyelids. Mohs micrographic surgery can be a valid alternative to assure negative excision margins in lentigo maligna melanomas located on the face.

- Lymph node dissection can be performed in three different settings. *Therapeutic lymphadenectomy* refers to lymph node excision when clinical involvement of lymph nodes (i.e., macrometastasis) is detected. There is no controversy about the advantages of therapeutic lymphadenectomy in terms of improving prognosis. The second type is prophylactic or *elective lymphadenectomy*. It refers to the excision of all lymph nodes located in the draining basin of the melanoma, even if nodes are not palpable. Several prospective studies have failed to show any improvement in survival in patients treated with this procedure. In the last decade, *selective lymphadenectomy* has gained acceptance as a form of treatment for intermediate thickness melanomas (1 to 4 mm Breslow thickness). It is agreed that the risk of lymph node involvement is very low for thin melanomas (<1.0 mm). At the other extreme, thick melanomas (>4.0 mm) have a high probability of already having spread beyond regional lymph nodes. Selective lymphadenectomy is based on the concept of sentinel lymph node (SLN). SLN is the first lymph node that receives the lymphatic drainage from a tumor. Morton and colleagues introduced the technique and demonstrated with 99% probability that the negativity of SLN for tumor implies that the rest of lymph nodes in that basin are also free of tumor cells, avoiding the necessity to perform a complete lymphadenectomy. Nevertheless, in spite of its wide acceptance due to its low morbidity, the issue of SLN is still undetermined, and there are no published studies about its influence on survival. It helps to stage patients, offers prognostic information, and is an important tool to allocate patients in trials for adjuvant treatment.

- Adjuvant therapy: In high-risk patients with lymph node involvement (stage III), high-dose interferon-α has demonstrated an improvement in disease-free and overall survival. Interferon-α is also deemed appropriate for patients with in-transit metastasis and for node-negative patients with primary melanomas deeper than 4 mm.

- Treatment for metastatic melanoma: When melanoma has disseminated systemically, treatment is highly unsatisfactory. There is no standard therapy and each case must be individually evaluated. Dacarbazine (DTIC) remains the standard for initial chemotherapy for metastatic melanoma. It has a documented response rate of 15 to 25%. Nevertheless, the median duration of response is 5 to 6 months, and only 5% achieved complete responses. A three-drug combination regimen with cisplatin, vinblastine, and dacarbazine (CVD) has produced responses in 40% however, most of them partial and of short duration. The combination of three chemotherapy drugs (dacarbazine, cisplatin, carmustine) plus the antihormonal agent tamoxifen is widely known as the Dartmouth regimen. The response rate to this regimen ranges between 40 and 50%, but again with the same disadvantages of partial and short lasting responses. Although combination regimens have achieved a better initial outcome, they are also associated with a high level of toxicity, and randomized trials with dacarbazine alone have not shown a significant difference in response rate or overall survival.

Temozolomide, a new alkylating agent with the potential to cross the brain–blood barrier, is being used in patients with brain metastases.

- In metastatic melanoma, surgery can be appropriate for those patients with limited, nonvisceral or pulmonary disease, as long as they have documented a reasonable period without disease progression. Patients with solitary brain metastasis may also benefit from surgical excision. Radiation therapy is an option as a palliative form of treatment for painful cutaneous lesions or for those large tumors that cause bleeding or neurologic or vascular compression. Palliative care is a reasonable option for elderly or debilitated patients with widespread, unsymptomatic disease, or for those who have not responded to other treatments.

- Biochemotherapy, a combination of chemotherapy and biologic response modifiers, is another alternative for metastatic melanoma. Several groups are investigating the combination of three chemotherapeutic agents (CVD) with interferon-α and interleukin-2. Concurrent therapy with both classes of agents have shown response rates ranging between 35 and 65%, with up to 30% of complete responses. The main disadvantage of biochemotherapy is its high toxicity, greater than chemotherapy.

- Several vaccines have been developed for the treatment of stage III or IV melanoma. The goal of this approach is to improve the cellular or humoral immune response against melanoma cells. The theoretical advantage of this therapy would be the lack of toxicity. Objective responses have been documented in several single-arm studies. Nevertheless, up-to-date vaccines have not demonstrated an improvement in the outcome of patients with metastatic melanoma in the context of phase III randomized studies.

REFERENCES

Anderson KW, Baker SR, Lowe L, Su L, Johnson TM. Treatment of head and neck melanoma, lentigo maligna subtype: A practical surgical technique. *Arch Facial Plast Surg.* 2001;3:202.

Balch CM, Buzaid AC, Soong SJ, et al. Final version of the American Joint Committee on Cancer Staging System for Cutaneous Melanoma. *J Clin Oncol.* 2001;19:3635.

Balch CM, Soong SJ, Gershenwald JE, et al. Prognostic factors analysis of 17,600 melanoma patients: Validation of the American Joint Committee on Cancer Melanoma Staging System. *J Clin Oncol.* 2001;19:3622.

Bataille V, Bishop JA, Sasieni P, et al. Risk of cutaneous melanoma in relation to the numbers, types, and sites of naevi: A case-control study. *Br J Cancer.* 1996;73:1605.

Dubois RW, Swetter SM, Atkins M, et al. Developing indications for the use of sentinel lymph node biopsy and adjuvant high-dose interferon alfa-2b in melanoma. *Arch Dermatol.* 2001;137:1217.

Gilchrest BA, Eller MS, Geller AC, Yaar M. The pathogenesis of melanoma induced by ultraviolet radiation. *N Engl J Med.* 1999;340:1341.

Goldstein AM, Tucker MA. Genetic epidemiology of cutaneous melanoma. A global perspective. *Arch Dermatol.* 2001;137:1493.

Lipsker DM, Hedelin G, Heid E, Grosshans EM, Cribier BJ. Striking increase of thin melanomas contrasts with stable incidence of thick melanomas. *Arch Dermatol.* 1999;135:1451.

Mayer J. Systematic review of the diagnostic accuracy of dermatoscopy in detecting malignant melanoma. *Med J Aust.* 1997;167:206.

Morton DL. Lymphatic mapping and sentinel lymphadenectomy for melanoma: Past, present and future. *Ann Surg Oncol.* 2001;8(9 Suppl):22S.

Sober AJ, Chuang TY, Duvic M, et al. Guidelines of care for primary cutaneous melanoma. *J Am Acad Dermatol.* 2001;45:579.

Terhune MH, Swanson N, Johnson TM. Use of chest radiography in the initial evaluation of patients with localized melanoma. *Arch Dermatol.* 1998;134:569.

20 CUTANEOUS LYMPHOMAS AND HISTIOCYTOSIS

Javier Alonso-Llamazares
Ramón M. Pujol

PRIMARY CUTANEOUS LYMPHOMA: CONCEPT AND CLASSIFICATION

- Cutaneous lymphomas are a heterogeneous group of malignant lymphoproliferative disorders that clinically originate in the skin. The majority of these cutaneous lymphomas are of T-cell origin (65%), whereas 20 to 25% are thought to originate from B-lymphocytes.
- The term primary cutaneous lymphoma has been used to define lymphomas arising in the skin without evidence of concurrent extracutaneous lymphoma for 6 months following initial presentation. A notable exception to this definition of primary and secondary cutaneous lymphoma is mycosis fungoides (MF), which is almost always presumed to represent a primary cutaneous lymphoma, even in cases that do not fulfill the aforementioned definition.
- Secondary cutaneous lymphomas are defined as those lymphomas that develop in the skin as secondary manifestation of primary extracutaneous lymphomas. Secondary cutaneous involvement is observed in 25 to 50% of cases of peripheral T-cell lymphoma and approximately 10% of systemic B-cell lymphomas.
- Primary cutaneous lymphomas often have distinct histomorphologic features and relatively indolent clinical behavior compared with their nodal counterparts of similar histologic subtype. According to clinical, histologic, immunohistochemical and prognostic data, primary cutaneous lymphomas can be divided into two main groups: primary cutaneous T-cell lymphomas (CTCL) and primary cutaneous B-cell lymphomas (CBCL; Table 20–1).

TABLE 20–1   Classification of Primary Cutaneous Lymphomas

TYPE (EVOLUTION)	5-YEAR SURVIVAL (%)
Primary cutaneous T-cell lymphomas	
Mycosis fungoides (indolent)	70
Sézary syndrome (aggressive)	11
Lymphomatoid papulosis (indolent)	100
CD30+ large T-cell lymphoma (indolent) Pleomorphic small/medium sized	85
Peripheral T-cell lymphoma (intermediate)	50 to 60
CD30− large cell lymphoma (aggressive)	10 to 20
Subcutaneous-panniculitic T-cell lymphoma[a] (variable)	
Intravascular T-cell lymphoma[a] (variable)	
Primary cutaneous angiocentric T/NK-cell lymphoma[a] (aggressive)	
Primary cutaneous B-cell lymphomas	
Marginal-zone cell lymphoma (indolent) (immunocytoma)	90
Follicle-center cell lymphoma (indolent)	95
Cutaneous plasmacytoma (indolent)	
Large B-cell lymphoma of the leg (intermediate)	50 to 60
Intravascular B-cell lymphoma[a] (variable)	<50

[a] Rare subtypes.

REFERENCES

Duncan LM. Cutaneous lymphoma. Understanding the new classification schemes. *Dermatol Clin.* 1999;17:569.

Sander CA, Flaig MJ, Kaudewitz P, et al. The revised European-American classification of lymphoid neoplasms (REAL): A preferred approach for the classification of cutaneous lymphomas. *Am J Dermatopathol.* 1999; 21:274.

Willemze R, Kerl H, Sterry W, et al. EORTC Classification for primary cutaneous lymphomas: A proposal from the cutaneous lymphoma study group of the European Organization for Research and Treatment of Cancer. *Blood.* 1997;90:354.

CUTANEOUS T-CELL LYMPHOMA

MYCOSIS FUNGOIDES/SÉZARY SYNDROME

EPIDEMIOLOGY

- Mycosis fungoides (MF) is the most common form of cutaneous T-cell lymphoma. It is a low-grade, mature T-cell malignancy with an estimated annual incidence of 0.29 per 100,000. It occurs almost exclusively in adults, with a peak of incidence in the sixth and seventh decades of life. The male to female ratio is 2:1.
- Sézary syndrome (SS), the leukemic variant of MF, is a much more rare disease. It occurs exclusively in adults.

PATHOPHYSIOLOGY

- MF is a monoclonal proliferation of malignant CD4-positive helper T lymphocytes with cerebriform nuclei that have a marked affinity for the skin, particularly the epidermis (epidermotropism). The disease may progress to systemic involvement (lymph nodes, peripheral blood cells, viscera) as they lose their affinity for the epidermis.
- The molecular mechanisms for epidermotropism are complex, multifactorial, and poorly understood. The homing mechanisms used by malignant T cells in MF appear to be similar to those used by inflammatory T cells. The malignant T-cell clone has a T-helper (Th)-2 cytokine profile. A possible role of Langerhans cells in perpetuating the lymphocyte epidermal affinity has also been postulated.
- In spite of several causative factors having been proposed, such as chronic antigenic stimulation [chemical exposure or cutaneous bacterial infections, medications or viral infections (retrovirus)], the etiology of MF/SS remains unknown. Moreover, no specific genetic defect has been identified.

CLINICAL FEATURES

- Mycosis fungoides (MF) has a long natural history, over years or sometimes decades, and develops in a multistep process from patches to more infiltrated plaques, and eventually tumors. Visceral disease is a late occurrence in MF.
- MF usually begins with persistent scaly, erythematous, patches often in non-sun-exposed areas. In early

stages, skin biopsy is frequently not diagnostic. The average time from the onset of skin lesions to diagnosis is 7 years.
- The plaque stage is entered gradually when the lesions become elevated and infiltrated. Plaques can arise from uninvolved skin. These lesions vary in shape and extension, may regress, remain stationary, or evolve into nodules and tumors. MF may also begin or evolve as exfoliative erythroderma.
- Tumors develop from preexisting plaques or erythroderma, or they may originate from normal skin. Necrosis and ulceration of plaques and tumors are common.
- Superficial enlarged and reactive lymph nodes may be detected in the plaque stage, (dermatopathic lymphadenopathy) and deep lymphadenopathy with visceral metastasis, such as to the spleen, lungs, or gastrointestinal tract, may occur during the tumor stage.
- Pagetoid reticulosis is a localized variant of mycosis fungoides that usually occurs in distal extremities and is characterized by marked epidermotropism with little underlying dermal infiltrate. Granulomatous slack skin is another peculiar clinical variant manifested by lax folds of skin in the axillae and groin, and histologically by elastolysis and a granulomatous inflammatory infiltrate.
- Sézary syndrome (SS), the leukemic variant of MF, is manifested by the triad of pruritic erythroderma, lymphadenopathy, and more than 1,000 atypical circulating mononuclear cells (Sézary cells)/mm. These cells are moderately large mononuclear cells with convoluted nuclei. Patients may have generalized pruritus, exfoliative dermatitis, ectropion, alopecia, nail dystrophy, peripheral edema, and thickening of the palms and soles. The disease generally is much more aggressive, progresses faster, and is more resistant to treatment than typical mycosis fungoides. There is a remarkable sparing of the bone marrow.

DIAGNOSIS AND DIFFERENTIAL

- The correct diagnosis requires evaluation of the clinical presentation and histopathologic features. Immunophenotyping, and T-cell gene rearrangement studies are techniques that may help to establish the diagnosis in early stages or in doubtful cases.
- Histopathologic examination varies with the stage of the disease. In early stages, the histopathologic features may not be diagnostic. In more advanced stages, a band-like dermal infiltrate consisting of small, medium-sized mononuclear cells with hyperchromatic

cerebriform nuclei without spongiosis is observed. Epidermal involvement with single-cell exocytosis or cellular aggregates of cerebriform cells in the epidermis (Pautrier's microabscesses) is highly characteristic.

- In tumor stages, the infiltrate is more monomorphous. Large, atypical cells with frequent mitoses often involve the entire dermis. Epidermotropism may be absent.

- MF/SS T cells may show an aberrant phenotype, lacking one or more mature T-cell markers, such as CD7, CD2, and CD5. In SS an aberrant phenotype CD3+, CD4+, CD7− or an elevated CD4/CD8 ratio are frequently detected in circulating atypical lymphocytes.

- Monoclonal rearrangement of the T-cell receptor genes by PCR-techniques are detected in 40 to 60% of patch stage lesions, 80% of plaques and 100% of tumors. A T-cell clone is detected from the peripheral blood in almost 100% of patients with SS.

- Clinically, the differential in patch-stage MF should be established with several chronic benign dermatoses, eczematous disorders, neurodermatitis, and contact dermatitis. When typical infiltrated plaques are present, the diagnosis is strongly suggested. MF tumor stage should be distinguished from leukemia cutis, cutaneous metastases or CD30+ cutaneous lymphoma. In patients having erythrodermic MF or Sézary syndrome, the differential diagnosis includes several diseases causing erythroderma, such as atopic dermatitis, drug reactions, and psoriasis.

- The evaluation of a patient with MF should include a complete history and physical examination, complete blood cell count, search for peripheral blood circulating Sézary cells, liver and renal biochemistry, immunophenotyping of peripheral blood lymphocytes, biopsy of enlarged lymph nodes (if present), chest x-ray films, and computed axial tomography of abdomen or pelvis (in advanced stages). Bone marrow biopsy is only performed in patients with tumor stage, SS, or in cases with a high suspicion of visceral disease.

- The single most important prognostic factor in mycosis fungoides is the extent of the disease, as reflected in the clinical stage. The TNM system of staging for MF is illustrated in Table 20–2.

TREATMENT

- There are many treatments for mycosis fungoides. Although permanent cures are unusual, complete remissions are common, especially in early-stage disease. Current management of CTCL usually involves a stepwise approach, beginning with conservative treatments. Treatment strategies can be divided into two categories: skin-directed treatments and systemic

TABLE 20–2   Staging of Cutaneous T-cell lymphoma (MF/SS): TNM Classification

T: Skin

T0: Lesions clinically and/or histopathologically suggestive of CTCL

T1: Limited plaques, papules, or eczematous patches covering <10% of skin surface

T2: Limited plaques, papules, or eczematous patches covering ≥10% of skin surface

T3: Tumors ≥1)
T4: Generalized erythroderma

N: Lymph nodes

N0: No palpable adenopathy, lymph node pathology negative for CTCL

N1: Palpable adenopathy, lymph node pathology negative for CTCL
N2: No palpable adenopathy, lymph node pathology positive for CTCL
N3: Palpable adenopathy, lymph node pathology positive for CTCL

B: Peripheral blood

B0: Atypical circulating cells not present (<5%)

B1: Atypical circulating cells present (>5%); record total white blood cell count, total lymphocyte count, and number of atypical cells/100 lymphocytes

M: Visceral organs

M1: No visceral organ involvement
M2: Visceral involvement (must have pathology confirmation and organ involved should be specified)

Stages:

IA	T1	N0	M0
IB	T2	N0	M0
IIA	T1, 2	N1	M0
IIB	T3	N0, 1	M0
III	T4	N0, 1	M0
IVA	T1–4	N2, 3	M0
IVB	T1–4	N0–3	M1

therapies. Treatments produce remissions, but cure is uncommon.

- Skin-directed treatments include psoralens plus ultraviolet light (PUVA), phototherapy with UVB, topical chemotherapy with mechloretamine (nitrogen mustard) or carmustine (BCNU) topical bexarotene, total skin electron-beam irradiation, and conventional irradiation of symptomatic skin lesions. No studies have demonstrated superiority of any topical therapy, and the decision on which therapy to choose depends on physician and patient preference. Skin-directed therapies are the first line of treatment and can be used in patch, plaque, and tumor stages.

- In patients with more advanced stages there can be a need for systemic therapy. Systemic therapy includes chemotherapy and other cytotoxic agents, extracorporeal photopheresis (ECP), interferon, oral retinoids (oral bexarotene), as well as other investigational biologic response modifiers. In patients with Sézary syndrome, conservative treatments with low-dose cytotoxic drugs (methotrexate, prednisone plus chlorambucil) or ECP are the treatments of choice.

REFERENCE

Diamandidou E, Cohen PR, Kurzrock R. Mycosis fungoides and Sézary syndrome. *Blood.* 1996;88:2385.

PRIMARY CUTANEOUS T-CELL LYMPHOMAS OTHER THAN MF/SS

PATHOPHYSIOLOGY

• The exact etiology of all of these subtypes of lymphomas is unknown.

CLINICAL FEATURES

• There is significant variability in the clinical appearances of this group of cutaneous T-cell lymphomas. The lesions range from a solitary erythematous or violaceous nodule to clustered nodules or infiltrated plaques and from subcutaneous lesions resembling panniculitis to multiple recurrent self-healing infiltrated papules. In some instances, clinical findings may allow the distinction of histologically similar processes.

DIAGNOSIS AND DIFFERENTIAL

• The diagnosis is established with a combination of clinical, histopathologic, immunohistochemical, and molecular genetic features. Clinicopathologic correlation is extremely important.
• A diffuse infiltrate of atypical lymphocytes of variable size extending from the superficial dermis into the subcutaneous fat is observed. Numerous mitoses are usually present. In some instances, an admixture of inflammatory cells is noted. The overlying epidermis may be ulcerated but more often exhibits marked pseudoepitheliomatous hyperplasia. Epidermotropism may be present.
• Immunophenotyping from skin biopsy specimens permit to determine a T-cell lineage (CD3+, CD2+, CD5+) and often shows the loss of some mature T-cell markers and/or the expression of characteristic lymphocyte activation markers (i.e., CD30 antigen).
• Genotypic analysis (Southern blot analysis/PCR) permits demonstration of a T-cell monoclonal cell population, especially in cases in which the diagnosis of lymphoma is suspected but not yet confirmed.
• The differential diagnosis of nodular lesions should include primary and secondary cutaneous B-cell lymphomas, leukemia cutis, or cutaneous metastases. Inflammatory subcutaneous nodules always obligate to rule out the different forms of panniculitis, and self-healing necrotic papules should be distinguished from pytiriasis lichenoides, insect bites, or folliculitis.

TREATMENT

• A majority of non-MF primary cutaneous T-cell lymphomas have a similar treatment algorithm. Solitary or localized tumors are usually treated with excision and/or radiation therapy. On the other hand, patients with multifocal or disseminated cutaneous lesions are usually treated with chemotherapy. In patients with CD30- large cell lymphoma, an aggressive treatment (chemotherapy) is recommended.

CD30+ PRIMARY CUTANEOUS T-CELL LYMPHOID PROLIFERATIONS (LYMPHOMATOID PAPULOSIS AND PRIMARY CUTANEOUS CD30+ T-CELL LYMPHOMA)

• This group of malignant T-cell disorders is characterized CD30 antigen expression by atypical lymphoid cells. They account for approximately 25% of the primary cutaneous T-cell lymphomas. There is a continuum spectrum extending from an indolent form [lymphomatoid papulosis (LyP)] to a more aggressive pole [primary cutaneous CD30+ T-cell lymphoma (PC-CD30+ TCL)]. Both diseases may coexist in individual patients. They may be clonally related and they often show overlapping clinical and/or histologic features.
• LyP is a chronic recurrent skin eruption characterized by the appearance of recurrent crops of reddish-brown papules and/or nodules that frequently crust or ulcerate and resolve, often leaving atrophic scars. The skin lesions have a lymphoma-like histology, but the clinical course is chronic and benign. The lesions regress spontaneously, typically within 3 to 6 weeks. Papules arise over the trunk and extremities for months to years. Progression to lymphoma is estimated to occur in approximately 10% of cases (MF, large anaplastic CD30+ T-cell lymphoma, T-immunoblastic lymphoma, and Hodgkin´s disease).
• PC-CD30+ TCL usually presents as rapidly growing, solitary or localized tumors and rarely papules. Multicentric cutaneous disease is seen in 20% of the cases. Occasionally, the lesions may show a complete or partial spontaneous regression, although cutaneous

relapses are common. Extracutaneous dissemination occurs in approximately 10% of the patients, mainly to regional lymph nodes and most frequently in patients with multicentric cutaneous disease. PC-CD30+ TCL is observed predominantly in adults/elderly and is rare in children.

- A correct diagnosis usually requires assessment of clinical, histologic, and phenotypic features.

- Histopathologic features of LyP are characterized by a wedge-shaped, dense, dermal perivascular lymphoid infiltrate composed of small, banal lymphocytes and large atypical CD30+ cells with Reed–Sternberg appearance (LyP type A). In other cases, a predominance of atypical cells with cerebriform nuclei is noted (LyP type B). In individual patients, both types of lesions may exist. Parakeratosis, acanthosis, and spongiosis may be present.

- PC-CD30+ TCL is characterized by sheets of large anaplastic lymphocytes, extending from the superficial dermis into the subcutaneous fat. Usually, more than 75% of the infiltrating lymphocytes display marked cellular anaplasia. The neoplastic cells often are large in size, but a medium-size cell variant has also been reported. Multinucleated atypical cells resembling Reed–Sternberg cells are usually observed, occasionally forming cohesive sheets.

- In both disorders (LyP and PC-CD30+ TCL), the atypical cells have a CD4+ phenotype. The large lymphocytes may show loss of some pan-T antigens. The Reed–Sternberg-like cells are usually CD30+, CD15−, CD45R−.

- Clonal rearrangements of T-cell receptor genes have been reported in 50% of lesions of LyP. Surprisingly, the presence of clonal rearrangements is not correlated with prognosis.

- In PC-CD30+ TCL, genotypic studies show clonal rearrangement of the T-cell receptor genes. The vast majority of primary cutaneous CD30+ lymphomas lack the t(2;5)(q23;q35) translocation.

- Patients with primary cutaneous form of CD30+ T-cell lymphoma have a favorable prognosis, with a 4-year survival rate of 90%.

- Most patients with LyP follow a benign course, but the disease is often of long duration. Low dose methotrexate (5 to 20 mg/week) and PUVA therapy are useful to reduce the number of skin lesions and recurrences. However, after treatment discontinuation, the disease continues its natural course. Therefore, treatment should be reserved for patients with large, numerous, and/or scarring skin lesions. Long-term follow-up is, therefore, recommended. For PC-CD30+ TCL, treatment guidelines are similar to the majority of non-MF T-cell cutaneous lymphomas (see below).

CD30 NEGATIVE CUTANEOUS LARGE T-CELL LYMPHOMA

- CD30 negative cutaneous large T-cell lymphomas are aggressive neoplasms with an overall survival of only 10 to 20%. The lesions are rapid-growing solitary or multiple plaques or nodules (d'emblée form of mycosis fungoides) not preceded by prior patches or plaques.

- Histologically, a nodular or diffuse infiltrate with more than 30% of large neoplastic atypical cells is observed. An aberrant CD4+ T-cell phenotype with minimal or absent CD30 expression is detected. Clonal TCR rearrangements are present in most cases.

SMALL TO MEDIUM SIZE PLEOMORPHIC T-CELL LYMPHOMA

- This entity is manifested clinically by one or several erythematous or violaceous nodules clinically distinct from mycosis fungoides.

- Skin biopsy specimens reveal a superficial and deep dermal proliferation of pleomorphic T cells with minimal or absent epidermotropism. The atypical infiltrate often extends into the subcutaneous fat. Histopathologic features may mimic MF tumor stage. Malignant T cells are usually CD4+ cells with an aberrant phenotype.

- Only a few series of these patients have been studied, however, this disease seems to have a good prognosis.

SUBCUTANEOUS PANNICULITIS-LIKE T-CELL LYMPHOMA

- Subcutaneous panniculitis-like T-cell lymphoma (SPLTCL) is an uncommon form of peripheral cytotoxic T-cell lymphoma that preferentially infiltrates subcutaneous tissue. Clinically, it is manifested by solitary or multiple subcutaneous nodules and plaques on the extremities and trunk of older adults.

- Systemic symptoms are variable. Some patients may present with hemophagocytic syndrome with pancytopenia, fever, and hepatosplenomegaly.

- The lymphomatous infiltrate is primarily confined to subcutis in a diffuse pattern resembling lobular panniculitis. Sheets of pleomorphic small to medium sized and large lymphocytes with irregular, hyperchromatic nuclei are observed. Mitotic features are often present. Phagocytosis of karyorrhectic nuclear debris and red blood cell fragments by reactive histiocytes is often, but not invariably present. Angioinvasion and coagulation necrosis are evident in some cases.

- The neoplastic cells commonly express one or more of the T-cell associated antigens CD3, CD45RO, CD43, as well as T-cell receptors αβ or γδ. An aberrant T-cell phenotype (i.e., loss of CD7, CD2, or CD5) may also be demonstrated. The neoplastic lymphocytes have either a CD8+ cytotoxic/suppressor or less commonly a CD4+ helper/inducer T-cell phenotype.
- The clinical evolution of SPLTCL is variable. Most patients have an aggressive clinical course with short-duration survival, with death usually secondary to intense hemophagocytic syndrome. Dissemination to lymph nodes and other organs is uncommon and usually occurs late in the clinical course. Some patients, however, have a protracted evolution with recurrent self-healing lesions without systemic involvement.

PRIMARY CUTANEOUS ANGIOCENTRIC NATURAL KILLER/T-CELL LYMPHOMA

- Angiocentric lymphoma natural killer (NK)/T cell lymphoma is an aggressive subtype of peripheral lymphoma and is characterized by the expression of the NK-cell antigen CD56. This lymphoma is frequently associated with Epstein–Barr virus infection. It is seen more frequently in Asian countries, Mexico, and Central and South America.
- These CD56+ lymphomas are divided into a nasal NK/T-cell lymphoma that commonly presents as mid-facial destructive disease and non-nasal NK/T-cell lymphomas that often arise in extranodal locations, including the skin.
- The non-nasal group is then subdivided into primary cutaneous and four types of secondary cutaneous lymphomas (nasal type, aggressive, blastoid, and other specific lymphoma types).
- Primary cutaneous angiocentric NK/T-cell lymphoma is a rare disease that is manifested by single or multiple papules, plaques, or nodules. A rapid progression to extracutaneous involvement (lymph nodes, bone marrow, spleen, and nasopharynx) has been reported.
- Histologically, it is characterized by an angioinvasive and angiodestructive pattern of infiltration, usually accompanied by extensive coagulation necrosis. The lymphomatous infiltrate typically involves the middle and lower dermis and superficial subcutis. There is a cytologic spectrum of small- or medium-sized cells to large transformed cells.

- Most angiocentric lymphomas express CD56, and less frequently CD16 and CD57 (NK-cell markers) and lack clonal rearrangement of the T-cell receptor gene. The neoplastic cells may express some T-cell associated antigens, most commonly CD2 or cytoplasmic CD3. The neoplastic cells also contain cytolytic effector proteins TIA-1, perforin, and granzyme B. A small subset of CD56+ angiocentric lymphomas are of true T-cell lineage as evidenced by the demonstration of clonal T-cell rearrangement. In contrast to secondary cutaneous involvement, in primary cutaneous forms, EBV is rarely detected by in situ hybridization techniques.
- The clinical course of angiocentric lymphomas is usually aggressive with a high relapse rate. Early visceral involvement is usually detected. Aggressive treatment (chemotherapy) is usually indicated.

REFERENCES

Kim BK, Nelson BP, Calonje E. Newly described cutaneous lymphomas. *Adv Dermatol.* 1999;15:397.

Siegel RS, Pandolfino T, Guitart J, et al. Primary cutaneous T-cell lymphoma: Review and current concepts. *J Clin Oncol.* 2000;18:2908.

PRIMARY CUTANEOUS B-CELL LYMPHOMAS

EPIDEMIOLOGY

- During the last 15 years, different diagnostic criteria regarding the classification of the different subtypes of P-CBCL have been proposed and still significant controversies regarding the definition of the some types of P-CBCL persist (especially primary cutaneous marginal-zone and primary cutaneous follicular lymphoma). This may explain the fact that the exact incidence of primary cutaneous B-cell lymphoma is still unknown. Primary cutaneous B-cell lymphoma seems to be slightly more common in females (2:1). The average age of onset is 59 years.

PATHOPHYSIOLOGY

- The mechanisms for the presence and persistence of malignant neoplastic B cells within the dermis are unknown. Malignant B cells may express skin-specific homing receptors. A possible role of antigen-presenting cells in the pathogenesis of P-CBCL has been postulated. Various infectious etiologies, such as virus (retrovirus) or *Borrelia burgdorferi*, have been occasionally related to isolated cases of P-CBCL.

- No specific genetic lesions have been identified in P-CBCL. The translocation t(14;18)(q32;q21) detected in 70 to 90% of nodal follicular lymphoma is only rarely detected in the primary cutaneous counterpart.

- Many similarities have been observed between P-CBCL and mucosa-associated lymphoid tissue (MALT) lymphomas. The possibility that the majority of P-CBCL, previously considered follicular lymphomas, really correspond to a marginal-zone lymphoma has been postulated.

CLINICAL FEATURES

- Most patients with primary cutaneous B-cell lymphoma have a similar clinical appearance. Specific cutaneous manifestations of cutaneous B-cell lymphomas usually present a flesh-colored, erythematous, or distinctive plum-colored, slightly infiltrated papules or nodules that often have a rubbery consistency on palpation. Occasionally, small, slightly infiltrated plaques or figurate lesions may surround the nodules and may precede for months to years the development of rapidly growing skin tumors.

- Lesions are most often located on the trunk, sometimes on the head, and, uncommonly, on the extremities. There are some regional predilection for various subtypes of tumors: follicular lymphomas more commonly arise on the scalp, marginal zone B-cell lymphomas occur on the trunk and extremities, and the aggressive large B-cell lymphoma usually arises on the lower leg. Nevertheless, all types of cutaneous B-cell lymphomas can occur at any cutaneous site of presentation.

- Most CBCL are indolent neoplasms. They tend to remain localized, they only rarely disseminate, and the prognosis is favorable in most cases. As a group, P-CBCL generally has a better prognosis than P-CTCL.

DIAGNOSIS AND DIFFERENTIAL

- The diagnosis of PCBCL is often difficult based on histopathologic criteria alone. Histologic findings of the various subtypes of PCBCL can be similar. However, each subtype has specific, characteristic findings that allow for distinct classification.

- Histologically, in early lesions, a patchy or nodular perivascular and periadnexal infiltrate in the superficial dermis is present, whereas in more advanced lesions, a more diffuse cellular infiltrate extending from the dermis into the subcutaneous fat, with or without the presence of reactive lymphoid follicles, is observed. The infiltrate tends to be bottom-heavy. There can be massive infiltration and destruction of adnexal structures. The epidermis is typically normal in appearance and there is usually an uninvolved zone of normal collagen separating lymphoid infiltrate from the normal epidermis, referred to as the grenz zone.

- The neoplastic cells usually express CD19, CD20, CD22, and CD79a. An aberrant B-cell immunophenotype, most commonly manifested by the coexpression of CD43 and CD20, can occasionally be observed. Monotypic expression of κ and λ immunoglobulin (Ig) light chains can often be demonstrated by immunohistochemistry in frozen or even in paraffin-embedded tissue. The demonstration of a monoclonal rearrangement of the Ig heavy-or light- chain by Southern blot and/or PCR gives additional support to the diagnosis.

- The differential diagnosis should always be established with reactive lymphoid hyperplasia, especially in those lymphomas that present prominent germinal center formation (follicular lymphoma and marginal-zone lymphoma)

- Once the diagnosis of PCBCL is established, a thorough history and physical examination should be performed to rule out systemic involvement. The patient should be questioned regarding B symptoms. A complete physical examination, including palpation of lymph nodes, liver and, spleen, should be undertaken. Staging procedures should include peripheral blood cell count with a chemistry panel (including lactate dehydrogenase, β2-microglobulin), chest x-ray, CAT scanning, and bone marrow biopsy.

TREATMENT

- Surgical excision or localized radiotherapy of primary or recurrent lesions is the treatment of choice. Solitary low-grade tumors may also be treated with the injection of high-dose steroids. Polychemotherapy is only recommended for patients with extensive cutaneous disease, in aggressive forms, or in cases with extracutaneous spread, usually in combination with radiotherapy.

PRIMARY CUTANEOUS MARGINAL-ZONE LYMPHOMA/IMMUNYCTOMA

- Marginal-zone B-cell lymphoma is a clinicopathologic entity with a predisposition to involve mucosal and epithelial extranodal sites. It has been described in the stomach, salivary glands, thyroid, breast, lung and trachea, uterine cervix, and, more recently, skin and subcutaneous tissue. Primary cutaneous marginal-zone lymphoma is probably the more frequent form of P-CBCL. In some classifications, it is grouped with primary cutaneous immunocytoma.

- Primary cutaneous marginal-zone lymphoma presents as solitary or multiple erythematous nodules, often on the trunk and extremities, of middle-aged individuals. In the event of dissemination, the tumor most commonly spreads to other extranodal sites.

- Histologically, primary cutaneous marginal-zone lymphoma is characterized by a diffuse or nodular infiltration of the reticular dermis and subcutis with relative sparing of the papillary dermis and epidermis. Small to medium lymphocytes with moderately abundant pale cytoplasm (monocytoid B cells), centrocyte-like cells, and large transformed blasts are seen in varying proportions. Well-formed or rudimentary reactive germinal centers are observed and rarely, follicular colonization by neoplastic lymphocytes may be evident. Variable degrees of plasma cell differentiation with monotypic immunoglobulin production are also present. There is a distinct compartmentalization of plasma cells in the subepidermal zone, at the periphery of the lymphoid aggregates, and interfollicular zones. Lymphoepitelial lesions, commonly seen in other extranodal sites, are infrequent or absent in the skin.

- The neoplastic cells are immunophenotypically CD20+, CD43 +/−, CD5−, and CD10−. Lymphoplasmacytoid and plasma cells express CD79a. The reactive germinal centers display polytypic light chain immunoglobulins and the T cells have a normal phenotype.

- In contrast to secondary immunocytomas, primary cutaneous marginal-zone B-cell lymphoma/immunocytoma has not been associated with an increased incidence of autoimmune disorders. The clinical course is favorable with a low mortality rate, but localized cutaneous relapses are relatively frequent.

PRIMARY CUTANEOUS FOLLICULAR LYMPHOMA

- Primary cutaneous follicular lymphoma (P-CFL) is a malignant cutaneous disease characterized by proliferations of lymphoid cells with a follicular pattern and germinal center cytology. Neoplastic cells are B cells (CD19, CD20, CD22) that express the classic markers of the germinal center, such as bcl-6 and CD10, and the presence of aggregates of follicular dendritic cells.

- Clinically, P-CFL is manifested by solitary or multiple plaques or nodules often involving the head and neck area.

- Histologically, the lesions are composed of dermal and, occasionally, subcutaneous confluent nodules showing tumoral follicles in the center of the lesion. A grenz zone may be observed. Neoplastic follicles are composed of centrocytes and centroblasts with an indistinct mantle zone. Peripheral reactive lymphoid follicles are occasionally present.

- Neoplastic cells are germinal center B-cells (CD20+, CD79a+, CD10+, bcl-6+, CD5−, and CD43−). Immunohistochemical stains for λ and κ light chains reveal light chain restriction of the neoplastic follicle centers. Cutaneous follicle center lymphomas express bcl-2 protein in less than 40 to 60% of cases. A network of CD21-positive follicular dendritic cells is also a diagnostic feature.

- Primary cutaneous follicle center lymphoma typically does not have associated translocation that is observed in nodal follicle center lymphoma. Clonal rearrangement of immunoglobulin genes is often detected.

- Different histologic and immunophenotypic criteria have been used to define this subtype of primary cutaneous lymphoma and a diagnostic overlap exists between marginal-zone lymphoma and follicle center lymphoma arising in the skin. Follicular colonization (invasion of reactive follicles by neoplastic marginal-zone B cells) is often observed in marginal-zone lymphoma. Some investigators have postulated that some of the lesions diagnosed as primary cutaneous follicle center lymphomas probably represent marginal-zone lymphomas with follicular colonization.

- The main differential diagnosis concerns B-cell pseudolymphomas with a follicular pattern of growth. The estimated 5-year survival rate is greater than 97%.

LARGE B-CELL LYMPHOMA OF THE LEG

- Diffuse large B-cell lymphoma involving the lower extremity has a less favorable prognosis than diffuse large cell lymphoma arising at other cutaneous sites.

- This entity is manifested by erythematous or violaceous nodules on one or both legs often with ulceration. Diffuse large B-cell lymphoma is more frequently observed in women and occurs late in life, with more than 80% of tumors occurring in patients older than 70 years.

- Histologically, a diffuse dermal infiltration by a proliferation of large B cells, predominantly centroblasts and immunoblasts, with scattering centrocytes, is observed.
- Monotypic surface immunoglobulin is identified along with a CD19+, CD20+, CD22+, CD79a+, CD5+ or −, bcl-2+ immunophenotype. Immunoglobulin genes have detectable clonal rearrangements. The translocation t(14;18) is usually absent.

INTRAVASCULAR B-CELL LYMPHOMA

- Intravascular B-cell lymphoma (IVBCL) is characterized by intravascular accumulations of large neoplastic B cells. The disease involves mainly the skin (32%) and central nervous system (42%), but virtually any organ may also be affected. Involvement of the central nervous system is associated with a poor outcome.
- Primary cutaneous IVBCL is usually manifested by indurated, violaceous plaques on the trunk and lower extremities, in many cases accompanied by pain and progressive swelling of the affected limb.
- Skin biopsy specimens reveal numerous dilated blood vessels in the dermis and subcutis, which are filled and often extended by a proliferation of large atypical mononuclear cells, which cause total or partial luminal occlusion.
- The tumor cells express pan-B antigens (CD20, CD19, CD22, CD79a) and monotypic immunoglobulins. Clonal rearrangement of immunoglobulin genes is present.
- A high index of suspicion is important in making this diagnosis because patients usually present with nonspecific central nervous system abnormalities and frequently have fever, malaise, weight loss, and evidence of antinuclear antibody rheumatoid factor, which suggest a rheumatology disorder.
- Patients with IVBCL have a poor prognosis and a 5 year-survival rate of less than 50% has been reported. Treatment is with combination chemotherapy.

PLASMACYTOMA

- Extramedullary plasmacytoma of the skin is an unusual proliferation of plasma cells that occurs without an underlying myeloma. Clinically, it is manifested as a solitary or multiple violaceous nodules. Progression to myeloma has been reported.

- Plasmacytomas appear as diffuse dermal nodules of mature plasma cells, multinucleate plasma cells, and occasional plasma cells with prominent eosinophilic macronucleoli and anaplastic nuclei. The plasma cells usually have the phenotype CD79a+, CD38+, CD43+, CD19−, CD20−, CD22−. Monotypic expression of immunoglobulin light chains is detected.

REFERENCE

Sander CA, Flaig MJ. Morphological spectrum of cutaneous B-cell lymphomas. *Dermatol Clin.* 1999;17:93.

CUTANEOUS PSEUDOLYMPHOMAS

- Pseudolymphoma of the skin is a term applied to a heterogeneous group of benign proliferations of lymphocytes, which simulate malignant lymphomas clinically and histologically. Depending on the predominant cell type in the infiltrate, cutaneous pseudolymphomas are divided into cutaneous T-cell pseudolymphomas (CT-PSL) and cutaneous B-cell pseudolymphomas (CB-PSL).

EPIDEMIOLOGY

- No data are available about the overall incidence or prevalence of this group of disorders. CB-PSL seems to be more frequent in males (2:1) and develops in early adult life (median age 34 years).

PATHOPHYSIOLOGY

- The exact pathogenic mechanisms that lead to the development of cutaneous pseudolymphomas are poorly understood. These conditions seem to represent an exaggerated immune response to antigens of various types.
- In most cases the etiology of cutaneous pseudolymphoma is unknown (idiopathic CT-PSL and CB-PSL). CT-PSLs include lymphomatoid drug reactions (anticonvulsivants, antihypertensives, etc.), lymphomatoid contact dermatitis, persistent nodular arthropod-bite reactions, nodular scabies, actinic reticuloid, and acral pseudolymphomatous angiokeratoma. CB-PSLs include idiopathic reactive lymphoid hyperplasia and reactive lymphoid hyperplasia secondary to tattoos,

Borrelia burgdorferi infection, post-herpes zoster, or after antigen-injections/punctures.

CLINICAL FEATURES

- Cutaneous B-cell pseudolymphoma is regarded as a distinct clinicopathologic entity, whereas, T-cell pseudolymphoma is a heterogeneous group of diseases, rather than an individualized clinical picture.
- The clinical picture of the different types of CT-PSL may be manifested as erythematous eruptions associated with fever and lymphadenopathy after anticonvulsivant drug intake, eczematous patches or plaques, as single or multiple red-brown nodules and infiltrated plaques, exfoliative erythroderma, or as a chronic, persistent, pruritic photosensitive eruption (actinic reticuloid).
- Clinically, CB-PSLs are manifested by asymptomatic, red-brown, violaceous or erythematous papules or nodules, which may vary in diameter from 3 mm to 5 cm or more. The lesions may be solitary or multiple, grouped, or widespread. Solitary lesions occur predominantly on the head, while the grouped or multiple lesions tend to involve the trunk and lower extremities, although any site can be involved. Lesions may heal spontaneously after months to many years.

DIAGNOSIS AND DIFFERENTIAL

- In some instances, the differential diagnosis between cutaneous pseudolymphomas and true lymphomas can be very difficult. The definitive diagnosis is based on a combination of clinical, histopathologic data, and in the majority of cases by the use of immunohistochemical techniques or gene rearrangement studies. Occasionally, the final diagnosis is only confirmed after a long-term follow-up period.
- T-cell pseudolymphomas histologically simulate primary cutaneous T-cell lymphomas. Two different histologic patterns have been described: a band-like pattern (MF-like) that simulates MF (lymphomatoid drug eruption, lymphomatoid contact dermatitis, actinic reticuloid), and a nodular pattern mimicking CTCL other than MF (nodular scabies, idiopathic CT-PSL). Immunohistochemical studies disclose a predominant T-cell phenotype CD4+ and occasionally CD8+ (actinic reticuloid). Mature T-cell markers (CD2, CD5, CD7) are preserved. TCR gene rearrangement studies disclose a T-cell polyclonal proliferation.

- Histologically, CB-PSL show a rather constant pattern. A dense, well-circumscribed symmetric nodular infiltrates are observed in upper parts of the dermis (top-heavy pattern). The lymphocytic infiltrate is separated from the uninvolved dermis by a grenz zone. The infiltrate often shows a perivascular and periadnexal accentuation but the surrounded structures are not destroyed. Follicular structures often can be observed and a regular network of CD21-expressing follicular dendritic cells can be seen within the follicular structures. In addition to the B-cell infiltrate, accompanying T-cells are also present between the nodular collections of B-cells. An admixture of "tingible body" macrophages, eosinophils, and plasma cells can also be observed. The most important factor identifying CB-PSL is the polytypic expression of the immunoglobulin light chains κ and λ and the lack of clonal rearrangement of immunoglobulin heavy or light chains.

TREATMENT

- In cases of cutaneous pseudolymphomas with an identified cause, removal or treatment of the causative agent (scabies, *Borrelia*, drugs) is mandatory.
- In idiopathic pseudolymphomas, the lesions can be chronic and persistent and may resolve spontaneously after several months or years. For localized persistent lesions, surgical excision or cryosurgery can be recommended. Topical or intralesional corticoesteroids can also be prescribed. In cases with multiple or generalized lesions, antimalarials, PUVA therapy, or cytotoxic agents have been used with variable success.

REFERENCE

Ploysangam T, Breneman DL, Mutasim DF. Cutaneous pseudolymphomas. *J Am Acad Dermatol.* 1998;38:877.

LEUKEMIA CUTIS

EPIDEMIOLOGY

- Patients with leukemia may present with a variety of cutaneous manifestations. Specific lesions resulting from infiltration of the skin by leukemic cells (leukemia cutis), and non-specific, which do not have tumor cells but are considered to be a cutaneous reaction to the malignancy.

- Specific cutaneous involvement seems to indicate advanced leukemia and is a marker of either rapid disease progression or the presence of extramedullary involvement. Specific cutaneous leukemic lesions have been reported in 18 to 31% of patients with acute monocytic leukemia, in 20 to 100% of patients with adult T-cell leukemia/lymphoma, in 10% of patients chronic lymphocytic leukemia, in 8% of hairy-cell leukemia, in 3% of acute lymphoblastic leukemia, and in 2 to 5% of patients with chronic granulocytic leukemia. Early cutaneous involvement is more frequent in acute myelomonocytic leukemia and monocytic leukemia (11%).

- Nonspecific cutaneous lesions are much more common than specific lesions (30 to 40%). Nonspecific cutaneous lesions have been divided into two groups: Lesions arising from marrow failure (anemia, thrombocytopenia, and neutropenia) and reactive or paraneoplastic cutaneous lesions. The first group includes cutaneous pallor, petechiae, mucosal bleeding, and multiple infectious disorders (fungal, viral, or bacterial). Reactive or paraneoplastic skin disorders include pruritus, erythema, nodosum, erythroderma, erythema multiforme, Sweet's syndrome, pyoderma gangrenosum.

PATHOPHYSIOLOGY

- The specific lesions of leukemia cutis result from infiltration of the epidermis, dermis, or subcutaneous tissue by neoplastic leukocytes or their precursors. Cutaneous involvement seems to result from specific tissue homing pattern of the leukemic cells. Leukemia cutis seems to be the result of cutaneous local proliferation of malignant cells.

- In adult T-cell lymphoma/leukemia (ATL), integration of human T-lymphotropic virus-1 (HTLV-1) proviral sequences have been demonstrated. ATL is the first human malignancy demonstrated to be of retroviral origin.

CLINICAL FEATURES

- Leukemia cutis may present as localized or widespread firm, rubbery erythematous, pink, or red-brown to purple papules or nodules (60%) or infiltrated plaques (26%), and rarely, macules, ulcers, ecchymoses, or diffuse erythroderma. The lesions can become purpuric when a marked thrombocytopenia is associated. Different leukemia subtypes produce similar lesions and a particular type of leukemia can produce clinically different lesions over the course of the disease. Rarely, leukemic infiltrates may localize at sites of trauma or inflammation.

- Some subtypes of leukemia seem to have a tendency to develop cutaneous specific lesions in particular areas: the face and extremities in acute and chronic lymphocytic leukemia, the trunk in granulocytic leukemia, and the entire body surface in monocytic leukemia. Hypertrophy of the gums has been reported to occur in 34% of patients with monocytic leukemia, in 8% with myeloblastic leukemia, and in 2% of patients with acute lymphoblastic leukemia. In acute or chronic myeloblastic leukemia, a characteristic cutaneous lesion, termed granulocytic sarcoma or chloroma (because the presence of the enzyme myeloperoxidase turns them a greenish hue), can be observed. This specific lesion involves the periostium of the orbital and cranial bones and, occasionally, the skin. Erythroderma, bullous lesions, and, rarely, follicular mucinosis have been reported in chronic lymphocytic leukemia.

- In ATL, cutaneous lesions may be similar to those observed in mycosis fungoides. Hepatosplenomegaly, lymphadenopathy, hypercalcemia, and significant bone marrow involvement are other characteristic features.

- Specific lesions may develop in the course of the disease, although sometimes may precede by months the detection of leukemic cells in the blood or bone marrow. The term aleukemic leukemia cutis is used for this uncommon event, which is seen more often in myeloid leukemia than in other leukemias.

DIAGNOSIS AND DIFFERENTIAL

- The diagnosis of leukemia cutis is based on the combination of clinical, hematologic, histopathologic, and immunohistochemical features. Specific skin infiltrates usually occur in patients when the diagnosis of leukemia is already established. In such cases, the diagnosis is often clinically suspected, and confirmed after obtaining a skin biopsy specimen for routine stains and special immunohistochemical techniques.

- Histologic examination reveals a patchy, superficial, and deep perivascular infiltrate or a dense interstitial or diffuse infiltrate of leukemic cells. The subcutis is frequently involved and there may be a zone of normal dermis between the epidermis and leukemic infiltrate.

- The diagnosis is established after the identification of the specific leukemic cell. The predominant cells in acute granulocytic leukemia (AGL) are myeloblasts and atypical myelocytes that typically infiltrate collagen bundles and the subcutaneous fibrous septa. In chronic myeloid leukemia, the cell population is more pleomorphic, with granulocytes in varying stages of maturation. In acute lymphocytic leukemia, the infiltrate is composed of medium to large blast cells with scanty cytoplasm. In acute monocytic leukemia, monomorphous atypical monocytoid cells of variable size are observed, whereas in chronic lymphocytic leukemia, an infiltrate of small- to medium-size lymphocytes is present. A dense, epidermotropic infiltrate of pleomorphic lymphocytes with hyperlobed nuclei is characteristic of ATL.

- Histochemical and immunohistochemical techniques may help to establish a definitive diagnosis. Chloroacetate esterase (Leder's stain) preferentially stains mature granulocytes and mast cells and generally does not stain monocytes. A panel of monoclonal antibodies can be used in acute and chronic leukemias that may help to establish the presence of markers of hematopoietic precursors (CD34, HLA-DR, TdT, CD45), B-lineage (CD19, CD20, CD22, CD79a), T-lineage (CD2, CD3, CD5, CD7), myeloid (CD13, CD33, CD15, CD117, MPO), or monocytic (CD14, CD68, CD64) cells. The immunophenotype of the specific cutaneous infiltrate must be concordant with that of the leukemic cell.

- Clinically, leukemic infiltration of the subcutaneous tissue may mimic erythema nodosum, whereas dermal infiltrates may resemble clinically mycosis fungoides or erythema annulare centrifugum. Some lesions may resemble urticaria or even pyoderma gangrenosum. In leukemic patients under cytotoxic treatment, the differential diagnosis of leukemia cutis should include infectious disorders (septic vasculitis and viral, fungal, and bacterial infections).

- Aleukemic leukemia cutis may adopt a clinical appearance similar to that of cutaneous lymphomas. Only the combination of clinical, histopathologic, and immunohistochemical features may establish a definitive diagnosis.

TREATMENT

- The management of leukemia cutis entails the treatment of the underlying leukemia. Local radiotherapy may be occasionally necessary for recurrent or resistant specific lesions.

REFERENCE

Ratnam KV, Khor CJL, Su WPD. Leukemia cutis. *Dermatol Clin.* 1994;12:419.

HISTIOCYTOSIS

- Since its inception in 1985, the Histiocyte Society has been active in studying these diseases and in clarifying a confusing literature. Classification and diagnostic criteria published in 1987 became recognized as the standard in the field. Information acquired since then justified reassessment and reclassification of histiocytic disorders based on cell lineage and biologic behavior.

- Histiocytes represent a group of immune cells that includes macrophages and dendritic cells. Macrophages, with predominantly antigen processing functions, and dendritic cells, with primarily accessory cell or antigen presenting functions, are considered as polar representatives of one common regulatory system. The ontogeny of histiocytes is currently incompletely understood, and knowledge is based on "in vitro" experiments. It seems that a group of cytokines play important roles in the differentiation toward several cell lines from a common CD34+ hemopoietic progenitor originating in the bone marrow.

- The cutaneous histiocytosis are best divided into the Langerhans cell histiocytosis (LCH) and non-Langerhans cell histiocytosis (NLCH). In the former group, the cells react with S100 and CD1a antibodies; while in the latter group, they express a variety of macrophage markers (Table 20–3).

LANGERHANS CELL HISTIOCYTOSIS

PATHOPHYSIOLOGY

- The Langerhans cell (LC) is a dendritic cell. It belongs to a group of nonphagocytic mononuclear cells that play a role in the trapping and processing of antigens for presentation to T lymphocytes.

- The LC arises from a CD34+ bone marrow precursor, and it seems that a number of cytokines including granulocyte-macrophage colony-stimulating factor (GM-CSF), interleukin (IL-4), and tumor necrosis factor (TNF-α) are involved in the maturation process toward LC lineage.

- The LC acquires its typical phenotype within the epidermis, therefore expressing CD1a, S100 protein and HLA-DR. It also shows esterase, acid phosphatase, and ATPase activity. It accounts for approximately 2% of the cells in the epidermis, representing a very slowly cycling cell population.

- Ultrastructurally, LC possesses many organelles, specifically the Birbeck granule, with a characteristic

TABLE 20–3   Cutaneous Histocytoses Classified by Marker Type

DISEASE/MARKER	S100	CD1a	BIRBECK	MACROPHAGE	MS-1
Langerhans cell histiocytosis	+	+	++	–	–
Congenital self-healing histiocytosis	+	+	+	–	
Indeterminate cell histiocytosis	+	+	–	+	
Sinus histiocytosis with massive lymphadenopathy	+	–	–	+	
Non-Langerhans cell histiocytosis	–	–	–	+	+

[a] MS-1 protein is specific for sinusoidal endothelial cells and dendritic perivascular macrophages.
[b] MS-1 protein is expressed by NLCH cells, but not by LCH cells, epithelioid cells, or palisading histiocytes.

TABLE 20–4   Classic Types of Langerhans Cell Histiocytosis

LCH TYPE/CLINICAL FEATURES	SKIN INVOLVEMENT	ORGAN INVOLVEMENT
Letterer–Siwe	Common and extensive; yellow-brown scaly papules on the scalp, face, trunk, and buttocks resembling seborrheic dermatitis	Acute form; fever, anemia, lymphadenopathy, osteolytic lesions, hepatosplenomegaly
Hand–Schüller–Christian	One third of the cases; lesions similar to the acute form, papulonodular lesions, or granulomatous ulcerations in intertriginous areas	Chronic form; classic triad; bone lesions, diabetes insipidus, and exophthalmos
Eosinophilic granuloma	Uncommon; noduloulcerative lesions in the mouth, perineal, perivulvar or retroauricular regions	Bone

rod or tennis-racquet shape. Similar dendritic cells without these granules are the so-called "indeterminate cells" (see Table 20–3).

- It is well known that upon stimulation by epicutaneous antigens, the LC migrates into the afferent lymphatics to the peripheral lymph nodes, where it presents the antigen to CD4+ T lymphocytes in the paracortical zone. The LC plays a very important role in the integrity and surveillance of the immune system within the skin. Therefore, it is responsible for contact allergic dermatitis reactions and graft-versus-host disease. Other than the skin, the Langerhans cell is normally found in other organs such as the lymph nodes and the thymus.

CLINICAL FEATURES

- Cutaneous LCH may be the initial presentation of the disease in up to 50% of the cases. The skin is uncommonly the only manifestation, and after a variable period of time, the disease may progress to other organ involvement. Cutaneous LCH, formerly known as histiocytosis X, represents a clinical spectrum of diseases, which include Letterer–Siwe disease, Hand–Schüller–Christian disease, and eosinophilic granuloma of bone, as well as intermediate and poorly elucidated forms.
- LCH is a rare disease with a prevalence of 0.5/100.000 children per year. Usually, Letterer–Siwe disease occurs in the first 2 years of life, Hand–Schüller–Christian disease in older children, and

eosinophilic granuloma in older children and adults (Table 20–4). There are many reports of patients with atypical presentations that do not conform these three classic patterns. For this reason, it is preferred to group all cases together as LCH, although when the diagnosis is made, the physician should still be aware of the classic types since the prognosis is quite different in each variant of the disease. The main prognostic factors seem to be the age of the patient, the type and number of disease sites, organ dysfunction, and the response to treatment. Postpituitary involvement might be a good prognosis factor. Therefore, children under the age of 2 years with multisystem disease and organ dysfunction have a mortality rate of at least 50%.

- In a few instances, patients with multiorgan involvement have experienced spontaneous remission. Thus, some investigators have speculated that LCH might be a reactive process rather than a malignant neoplastic disorder. Against this concept, immunohistochemical studies demonstrate the presence of proliferating cell nuclear antigen (PCNA) in many cases, which supports the neoplastic theory.
- Congenital "self-healing" LCH, is a rare variant of the disease, also called Hashimoto–Pritzker disease. Cutaneous lesions generally start in the neonatal period, with numerous firm, red-violaceous or brownish papulonodular lesions, up to 1 cm in diameter, scattered over different areas of the body. Characteristically, lesions regress by 3 months of age, relapse and systemic involvement are unexpected but long-term follow-up is advisable.

DIAGNOSIS AND DIFFERENTIAL

- The diagnosis of LCH is based on cytohistologic criteria defined by the Writing Group of the Histiocyte Society (1987). Three levels are specified:
  1. A presumptive diagnosis is made on the characteristic histologic features.
  2. A probable diagnosis is made on the finding of S100, peanut agglutinin (PNA), or α-mannosidase positive cells.
  3. A definitive diagnosis depends on the finding of CD1a+ cells or the demonstration of Birbeck granules within lesional cells on electron microscopy.
- Histopathologically, LCH is characterized by clusters and sheets of ovoid cells, 15 to 25 μm in diameter, that show an abundant eosinophilic cytoplasm and a reniform nucleous ("coffee-bean" nucleus). The cells are usually found immediately beneath the epidermis and rarely extend deep into the reticular dermis, except in nodular lesions. Focally, the cells invade the upper epidermis, where isolated cells or clusters of small aggregates may be observed. Occasionally, few xanthomized cells are found in the papillary dermis more often in the chronic forms. Binucleate cells and a few scattered mitoses are also present. There is a variable admixture of other inflammatory cells, depending on the type of lesion and the clinical variant of the disease. Therefore, in Letterer–Siwe disease, the infiltrate is largely composed of LC, with the admixture of relatively few neutrophils, eosinophils, and lymphocytes. In eosinophilic granuloma, the presence of eosinophils usually obscures other inflammatory cells. Multinucleate giant cells may be prominent in both eosinophilic granuloma and Hand–Schüller– Christian disease. The histologic picture in congenital self-healing histiocytosis is similar to other variants of LCH, although characteristically, the infiltrate is dense and is located in the mid and lower dermis. Epidermotropism is rare, and the presence of multinucleate giant cells is a constant finding. The immunophenotype is typical for LC, in contrast, electron microscopy demonstrate in less than 25% the presence of Birbeck granules (see Table 20–3).
- Immunohistochemical markers for LCH include CD1a, S100, and HLA-DR. The cells are negative for Mac-387, which stains cells of the monocyte–macrophage system but not dendritic cells. The cells do not express CD34 or MS-1, a marker for sinusoidal endothelial cells and dendritic perivascular macrophages, expressed by the NLCH.

TREATMENT

- A large number of treatments have been proposed for cutaneous LCH. Common sense is mandatory, and it is advisable to start a regime with fewest side effects and progress to more aggressive treatments depending on clinical response. Briefly different options that have been used with a variable success in the therapy of cutaneous LCH are summarized as follows.
- Surgery has been shown of limited value, usually performed as a diagnostic procedure in small, isolated skin lesions.
- Potent topical steroids may be of value in the short-term treatment due to the risk of systemic absorption and cutaneous side effects.
- PUVA can be a very effective form of therapy for cutaneous LCH, and if available, might be the first-line treatment of choice.
- Topical nitrogen mustard (mechloretamine) and carmustine, well-recognized therapeutic options for cutaneous T-cell lymphoma, are also effective for cutaneous LCH, although with some side effects. It might be regarded as the treatment of choice in the outpatient setting.
- Systemic steroids are of limited value in cutaneous LCH, since it has been observed that the skin does not usually respond well to this regime and the risk/benefit ratio is poor.
- Radiotherapy is of value in recalcitrant areas, particularly at sites of sinuses overlying lymph nodes or bone involvement.
- Trimethoprim-sulfamethoxazole has been shown to be a very interesting and safe approach for the treatment of cutaneous LCH and it is worth trying. Multisystem disease though shows a variable and usually poor response.
- Thalidomide has been used successfully in some patients with LCH, however, the risk of neuropathy with prolonged treatment limits its use.
- Isotretinoin has an immunomodulatory effect on LC. It has been used with success in a few cases of pure cutaneous involvement. At this point, it seems to be a promising therapeutic option.
- 2-Chlorodeoxyadenosine, a purine analogue also used in the treatment of hairy cell leukemia, will probably be of only limited value because relapse after therapy is common.
- Intralesional interferon β and intravenous interferon α should be regarded as a second-line therapy if other regimes are not effective.
- Cyclosporine is of limited value in cutaneous disease because relapse while on treatment or relapse afterward is often seen.

- Etoposide (VP16), a semisynthetic epipodophyllotoxin derivative used in the treatment of malignancies of the macrocyte–monophage lineage, should only be considered in patients with recalcitrant and symptomatic long-standing LCH of the skin.
- Methotrexate intravenously in low doses (20 mg weekly) has been recently seen to be a very effective treatment for pure cutaneous involvement in one case report.

REFERENCES

Favara BE, Feller AC, Pauli M. Contemporary classification of histiocytic disorders. The WHO committee on histiocytic/reticulum cell proliferations. Reclassification Working Group of the Histiocyte Society. *Med Pediatr Oncol.* 1997; 29:157.

Munn S, Chu AC. Langerhans cell histiocytosis of the skin. *Hematol Oncol Clin North Am.* 1998;2:269.

Weedon D. Cutaneous infiltrates non-lymphoid. In: Weedon D, ed. *Skin Pathology.* New York:Churchill-Livingstone, 1997; 865.

NON-LANGERHANS CELL HISTIOCYTOSIS

PATHOPHYSIOLOGY

- The histiocytoses include a variety of disorders that may be categorized based on their clinical features, histologic pattern, and immunohistochemical analysis of the predominant cells. Many diseases may produce cutaneous histiocytic infiltrates, including metabolic disorders, infectious diseases, Hodgkin's lymphoma, and foreign body reactions. However, this chapter includes in this group those idiopathic processes of unknown cause and unclear classification.
- Most of the disorders in this group have macrophage markers and lack LC features. The monocyte–macrophage is also bone-marrow derived, circulates, and then migrates to the skin where it is phagocytic. Macrophages can be labeled with a variety of markers including factor XIIIa (early lesions), CD11B, CD11C, and CD14B antibodies. Three recently delineated antibodies, Mac-387, HAM56 (developed lesions), and CD68, are currently regarded as markers of the macrophage subset of histiocytes, although Mac-387 is a low-sensitive marker. Lysozyme may also be present, and MS-1, a high-molecular weight extracellular protein is specific for sinusoidal endothelial cells and dendritic perivascular macrophages. It is expressed by the cells of these histiocytic processes but not by the LC or the palisading histiocytes of granuloma annulare.

CLINICAL FEATURES AND DIAGNOSIS AND DIFFERENTIAL

INDETERMINATE CELL HISTIOCYTOSIS

- The indeterminate cell is a class of dendritic cell found in the dermis. It is related to the LC but lacks Birbeck granules and displays some macrophage markers. It is believed that indeterminate cells are most likely a stage in LC development. Very few cases have been reported, but most patients present with generalized papules or nodules similar in appearance to generalized eruptive histiocytomas.
- On histologic examination, there is a monomorphous infiltrate of mononuclear and, occasionally, multinucleate, histiocytes. The cells express factor XIIIa, CD68, HAM56, S100 protein, and CD1a.

SINUS HISTIOCYTOSIS WITH MASSIVE LYMPHADENOPATHY

- The eponymous designation Rosai–Dorfman disease is more appropriate, because it is recognized that some cases may present with extranodal lesions, including lesions in the skin that may be the only manifestation of the disease. The typical presentation consists of painless cervical lymphadenopathy, accompanied by fever, anemia, an elevated erythrocyte sedimentation rate, and usually, polyclonal hypergammaglobulinemia. The average age of onset is around 20 years, and the skin is the most common extranodal site of involvement. Cutaneous lesions are usually multiple, and consist of large nodular lesions and erythematous or xanthomatous plaques predominantly located on the eyelids and malar regions. Usually, the disease runs a benign course, however, it sometimes is associated with significant morbidity.
- The pathologic changes in the lymph nodes are characteristic, showing expansion of the sinuses by large foamy histiocytes admixed with plasma cells. Cutaneous lesions are not specific. A dense dermal infiltrate of histiocytes, with scattered multinucleate cells, Touton cells, and neutrophils, may be present. Plasma cells are a constant finding, sometimes accompanied by dense lymphoid nodules. Phagocytosis of plasma cells and lymphocytes (emperipolesis), fibrosis, and focal necrosis may also be observed. The histiocytes are S100 positive, CD1a negative, and express macrophage and monocyte markers.

JUVENILE XANTHOGRANULOMA

- Clinically, it is a process more common in children under 1 year of age, but cases observed in adolescence or adult life also occur. Solitary or multiple red-brown papulonodules, up to 1 cm in diameter or larger, are found predominantly on the head and neck regions, upper part of the trunk, and proximal parts of the limbs. Spontaneous involution after months or years is a common event seen in these patients. In some cases, there is associated ocular problems, mainly glaucoma or an asymptomatic retinal mass. Involvement of other organs, such as the central nervous system, kidneys, lungs, and bones, is exceedingly rare. For instance, there may be an overlap with Erdheim–Chester disease, which shows features of sclerotic bone lesions and xanthogranulomatous soft tissue inflammation. Juvenile xanthogranuloma has been reported in association with neurofibromatosis type 1, sometimes with associated chronic myelogenous leukemia.
- The histopathology shows a nodular, poorly demarcated, dense infiltrate of small histiocytes involving the dermis. Sometimes, the infiltrate may be seen in the upper subcutis and, rarely, deeper into skeletal muscle. The cells are polygonal or spindle-shaped; in the early stage, a monomorphous appearance with foamy cells is observed. In late stages, varying numbers of Touton cells are present. There is also an admixture of inflammatory cells, such as lymphocytes, neutrophils and eosinophils; interstitial fibrosis may be seen in older lesions. The histiocytes are usually positive for fat stains, CD68, HAM56, cathepsin B, vimentin, lysozyme, α1-antichymotrypsin, factor XIIIa, but negative for Mac-387, smooth muscle actin, CD34, and S100 protein.

XANTHOMA DISSEMINATUM

- Patients typically have grouped yellow-brown papules in the flexural areas, especially the axilla, lateral neck, and periocular region. There have been attempts to classify this condition into three clinical presentations: persistent form, self-healing form (rare), and progressive form with systemic organ dysfunction. Oral involvement is common, and there is associated diabetes insipidus in about 40% of patients. Other organ involvement is rare.
- Pathologic features in well-established lesions consist on infiltrates of histiocytes, foam cells, fibroblasts, Touton cells, and a variable admixture of inflammatory cells. Immunohistochemical characterization of the infiltrate has demonstrated positive stain for HLA-DR but negative for S100. Cells express macrophage markers and staining with Mac-387 is variable.

NECROBIOTIC XANTHOGRANULOMA

- This entity is a rare, chronic disorder characterized by the presence of multiple erythematoviolaceous nodules and large indurated plaques, usually located on the periorbital area, but other areas on face. The trunk and limbs may also be involved. Associated paraproteinemia is a constant finding in these patients. Ocular impairment is common, and cardiac and laryngeal involvement has also been reported.
- Histopathologically, there are hyaline and granulomatous foci composed by histiocytes, foamy cells, and multinucleated giant cells, scattered throughout the dermis and subcutis. The process is more cellular, and has more atypical and prominent giant cells than necrobiosis lipoidica. The histiocytes do not stain for S100 protein.

BENIGN CEPHALIC HISTIOCYTOSIS

- Patients are typically young children who have small tan papules on the cheeks and forehead. Usually, lesions resolve spontaneously during childhood without scarring. Clinically, the differential with warts is often difficult to make. Currently, the view is that this condition is part of the spectrum of juvenile xanthogranuloma.
- Histopathologic findings show a diffuse infiltrate of histiocytes in the papillary dermis closely related to the epidermis. Occasional multinucleate cells are observed and xanthomization can be seen in older lesions. The histiocytes are negative for S100 protein and CD1a, but positive for macrophage markers.

PROGRESSIVE NODULAR HISTIOCYTOSIS

- This rare disorder probably represents the multiple form of the spindle-cell variant of xanthogranuloma. It is defined by the presence of two distinct types of lesions: superficial xanthomatous papules and indurated erythematous nodules.
- The histopathology of a nodular lesion resembles the changes observed in a dermatofibroma, with the presence of histiocytes, foam cells, and spindle-shaped cells, sometimes arranged in a storiform pattern. Cells express macrophage markers, but not CD34 and S100 protein and staining is variable for Mac-387.

GENERALIZED ERUPTIVE HISTIOCYTOMA

- It is defined as the sudden appearance of multiple papules, which on histologic examination show a histiocytic infiltrate. It has been described in association with underlying malignancy or other systemic disorders. The current view is that this condition is the early stage of different NLCH disorders.
- Pathologic features of this process consist of the presence of an infiltrate in the superficial and mid dermis,

where histiocytes are intermingled with few lymphocytes and fibroblasts. Histiocytes express macrophage markers, including the MS-protein, also positive in other NLCH conditions, and do not stain for S100 protein and CD1a.

MULTICENTRIC RETICULOHISTIOCYTOSIS

- It is a rare systemic disorder of unknown cause characterized by an asymptomatic papulonodular skin eruption, associated with a severe and destructive arthropathy of the interphalangeal joints of the hands. Lesions usually arise on the face and distal parts of the upper extremities. Onset is generally observed in adult females, and an underlying neoplasia may be seen in up to one fourth of the cases.
- The histopathology usually show a subepidermal grenz zone of uninvolved collagen that separates a circumscribed, nonencapsulated dermal infiltrate of mononuclear and multinucleate histiocytes that are the hallmark of the disease, because of its huge size and the presence of multiple nuclei. Immunohistochemical stains are characteristic for macrophage lineage, except for Mac-387 that is usually negative.

RETICULOHISTIOCYTOMA

- Reticulohistiocytomas are nodular lesions 0.5 to 2 cm in diameter, with similar histology to multicentric reticulohistiocytosis but without associated arthritis or systemic involvement.

HEMOPHAGOCYTIC SYNDROME

- Among the macrophage-related histiocytic disorders, the hemophagocytic syndromes or macrophage activation syndromes are the most prevalent and significant in terms of morbidity and mortality. Diagnostic criteria, defined by the Histiocyte Society are: fever of otherwise undetermined etiology, splenomegaly, cytopenias, hypofibrinogenemia, or hypertriglyceridemia and hemophagocytosis displayed in bone marrow, spleen, lymph node or other tissue. The most common cutaneous manifestations are panniculitis and purpura. In the past, this condition was known as malignant histiocytosis, but now two forms of the disease are known to exist. The familial form or primary hemophagocytic lymphohistiocytosis may occur in a familial setting or as a sporadic event in a first-affected child in a family with a putative recessive gene that is not yet determined. Often, this form is elicited by viral infections, but it is important to distinguish the familial form from the latter since the prognosis in the primary is lethal without bone marrow transplantation. In the secondary (infection-associated disorder) form, a treatment may not be needed. A secondary form of this syndrome has been associated with viral infections and T-cell lymphomas, especially in the immunocompromised host.
- The most consistent histopathologic feature is a proliferation of mature histiocytes that exhibit prominent erythrophagocytosis and cytophagocytosis. The histiocytic cells show positive reactions for KP-1 (CD68) and negative with MAC-387, factor XIIIa, and S100; lymphoid markers are negative. It seems that the phagocytic histiocytes are reactive and stimulated by T-cell lymphocytes, either neoplastic or in response to viral infection. Cytokines may play a very important role in the clinical and histopathologic findings observed in these syndromes.

REFERENCE

Zelger BW, Sidoroff A, Orchard G, et al. Non-Langerhans cell histiocytoses. A new unifying concept. *Am J Dermatopathol.* 1996;8:490.

21 DERMAL AND SUBCUTANEOUS TUMORS

Francisco Jimenez-Acosta
Enrique Poblet

VASCULAR TUMORS

- In this chapter discussion, it is common to include not only neoplasms, but also reactive proliferations, malformations, hyperplasias, hamartomas, and dilatation of preexisting vessels. The controversies generated about the histogenesis and the true nature of many of the vascular anomalies that have been classically included in the group of vascular tumors have produced numerous classifications and a plethora of terminology.

CONGENITAL HEMANGIOMA (STRAWBERRY NEVUS)

EPIDEMIOLOGY

- According to cellular kinetics and clinical behavior, the congenital vascular anomalies can be classified into two major categories: hemangiomas and vascular malformations (Table 21–1).
- Hemangiomas are the most common tumors of infancy. The incidence in the general newborn population is between 1 and 2.6%. They occur four times more frequently in females than males, and are especially common among those infants born prematurely.

PATHOPHYSIOLOGY

- Hemangiomas are characterized by a rapid growth phase (the proliferative phase) marked by endothelial

TABLE 21–1 Classification of Vascular Anomalies

PROLIFERATIVE	NONPROLIFERATIVE
Hemangioma	Vascular malformations
Superficial	Capillary
Deep (subcutaneous)	Venous
Compound or mixed	Lymphatic
Visceral	Arterial
	Combined

proliferation and hypercellularity, followed by slow regression (the involuting phase). Proliferation is characterized by increased levels of two angiogenic proteins (basic fibroblast growth factor and vascular endothelial growth factor) and enzymes involved in remodeling of extracellular matrix. Involution is characterized by endothelial apoptosis and downregulation of angiogenesis.

CLINICAL FEATURES

- Infantile capillary hemangiomas appear between the third and the fifth week of life as a small erythematous macular patch or localized telangiectasia. The most common locations are the head and neck.
- Hemangiomas increase rapidly in size for several weeks up to 1 year, and then start to regress from 1 to 10 years of age. Complete spontaneous resolution of the hemangioma occurs in about 75% of the patients by the time they have reached the age of 7 years. However, 20 to 40% of patients have residual changes of the skin, and very large superficial hemangiomas of the face often leave disfiguring scars.
- The clinical appearance is dictated by the depth of proliferation and the stage of evolution. Lesions may be superficial, deep, or combined. Typical superficial hemangioma looks like a bright, red, slightly elevated plaque, ranging from a few millimeters to several centimeters in diameter. If the hemangioma involves the deep dermis and subcutaneous tissue, it looks like a soft mass with a slightly bluish color. Deep hemangiomas have been incorrectly labeled "cavernous" hemangioma.
- Possible complications of common hemangiomas include ulceration and bleeding. Ulceration may result in secondary infection, pain, and/or scarring. Bleeding is more likely to occur in ulcerated hemangiomas, and can generally be controlled by applying local pressure.
- Twenty percent of affected infants have more than one hemangioma. An infant with multiple cutaneous hemangiomas should be assessed for visceral involvement, especially hemangiomas in the liver, gastrointestinal tract, and brain (disseminated neonatal

hemangiomatosis). Visceral hemangiomas are associated with high morbidity and mortality rates, particularly hepatic lesions with a high-flow pattern, which can cause cardiac failure and anemia.

- While most hemangiomas remain uncomplicated, certain unique presentations may be cause for concern, requiring further evaluation and therapy. Periorbital hemangiomas may lead to permanent visual sequelae, including blindness, and warrant early examination by an ophthalmologist. Infants with cervicofacial hemangiomas in a beard distribution are at risk for simultaneous symptomatic hemangiomas of the upper airway (subglottic area), often requiring tracheostomy. Hemangiomas of the lumbosacral region may be markers for occult spinal malformations and anomalies of the anorectal and urogenital regions.

- Infants with large, plaque-like facial hemangiomas should be evaluated for PHACES syndrome, which stands for: posterior fossa malformations, (most commonly of the Dandy–Walker variant); hemangiomas; cerebrovascular arterial anomalies; cardiac anomalies and coarctation of the aorta; eye abnormalities; and sternal cleft and/or supraumbilical raphe.

- Kasabach–Merritt syndrome refers to the development of life-threatening thrombocytopenia and bleeding as a result of platelet trapping within a vascular tumor. Once thought to be a complication of the common hemangioma, this syndrome is now known to be associated with two histologically benign but aggressive vascular tumors of infancy, namely kaposiform hemangioendothelioma and tufted angioma.

DIAGNOSIS AND DIFFERENTIAL

- The differential diagnosis of a congenital hemangioma is a congenital vascular malformation. Hemangiomas grow rapidly during the first year of life and spontaneously regress. In contrast, vascular malformations are present at birth, do not regress, and enlarge very slowly, commensurately with the growth of the child.

- If necessary, computed tomography with dye injection and magnetic resonance may be used for the differential diagnosis. Magnetic resonance studies can detect extension and involvement of other organs, and is indicated for all patients with hemangiomas in the midline region. Ultrasonography with Doppler demonstrates the high-flow pattern characteristic of hemangiomas.

- In infants with multiple hemangiomas, an abdominal ultrasonography with Doppler and imaging studies should be obtained to rule out visceral involvement.

TREATMENT

- Clinicians must follow hemangiomas carefully and tailor their approach to the specific characteristics of each case. Most infantile capillary hemangiomas are banal superficial tumors, regress spontaneously, and do not require intervention. However, the rate of involution is highly variable, as is the resulting cosmetic deformity. Addressing the psychosocial implications, especially of facial hemangiomas, is an essential part of providing complete care for patients and their families. The difficulty and challenge in managing these lesions is determining at what point the physician should intervene, and with what treatment modality.

- Careful observation with no intervention (watchful waiting) should be reserved only for nonfacial or cosmetically insignificant hemangiomas. Hemangiomas causing problems always require early intervention and treatment with a multidisciplinary approach.

- Therapies most commonly used include intralesional and oral corticosteroids, laser therapy, surgical excision, interferon alfa, and embolizations.

- For problematic or endangering hemangiomas, the first-line treatment is corticosteroids. Intralesional triamcinolone (10 mg/mL) can be injected monthly into a small, well-localized hemangioma that distorts the facial structures, impinges on the vision, or ulcerates. For large or multiple hemangiomas, corticosteroids are administered orally, beginning at 2 to 4 mg/kg/day. The dosage is tapered slowly until late infancy, when regression begins. The overall response rate is over 80 to 90% with either stabilization or accelerated regression.

- The second-line treatment for endangering or life-threatening hemangiomas that have not responded to corticosteroid therapy is interferon alfa, administered subcutaneously daily at 3 million units/m^2, until regression is under way. Toxicities include low-grade fever, elevation of transaminase, neutropenia, anemia, and spastic diplegia (5% of patients), which is usually reversible with the termination of the drug.

- Pulsed dye laser (595 nm) can be used for superficial hemangiomas in the rapid proliferation phase. Hemangiomas should be treated as soon as possible, before the lesions reach an exponential growth phase. Deep hemangiomas do not benefit from pulsed dye laser, because of its limited penetration into the tissue (1 mm). Pulsed dye laser is useful for controlling the pain and promotes epithelization of ulcerated hemangiomas. It can also improve the residual telangiectases after involution.

- Indications for surgical debulking during the growing phase include patients with hemangiomas that are blocking the airway or vision and do not respond to medical treatment. In cases without medical complications, the benefits and risks of a surgical approach must be weighed carefully, since the scar may be worse than the results of spontaneous regression. Surgical intervention can be considered for correction of the subcutaneous residual deformity after regression of the hemangioma.

- Embolization is sometimes used as an adjunct to control high-output heart failure that is caused by either an intrahepatic hemangioma or a large cutaneous tumor.
- Ulcerations can be treated with local wound care (topical antibiotics and biooclusive dressings).

VASCULAR MALFORMATIONS

EPIDEMIOLOGY

- Vascular malformations are subdivided anatomically and rheologically into slow-flow lesions (i.e., capillary malformation, lymphatic malformation, venous malformation) and fast-flow lesions (i.e., arterial malformation, such as aneurysm, ectasia, stenosis, fistulas, and arteriovenous malformation).
- The most typical cutaneous vascular malformation is a capillary malformation known as port-wine stain. It is estimated to occur in 3 out of 1000 newborns.

PATHOPHYSIOLOGY

- Vascular malformations are developmental defects, probably caused by dysregulation in the signaling that regulates proper formation of the vascular tree. The dysmorphic channels exhibit a normal rate of endothelial turnover.

CLINICAL FEATURES

- By definition, vascular malformations are present at birth, but certain vascular malformations go undetected, only to manifest during adolescence or adulthood.
- Port-wine stain presents at birth as a flat, well-defined, pink to red macular lesion. It is usually unilateral and can occur anywhere on the body, but most commonly in the head and neck region. As a vascular malformation, port-wine stain grows proportionally with the child and does not have a tendency to resolve. Left untreated, the color of the port-wine stain darkens with age and small papules can appear on its surface.

TABLE 21–2   Syndromes Associated with Vascular Malformations

SYNDROME	CLINICAL FINDINGS
Sturge–Weber syndrome	Port wine stain upper trigeminal dermatome; leptomeningeal angiomatosis; epilepsy (80%); others: glaucoma, mental retardation
Klippel–Trenaunay syndrome	Capillary, lymphatic, venous malformation; limb hypertrophy
Parkes–Weber syndrome	Capillary-lymphatic-venous malformation of upper limb; arteriovenous shunting
Maffucci syndrome	Exophytic venous anomalies of the upper limbs, with multiple bony exostoses and enchondromas
Blue rubber bleb syndrome	Multiple compressive vascular tumors of the skin and gastrointenstinal tract; gastrointestinal bleeding and anemia

- Venous malformations present in a wide spectrum, from isolated skin varicosities or ectasias, to localized spongy masses, to complex lesions involving multiple tissues and organs. Venous malformations are soft and compressible and the overlying skin/mucosa have a bluish hue.
- Syndromes associated with vascular malformations are listed in Table 21–2.

DIAGNOSIS AND DIFFERENTIAL

- Physical examination and clinical history permit the correct diagnosis in most patients. Port-wine stains should not be confused with a banal macular stain of infancy, commonly located in the glabella, eyelids, and nuchal regions, known as the "angel's kiss" or "salmon patch." This stain affects over one third of all newborns, fades within the first year of life, and is considered more of a physiologic phenomenon than a true dermatopathologic lesion.
- Magnetic resonance and ultrasonography with Doppler studies may be required in order to determine extension to deep levels and the flux of a given malformation.
- Children with port-wine stains on the upper trigeminal area should be referred to the ophthalmologist to rule out glaucoma. Imaging studies should be performed in order to detect neurologic calcifications adjacent to leptomeningeal angiomas.

TREATMENT

- Pulsed dye laser is the treatment of choice for port-wine stains. The wavelength of the laser

(595 nm) and the duration of the pulse (1.5 ms) are chosen to produce thermal injury that remains confined to the targeted vasculature. Multiple monthly sessions may be needed to achieve the best possible clearance.

ACQUIRED CAPILLARY HEMANGIOMA (CHERRY OR RUBY SPOTS, SENILE HEMANGIOMAS)

CLINICAL FEATURES

- Asymptomatic, multiple, small, bright red and smooth papules that arise in middle age, and are nearly always present in the elderly. Most commonly on the skin of the trunk.

DIAGNOSIS AND DIFFERENTIAL

- Easily diagnosed clinically by their small size and distribution.
- Microscopically, lesions show aggregates of dilated capillaries located in the superficial dermis.

TREATMENT

- Pulsed dye laser, electrodessication, cryotherapy, or shaving excision are indicated for cosmetic reasons.

TELANGIECTASIA

PATHOPHYSIOLOGY

- Permanent, abnormal dilatations of venules, capillaries, and precapillay arterioles of the subpapillary plexus.
- Telangiectasia may be associated with a number of different clinical conditions (Table 21–3).

CLINICAL FEATURES

- According to morphology, telangiectasia may be classified as punctate, spiderlike, matted, or linear.
- *Spider telangiectasia* have a central puctum from which fine vessels radiate. They are frequently associated with pregnancy and cirrhosis. Usual locations are the face, neck, and upper thorax.
- In *generalized essential telangectasia,* blood vessels become dilated over extensive areas of the body. More

TABLE 21–3   Etiologic Classification of Telangiectasia

Associated to hereditary syndromes
  Rendu–Osler–Weber disease
  Ataxia–telangiectasia
  Cockayne syndrome
  Bloom's syndrome
  Rothmund–Thomson syndrome (congenital poikiloderma)

Associated with systemic diseases
  Connective tissue diseases; lupus, dermatomyositis, scleroderma
  Hepatic cirrhosis
  Hormonal conditions: pregnancy, corticoids, or estrogen therapy

Associated with primary dermatoses
  Rosacea
  Mastocytosis
  Poikiloderma of Civatte

Physical causes
  Sun damage
  Radiodermitis
  Trauma

Primary telangiectasia
  Generalized essential telangiectasia
  Unilateral nevoid telangiectasia

common in women, telangiectases appear on the lower extremities and progress symmetrically to the trunk and arms.
- In *unilateral nevoid telengiectasia* the lesions have a unilateral dermatomal distribution, especially the trigeminal and the third and fourth cervical nerves. It may be congenital or acquired. Estrogen, alcohol, and liver disease have a major role.
- *Rendu–Osler–Weber disease* or *hereditary hemorrhagic telangiectasia* is a dominantly inherited disease with telangiectases on the skin, mucous membranes, and gastrointestinal tract, and aneurysms, and arteriovenous malformations. Cutaneomucosal telangiectases do not begin to appear until the adolescence and are typically present on the lips, tongue, nasal mucosa, conjunctiva, fingers, and toes. Recurrent episodes of epistaxis are characteristic. The prognosis is conditioned by the risk of hemorrhage of other organ systems.

TREATMENT

- Cutaneous telangiectasia can be eliminated with lasers, especially the pulsed dye laser or the long pulsed Nd-YAG laser.
- Cryotherapy or electrosurgery can destroy telangiectasia but may leave residual scars.
- Linear telangiectasia on the legs can be treated with infiltration of sclerosing agents.

ANGIOKERATOMA

PATHOPHYSIOLOGY

- Angiokeratomas are considered to be acquired telangiectasias in combination with hyperkeratosis (thickening of epidermal stratum corneum).

CLINICAL FEATURES

- Well-circumscribed, dark red, scaly papules of at least 0.5-mm diameter, they are asymptomatic, but may bleed if traumatized.
- Five clinical types are recognized: (1) the Mibelli type, characterized by the presence of angiokeratomas on the dorsa of fingers and toes; (2) the Fordyce type, involving the scrotum and vulva; (3) angiokeratoma corporis diffusum, with generalized and systemic lesions associated with Fabry's disease (α-galactosidase A deficiency); (4) angiokeratoma circumscriptum, showing groupings of angiokeratomas on an extremity, and (5) the solitary or multiple type, occurring anywhere on the skin.

DIAGNOSIS AND DIFFERENTIAL

- Clinical differential diagnoses include acquired hemangiomas, warts, nevus, and even melanoma.
- Histologically, angiokeratomas show marked dilatation of blood vessels in the papillary dermis, intimately associated with an overlying acanthotic thick epidermis.

TREATMENT

- Surgical excision may be indicated in symptomatic lesions as well as for diagnostic or cosmetic reasons.

PYOGENIC GRANULOMA (CAPILLARY HEMANGIOMA, BOTRIOMYCOMA)

PATHOPHYSIOLOGY

- Pyogenic granuloma has been regarded as a reactive vascular lesion that arises as exuberant granulation tissue in response to trauma or as a true benign vascular tumor.

CLINICAL FEATURES

- Pyogenic granuloma is a rapidly growing, solitary, dark red nodule 5 to 10 mm in diameter. It bleeds easily with minor trauma.
- Appears anywhere on the skin, but it is most commonly seen on the fingers and on the face. The gingiva is another common site, with pregnancy often acting as a precipitating factor.

DIAGNOSIS AND DIFFERENTIAL

- The diagnosis is made clinically. In special settings, a biopsy is necessary to rule out a nodular melanoma, Kaposi's sarcoma, and bacillary angiomatosis.
- The histology shows a proliferation of capillaries with a lobular arrangement. The overlying epidermis is usually flattened, forms a peripheral collarette, and is often eroded.

TREATMENT

- Pulsed dye laser, electrodessication, cryotherapy, or surgical removal.

VENOUS LAKE

CLINICAL FEATURES

- A venous lake is a dilated vein or venules in the superficial dermis. Clinically, it presents as dark blue, soft, raised lesions commonly found on the lips, ears, and face of elderly individuals.

TREATMENT

- Pulsed dye laser (treatment of choice), cryotherapy, or surgical excision.

GLOMUS TUMOR

PATHOPHYSIOLOGY

- Benign neoplasm that arise from modified smooth muscle cells, the glomic cells, normally found in specialized arteriovenous shunts, present in acral sites, especially the fingertips.
- Glomus tumors can be solitary or multiple. Multiple glomus tumors, also known as glomangiomas, may be dominantly inherited.

CLINICAL FEATURES

- Solitary glomus tumor is a painful lesion appearing as a small purple nodule with a marked predilection for the extremities, especially the nail bed. Lancinating pain can follow gentle touch or exposure to cold.

DIAGNOSIS AND DIFFERENTIAL

- Microscopically, the glomus tumor consists of convoluted vascular channels, the walls of which contain glomus cells.
- Glomus tumor is included into the spectrum of painful cutaneous tumors along with angiolipoma, neurilemmoma, ecrine spiradenoma, and leiomyoma.

TREATMENT

- Surgical excision is the treatment of choice. In patients with multiple lesions, excision should be restricted to the painful lesions.

LYMPHANGIOMA

PATHOPHYSIOLOGY

- The term lymphangioma describes localized malformations of lymphatic vessels. The two main types are lymphangioma circumscriptum (superficial lymphatic malformation) and cystic hygroma (cystic lymphatic malformation).

CLINICAL FEATURES

- The lesions are usually present at birth or appear early in life.
- In lymphangioma circumscriptum, one or several patches with translucent vesicles are present. Cystic hygroma presents as multilocular cysts, typically in the neck or axilla.

DIAGNOSIS AND DIFFERENTIAL

- Histologically, lymphangiomas show cystically dilated lymph vessels lined by a single layer of endothelium.

TREATMENT

- Small and superficial lesions may be effectively treated by surgery, cryotherapy, or laser therapy. Recurrences are common.

KAPOSI'S SARCOMA

EPIDEMIOLOGY

- Kaposi's sarcoma is a malignant tumor of vascular endothelium.
- Four distinct epidemiologic variants are recognized: (1) classical type; (2) endemic African type; (3) iatrogenic or transplant-related type, and (4) epidemic type associated with acquired immunodeficiency syndrome (AIDS).
- The classical type of Kaposi's sarcoma was first described by the Hungarian dermatologist Moritz Kaposi in 1872. It is a rare type of cancer, affecting elderly male patients with an increased incidence in Eastern European and Mediterranean countries.
- Transplant-related Kaposi's sarcoma constitutes approximately 6% of all cancers in solid-organ transplant recipients. Affects mainly patients receiving chronic immunosuppressive therapy, such as azathoprine, cyclosporine, or corticosteroids to prevent organ rejection.
- AIDS-related Kaposi's sarcoma is seen predominantly in men who acquire human immunodeficiency virus (HIV) infection through unprotected sex with men. The first cases were reported in 1981 in homosexual men living in California and New York. Since then, approximately 15 to 25% of men infected with HIV in the United States have been diagnosed with Kaposi's sarcoma.

PATHOPHYSIOLOGY

- The human herpesvirus type 8 (HHV-8) is the etiologic virus in the pathogenesis of Kaposi's sarcoma, along with aberrant cytokine expression, production of multiple angiogenic peptides, and immune dysregulation. The specific mechanism by which HHV-8 participates in the oncogenic process is unclear.
- Patients with AIDS-related Kaposi's sarcoma are uniformly co-infected with HIV and HHV-8. The HIV contributes to the pathogenesis of Kaposi's sarcoma by inducing the immunosuppression necessary for the clinical expression of disease. HHV-8 appears to be sexually transmitted. The rate of seropositivity to HHV-8 in men increases with the number of male sexual contacts, but is minimal in exclusively heterosexual men.
- Two cellular types compose the histologic lesions of Kaposi's sarcoma: a vascular and a spindle-cell component (Kaposi's sarcoma cells). The origin of the spindle cells is controversial, but sequences of HHV-8 have been amplified from them. Kaposi's sarcoma cells secrete factors that induce proliferation and

migration of endothelial cells, including angiogenic factors basic fibroblast growth factor, vascular endothelial growth factor, and cytokines.

CLINICAL FEATURES

- The classic variant of Kaposi's sarcoma presents as blue-red macules and papules that may coalesce, forming large plaques involving the distal portion of lower extremities. The course is progressive, but usually the lesions remain stable for many years. In only 10% of the cases, visceral lesions occur.
- The earliest cutaneous lesions of AIDS-related Kaposi's sarcoma are small zones of apparent intracutaneous hemorrhage similar to petechiae or ecchymoses (patch stage). Cutaneous lesions may occur at any site but usually begin on the head and neck area, upper torso, or extremities. In contrast with the classic type, AIDS-related Kaposi's sarcoma can rapidly progress and disseminate. Lesions become raised to form violaceous plaques (plaque stage), nodules, and tumors (nodular stage). At the time of initial diagnosis, 20% of patients have lesions in the oral mucosa, especially on the palate or gingiva.
- Visceral involvement occurs in over 50% of AIDS-related Kaposi's sarcoma. The gastrointestinal tract is the most common extracutaneous site, and may present with abdominal pain, weight loss, or diarrhea, which may be bloody. Pulmonary Kaposi's sarcoma is the second most common site of extracutaneous involvement, and is the most life-threatening form of the disease. Patients may present with shortness of breath, cough, and hemoptysis.

DIAGNOSIS AND DIFFERENTIAL

- It is important to confirm the clinical diagnosis with a skin biopsy because several other entities, such as bacillary angiomatosis, vasculitis, ecchymosis or pigmentary purpuras, may look similar.

- In the early patch stage, the microscopic specimens show dilated, anastomosing, thin-walled vascular spaces in the dermis, dissecting the collagen. In plaque-like and nodular lesions, a proliferation of spindle cells is present peripheral to the layer of endothelial cells. The stroma contains numerous erythrocytes and deposits of hemosiderin. A characteristic histopathologic finding, although nonspecific, is the presence of the so-called "hyalin globules," which probably represent degenerated erythrocytes phagocytized by neoplastic cells. When the spindle-cell component predominates, Kaposi's sarcoma may be difficult to differentiate from other spindle-cell neoplasms. In these cases, the positive staining of Kaposi's sarcoma spindle cells with the anti-CD34 antibody is helpful (Table 21–4).
- A chest x-ray, routine blood tests, CD4+ T-lymphocyte cell count, and HIV viral load may help stratify patients into good or poor prognostic groups.
- Bronchoscopy to establish pulmonary involvement is indicated for patients with abnormal chest x-ray. Symptomatic gastrointestinal involvement is best evaluated with endoscopy.

TREATMENT

- While not presently curable, multiple treatment options exist and must be considered according to the extension of the disease and specific needs of the patient.
- The use of highly active antiretroviral therapy aimed at controlling the underlying HIV infection has been associated with a dramatic decrease in the incidence of Kaposi's sarcoma, and may also be effective in the treatment of existing disease.
- Localized lesions of Kaposi's sarcoma can be treated with 0.1% alitretinoin topical gel, intralesional injection of vinblastine, local radiation, or cryotherapy. Alitretinoin gel is administered by the patient twice daily. Most patients require 4 to 8 weeks of treatment

TABLE 21–4   Immunohistochemical Identification of Malignant Dermal Tumors and Spindle-cells Neoplasms

	CYTOKERATIN	S100	FVIII	CD31	CD34	DESMINE
Kaposi's sarcoma	–	–	+/–	+/–	+	–
Angiosarcoma	–	–	+/–	+	+/–	–
DFSP	–	–	–	–	+	–
AFX	–	–	–	–	–	–
Lieomyosarcoma	–	–	–	–	–	+
Squamous carcinoma (spindle type)	+	–	–	–	–	–
Melanoma (spindle type)	–	+	–	–	–	–

DFSP = Dermatofibrosarcoma protuberans; AFX = Atypical fibroxanthoma.

before response is noted. Intralesional injections of vinblastine result in response rates of 70 to 90%.

- Patients with extensive mucocutaneous or symptomatic visceral disease can be treated with systemic chemotherapy. New liposomal anthracyclines (daunorubicin and doxorubicin) have replaced the conventional combination chemotherapy (bleomycin and vincristine) as first-line therapy for advanced disease. Liposomal daunorubicin (40 mg/m^2 every 2 weeks) or liposomal doxorubicin (20 mg/m^2 every 3 weeks), used as single agents, have demonstrated equivalent or better response rate with a much lower toxicity profile.
- Pathogenic-based therapies with various antiangiogenic peptides and specific antiviral approaches aimed at HHV-8 are currently under investigation.

ANGIOSARCOMA

CLINICAL FEATURES

- Angiosarcoma is a relatively rare malignant vascular tumor.
- Angiosarcoma of the scalp and face of the elderly starts rather innocuously with erythematous or purple macules or plaques on the scalp or the face. Nodules, ulceration, and edema, especially of the eyelids, develop. Cervical lymph node and hematogenous metastasis are frequent, especially to the lungs, spleen, and liver.
- Angiosarcoma may also arise secondary to persistent chronic lymphedema, referred to as *Stewart–Treves syndrome*. Most commonly the severe edema is secondary to previous ipsilateral mastectomy for breast carcinoma. Clinical lesions consist of subcutaneous nodules of a bluish color. The nodules increase in number and size quite rapidly and may undergo ulceration. Metastasis, especially to the lungs, is the main cause of death.

DIAGNOSIS AND DIFFERENTIAL

- A biopsy is needed to make the diagnosis because clinical initial lesions of angiosarcoma can resemble a cellulitis, hematoma, or chronic lymphedema.
- Microscopically, angiosarcomas of the skin are localized in the dermis, but often infiltrate subcutaneous tissue or deeper structures. Well-differentiated areas show marked vascular formation with vessels that "dissect" between collagen fibers. The cells lining the abnormal vessels are enlarged with nuclear atypia and sparse mitotic figures.

- Poorly differentiated angiosarcomas may simulate other malignant tumors, especially poorly differentiated carcinoma or malignant melanoma. In these cases, additional electron microscopy or immunohistochemical studies may be necessary for the differential diagnosis.
- Immunohistochemistry of angiosarcomas show vimentin positivity and cytokeratin negativity, a staining pattern that allows differentiation from poorly differentiated carcinomas (cytokeratin positive). The staining with endothelial markers (factor VIII-related antigen and, especially, anti CD31 antibody) confirms the vascular nature of the angiosarcoma (see Table 21–4).

TREATMENT

- The prognosis is very poor. Early and aggressive surgical management and radical wide-field electron beam radiation therapy may be of benefit in some patients.

REFERENCES

Aboulafia DM. Kaposi's sarcoma. *Clin Dermatol.* 2001; 19:269.

Dinehart SM, Kincannon J, Geronemus R. Hemangiomas: Evaluation and treatment. *Dermatol Surg.* 2001;27:475.

Levine Am, Tulpule A. Clinical aspects and management of AIDS-related Kaposi's sarcoma. *Eur J Cancer.* 2001; 37:1288.

Martin JN, Ganem DE, Osmond DH, et al. Sexual transmission and the natural history of human herpesvirus 8 infection. *N Engl J Med.* 1998;338:948.

Metry DW, Hebert AA. Benign cutaneous vascular tumors of infancy: When to worry, what to do. *Arch Dermatol.* 2000; 136:905.

Mulliken JB, Fishman SJ, Burrows PE. Vascular anomalies. *Curr Probl Surg.* 2000;37:517.

Mulliken JB, Glowacki J. Hemangiomas and vascular malformations in infants and children: A classification based on endothelial characteristics. *Plast Reconstr Surg.* 1982; 69:412.

Poblet E, Gonzalez-Palacios F, Jimenez FJ. Different immunoreactivity of endothelial markers in well and poorly differentiated areas of angiosarcomas. *Virchows Arch.* 1996;428:217.

Poetke M, Philipp C, Berlien HP. Flashlamp-pumped pulsed dye laser for hemangiomas in infancy: Treatment of superficial vs mixed hemangiomas. *Arch Dermatol.* 2000; 136:628.

Requena L, Sanguenza OP. Cutaneous vascular proliferations. Part III. Malignant neoplasms, other cutaneous neoplasms with significant vascular component, and disorders erroneously considered as vascular neoplasms. *J Am Acad Dermatol.* 1997;38:143.

Requena L, Sanguenza OP. Cutaneous vascular proliferations. Part II. Hyperplasias and benign neoplasms. *J Am Acad Dermatol.* 1997;37:887.

Williams III EF, Stanislaw P, Dupree M, Mourtzikis K, Mihm M, Shannon L. Hemangiomas in infants and children: An algorithm for intervention. *Arch Facial Plast Surg.* 2000;2:103.

FIBROHISTIOCYTIC TUMORS

FIBROUS PAPULE

CLINICAL FEATURES

- A very common lesion occurring nearly always on the face, especially on the nose, in mature persons.
- Asymptomatic, small, dome-shaped papules. In most cases, they are skin-colored, but they may be reddish.
- Patients with tuberous sclerosis may have hundreds of them located on the nose and cheeks (angiofibromas/adenoma sebaceum).

DIAGNOSIS AND DIFFERENTIAL

- The differential diagnosis includes an intradermal nevus, sebaceous hyperplasia, and basal cell carcinoma.

TREATMENT

- For cosmetic reasons, a fibrous papule can be removed by superficial shaving excision, electrodesiccation, dermabrasion, or CO_2 laser.

ACROCHORDON (SKIN TAGS)

CLINICAL FEATURES

- Pedunculated, asymptomatic, small lesions that occur mainly in flexural regions (neck, axilla, and groin).
- They appear with advancing age and more frequently in obese individuals.

TREATMENT

- For cosmetic reasons, acrochordons can be easily eliminated with scissors or electrodesiccation.

KELOID

PATHOPHYSIOLOGY

- Keloids are cosmetically unacceptable, thickened scars that result from an abnormal healing response to injury. Although the exact cause of formation is unknown, there are predisposing factors such as heredity, race (more common in black patients), and location (more common on the earlobes, shoulders, upper back, and chest).
- Among theories regarding the etiology of keloids are decreased apoptosis in keloidal fibroblasts, increased levels of plasminogen activator inhibitor 1, and tissue hypoxia. Fibroblasts from keloids have been shown to have a greater capacity to proliferate. Transforming growth factor beta types 1 and 2, which stimulate fibroblasts, are also increased in keloidal scars.

CLINICAL FEATURES

- Most keloids appear weeks to months after minor trauma or surgical scars. Rarely, keloids can also occur spontaneously.
- A keloid is characterized by the overgrowth of a dense fibrous tissue that extends beyond the borders of the original wound. In contrast, a hypertrophic scar is a thick scar that remains confined to the borders of the original wound.
- A keloid can be pruritic or painful, does not regress spontaneously, and tends to recur after excision.

TREATMENT

- There is no universally effective method of treatment for keloids and hypertrophic scars. A variety of therapies can be tried with variable success.
- Intralesional steroid injection can produce flattening the keloid scar and remains the mainstay of therapy (40 mg/mL of triamcinolone every 2 to 4 weeks). Surgical excision alone has an excessively high recurrence rate (50 to 80%).
- Other therapies for keloids are listed in Table 21–5.

DERMATOFIBROMA

PATHOPHYSIOLOGY

- The positive immunohistochemical staining with factor XIIIa suggest that this tumor could derive from the dermal dendrocyte (mononuclear dendritic cells normally present in papillary dermis).

TABLE 21–5   Treatment of Keloids

Intraleslional steroids
Excision followed by intralesional steroid[a]
Radiation combined with surgical excision[b]
Cryotherapy alone or in combination with intralesional steroid injection
Pulsed dye layer[c]
Silicone gel dressing (12 hr/day for 2 to 4 months)[d]
Intralesional 5-fluorouracil (50 mg/ML once weekly)
Intralesional bleomycin

[a] Reduces the recurrence rate of the surgery alone.
[b] Should be performed within 10 days of the surgery and is of no additional benefit when performed before surgery. It prevents recurrence in 75% of cases at 1-year follow-up.
[c] Improves symptoms, color, and reduces height of keloids.
[d] Most useful for hypertrophic scars.

CLINICAL FEATURES

• The dermatofibroma is one of the most common benign cutaneous tumors. It is more frequent in adults, and 80% of cases occur on the extremities.
• Dermatofibromas are asymptomatic, brown, firm papules, 5 to 10 mm in diameter. Some lesions are dome-shaped, while others appear depressed.

DIAGNOSIS AND DIFFERENTIAL

• A simple maneuver to help confirm the diagnosis is to apply lateral compression, which causes the central portion of the dermatofibroma to "dimple."
• The clinical differential diagnosis includes scar, nevus, and dermatofibrosarcoma protuberans (in larger lesions).
• In certain cases, a biopsy may be necessary to confirm the diagnosis. Histology shows a proliferation of spindled fibroblasts arranged as intersecting fascicles. Large bundles of collagen are typically present at the periphery of the lesion.

TREATMENT

• Treatment is not necessary. When required, simple excision is the treatment of choice.
• Small lesions may respond to cryotherapy.

DERMATOFIBROSARCOMA PROTUBERANS

PATHOPHYSIOLOGY

• Dermatofibrosarcoma protuberans (DFSP) is a cutaneous fibrocytic tumor of intermediate malignancy with an infiltrative growth pattern, a high rate of recurrence after simple excision, and a low potential for metastasis. This tumor has been considered a fibroblastic, histiocytic, and even a neural tumor. To date, there is no general consensus concerning its histogenesis.

CLINICAL FEATURES

• Clinically DFSP appears as an asymptomatic indurated plaque or nodule that may be violaceous, red-brown, or flesh colored. It appears more frequently during early and mid-adult life, and may occur at almost any site, although most frequently on the trunk and proximal extremities.

DIAGNOSIS AND DIFFERENTIAL

• At the initial stage, DFSP may simulate a dermatofibroma, scar, a plaque of morphea, or a sclerodermiform basal cell carcinoma.
• Histologically, the tumor is composed of a uniform population of plump fibroblasts arranged in a distinct and often monotonous pattern that is called "storiform pattern." Cells are only slightly atypical. Because dermatofibrosarcoma protuberans shows a deceptively bland appearance, especially at the periphery, it has to be differentiated from dermatofibroma. However, this is a deceptive appearance, because tumor fascicles infiltrate the dermis, hypodermis, and sometimes the underlying skeletal muscle.
• DFSP shows a positive staining for CD34 and negative for FXIIIa, which helps to distinguish it from dermatofibroma.

TREATMENT

• DFSP has a very high recurrence rate after simple surgical excision. Even wide, local excision, with 3-cm margins, give a 20% rate of local recurrence.
• Mohs micrographic surgery, due to its precise margin control, appears to be the current preferred treatment of choice.

ATYPICAL FIBROXANTHOMA

PATHOPHYSIOLOGY

• Atypical fibroxanthoma (AFX) is a malignant and pleomorphic tumor that usually occurs on sun-damaged skin of elderly individuals. It is currently

considered the superficial or cutaneous variant of the malignant fibrous histiocytoma of soft tissue.
- The immunohistochemical profile of AFX indicates a fibroblastic rather than a histiocytic differentiation.

CLINICAL FEATURES

- AFX are tumors usually less than 2 cm in diameter, with a short history of rapid growth. They appear as solitary lesion, often ulcerated, on markedly sun-damaged or X-irradiated skin of the head and neck of elderly patients. Occasionally, atypical fibroxanthoma arises on nonexposed sites in younger individuals, and in children with xeroderma pigmentosum.
- AFX tend to recur locally, and has a low but definitive potential for metastasis, most commonly to regional lymph nodes.

DIAGNOSIS AND DIFFERENTIAL

- A biopsy is needed for diagnosis. The tumor is composed of pleomorphic histiocyte-like cells, with bizarre nuclei, or fusiform cells, showing mitotic figures, including abnormal forms.
- Immunohistochemical staining is helpful in distinguishing atypical fibroxanthoma from other spindle-cell or pleomorphic neoplasms. Atypical fibroxanthoma is positive for vimentin but negative for both keratin and S100 protein, thereby excluding squamous cell carcinoma (keratin positive and S100 negative) and malignant melanoma (keratin negative and S100 positive).

TREATMENT

- Wide local excision is indicated. In recent years, several series of investigations have reported successful treatment with Mohs micrographic surgery.

REFERENCES

Guillén DR, Cockerell CJ. Cutaneous and subcutaneous sarcomas. *Clinics Dermatol.* 2001;19:262.

Ratner D, Thomas CO, Johnson TM, et al. Mohs micrographic surgery for the treatment of dermatofibrosarcoma protuberans. *J Am Acad Dermatol.* 1997;37:600.

Shaffer JJ, Taylor SC, Cook-Bolden F. Keloidal scars: A review with critical look at therapeutic options. *J Am Acad Dermatol.* 2002;46:S63.

Youssef N, Vabres P, Buisson T, Brousse N, Fraitag S. Two unusual tumors in a patient with xeroderma pigmentosum: Atypical fibroxanthoma and basosquamous carcinoma. *J Cutan Pathol.* 1999;26:430.

TUMORS OF FAT

LIPOMA

PATHOPHYSIOLOGY

- Lipomas are very common benign tumors of the fat. The observation that some cases are familial suggests that their development is under genetic control. Multiple lipomatosis, a familiar form of lipomas, is autosomal dominant.

CLINICAL FEATURES

- Lipomas present in the adult population as soft, mobile tumors of the subcutaneous fat. They are mainly located on the trunk and extremities. Although usually solitary, lipomas may be multiple and can range from a few millimeters to 20 or more centimeters.
- Lipomas are usually asymptomatic tumors. A painful lipoma is always suggestive of an angiolipoma.
- Madelung's disease is a form of multiple lipomatosis in which the lesions are poorly circumscribed and congregate especially around the neck and occiput.

DIAGNOSIS AND DIFFERENTIAL

- The diagnosis of lipoma is usually clinical, but may be confused with epidermoid cysts, other benign fatty tumors, and liposarcomas.
- Histologically, there is a proliferation of normal-appearing fat cells in the subcutaneous tissue. Histologic variations of lipomas include the angiolipoma, the spindle-cell lipoma, and the pleomorphic lipoma.

TREATMENT

- Surgical excision if desired.

LIPOSARCOMA

PATHOPHYSIOLOGY

- Cutaneous liposarcomas are very rare malignant tumors. They may arise in the subcutaneous fat or may result from the infiltration of a tumor localized in deeper tissues.

- Liposarcoma takes its origin from primitive mesenchymal cells rather than from mature cells. Liposarcoma developing in previous lipomas is an extraordinary event, and for practical purposes, it is better not to consider this possibility.

CLINICAL FEATURES

- Liposarcoma is a tumor of adults, more common between 40 to 60 years of age.
- The tumor usually presents as a large, lobulated mass greater than 10 cm in diameter with poorly defined margins. It enlarges rapidly and is painful. There is a predilection for the lower leg.

DIAGNOSIS AND DIFFERENTIAL

- Clinically, liposarcomas may be confused with lipomas and other soft tissue sarcomas.
- The microscopic diagnosis of liposarcoma is characterized by the presence of lipoblasts. Malignant lipoblasts are cells with lipid droplets in the cytoplasm and hyperchromatic nucleus that is indented by the cytoplasmic vacuoles. Histologically, liposarcomas are subclassified as well-differentiated, myxoid, pleomorphic, and round cell liposarcoma. Myxoid and well-differentiated liposarcomas have a more favorable prognosis.

TREATMENT

- Radical surgical excision is the treatment of choice.

REFERENCE

Mentzel T. Cutaneous lipomatous neoplasms. *Semin Diagn Pathol.* 2001;18:250.

Smooth Muscle Tumors

SMOOTH MUSCLE HAMARTOMA

PATHOPHYSIOLOGY

- Smooth muscle hamartoma represents a developmental defect characterized by an overgrowth of smooth muscle.

CLINICAL FEATURES

- Smooth muscle hamartomas are usually present at birth or they may arise in childhood.
- They appear as a single patch, usually associated with hyperpigmentation and hypertrichosis. Sometimes, small follicular papules are present throughout the patch.

DIAGNOSIS AND DIFFERENTIAL

- Histologically, thick and well-defined bundles of smooth muscle are present in the dermis.

TREATMENT

- This is a benign condition and treatment is not needed except for cosmetic purposes. The hypertrichosis can be eliminated with hair removal lasers.

LEIOMYOMA

PATHOPHYSIOLOGY

- Leiomyomas of the skin are benign tumors that may arise from the arrector pili muscle (piloleiomyoma), the smooth muscle of blood vessels (angioleiomyoma), or the smooth muscle of the vulvar, dartoic, or mamillary muscles (genital leiomyomas). The most common type of presentation is that of multiple piloleiomyomas.

CLINICAL FEATURES

- Piloleiomyomas may be solitary or multiple. Solitary piloleiomyomas are usually larger, measuring up to 2 cm in diameter. Multiple piloleiomyomas are small (less than 1 cm), firm, red or brown nodules, that may be grouped or show a linear arrangement. Multiple piloleiomyomas may be associated with bone exostoses and colonic polyposis (Gardner syndrome).
- Piloleiomyomas are typically tender and may give rise to occasional attacks of spontaneous pain.
- Genital leiomyomas are solitary asymptomatic tumors located on the labia majora, the scrotum, or the nipples.

DIAGNOSIS AND DIFFERENTIAL

- The diagnosis is made by biopsy. The tumors are formed by interlacing bundles of smooth muscle cells that extend in various directions. The bundles are composed of elongated muscle cells, with a centrally located, oval, blunt-edged nuclei.

- Leiomyomas may simulate neural tumors. Immuno-histochemical techniques are useful for the differential diagnosis: desmine or alfa smooth muscle actine in muscular tumors, and S-100 protein in neural tumors.

TREATMENT

- Surgical excision may be indicated in symptomatic cases.

LEIOMYOSARCOMA

PATHOPHYSIOLOGY

- Superficial leiomyosarcoma is a rare, malignant, smooth muscle neoplasm that comprises 2% of all soft tissue sarcomas. Superficial leiomyosarcomas have been subdivided into cutaneous (dermal) and subcutaneous forms because of their different clinical and prognostic implications. The cutaneous form is believed to derive from the arrector pili or genital dartoic muscles, whereas the subcutaneous type is thought to arise from the smooth muscle wall of blood vessels.
- Interestingly, these tumors have been anecdotally associated with a history of various types of trauma.

CLINICAL FEATURES

- Leiomyosarcomas are more common in middle-aged to elderly patients. The extremities, especially the thighs, are the main location of these tumors.
- Dermal leiomyosarcomas present as painful, firm nodules, less than 2 cm in diameter, that tend to depress or ulcerate the overlying skin. Subcutaneous leiomyosarcomas are larger and deep-seated, and do not affect the overlying skin.
- The risk of metastasis for dermal tumors is small (5 to 10%), but for subcutaneous tumors, it is about 50 to 60%. Metastasis may appear many years after the surgical excision of the primary tumor.
- The presence of multiple superficial leiomyosarcomas should always suggest the possibility of metastasis from another soft tissue site, mainly the retroperitoneum.

DIAGNOSIS AND DIFFERENTIAL

- Leiomyosarcomas are commonly misdiagnosed as epidermal cyst, dermatofibromas, or a variety of dermal and subcutaneous nodules.

- The diagnosis is made by the histologic findings. Microscopically, tumor fascicles infiltrate the dermis or hypodermis. The fascicles are more cellular than the fascicles of leiomyomas. Nuclear atypia and mitotic figures are variable. Poorly differentiated tumors may be so anaplastic that the diagnosis can be established only with electronmicroscopy or immuno-histochemistry. Immunohistochemical staining shows positivity for desmin or alfa smooth muscle actin in almost all dermal leiomyosarcomas.

TREATMENT

- The current recommendation is wide surgical excision with 3 to 5 cm margins including subcutaneous tissue and fascia. Local recurrences are common, even after wide excisions.
- Mohs micrographic surgery can be useful but more studies with long-term follow-up are needed to determine the recurrence rate.

REFERENCE

Holst VA, Junkins-Hopkins JM, Elenitsas R. Cutaneous smooth muscle neoplasms: Clinical features, histologic findings, and treatment options. *J Am Acad Dermatol.* 2002; 46:477.

NEURAL TUMORS

- Cutaneous neural tumors can be classified into two major groups: (1) those derived from any of the structures that compose the peripheral nerves (axons and nerve sheath cells), and (2) those derived from ectopic or heterotopic neural tissue (Table 21–6).

TABLE 21–6   Classification of Cutaneous Neural Tumors

Tumors of peripheral nerves
   Neuromas
      Palisaded, encapsulated type
      Traumatic type
   Neurofibroma
   Schwannoma
   Neurothekoma (nerve sheath mixoma)

Tumors of ectopic/heterotopic neural tissue
   Nasal glioma
   Extracranial meningioma
   Neuroectodermal tumors

NEUROMA

PATHOPHYSIOLOGY

- Neuromas are benign tumors of peripheral nerves.
- Traumatic neuromas are traumatically induced proliferation of axonal elements, and not true neoplasms. Traumatic neuromas include the amputation neuromas, the rudimentary supernumerary digits, and the so-called Morton's neuromas. Rudimentary supernumerary digits are probably the result of autoamputation of a supernumerary digit in utero.
- Multiple endocrine neoplasia syndrome (type 2b) is inherited as an autosomal dominant trait and characterized by multiple mucosal neuromas, medullary carcinoma of the thyroid, and pheochromocytoma.

CLINICAL FEATURES

- Traumatic neuromas present as firm, often painful, nodules at sites of a previous injury to peripheral nerves.
- Palisaded encapsulated neuromas are solitary, painless, flesh-colored nodules, generally located on the face.
- Neuromas in multiple endocrine neoplasia are one of the earliest clinical manifestations of the syndrome. Neuromas appear as multiple, small nodules on the lips, tongue, eyelids, and oral mucosa.

DIAGNOSIS AND DIFFERENTIAL

- Neuromas are often mistaken for cysts, intradermal nevi, or neurofibromas.
- Histologic examination is diagnostic. Microscopic examination shows bundles of axons and neural supporting cells that form structures similar to peripheral nerves, extending in various directions, with intermingled connective tissue.
- True neuromas have a 1:1 axon to Schwann cells ratio, whereas in neurofibromas and schwannomas, proliferating Schwann cells by far outnumber axons.

TREATMENT

- Surgical excision.

NEUROFIBROMA

PATHOPHYSIOLOGY

- Neurofibroma is a benign proliferation of Schwann cells and fibroblasts associated with a minor component of axons and embedded in collagenous tissue.

- Neurofibromas may appear as a solitary lesions or as part of a syndrome (neurofibromatosis of Von Recklinghausen).
- Neurofibromatosis type 1 (NF1) has a prevalence of 1/2500 to 1/7800. It can arise as an autosomal dominant condition (gene on chromosome 17q) or by spontaneous mutation. The NF1 gene is usually classified as a tumor suppressor gene, but it is not yet known how NF1 gene mutations cause many of the nontumor manifestations of the disorder. The NF1 protein, neurofibromina, is expressed early during embryonic development with high levels of expression in the brain, suggesting that it plays an important role in regulating the orderly differentiation of central nervous system neurons.

CLINICAL FEATURES

- Solitary neurofibromas generally arise in adulthood. Individual lesions are flesh-colored, soft papules, nodules, or pedunculated tumors.
- NF1 is characterized by café-au-lait macules, cutaneous neuromas, and neurofibromas. Three types of neurofibromas can be found: cutaneous, subcutaneous, and plexiform. The presence of more than six café-au-lait macules exceeding 1.5 cm in diameter is considered indicative of neurofibromatosis type 1. Freckle-like pigmentation of the axilla is a pathognomonic sign that may be present since childhood.
- Systemic manifestations of NF1 include hamartomas of the iris (Lisch nodules), optic nerve glioma, skeletal manifestations (pseudoarthrosis of the tibia, kyphoscoliosis), and higher risk for malignant tumors.

DIAGNOSIS AND DIFFERENTIAL

- Neurofibromas may be clinically confused with acrochordons and melanocytic nevi.
- Histologic study of the lesions may be necessary for differential diagnosis.

TREATMENT

- Solitary neurofibromas may be treated with surgical excision.

SCHWANNOMA (NEURILEMMOMA, NEURINOMA)

PATHOPHYSIOLOGY

- Schwannomas are benign proliferations of Schwann cells.

- Schwannomas may appear as a solitary, sporadic tumors or may be associated with neurofibromatosis type 2 (NF2).
- The mutated gene of NF2 has been identified in the long arm of chromosome 22 (22q12) and encodes a tumor suppressor protein named merlin. This protein may act as a membrane-associated molecular switch that regulates cell–cell and cell–matrix signals transduced by cell surface receptors.

CLINICAL FEATURES

- Neurilemmomas are solitary, smooth-surfaced dermal or subcutaneous tumors that appear on the head, neck, or extremities.

DIAGNOSIS AND DIFFERENTIAL

- The diagnosis is microscopic. The tumors are encapsulated, showing a biphasic pattern, consisting of hypercellular (Antoni A) and hypocellular (Antoni B) areas. A highly characteristic feature are the Verocay bodies that consist of a parallel arrangement of the nuclei in two rows, enclosing homogeneous collagen between them.

TREATMENT

- Surgical excision.

NASAL GLIOMA

PATHOPHYSIOLOGY

- Nasal glioma represents an intrauterine herniation of the brain tissue.

CLINICAL FEATURES

- Nasal glioma is present at birth as a firm 2 to 3-cm nodule located near the root of the nose. The nodule is smooth with a red-purple coloration.

DIAGNOSIS AND DIFFERENTIAL

- The typical location and its clinical appearance should suggest the diagnosis, although may simulate a congenital hemangioma.

TREATMENT

- Surgical intervention should always be preceded by a radiologic and neurosurgical consultation.

GRANULAR CELL TUMOR

PATHOPHYSIOLOGY

- The tumoral cells of the granular cell tumor are considered a variant of Schwann cells, and the characteristic cytoplasmic granules are lysosomes.

CLINICAL FEATURES

- Granular cell tumor is a solitary and small lesion (under 2 cm in diameter), mainly located on the head and neck areas. Thirty percent of these tumors are confined to the tongue.
- Tumor recurrences and malignant granular cell tumors with metastatic potential is a very uncommon event (3% of the cases).

DIAGNOSIS AND DIFFERENTIAL

- The diagnosis is made microscopically. Neoplastic cells show abundant, pale-staining cytoplasm filled with eosinophilic granules that are S100 positive.

TREATMENT

- Surgical excision.

REFERENCES

Gutmann DH. The neurofibromatosis: when less is more. *Hum Mol Genet.* 2001;10:747.
Riccardi M. Neurofibromatosis: Past, present, and future. *N Eng J Med.* 1991;324:1283.

22 HAIR AND NAILS

Francisco Jimenez-Acosta
Martin N. Zaiac

- Hair follicles vary considerably in size and shape depending on their location, but they all have the same basic structure. Roughly 5 million hair follicles cover the human body at birth. After birth, no additional follicles form, although the size of the follicles and hairs can change with time, primarily under the influence of androgens. Hair is composed of keratin proteins, which form the hair shaft. Three types of hair are recognized. Lanugo is the prenatal hair that is fine, soft and silky. Vellus hair replaces lanugo hair in post-natal life. It is spread over the body surface. It is soft, unmedullated and rarely exceeds 2 cm in length. Terminal hair is longer, coarser, medullated, and pigmented. Before puberty, terminal hairs are limited to the scalp, eyebrows, and eyelashes. After puberty, secondary sexual terminal hair develops from vellus hair in response to androgens.

- The precise spacing and distribution of the follicles are established by genes. The genes are expressed very early in the morphogenesis of the follicles. Under appropriate magnification, an observer will see that the majority of human hair shafts emerge from the scalp in 2- and 3-hair groupings. These groupings are the visible superficial portion of a distinctive histologic structure, known as the follicular unit. Follicular units are composed of approximately two to four terminal hairs and their associated sebaceous glands and arrector pili muscles, surrounded by a circumferential band of adventitial collagen. Although there is considerable racial variation, the follicular unit density on the scalp ranges between 65 and 100 follicular units per cm^2. The absolute number of follicular units per given area remains relatively constant, and it is the proportion of natural hair groupings that determines the patient's hair density.

- Hair follicle cycling: Each hair follicle perpetually goes through consecutive cyclical periods of growth (anagen), involution (catagen), rest (telogen), and shedding (exogen). The follicle, although it is largely epithelial in origin, contains at its base a ball of specialized dermal cells, the dermal papilla, which play a crucial part in the regulation of successive cycles of hair growth. At the onset of the growth phase, signals from the dermal papilla are thought to instruct epithelial stem cells residing in the bulge region of the follicle to divide transiently. The bulge is a portion of the outer root sheath of the hair follicle located at the region of the insertion of the arrector pili muscle. At the end of anagen phase, hair growth ceases, and the catagen phase begins. During catagen phase, hair follicles go through a process of involution that largely reflects a burst of programmed cell death (apoptosis) in the majority of follicular keratinocytes. Toward the end of the catagen stage, the dermal papilla condenses and moves upward, coming to rest underneath the hair follicle bulge. During the telogen stage, the hair shaft matures into a club hair, a fully keratinized dead hair that is eventually shed from the follicle, usually during combing or washing. Most people lose 50 to 150 club scalp hairs per day.

- Hair follicles in different areas of the body produce hairs of different length, with the length proportional to the duration of the anagen cycle. For example, scalp hair follicles stay in the anagen stage for 2 to 8 years and produce long hairs. Eyebrow hair follicles do so for only 2 to 3 months and produce short hairs. On average, 90% of scalp hairs are in the anagen phase at any one time, 1% will be in catagen, and 5 to 15% in telogen. The catagen phase lasts several weeks. The telogen stage lasts for 2 to 3 months before the scalp follicles reenter the anagen stage and the cycle is repeated.

- Alopecia, a generic term for hair loss, results from a diminution of visible hair. The most common forms of alopecia are androgenetic alopecia, telogen effluvium, alopecia areata, and chemotherapy-induced alopecia.

- Some types of inflammatory alopecias (such as those caused by lichen planopilaris and discoid lupus erythematosus) are scarring and permanent. Other types (such as alopecia areata) are nonscarring and reversible. In scarring alopecias, the inflammation usually involves the superficial and mid-portion of the follicle, including the bulge area, suggesting that the stem cells necessary for the regeneration of the follicle are damaged irreversibly.

REFERENCES

Bernstein RM, Rassman WR, Szaniawski W, Halperin AJ. Follicular transplantation. *Int J Aesth Rest Surg.* 1995;3:119.

Headington JT. Transverse microscopy anatomy of human scalp. *Arch Dermatol.* 1984;120:449.

Jimenez F, Ruifernández JM. Distribution of human hair follicular units. *Dermatol Surg.* 1999;25:294.

Lyle S, Christofidou-Solomidou M, Liu Y, Elder DE, Albelda S, Cotsarelis G. The C8/144B monoclonal antibody recognizes cytokeratin 15 and defines the location of human hair follicle stem cells. *J Cell Sci.* 1998;111:3179.

Millar SE. Molecular mechanisms regulating hair follicle development. *J Invest Dermatol.* 2002;118:216.

Stenn KS, Paus R. Controls of hair follicle cycling. *Physiol Rev.* 2001;81:449.

ANDROGENETIC ALOPECIA

- Androgenetic alopecia (AGA), or common baldness, is the most common form of human hair loss. It is characterized by the progressive thinning of scalp hair in genetically susceptible individuals.

EPIDEMIOLOGY

- In general, more than 50% of men by the age of 50 years, and 50% of women by the age of 60 years have AGA. The proportion of men with moderate to extensive male pattern alopecia increases with increasing age, ranging from 16% for men 18 to 29 years of age to 53% of men 40 to 49 years of age. Female pattern alopecia is also quite common, reaching almost 30% in women over 30 years of age. There are racial differences in the prevalence of male pattern hair loss; for example, Caucasian men are four times more likely to develop premature balding than black men.

PATHOPHYSIOLOGY

- AGA is characterized by a stepwise miniaturization of hair follicles and a progressive shortening of the anagen phase with an increase in the telogen/anagen ratio. Miniaturization results in the conversion of large (terminal) hairs into small barely visible depigmented (vellus) hairs. The miniaturization involves a progressive reduction in the size of the follicle, dermal papilla, and hair shaft with each successive cycle. Nonetheless, hair follicles are still present and cycling, even in bald scalps. On the other hand, as telogen hairs are more easily plucked than anagen hairs, the increased telogen count explains the increased hair shedding commonly noticed during washing and combing the hair.

- Androgens (testosterone) and a genetic predisposition are required for AGA to develop in men. A balding scalp is characterized by increased concentrations of dihydrotestosterone (DHT), the most active metabolite of testosterone, as well as an increased expression of the androgen receptor. Moreover, men with a genetic deficiency of type II 5α-reductase, the enzyme that converts testosterone to DHT, do not experience male pattern hair loss. Paradoxically, the influence of androgens on hair is site specific. Prepubertal pubic, axillary, and beard vellus hair react to androgens by growing into terminal hairs. The same androgens miniaturize the pigmented terminal hairs on the scalp. There is no explanation for these different effects.

- In women, however, there is no consensus on whether hair loss is truly androgen dependent. Differences in local sex steroid metabolism have been found between women and men with AGA that could explain the different clinical presentation of AGA in men and women. For example, the content of 5α reductase in the frontal hair follicles is threefold less than in the frontal hair follicles of men with AGA. However, other reports indicate that AGA in women may occur even in the absence of androgens. Based on this evidence, it seems appropriate to replace the term androgenetic alopecia in women by the term female pattern hair loss.

- The mode of inheritance of the genetic predisposition of AGA remains controversial. It appears that it is determined by a number of genes in a polygenic fashion. An association between the androgen receptor gene and male pattern baldness has been described recently.

CLINICAL FEATURES

- Androgenetic alopecia in men (male pattern hair loss) is a focal hair loss process, with alopecia largely limited to the top of the scalp with typical frontotemporal recessions. The patterns of hair loss in men with AGA have been described by Hamilton and Norwood. The onset of AGA is usually gradual and the condition slowly develops over the years. The hairs become smaller in diameter (vellus type), are shorter, and in a given area, less density can be observed and quantified. The age of onset of male pattern hair loss in men is primarily puberty through the fourth decade, with variation both in the rapidity and the final degree of hair loss. Rarely, some men develop androgenetic alopecia with a typical female pattern of hair loss.

- AGA in women may present as two patterns: a female pattern consisting of a progressive loss of hair density in a uniform pattern over the top of the scalp with preservation of the frontal hairline (Ludwig pattern), and a pattern similar to male pattern baldness with bitemporal recessions. The vast majority of women with AGA present with the female pattern, beginning in the late 20s and peaking after 50 years of age.
- In many patients, AGA is experienced as a stressful condition that diminishes body image satisfaction. Deleterious effects on self-esteem are more apparent among women than men.

DIAGNOSIS AND DIFFERENTIAL

- The pattern of hair loss in men with AGA is characteristic and the diagnosis is relatively straightforward, whereas in women, the pattern of hair loss, especially in the early stages, can be mimicked by several other conditions such as chronic telogen effluvium, drug-induced hair loss, iron deficiency, or thyroid disease (Table 22–1).
- Patients with AGA usually have a positive family history for the disease. The hair pull test consists of gently grasping a group of 25 to 50 hairs and pulling to the ends of the hair with gentle constant traction. The hair pull in active telogen effluvium shows a marked increase in telogen hairs in multiple areas of the scalp, whereas the pull test in AGA may show a mild increase in telogen hairs only in involved areas, that is, the top of the scalp.
- Laboratory tests are generally unnecessary in men with AGA. Women with bitemporal recessions, as seen in male pattern baldness, must be questioned about the regularity of their menses and the presence of hirsutism to rule out hyperandrogenism. On the other hand, women with AGA in a Ludwig pattern usually do not show abnormalities in circulating androgens, but should be checked for iron deficiency (serum iron and serum ferritin) and thyroid function

TABLE 22–1   Diffuse Hair Loss: Differential Diagnosis

Acute telogen effluvium
Chronic telogen effluvium
Drug-induced hair loss (including chemotherapy)
Early androgenetic alopecia
Diffuse alopecia areata
Iron deficiency
Starvation, malabsortion, crash diet
Hypothyroidism and hyperthyroidism
Acute lupus erythematosus
Syphilis

tests (TSH and free T_4), to rule out other causes of diffuse hair loss.

TREATMENT

- Currently, medical treatments can slow or halt the progression of hair loss, with improvement in some cases. For early male pattern baldness, finasteride, a highly specific inhibitor of the type II 5α-reductase enzyme, is the treatment of choice. It is taken at a dosage of 1 mg/day orally and continuous administration is necessary to maintain the benefits. After 2 years of treatment, 83% of patients show unchanged or increased hair counts from baseline, compared to 28% of those on placebo. Not all patients, however, respond to finasteride; at 12 months, 14% of treated individuals have an absolute reduction in hair numbers, compared with 58% of untreated men. Some patients on finasteride report reversible adverse effects on sexual function (decreased libido). Finasteride is contraindicated in women who are or may become pregnant.
- Minoxidil (2 to 5% solution), 1 mL twice daily, is also used in AGA but the results are more disappointing than finasteride. Minoxidil is a potent antihypertensive drug, due to its vasodilatory effect. However, the mechanism of action on hair growth is not known, but is probably related to its properties as a potassium channel agonist. Topical minoxidil increases the duration of the anagen phase, leading to production of hairs that are progressively thicker and longer.
- For female pattern hair loss, the most effective approach is the combination of an oral antiandrogen therapy with 5% minoxidil solution. The antiandrogen therapy uses an oral estrogen (oral contraceptive) in combination with the antiandrogenic progestin, cyproterone acetate. Dosage of cyproterone acetate is 50 to 100 mg/day administered in the first 10 days of the menstrual cycle. As an alternative, spironolactone (100 to 200 mg/day) or flutamide can be used. Finasteride has not been formally evaluated in premenopausal women because of its teratogenic potential.
- Hair transplantation is a very effective treatment to cover balding areas. It is especially useful in moderate and advanced cases of androgenetica alopecia. The basis of hair transplantation is the tendency of hair-bearing autografts to maintain those characteristics of the donor site (donor dominance). Hair grafts are excised from the occipital donor scalp and inserted into the receptor balding area. It is estimated that the survival rate of these grafts is around 90 to 100%. Recent techniques using small grafts (follicular units)

achieve very impressive, natural, and undetectable results.

REFERENCES

Cash TF. The psychosocial consequences of androgenetic alopecia: A review of the research literature. *Br J Dermatol.* 1999;141:398.

Ellis JA, Stebbing M, Harrap SB. Polymorphism of the androgen receptor gene is associated with male pattern baldness. *J Invest Dermatol.* 2001;116:452.

Kaufman KD, Olsen EA, Whiting D, et al. Finasteride in the treatment of men with androgenetic alopecia. *J Am Acad Dermatol.* 1998;39:578.

Limmer BL. Elliptical donor stereoscopically assisted micrografting as an approach to further refinement in hair transplantation. *J Dermatol Surg Oncol.* 1994;20:789.

Norwood OT. Incidence of female androgenetic alopecia (female pattern alopecia). *Derm Surg.* 2001;27:53.

Olsen E. The diagnosis of androgenetic alopecia. *Dermatol Therapy.* 1998;8:18.

Rhodes T, Girman CJ, Savin RC et al. Prevalence of male pattern hair loss in 18–49 year old men. *Derm Surg.* 1998;24:1330.

Sawaya ME, Price VH. Different levels of 5α reductase type I and II, aromatase and androgen receptor in hair follicles of women and men with androgenetic alopecia. *J Invest Dermatol.* 1997;109:296.

Sinclair RD, Dawber RPR. Androgenetic alopecia in men and women. *Clin Dermatol.* 2001;19:167.

TELOGEN EFFLUVIUM

EPIDEMIOLOGY

- Telogen effluvium (TE) is a self-limiting diffuse hair loss that occurs around 3 months after a triggering event. An acute and chronic form can be differentiated. By definition, acute TE resolves within 3 to 6 months. When the hair shedding continues beyond 6 months, it is called chronic TE.
- Acute TE is a common cause of diffuse hair loss. Numerous potential triggers have been implicated including severe febrile illness, pregnancy, chronic systemic illness, a change in medication, a crash diet, accidental trauma, surgical operations, and emotional stress. Pregnancy is probable the most common cause. It is estimated that TE occurs in a third to a half of all pregnant women following childbirth.
- Chronic TE has been related to stress and to nutritional imbalance involving iron and the essential amino acid L-lysine.

PATHOPHYSIOLOGY

- Telogen effluvium results from the sudden synchronous entry of many anagen follicles into telogen and then exogen (the shedding) phase.

CLINICAL FEATURES

- Acute TE manifests as an excessive and diffuse shedding of hair that occurs 2 to 3 months after a triggering event. Often, patients do not relate these events and become anxious that they are going to go bald. Acute TE usually lasts 2 to 6 months and is followed by complete recovery.
- Chronic TE is a common cause of hair loss in middle-aged women. It predominantly affects women between 30 to 50 years of age. Patients report persistent and severe shedding of hair that tends to run a fluctuating course for several years. They often report thinning and recession of hair in the temples that may fluctuate in intensity. However, on examination, these patients do not have noticeable thinning and usually have a full, thick head of hair.

DIAGNOSIS AND DIFFERENTIAL

- A detailed clinical history may identify a triggering event in acute TE.
- The hair pull test is strongly positive (numerous telogen hairs are extracted with ease) in acute TE and less marked in the chronic form. In acute TE the trichogram from a hair pluck sample shows that more than 25% are telogen hairs.
- A full blood count, iron studies, and thyroid function tests should be performed. Patients with chronic TE usually have depleted iron stores (as assessed by serum ferritin).
- The differential diagnosis of chronic TE with early androgenetic alopecia in women may be very difficult. As the prognosis and treatment of these two conditions are different, these women may benefit from having a scalp biopsy before starting on long-term antiandrogen therapy for androgenetic alopecia.

TREATMENT

- Reassuring patients with acute TE that the increased shedding is temporary and the hair will regrow is sufficient. In severe cases, however, some patients require a wig while awaiting regrowth.

- In the majority of patients with chronic TE, the hair shedding eventually stabilizes and the patient retains a cosmetically acceptable amount of hair.
- In patients with nutritionally induced hair loss, either a change in dietary habits or taking the appropriate supplement will correct this widespread problem.

REFERENCES

Rushton DH, Norrris MJ, Dover R, Busuttil N. Causes of hair loss and the developments in hair rejuvenation. *Int J Cosm Sci.* 2002;24:17.

Whiting DA. Chronic telogen effluvium: Increased scalp hair shedding in middle-aged women. *J Am Acad Dermatol.* 1996;35:899.

Chemotherapy-Induced Alopecia

PATHOPHYSIOLOGY

- Chemotherapy disrupts the proliferation of matrix keratinocytes in the anagen bulb that produces the hair shaft. This forces anagen follicles to enter a dystrophic catagen stage in which the integrity of the hair shaft is compromised and the hair then breaks and falls out.

CLINICAL FEATURES

- Because more than 90% of scalp follicles are in anagen at any one time, these hairs are rapidly lost after chemotherapy. The hair loss is rapid and extensive (anagen effluvium). However, hair does eventually regrow, presumably because the cycling follicular stem cells are relatively unaffected by chemotherapy and generate a new hair follicle and hair shaft.

TREATMENT

- The most widely applied method to prevent chemotherapy-induced alopecia is the cooling of the scalp by a variety of techniques ranging from ice packs applied to the entire scalp to more sophisticated methods that use cryogel caps, caps connected to a cooling device, or cold air. These methods are based on the rationale that by cooling the scalp, vasoconstriction is

produced, thus reducing the amount of the drug delivered to the hair follicle.
- Davis and collaborators showed that the inhibition of the cell cycle regulator cyclin-dependent kinase 2 (CDK2) using a novel, topically applied CDK2 inhibitor prevents chemotherapy induced alopecia in rats.

REFERENCES

Davis ST, Benson BG, Bramson N, et al. Prevention of chemotherapy-induced alopecia in rats by CDK inhibitors. *Science.* 2001;291:134.

Katsimbri P, Bamias A, Pavlidis N. Prevention of chemotherapy induced alopecia using an effective scalp cooling system. *Eur J Cancer.* 2000;36:766.

Alopecia Areata

EPIDEMIOLOGY

- Alopecia areata (AA) presents with patchy hair loss. It is more common than originally supposed and the lifetime risk of developing AA is 1.7%. It affects both genders and can occur at any age, but the peak incidence appears to be between 15 and 29 years.
- There is a positive family history in 10 to 20% of affected individuals.

PATHOPHYSIOLOGY

- Alopecia areata is an autoimmune disorder in which cells of the anagen hair bulb are attacked by lymphocytes. As a result, the growth of the hair is impaired and the shaft is subsequently narrowed and tends to break off at the skin surface. It is a T-cell-mediated disease. Possible targets of the immune attack include matrix keratinocytes, dermal papilla cells, and melanocytes. The hair loss is potentially reversible because the inflammatory process spares the stem-cell rich bulge area.

CLINICAL FEATURES

- Alopecia areata can affect any hair-bearing area, but the scalp is more commonly affected. The characteristic initial lesion is a circumscribed, totally bald, smooth patch. Often, it is noticed by chance by a friend or hairdresser. The presence of broken, short hairs that taper proximally (exclamation point hairs) within the plaque is a characteristic sign. A positive pull test at the margins of the patch indicates active disease.

- The course of the disease is varied. The intial patch may regrow within a few months, or further patches may appear after an interval of several weeks. Alopecia areata involving more than 40% scalp hair is seen in 11% of patients, while alopecia totalis (100% loss of scalp hair) or alopecia universalis (100% loss of body hair) occurs in about 7% of patients. Patients with alopecia totalis/universalis usually have a poorer prognosis, especially if it is a long-standing condition.
- Nail dystrophy (pitting, Beau's lines, etc.), as well as several autoimmune diseases, such as atopy, thyroid disease, and vitiligo, have been associated with AA. The presence of atopy and onset at a young age are associated with more extensive forms.

DIFFERENTIAL DIAGNOSIS

- The diagnosis of AA is made on clinical grounds. Other causes of patchy alopecia that may be confused with AA include tinea capitis, trichotillomania, and scarring alopecia.

TREATMENT

- Knowing the fact that AA is a benign and usually self-limited condition allows some patients to decide not to attempt treatment and let nature run its course. Fifty percent of patients will regrow their hair entirely within 1 year with or without treatment. The initial regrowth is often white hair, followed by repigmentation.
- The most commonly used treatments are corticosteroids, minoxidil 5% solution, anthralin cream, and topical immunotherapeutic agents.
- For adults with less than 50% scalp involvement, the first option is intralesional corticosteroid, followed by minoxidil solution and anthralin cream. For adults with more than 50% scalp involvement, topical immunotherapy and phototherapy with PUVA are added options. For patients less than 10 years of age, the options are corticoisteroid creams, minoxidil, and anthralin.
- Intralesional triamcinolone (2.5 to 5 mg/mL once a month) is the treatment of choice for localized patches. Less than 0.1 mL is injected intradermally per site and injections are spread out to cover the affected areas for a maximum volume of 2 to 3 cc. The use of systemic steroids is controversial, and

should be limited to halt the progression of active extensive AA.

- Topical immunotherapy consists of the induction of an allergic contact dermatitis by topical application of potent contact allergens. Commonly used are diphencyprone and squaric acid dibutylester. Treatment with diphencyprone is done once a week. The patient is first sensitized directly on the scalp with a 2% concentration on a small area (2×2 cm^2). The following week, the lowest concentration (0.0001%) is applied. Then, the concentration is increased slowly every week as needed until a mild, tolerable allergic contact dermatitis is elicited. Initial regrowth should not be expected before 12 weeks of treatment. The success rate is about 30 to 50%.

REFERENCES

Bolduc Ch, Shapiro J. The treatment of alopecia areata. *Dermatol Therapy.* 2001;14:306

Shapiro J, Madani S. Alopecia areata: Diagnosis and management. *Int J Dermatol.* 1999;38(suppl 1):19.

SCARRING ALOPECIAS

EPIDEMIOLOGY

- Scarring, or cicatricial, alopecia is the result of the destruction and fibrosis of hair follicles. Scarring alopecia is divided into primary and secondary types. In the primary type, the hair itself is the principal target for destruction. In secondary scarring alopecia, the follicle is an "innocent bystander" and is destroyed in a nonspecific manner. Causes (Table 22–2) of primary scarring alopecia include discoid lupus, lichen planopilaris, frontal fibrosing alopecia, dissecting

TABLE 22–2   Scarring Alopecias: Differential Diagnosis

Lichen planopilaris
Discoid lupus erythematosus
Central centrifugal scarring alopecia
    Folliculitis decalvans
    Tufted folliculitis
    Follicular degeneration syndrome
    Acne keloidales
Dissecting cellulites
Frontal fibrosing alopecia[a]
Unclassified type (pseudopelade)

[a]Frontal Fibrosing Alopecia may be a variant of Lichen Planopilaris. Modified from Sperling LC, Solomon AR, Whiting DA. *Arch Dermatol.* 2000;136:235.

cellulitis, acne keloidalis, central centrifugal scarring alopecia, and pseudopelade. Examples of secondary scarring alopecia include cutaneous sarcoid, morphea, scleroderma "en coup de sabre," necrobiosis lipoidica, lupus vulgaris, and a host of other destructive cutaneous diseases. In addition to the primary and secondary forms of scarring alopecia, certain nonscarring hair diseases demonstrate a biphasic pattern, in which nonscarring hair loss is seen early in the course of the disease, but after many years of continuous active disease, permanent dropout of follicles occurs. Examples of this phenomenon include androgenetic alopecia, alopecia areata, and traction alopecia.

- The most common form of primary scarring alopecia diagnosed in clinical practice (32.4% of cases) is pseudopelade. Pseudopelade is a broad term that encompasses a range of idiopathic, noninflammatory, irregular, scarring alopecias. Its existence as an individual clinical entity is doubted by many because many different entities causing scarring alopecia gradually burn out and become indistinguishable from pseudopelade. For instance, some patients originally diagnosed as having pseudopelade are later reclassified as having lichen planopilaris or discoid lupus.

PATHOPHYSIOLOGY

- In scarring alopecias, the inflammation occurs high up in the follicle, involving the stem-cell rich bulge area. The resultant destruction of this area inactivates further follicular cycling and leads to a permanent loss of the follicle.
- Recently, it has been suggested that the primary pathology of many obscure scarring alopecias may be an aberrant functioning of the sebaceous gland, which appears necessary for normal detachment of the inner root sheath from the hair shaft, causing follicle rupture followed by a fibrotic healing process.

CLINICAL FEATURES

- Cicatricial alopecia presents as areas of hair loss in which the underlying scalp is scarred, sclerosed, or atrophic. It is usually circumscribed but may be widespread. A large list of entities can present as a scarring alopecia. In early stages, the underlying disease is usually diagnosable, but in late stages, only scarring may be evident.
- Pseudopelade of Brocq occurs mainly in young to middle-aged women. The patient discovers discrete asymptomatic areas of alopecia. The patches are smooth, soft, and slightly depressed, without any evidence of folliculitis. They tend to be round or oval, and may coalesce to form irregular bald patches.
- Classical lichen planopilaris usually affects adult women. Hyperkeratotic follicular papules with perifollicular erythema are the hallmarks of this conditions. It produces atrophic polygon-shaped patches of alopecia with the activity at the margins of the lesions and a lack of clinical reactivity in the center. A significant number of cases occur with lesions of cutaneous lichen planus. Graham–Little syndrome describes the combination of lichen planopilaris with a keratosis pilaris-like appearance of patchy areas of alopecia on eyebrows, axillary, and pubic areas.
- Chronic cutaneous discoid lupus erythematosus can cause cicatricial alopecia. Initial lesions are often itchy and sensitive. Typical lesions show follicular plugging, erythema, and dyspigmentation. Subcutaneous and acute systemic lupus may be a cause of diffuse hair loss, but rarely cause scarring.
- Frontal fibrosing alopecia is a recently described entity that occurs more frequently in postmenopausal women. The clinical appearance is very distinctive. The patient experiences a progressive recession of the frontal and temporal hairlines in a symmetric pattern. In some patients, the condition affects the occipital hair. Most patients also report alopecia of the eyebrows. This disease is much more common than described in the literature, and many women are probably misdiagnosed as androgenetic alopecia. Based on histologic similarities, some investigators believe that frontal fibrosing alopecia is a localized variant of lichen planopilaris.
- Central centrifugal scarring alopecia (CCSA) is a recently described term that encompasses a group of diseases that share a similar clinical pattern of hair loss: (1) hair loss centered on the crown or vertex; (2) chronic and progressive disease; (3) symmetrical expansion with the most active disease at the periphery; and (4) both clinical and histologic evidence of inflammation in the active peripheral zone. Clinical subsets of CCSA include the follicular degeneration syndrome, folliculitis decalvans, and tufted folliculitis. Folliculitis decalvans is characterized by crops of pustules that surround multiple, slowly expanding round or oval areas of alopecia on the scalp. The lesions may coalesce into a large central area of scarring alopecia. Episodes of folliculitis can occur for years. Tufted folliculitis presents as circumscribed inflamed areas of scalp with alopecia and residual tufted hairs. Each tuft consists of 10 to 15 hairs converging toward a single orifice in the epidermis. Tufted folliculitis can be found as an end stage in

several forms of scarring alopecia. The tufting occurs because the infundibular epithelia of damaged follicles heal with the formation of a large common infundibulum.

- Dissecting cellulitis (perifolliculitis capitis abscedens and suffodiens) presents as multiple, indurated, scalp inflammatory nodules that eventually break through the skin with purulent drainage. The disease can wax and wane for many years, but eventually it will result in fibrosis, sinus tract formation, hypertrophic scarring, and permanent hair loss. The disease may occur alone or in conjunction with hidradenitis suppurativa and acne conglobata, forming the "follicular occlusion triad."

DIAGNOSIS AND DIFFERENTIAL

- A patient with scarring alopecia should be clinically and histologically evaluated to classify the condition under a specific entity. However, clinical and histologic features may overlap, and the greater the overlap, the greater the diagnostic difficulty.
- The ideal biopsy specimen for evaluation of a scarring alopecia is two 4-mm punch biopsies, one sectioned horizontally to allow hair counts, and the other vertically. The biopsies should be done from actively inflamed areas as early as possible to establish the diagnosis. The horizontal or transverse sectioning allows an examination of most of the follicles contained in the biopsy. However, the interpretation of a horizontal biopsy is difficult, requiring considerable experience with the microscopic anatomy of horizontal sections.
- Bacterial and fungal infections should be excluded in all cases. The biopsy may show the typical histologic changes of discoid lupus and lichen planopilaris. If direct immunofluorescence demonstrates deposition of immunoreactants at the dermoepidermal junction, the diagnosis of discoid lupus is further supported.

TREATMENT

- Early diagnosis is necessary to initiate treatment before irreversible scarring takes place.
- Intralesional triamcinolone (10 mg/mL) repeated every 4 weeks is the treatment of choice for active plaques of discoid lupus and lichen planopilaris. Other agents that can be tried include topical and oral corticosteroids, antimalarials, retinoids (isotretinoin, acitretin), and immunosuppressive drugs.
- Topical antibiotics, such as mupirocin, as well as a long-term dosage of oral antibiotics, especially rifampin and sulfamethoxazole/trimethoprim, can be used in active cases of neutrophilic scarring alopecias, such as folliculitis decalvans, dissecting cellulitis, and tufted folliculitis.
- No effective treatment is known for frontal fribrosing alopecia, and some patients end up wearing a hair piece.
- Surgical treatment: only nonactive, stable patches can be treated surgically. Small scarring patches can be excised. In the setting of multiple or stable larger plaques, a hair transplant surgeon should evaluate the possibility of hair transplantation and/or tissue expansion followed by excision.

REFERENCES

Cotsarelis G, Miller SE. Towards a molecular understanding of hair loss and its treatment. *Trends Mol Med*. 2001;7:293.

Headington JT. Transverse microscopic anatomy of the human scalp: A basis for morphometric approach to disorders of the hair follicle. *Arch Dermatol*. 1984;120:449.

Kossard S, Lee MS, Wilkinson B. Postmenopausal frontal fibrosing alopecia: A frontal variant of lichen planopilaris. *J Am Acad Dermatol*. 1997;36:59.

Sperling LC. Scarring alopecia and the dermatopathologist. *J Cut Pathol*. 2001;28:333.

Sperling LC, Solomon AR, Whiting DA. A new look at scarring alopecia. *Arch Dermatol*. 2000;136:235.

Stenn KS. Insights from the *Asebia* mouse: A molecular sebaceous gland defect leading to cicatricial alopecia. *J Cutan Pathol*. 2001;28:445.

Whiting DA. Cicatricial alopecia: Clinico-pathological findings and treatment. *Clin Dermatol*. 2001;19:211.

HIRSUTISM

EPIDEMIOLOGY

- Hirsutism is defined as the growth of terminal hairs in females in a male-like pattern. Hypertrichosis is defined as a uniform excess hair growth over the body, but the hair shafts tend to be fine and uniform. Hypertrichosis is most commonly familial or caused by metabolic disorders or medications (Table 22–3).
- The prevalence of hirsutism is difficult to assess. The perception of hirsutism is subjective, and significant racial and ethnic differences in normal hair growth patterns exist. The scoring system used to determine the degree of hirsutism is the Ferriman–Gallwey scale. Based on this scale, approximately 5 to 10% of women suffer from hirsutism.

TABLE 22–3 Causes of Hypertrichosis

Familiar
    Metabolic disorders
    Thyroid diseases
    Anorexia nerviosa
    Porphyria
Medications
    Phenytoin
    Minoxidil
    Cyclosporine
Malignancies

PATHOPHYSIOLOGY

- Hirsutism is usually a sign of endocrine disorders characterized by hyperandrogenemia. Increased androgen levels can be originated in adrenal glands (androgen-producing tumors, congenital adrenal hyperplasia), pituitary gland (Cushing's disease, acromegaly, hyperprolactinemia), or ovary (polycystic ovary syndrome, ovarian tumors).
- The most common hormonal cause of hirsutism is polycystic ovary syndrome (PCOS), affecting 1 to 4% of the female population of reproductive age.
- A partial deficiency of the enzyme 21β hydroxylase leads to a late onset congenital adrenal hyperplasia that presents with postpubertal hirsutes (3 to 6% of women presenting with hirsutism).
- A proportion of hirsute women (approximately 20%) are classified under idiopathic hirsutism, a term that should be applied only to patients with normal ovulatory function and no detectable hormonal abnormality. The pathophysiology of idiopathic hirsutism is presumed to be a primary increase in skin 5α-reductase activity, and possibly an alteration in androgen receptor function.

CLINICAL FEATURES

- Seborrhea, acne, and alopecia, all manifestations of androgen excess, may exist singly or in combination in different women with hirsutism (the SAHA syndrome). Although all four signs of SAHA syndrome are only present in approximately 20% of the patients, knowledge of it is important for recognizing hormonal disorders involving androgen metabolism.
- Polycystic ovary syndrome (PCOS) has a wide spectrum of clinical features. The classic clinical presentation is a woman with oligomenorrhea or amenorrhea with symptoms of hyperandrogenism (hirsutism, acne, or alopecia). However, the advent of high-resolution pelvic ultrasonography has allowed the detection of polycystic ovaries in women with mild to moderate hirsutism and normal menses. Some

young women also display a particular metabolic pattern including an atherogenic lipid profile, glucose intolerance, and an increased fasting insulin level, which is known to be closely linked with an insulin-resistant state. These patients are usually obese, can develop acanthosis nigricans, and are at risk of developing type 2 diabetes mellitus and cardiovascular disease.
- Androgen-secreting tumors are very rare, and the best clue to their existence is the recent onset of anovulation, a rapidly progressive hirsutism outside of the peripubertal period, and elevated free testosterone levels above 200 ng/dL.

DIAGNOSIS AND DIFFERENTIAL

- No single test is diagnostic of PCOS. Biochemical markers include a raised LH and normal FSH (quite specific but not very sensitive), and normal or a mild elevation of free testosterone (not greater than 200 ng/dL), and possibly dehydroepiandrosterone sulfate (DHEAS). Hyperinsulinemia (fasting insulin) is observed in more than half of the PCOS patients. Pelvic ultrasonography will define the polycystic ovarian morphology, but the presence of polycystic ovaries does not necessarily mean that the patient has PCOS.
- By definition, patients with idiopathic hirsutism have normal circulating androgens, and a normal ovulatory function, verified by either daily basal body temperature charting and/or a luteal phase (day 20 to 24 of the menstrual cycle) progesterone level. It should be remembered that a history of regular menses is not sufficient to exclude ovulatory dysfunction, since up to 40% of eumenorrheic hirsute women are anovulatory.
- In addition, serum 17-hydroxyprogesterone level should be measured to exclude 21-hydroxylase-deficient congenital adrenal hyperplasia. Menstrual cycles in these patients may be normal, and differentiation depends on endocrine studies.

TREATMENT

- Although hirsutism is more a cosmetic problem than a disease, the presence of hirsutism is extremely distressing to patients, with a significant negative impact on their psychosocial development. The current approach in the treatment of hirsutism is the combination of laser hair removal along with judicious use of medications.
- Patients with hirsutism respond, at least partially, to antiandrogen or 5α-reductase inhibitor therapy

TABLE 22–4 Hormonal Treatment of Hirsutism

Andogen suppression
  Oral contraceptive pills
  GnTR agonists
  Ketoconazole
  Glucocorticoids

Antiandrogens
  Cyproterone acetate
  Spironolactone
  Flutamide

5α-reductase inhibitors
  Finasteride

Insulin-lowering agents
  Metformin
  Thiazolidinediones
  D-Chiro-inositol

(Table 22–4). Typically, 9 to 12 months of treatment are needed to judge the efficacy of a given treatment on hair growth. Oral contraceptive pills (combination estrogen-progestin therapy) reduce hirsutism by decreasing circulating androgen levels through suppression of circulating LH and stimulation of sex hormone binding globulin (SHBG). Androgen receptor blockers include spironolactone, flutamide, and cyproterone acetate. Their efficacy in hirsutism is very similar. Spironolactone is used at a daily dosage of 100 mg/day, and side effects include menstrual irregularity, dyspepsia, and breast tenderness. Patients should be monitored for hyperkalemia, hypotension, and liver dysfunction. Flutamide is used at a dose of 125 to 250 mg twice daily, and monitoring serum markers of hepatic functions at regular intervals is recommended due to the possibility of hepatotoxicity. Cyproterone acetate is used at a dose of 50 to 100 mg /day from the 5th to 15th day of the menstrual cycle, and combined with an oral contraceptive pill. Side effects include irregular uterine bleeding, headache, weight gain, and decreased libido. Finasteride, a 5α-reductase inhibitor, can be used for treating women with hirsutism at a dose of 5 mg/day. All agents must be used with adequate contraception in women to prevent the possibility of genital ambiguity in a male fetus.

• There is considerable interest in the possible role of insulin-lowering agents in the therapy of hyperandrogenism. It has been demonstrated that caloric restriction in obese women with PCOS will improve hirsutism and the chances of ovulation, as well as reduces the risk of diabetes mellitus. Other medications used to lower insulin levels in PCOS include metformin, thiazolidinediones, and D-chiro-inositol.

• Glucocorticoid therapy (prednisone in doses of 5 to 10 mg/day) can be helpful in women with hyperandrogenism from an adrenal source, such as in congenital adrenal hyperplasia.

• Mechanical means of removing unwanted hairs should be always considered in combination to medical management of the hirsute patient. Various options are available including shaving, waxing, plucking, electrology, and laser depilation. Currently, laser therapy is the most effective method to achieve long-term and even permanent hair removal. Unfortunately, not all commercially available lasers achieve the same results. The 800-nm diode laser, the long-pulsed alexandrite laser, the long-pulsed ruby laser, and the long-pulsed Nd:YAG laser are currently the most effective devices. They directly damage the hair follicles based on the theory of selective photothermolysis. A number of variables have a great influence on the expected results: the thickness of the hair, the skin and hair color, the fluence (energy/cm^2), the skin area to be treated, and the number of sessions received by the patient.

• Topical eflornithine (15% cream), an inhibitor of the enzyme ornithine decarboxylase that is thought to inhibit keratin protein synthesis in hair follicles, has been superior to placebo in reducing hair growth. Unfortunately, hair growth seems to return to pretreatment rate 8 weeks after stopping treatment.

REFERENCES

Azziz R, Carmina E, Sawaya ME. Idiopathic hirsutism. *Endocr Rev.* 2000;21:347.

Balfour JA, McClellan K. Topical eflornithine. *Am J Clin Dermatol.* 2001;2:197.

Campos VB, Dierickx CC, Farinelli WA, Lin TY, Manusjiatti W, Anderson RR. Hair removal with an 800-bm pulsed diode laser. *J Am Acad Dermatol.* 2000;43:442.

Dierickx CC, Grossman MC, Farinelli WA, Anderson RR. Permanent hair removal by normal-mode ruby laser. *Arch Dermatol.* 1998;134:837.

Ferriman D, Gallwey JD. Clinical assessment of body hair growth in women. *J Clin Endocrinol Metab.* 1961;21:1440.

Orfanos CE, Adler YD, Zouboulis CC. The SAHA syndrome. *Horm Res.* 2000;54:251.

Pugeat M, Ducluzeau PH, Mallion-Donadieu M. Association of insulin resistance with hyperandrogenemia in women. *Horm Res.* 2000;54:322.

NAILS

• The development of nails through evolution has allowed humans to use fingers as precise tools. The nails are located at the distal ends of the fingers and toes and enhance the capacity for fine movement and tactile sensation. The nail is more than a cosmetic unit; it can also serve as a tool for diagnosing underlying systemic and cutaneous disease.

- The nail is divided into four distinct structures, which compose the nail unit. The nail unit structures are the proximal nail fold, nail matrix, nail bed, and hyponychium. The proximal nail fold is an extension of the overlying epidermis and produces a thin layer of stratum corneum, which adheres to the nail plate and is known as the cuticle. The cuticle acts as a barrier to protect the nail unit from environmental irritants. Loss of the cuticle leads to paronychia. The nail bed begins at the distal end of the matrix and continues to the hyponychium. The nail bed adheres to the nail plate in a unique interconnecting manner such that it grows distally and at the same rate as the nail plate. The hyponychium is the most distal component of the nail unit. It is the transition to the normal epidermis of the digit and ends at the distal groove. The matrix is the most important component of the nail unit; it is responsible for the production of the nail plate. The nail plate is composed of hard keratin and is the end product of differentiation of the matrix. Conditions affecting the matrix will lead to abnormal nail plate formation. The lunula is the whitish half moon pattern, which is the visible portion of the matrix seen through the translucent nail plate and represents the distal matrix.
- The scope of this section is to focus on the nail findings most commonly seen. The terms listed in Table 22–5 are the definitions used when describing nails.

TABLE 22–5 Glossary of Terms Relating to Nails

Anonychia: Absence of nail plate or nail unit

Hyponychium: Distal component of the nail unit after the nail bed

Koilonychia: Spoon-shaped nail plate

Leukonychia: Whitening of the nail plate

Lunula: Half-moon pattern of distal matrix that is visible

Median nail dystrophy: Medial split in the nail plate

Onychalgia: Nail unit pain

Onychauxis: Hypertrophied nail plate

Onychogryposis: Curved pattern nail plate growth like a ram's horn

Onycholysis: Distal separation of the nail plate from the nail bed

Onychomadesis: Proximal separation of the nail plate from the matrix

Onychomycosis: Fungal infection of the nail unit

Onychophagia: Nail biting

Onychorrhexis: Longitudinal striations of the nail plate

Onychoschizia: Distal splitting of the nail plate parallel to the nail bed

Onychotillomania: Compulsive pulling or picking of nail

Paronychia: Inflammation or infection of the nail unit

Trachyonychia: Rough nails

Unguium incarnates: Ingrown nail

PAPULOSQUAMOUS AND INFLAMMATORY DISEASES

PSORIASIS

EPIDEMIOLOGY

- Psoriasis is the most common of the papulosquamous skin diseases affecting the nails. Psoriatic nail disease occurs approximately in 50% of patients with psoriasis. Over a lifetime, between 80 to 90% of patients with psoriasis will suffer nail disease.
- Children and adults as well as any ethnic group can be affected.

PATHOPHYSIOLOGY

- Psoriatic nail is characterized by a hyperproliferation of keratinocytes in conjunction with an inflammatory process that causes abnormal keratinization in the matrix, which in turn, produces pits in the nail plate. As a result of increased cell proliferation, thickened plaques of stratum corneum develop, which in the nail bed becomes subungual debris or the development of defects in the nail plate.

CLINICAL FEATURES

- Nail involvement may be single, multiple, or affect all nails. Disease may be present with or without skin involvement. Clinical features can improve or worsen over time. As in plaque-type psoriasis, nail psoriasis can be affected by the Koebner phenomenon. Patients with severe nail involvement have difficulties in self-esteem.
- The main clinical features, in order of frequency, are pitting, discoloration of the nail, onycholysis, subungual hyperkeratosis, and splinter hemorrhages. Clinical features depend on the location in the nail unit where the disease is active.
- Pits may vary from few to many and are pin-head size depressions to large punched out areas affecting the nail plate. Pits originate from focal psoriasis of the proximal matrix. Discoloration, or the "oil drop sign," represents the psoriatic lesion in the nail bed producing a reddish brown color. Subungual hyperkeratosis is a nail bed and hyponychium condition and leads to onycholysis. Psoriatic nails may become thickened and yellow, and the distal digits can become painful. Splinter hemorrhages in the nail bed occur secondary to minor traumatic events.

- Patients with nail involvement may have moderate to severe debilitating psoriatic arthritis.

DIAGNOSIS AND DIFFERENTIAL

- The diagnosis is made based on the clinical findings and family history of psoriasis. Classic skin lesions of psoriasis can be found along with the typical nail changes described. Nail clipping or full-thickness nail unit biopsy show changes of psoriasis or nail plate findings of confluent parakeratosis with neutrophils.
- The differential diagnosis includes other causes of pitting as seen in alopecia areata, lichen planus, pityriasis rubra pilaris, as well as other causes of nail thickening, such as onychomycosis, yellow nail syndrome, Darier's disease, and pachyonychia congenita.

TREATMENT

- For the most part unsatisfactory. Patients should be counseled to keep nails short, avoid trauma to the nails, and avoid possible contact irritants.
- Intralesional corticosteroid at low doses (2.5 mg/mL) into the nail matrix is the most effective therapy but requires a highly motivated patient because of the pain associated with the injections. Topical therapy requires removal of the nail plate for any improvement, because the ointments cannot penetrate the nail plate. Topical steroids, 5-FU, and retinoic acid have been tried.
- PUVA therapy (using a hand/foot unit) can be helpful but requires multiple treatments per week and good compliance. Excellent results have been seen with the use of systemic medications employed for diffuse psoriasis, such as methotrexate, cyclosporin, and retinoids. Severity of disease must justify the use of these agents.

LICHEN PLANUS

EPIDEMIOLOGY

- Incidence of involvement of nails among patients with lichen planus has been reported to be between 1 and 10%.

CLINICAL FEATURES

- Lichen planus may affect one, multiple, or all nails, and may occur with or without typical skin lesions. It usually starts as a small focus in the matrix creating a longitudinal red line distally. The focus of disease produces thinning of the nail plate leading to a distal split. This distal point of the nail plate is very fragile, and eventually becomes a complete split and the formation of pterygium between the matrix and the proximal nail fold occurs. With broad involvement of the matrix, complete nail loss can occur. Pterygium, which in Latin means wing shaped, is the end-stage scar process. The nail plate looks like two wing patterns with a central longitudinal scar. If pterygium occurs, the nail plate will be permanently disfigured.
- Other clinical features of lichen planus include longitudinal ridging, pitting, and nail plate thinning. When disease affects the nail bed, subungual hyperkeratosis is seen.

DIAGNOSIS AND DIFFERENTIAL

- The diagnosis is made by the clinical features as described above along with evidence of skin lesions of lichen planus. The differential includes onychomycosis and psoriasis.
- Biopsy of the nail unit shows a dense, band-like lymphocytic infiltrate with epidermotropism, hydropic degeneration of basal cells, the development of a stratum granulosum with keratohyalin granules, and a saw-tooth appearance of the rete ridges.

TREATMENT

- Early intervention must be made to avoid pterygium formation. High-potency topical steroids or intralesional corticosteroids into the matrix as early as possible may be helpful to avoid scarring. If injections are not tolerated, oral prednisone can be used.

TRACHONYCHIA (TWENTY-NAIL DYSTROPHY)

EPIDEMIOLOGY

- Thought to be associated with lichen planus or psoriasis. Sixteen percent of patients with twenty-nail dystrophy have lichen planus. Trachonychia has been reported as familial, congenital, or acquired and idiopathic.

CLINICAL FEATURES

- It is seen mostly in children; however, it can affect adults. The nail plate surface appears rough with a yellowish-grey opaque color. The nails become brittle and split at the free edge. One, several, or all twenty nails can be affected.

DIAGNOSIS AND DIFFERENTIAL

- The diagnosis can be made by the clinical findings. The biopsy can show changes of lichen planus, psoriasis, or changes consistent with spongiotic dermatitis. The differential includes lichen planus, psoriasis, and chronic paronychia.

TREATMENT

- It may resolves spontaneously. Oral biotin and intralesional or oral steroid has been reported to be effective.

PARONYCHIA

PATHOPHYSIOLOGY

- Loss or damage to the cuticle exposes the proximal nail fold to irritants, such as chemicals, solvents, foodstuff products, and prolonged water exposure, leading to paronychia. Seen mostly among people who have their hands in wet conditions, for example, bartenders, dishwashers, chefs, and hospital and hair salon personnel.
- Paronychia can also be caused by overly aggressive manicuring of the cuticle or by habitual pulling of a "hang nail" leading to the loss of barrier protection of the cuticle.

CLINICAL FEATURES

- Paronychia presents as an inflammation, redness, swelling, and pain around the proximal and lateral nail folds. Two types are seen: acute and chronic paronychia. In acute paronychia, there is rapid onset of inflammation, redness, pain, and a small pustule may develop which can enlarge to form an abscess. Chronic paronychia is a more insidious process. A boggy appearance of the periungual skin is seen along with cracking, fissuring, and nail plate defects.

DIAGNOSIS AND DIFFERENTIAL

- The diagnosis is made by the clinical features along with a history of exposure to some irritants or predisposing conditions as described. The differential includes contact dermatitis and eczema. If the episodes are frequent and involve the same digit, a herpes virus infection should be ruled out.

TREATMENT

- The most important element is to eliminate the predisposing cause and follow strict avoidance of potential irritants and moisture. Use of thick, emollient creams to form a barrier from the environment are useful. Patient education is a must for those working in predisposing jobs.
- Acute paronychia: Incision and drainage of the pustule or abscess, culture of the purulent material if infection is suspected, accompanied by a course of antibiotics.
- Chronic paronychia: If the area appears infected, culture for correct antibiotic course. Most chronic paronychia mimic chronic contact dermatitis and respond to topical or intralesional steroids.

ONYCHOLYSIS

EPIDEMIOLOGY

- Onycholysis is defined as the separation of the nail plate from the underlying nail bed. It can affect anyone, although is more common in women. It occurs more frequently in the fingernails than in toenails.
- The exact cause is unknown; however, many factors have been identified including self-manipulation, occupational causes, as well as drug reactions.

CLINICAL FEATURES

- Separation begins distally at the hyponychium and progresses proximally. After the space develops, the nail plate develops a yellowish opaque color.
- The course is chronic, and patients must be continuously educated and advised that reversal is slow. Secondary infections with Candida and Pseudomonas species are common.

DIAGNOSIS AND DIFFERENTIAL

- The diagnosis is made by the clinical features and exclusion of onychomycosis and psoriasis.

TREATMENT

- The most important element is to eliminate the predisposing cause and follow strict avoidance of potential irritants and moisture. Proper nail hygiene, keeping nails short, and using a hair dryer on a low setting to dry out the moisture trapped under the nail plate.

REFERENCES

Burge SM, Wilkinson JD. Darier–White disease: A review of the clinical features of 163 patients. *J Am Acad Dermatol.* 1992;27:40.

Daniel CR, Daniel MP, Daniel CM, et al. Chronic paronychia and onycholysis. A thirteen-year experience. *Cutis.* 1996; 58:397.

Daniel DR III. Onycholysis: An overview. *Semin Dermatol.* 1991;10:34.

Farber EM, Nall L. Nail psoriasis. *Cutis.* 1992;50:174.

Scher RK, Fischbein R, Ackerman AB. Twenty-nail dystrophy. A variant of lichen planus. *Arch Dermatol.* 1978;114:612.

Tosti A, Fanti PA, Morelli R, et al. Trachyonychia associated with alopecia areata. A clinical and pathological study. *J Am Acad Dermatol.* 1991;25:266.

Zaias N. Psoriasis of the nail. A clinical-pathology study. *Arch Dermatol.*1969;99:567.

Zaias N, Ackerman AB. The nail in Darier–White disease. *Arch Dermatol.* 1973;107:193.

INFECTIONS

- There are many infections that involve the nail unit. The most common are fungal infections, known as onychomycosis. Onychomycosis is defined as an infection of the nail unit by fungal organisms, specifically dermatophytes, yeasts, or moulds. Bacterial infections, most commonly pseudomonal, as well as viral disease (human papilloma virus and herpes virus) can also affect the nail.

ONYCHOMYCOSIS

EPIDEMIOLOGY

- Invasion of the nail unit by dermatophyte, yeast, or mold. Affects approximately 15 to 30% of the population. It occurs in both children and adults. In 90 to 96%, a dermatophyte is the causative agent, and *Trychophyton rubrum* is the most common organism involved.

CLINICAL FEATURES

- The clinical features can be divided into four types: distal subungual (DSO), superficial white (SWO), proximal subungual white (PSWO), and chronic mucocutaneous onychomycosis. DSO, SWO, and PSWO are caused by dermatophytes. Mucocutaneous onychomycosis is caused by *Candida albicans*.

DISTAL SUBUNGUAL ONYCHOMYCOSIS

- This is the most common type. *Trychophyton rubrum* is the most common organism involved followed by *Trychophyton mentagrophytes*. Nail bed hyperkeratosis and yellow-brown discoloration are typical signs. Subungual debris accumulates and crumbling of the nail plate causes nail plate defects. DSO can be seen associated with tinea pedis or tinea manum. Distal invasion of dermatophyte occurs from the glabrous skin into the nail bed.

SUPERFICIAL WHITE ONYCHOMYCOSIS

- The second most common type of onychomycosis. *Trychophyton mentagrophytes* is the most common organism involved. Powdery, white clinical appearance on the dorsal superficial nail plate, which flakes off easily.

PROXIMAL WHITE SUBUNGUAL ONYCHOMYCOSIS

- *Trychophyton rubrum*, the most common organism involved, invades the proximal subungual nail plate through the proximal nail fold. Clinically, it produces leukonychia and sometimes subungual debris. This variant is seen in immunocompromised conditions and is a marker for HIV disease.

PRIMARY CANDIDAL ONYCHOMYCOSIS

- Is seen only in patients with chronic mucocutaneous candidiasis. It results in total destruction of the nail plate by invasion of Candida species.

DIAGNOSIS AND DIFFERENTIAL

- Clinical features can make the diagnosis; however, confirmation is obtained with direct microscopic examination of a KOH preparation, culture, or a biopsy of the nail plate. The differential diagnosis includes psoriasis, lichen planus, and chronic paronychia.

TREATMENT

- All types respond to oral antifungals. Topical antifungals are only effective for superficial white onychomycosis.
- The new generation antifungals are more effective and have better patient compliance and safety profile. Terbinafine is taken, 250 mg a day, for 3 months. Itraconazole is taken, 200 mg twice a day, for 1 week

out of every month for 3 months. Fluconazole is effective for Candida but not recommended for dermatophyte infections.

PSEUDOMONAL INFECTION

EPIDEMIOLOGY

- *Pseudomonas aeruginosa* is a gram-negative bacterium that can invade the nail unit. It is common in nails with onycholysis.

CLINICAL FEATURES

- It is easily recognized by a dark green discoloration of the nail that develops under the nail plate. The green pigment is pyocyanin produced by Pseudomonas.

DIAGNOSIS AND DIFFERENTIAL

- The diagnosis is made by the green color under the nail plate. The differential includes onycholysis, onychomycosis, and psoriasis.

TREATMENT

- Clipping the nail plate removes the environment in which the bacteria likes to grow. Vinegar soaks or dilute bleach have been reported to be helpful. Oral antibiotics effective against Pseudomonas can be used.

VIRAL INFECTION

EPIDEMIOLOGY

- Human papilloma virus (HPV) and herpes simplex virus can invade the nail unit. It can affect anyone, but is more common in immunosupressed patients.

CLINICAL FEATURES

- Raised, verrucous papules with black dots are clinical signs of periungual verrucae (HPV infection). Painful, red, recurring episodes sometimes, with groups of small vesicles, are the clinical signs of herpetic disease.

DIAGNOSIS AND DIFFERENTIAL

- The diagnosis for both conditions can be made by the clinical features and history. With verrucae, if treatments are not successful, a biopsy should be performed to rule out a squamous cell carcinoma.

TREATMENT

- Periungual verrucae can be treated in the same fashion as those in other areas of the body, with topical salicylic acid, liquid nitrogen, and electrodessication. Pulsed dye laser and intralesional bleomycin can be used for recalcitrant cases.
- Herpes infection is treated with oral antivirals.

REFERENCES

Bauer MF, Cohen BA. The role of *Pseudomonas aeruginosa* in infection about the nails. *Arch Dermatol.* 1957; 75:394.

Chang T, Gorbach SL. Primary and recurrent herpetic whitlow. *Int J Dermatol.* 1977;16:752.

BENIGN TUMORS

KOENEN'S TUMOR

- Also known as periungual fibromas, they are found in 50% of patients with tuberous sclerosis. They appear as small, round, flesh-colored, asymptomatic papules, which arise out of the nail folds. They can be easily removed surgically.

GLOMUS TUMORS

- 75% of all glomus tumors occur in the hand, especially the fingertips in the subungual area. They appear as pink to bluish, red nodule through the nail plate in the nail bed, which does not blanch. Intense, often-pulsating pain is elicited by minimal pressure and changes in temperature. Glomus tumor can cause nail plate deformities, most commonly ridging and fissure formation. Treatment is surgical removal.

EXOSTOSIS

- Outgrowths of normal bone or calcified cartilaginous tissues that project out of the skin. They develop most commonly after trauma but may occur spontaneously, causing nail plate deformities. Exostosis may be painful. The diagnosis is made on clinical findings and confirmed by x-ray. The differential includes other neoplasms, and verrucae. The exostoses can be surgically removed.

DIGITAL MYXOID OR MUCOUS CYST

- Also called distal interphalangeal joint ganglion, this tumor results from a communication of the distal joint space and the cyst at the skin level. The clinical presentation is a soft, sometimes tender, nodular lesion around the proximal nail fold. It can be pink to red in color. If the cyst is adjacent to the matrix, a nail plate defect can be seen. If a 27-gauge needle is used to pierce the cyst, a clear gelatinous material exudes. Treatment with intralesional steroids can be helpful, but most of the time, surgical intervention is required and even then, these cysts have a tendency to recur.

LONGITUDINAL PIGMENTED MELANONYCHIA

- Brown, or black longitudinal streaks within the nail plate. This entity is very common in darkly pigmented persons, African Americans, Hispanics, and other ethnic groups. The thumbs and index fingers are most frequently involved. The pigmentation results from increased melanin deposition in the nail plate due to a benign pigmented nevus, malignant melanoma, trauma, or secondary to many medications. If the band is uniform in color and has been present for some time, it is more likely to be benign. If the band is irregular, composed of different colors, and continuous onto the proximal nail fold (Hutchinson's sign), it is highly suspicious for melanoma. The diagnosis is made by biopsy. The differential includes melanoma, pigmented squamous cell carcinoma, benign nevi, drug reaction, trauma, and genetic and ethnic patterns. Treatment involves surgical removal of the lesion if suspicious for malignancy; otherwise, it can be observed.

MALIGNANT TUMORS

MELANOMA

EPIDEMIOLOGY

- Malignant melanoma of the nail unit is rare and accounts for less then 10% of all melanomas.

Approximately 1 to 3% of melanomas in Caucasians and 15 to 20% of melanomas in African Americans are located in the nail unit.

CLINICAL FEATURES

- It is similar to that of longitudinal pigmented bands. The rapid growth, irregular patterns, variations in color, the development of nodules that cause nail plate defects, and the development of pigment in the proximal nail fold (Hutchinson's sign) all suggest melanoma.
- Most nail unit melanomas are located on the thumbs and great toes. About 25% of melanomas are amelanotic. The tumors are often asymptomatic. Pain and bleeding are unusual. Periungual infection, ulceration of the nail bed, and granulation tissue occur in about one third of the patients.

DIAGNOSIS AND DIFFERENTIAL

- The diagnosis is made by the clinical presentation and biopsy. The differential diagnosis includes chronic paronychia, onychomycosis, pyogenic granulomas, subungual hematomas, benign nevi, and any other nonhealing condition of the nail unit.

TREATMENT

- Treatment is surgical and has a good prognosis for lesions less than 0.76 mm of vertical growth. Prognosis is poor if lesions are invasive.

SQUAMOUS CELL CARCINOMA

PATHOPHYSIOLOGY

- Squamous cell carcinomas of the nail unit are usually linked to infections with human papilloma virus types 16, 34, and 35. Other reported causes include arsenic poisoning, and x-ray exposure.

CLINICAL FEATURES

- Usually, nonaggressive verrucous papules in the nail unit, which do not heal and progress slowly. In situ carcinoma occasionally will become invasive if not treated. They are seen more commonly on fingers than toes.

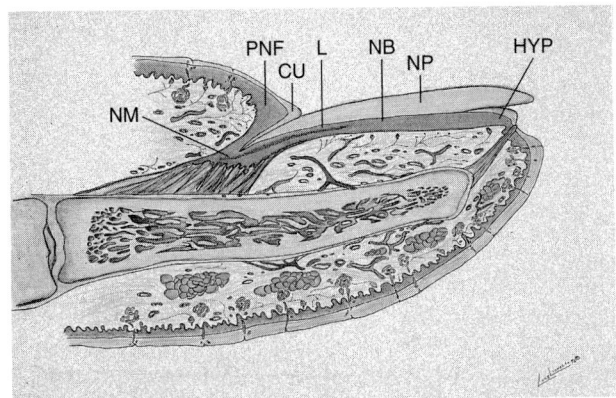

FIGURE 22.1 Diagrammatic drawing of a normal nail. PNF, proximal nail fold; NM, nail matrix; NB, nail bed; NP, nail plate; HYP, hyponychium; CU, cuticle; L, lunula region.

• The slow growth delays the diagnosis. The differential is that of normal verrucae, chronic inflammatory conditions like infections, pyoderma gangrenosum, and subungual exostosis.

TREATMENT

• Mohs surgery is the treatment of choice. If bone is involved, then amputation is commonly required.

REFERENCES

Ashinoff R, Junli J, Jacobson M, et al. Detection of HPV DNA in squamous cell carcinoma of the nail bed and finger determined by polymerase chain reaction. *Arch Dermatol.* 1991;127:1813.

Camirand P, Giroux JM. Subungual glomus tumor. *Arch Dermatol.* 1970;102:677.

Guitart J, Bergfeld WF, Tuthull RJ, et al. Squamous cell carcinoma of the nail bed: A clinicopathological study of 12 cases. *Br J Dermatol.* 1990;123:215.

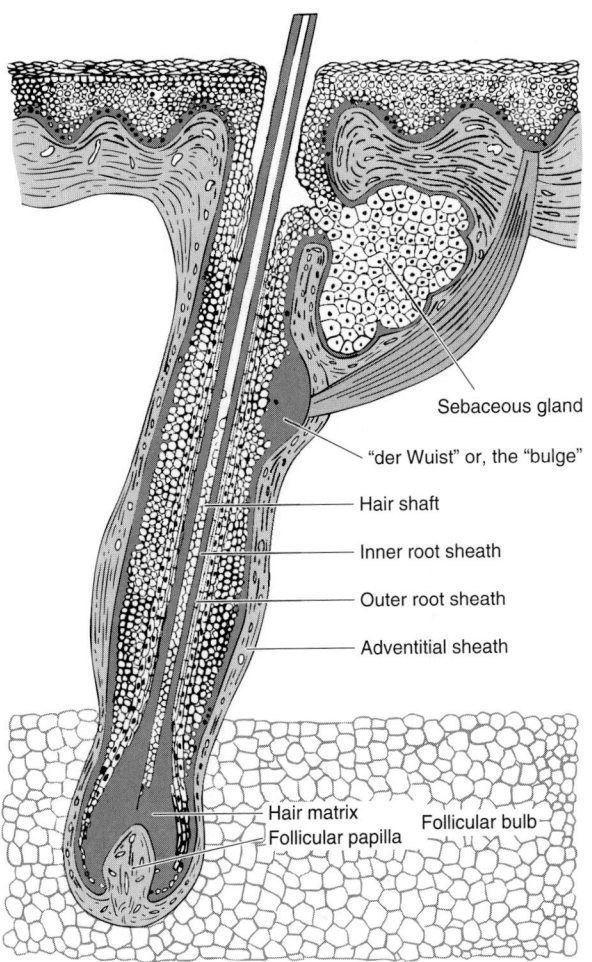

FIGURE 22.2 Diagrammatic representation of the adult human hair follicle. The follicle, an invagination of the surface epidermis, is characterized by an infundibulum that communicates directly with the epidermis and extends to the opening of the sebaceous gland. The portion directly beneath the sebaceous gland and terminating at the bulge is the isthmus. The lowermost portion of the hair follicle is the transient region which begins just beneath the bulge and terminates at the lowermost part of the follicle. The follicular bulb, the lowermost part of the follicle, consists of matrix keratinocytes and specialized mesenchymal cells known as the *follicular papilla*. The follicular papilla is contiguous with the adventital sheath, which lines the entire follicle. (*Courtesy of Michael Joffreda, MD*)

INDEX